# DIABETIC RETINOPATHY

WK 835 CUN  £84

# DIABETIC RETINOPATHY

## José Cunha-Vaz
*University of Coimbra, Portugal*

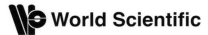

**World Scientific**

NEW JERSEY · LONDON · SINGAPORE · BEIJING · SHANGHAI · HONG KONG · TAIPEI · CHENNAI

*Published by*

World Scientific Publishing Co. Pte. Ltd.

5 Toh Tuck Link, Singapore 596224

*USA office:* 27 Warren Street, Suite 401-402, Hackensack, NJ 07601

*UK office:* 57 Shelton Street, Covent Garden, London WC2H 9HE

**Library of Congress Cataloging-in-Publication Data**
Diabetic retinopathy / [edited by] José Cunha-Vaz.
    p. ; cm.
  Includes bibliographical references and index.
  ISBN-13: 978-981-4304-43-6 (hardcover : alk. paper)
  ISBN-10: 981-4304-43-3 (hardcover : alk. paper)
  1. Diabetic retinopathy.  I. Cunha-Vaz, José G.
  [DNLM: 1.  Diabetic Retinopathy.  WK 835]
  RE661.D5D523 2010
  617.7'35--dc22

                    2010043318

**British Library Cataloguing-in-Publication Data**
A catalogue record for this book is available from the British Library.

Typeset by Stallion Press
Email: enquiries@stallionpress.com

Printed by FuIsland Offset Printing (S) Pte Ltd. Singapore

*To my wife*
*Teresa Maria*

# Preface

Diabetic retinopathy remains the leading cause of low vision and blindness in people of working age in Europe and USA. At the same time that there has been continuous improvement in the management and treatment of diabetic retinal disease. Projections for the next decade indicate that number of persons with diabetes will increase over the next twenty to thirty years by 35% creating a real challenge to the public health capacity to care for patients with diabetic retinopathy and persons at risk for this complication.

For over forty years I have been particularly involved in the study of diabetic retinopathy. Since my earlier training days under the guidance of Norman Ashton, in London, I have always been focusing on the "whys" and "hows" of diabetic retinopathy. The goal was always to improve our understanding of its development and progression. Since London I worked for extended periods of time in Coimbra, Portugal and in Chicago, USA, at the University of Illinois Eye and Ear Infirmary. Translational research by combining laboratory with clinical research has been my main interest and a great source of personal enjoyment. This, I believe is clearly reflected in this book. For the same reasons it deals primarily with nonproliferative retinopathy in diabetes type 2, the most frequent form of diabetic retinal disease and the disease stage where the mechanisms of the retinal pathology can be more clearly correlated with the systemic disease.

I believe strongly that improved understanding of diabetes in general is fundamental for the management of retinal disease and that an open and permanent communication between the ophthalmologist and the diabetologist is crucial for the best care to our patients with diabetic retinopathy. This is why the first chapter book includes the approved guidelines for management of diabetes and its complications.

This book is the result of a challenge by a colleague of mine, Manuel Sanchez Salorio, of Santiago de Compostela, Spain.

I hope sincerely that it may contribute by offering a balance between original thought and proven clinical practice. It would give me great pleasure if the readers, particularly young ones, find in this book concepts that stir in theirs minds new perspectives for improved understanding and management of diabetic retinopathy. This means that our patients will have better options and that their sight will have more chances to be preserved in spite of their diabetes.

Finally, I would like to thank all the authors that contributed to this book.

My personal thanks go also to the persons who helped me review and check all the details involved in the preparation of the book, namely, Alda Gonçalves, Cristina Ramos and Catarina Neves.

# Contents

# List of Contributors

**José Rui Faria de Abreu**
Assistant Professor of Ophthalmology and Consultant Ophthalmologist
Ophthalmology Department, University Hospital of Coimbra
Coimbra, Portugal

**Alda Ambrósio**
Senior Researcher
Clinical and Molecular Genetics Unit
National Institute of Legal Medicine
Institute of Biomedical Research in Light and Image (IBILI)
Faculty of Medicine of the University of Coimbra
Coimbra, Portugal

**António Francisco Ambrósio**
Senior Researcher
Division of Retinal Dysfunction
Centre of Ophthalmology and Vision Sciences of the University of Coimbra
Institute of Biomedical Research in Light and Image (IBILI)
Faculty of Medicine of the University of Coimbra
Coimbra, Portugal

**Rui Bernardes**
Director
Centre of New Tecnologies for Medicine
Association for Innovation and Biomedical Research on Light and Image (AIBILI)
Assistant Professor of Biophysics/Biomathematics
Faculty of Medicine of University of Coimbra
Coimbra, Portugal

**Miguel Castelo Branco**
Assistant Professor of Biophysics
Institute of Biophysics and Biomathematics
Visual Neuroscience Laboratory
Faculty of Medicine of the University of Coimbra
Director
Institute of Biomedical Research in Light and Image (IBILI)
Faculty of Medicine of the University of Coimbra
Coimbra, Portugal

**José Cunha-Vaz**
Emeritus Professor of Ophthalmology
University of Coimbra
President
Association for Innovation and Biomedical Research on Light and Image (AIBILI)
Coimbra, Portugal

**Lilianne Duarte**
Consultant Ophthalmologist
Association for Innovation and Biomedical Research on Light and Image (AIBILI)
Coimbra, Portugal

**João Figueira**
Consultant Ophthalmologist
Department of Ophthalmology, University Hospital of Coimbra
Association for Innovation and Biomedical Research on Light and Image (AIBILI)
Coimbra, Portugal

**Francisco Gomez-Ulla**
Professor of Ophthalmology
University Hospital of Santiago
Unit of Medical Retina and Ocular Diabetes
University of Santiago de Compostela
Technological Institute of Ophthalmology
Santiago Compostela, Spain
Ophthalmology Hospital of Santa Teresa
La Coruna, Spain

**José Carlos Pastor Jimeno**
Professor of Ophthalmology
University of Valladolid
Director of Instituto Universitário de Oftalmologia Aplicada (IOBA)
Chief of Department of the University Hospital
Valladolid, Spain

**Ermelindo Leal**
Researcher
Centre of Ophthalmology and Vision Sciences of the University of Coimbra
Institute of Biomedical Research in Light and Image (IBILI)
Faculty of Medicine of the University of Coimbra
Coimbra, Portugal

**Conceição Lobo**
Assistant Professor of Ophthalmology and Consultant Ophthalmologist
Faculty of Medicine of University of Coimbra and Department of Ophthalmology
University Hospital of Coimbra
Association for Innovation and Biomedical Research on Light and Image (AIBILI)
Coimbra, Portugal

**Paulo Pereira**
Director
Centre of Ophthalmology and Vision Sciences of the University of Coimbra
Institute of Biomedical Research in Light and Image (IBILI)
Faculty of Medicine, University of Coimbra
Vice-Director
Faculty of Medicine, University of Coimbra
Coimbra, Portugal

**Luisa Ribeiro**
Director and Consultant Ophthalmologist
Clinical Trial Centre, Association for Innovation and Biomedical Research on Light and Image (AIBILI)
Coimbra, Portugal

# Chapter 1

# Standards of Medical Care in Diabetes — 2009

## American Diabetes Association

Diabetes is a chronic illness that requires continuing medical care and patient self-management education to prevent acute complications and to reduce the risk of long-term complications. Diabetes care is complex and requires that many issues, beyond glycemic control, be addressed. A large body of evidence exists that supports a range of interventions to improve diabetes outcomes.

These standards of care are intended to provide clinicians, patients, researchers, payors, and other interested individuals with the components of diabetes care, treatment goals, and tools to evaluate the quality of care. While individual preferences, comorbidities, and other patient factors may require modification of goals, targets that are desirable for most patients with diabetes are provided. These standards are not intended to preclude more extensive evaluation and management of the patient by other specialists as needed. For more detailed information, refer to references (American Diabetes Association, 2003; 2008a; 2008b).

The recommendations included are screening, diagnostic, and therapeutic actions that are known or believed to favorably affect health outcomes of patients with diabetes. A grading system (Table 1), developed by the American Diabetes Association (ADA) and modeled after existing methods, was utilized to clarify and codify the evidence that forms the basis for the recommendations. The level of evidence

(Excerpts from *Diabetes Care*, Vol. 32, Suppl. 1, 2009).

that supports each recommendation is listed after each recommendation using the letters A, B, C, or E.

## 1.1. Classification and Diagnosis

### 1.1.1. Classification

In 1997, ADA issued new diagnostic and classification criteria (Expert Committee on Diagnosis and Classification of Diabetes Mellitus, 1997); in 2003, modifications were made regarding the diagnosis of impaired fasting glucose (Expert Committee on Diagnosis and Classification of Diabetes Mellitus, 2003). The classification of diabetes includes four clinical classes:

- type 1 diabetes (results from $\beta$-cell destruction, usually leading to absolute insulin deficiency)
- type 2 diabetes (results from a progressive insulin secretory defect on the background of insulin resistance)
- other specific types of diabetes due to other causes, e.g. genetic defects in $\beta$-cell function, genetic defects in insulin action, diseases of the exocrine pancreas (such as cystic fibrosis), and drug or chemical-induced (such as in the treatment of AIDS or after organ transplantation)
- gestational diabetes mellitus (GDM) (diabetes diagnosed during pregnancy)

**Table 1  ADA Evidence Grading System for Clinical Practice Recommendations**

| Level of Evidence | Description |
| --- | --- |
| A | Clear evidence from well-conducted, generalizable, randomized controlled trials that are adequately powered, including:<br>• Evidence from a well-conducted multicenter trial<br>• Evidence from a meta-analysis that incorporated quality ratings in the analysis<br>Compelling nonexperimental evidence, i.e. "all or none" rule developed by the Centre for Evidence-Based Medicine at Oxford<br>Supportive evidence from well-conducted randomized controlled trials that are adequately powered, including:<br>• Evidence from a well-conducted trial at one or more institutions<br>• Evidence from a meta-analysis that incorporated quality ratings in the analysis |
| B | Supportive evidence from well-conducted cohort studies, including:<br>• Evidence from a well-conducted prospective cohort study or registry<br>• Evidence from a well-conducted meta-analysis of cohort studies |
| C | Supportive evidence from a well-conducted case-control study<br>Supportive evidence from poorly controlled or uncontrolled studies<br>• Evidence from randomized clinical trials with one or more major or three or more minor methodological flaws that could invalidate the results<br>• Evidence from observational studies with high potential for bias (such as case series with comparison to historical controls)<br>• Evidence from case series or case reports |
| E | Conflicting evidence with the weight of evidence supporting the recommendation<br>Expert consensus or clinical experience |

Some patients cannot be clearly classified as type 1 or type 2 diabetes. Clinical presentation and disease progression vary considerably in both types of diabetes. Occasionally, patients who otherwise have type 2 diabetes may present with ketoacidosis. Similarly, patients with type 1 may have a late onset and slow (but relentless) progression of disease despite having features of autoimmune disease. Such difficulties in diagnosis may occur in children, adolescents, and adults. The true diagnosis may become more obvious over time.

### 1.1.2. Diagnosis of Diabetes

Current criteria for the diagnosis of diabetes in nonpregnant adults are shown in Table 2. Three ways to diagnose diabetes are recommended at the time of this statement, and each must be confirmed on a subsequent day unless unequivocal symptoms of hyperglycemia are present. Although the 75-g oral glucose tolerance test (OGTT) is more sensitive and modestly more specific than the fasting plasma glucose (FPG)

**Table 2  Criteria for the Diagnosis of Diabetes**

1. FPG ≥126 mg/dl (7.0 mmol/l). Fasting is defined as no caloric intake for at least 8 h.*

   OR

2. Symptoms of hyperglycemia and a casual (random) plasma glucose ≥ 200 mg/dl (11.1 mmol/l). Casual (random) is defined as any time of day without regard to time since last meal. The classic symptoms of hyperglycemia include polyuria, polydipsia, and unexplained weight loss.

   OR

3. 2-h plasma glucose ≥ 200 mg/dl (11.1 mmol/l) during an OGTT. The test should be performed as described by the World Health Organization using a glucose load containing the equivalent of 75-g anhydrous glucose dissolved in water.*

*In the absence of unequivocal hyperglycemia, these criteria should be confirmed by repeat testing on a different day (5).

to diagnose diabetes, it is poorly reproducible and difficult to perform in practice. Because of ease of use, acceptability to patients, and lower cost, the FPG has been the preferred diagnostic test. Though FPG is less sensitive than the OGTT, the vast majority of people who do not meet diagnostic criteria for diabetes by FPG but would by OGTT will have an A1C value well under 7.0% (Davidson *et al.*, 1999).

Though the OGTT is not recommended for routine clinical use, it may be useful for further evaluation of patients in whom diabetes is still strongly suspected but who have normal FPG or IFG (impaired fasting glucose) (see Section 1.1.3).

The use of the A1C for the diagnosis of diabetes has previously not been recommended due to lack of global standardization and uncertainty about diagnostic thresholds. However, with a worldwide move toward a standardized assay and with increasing observational evidence about the prognostic significance of A1C, an Expert Committee on the Diagnosis of Diabetes was convened in 2008. This joint committee of ADA, the European Association for the Study of Diabetes, and the International Diabetes Federation will likely recommend that the A1C become the preferred diagnostic test for diabetes. Diagnostic cut-points are being discussed at the time of publication of this statement. Updated recommendations will be published in *Diabetes Care* and will be available at diabetes.org.

### 1.1.3. Diagnosis of Prediabetes

Hyperglycemia not sufficient to meet the diagnostic criteria for diabetes is categorized as either impaired fasting glucose (IFG) or impaired glucose tolerance (IGT), depending on whether it is identified through the FPG or the OGTT:

- IFG = FPG 100 mg/dl (5.6 mmol/l) to 125 mg/dl (6.9 mmol/l)
- IGT = 2-h plasma glucose 140 mg/dl (7.8 mmol/l) to 199 mg/dl (11.0 mmol/l)

IFG and IGT have been officially termed "prediabetes." Both categories of prediabetes are risk factors for future diabetes and for cardiovascular disease (CVD) (Nathan *et al.*, 2007).

## 1.2. Testing for Prediabetes and Diabetes in Asymptomatic Patients

**Recommendations**

- Testing to detect prediabetes and type 2 diabetes in asymptomatic people should be considered in adults of any age who are overweight or obese (BMI $\geq$25 kg/m$^2$) and who have one or more additional risk factors for diabetes (Table 3). In those without these risk factors, testing should begin at age 45 years. (B)
- If tests are normal, repeat testing should be carried out at least at 3-year intervals. (E)
- To test for pre-diabetes or diabetes, an FPG test or 2-h OGTT (75-g glucose load) or both are appropriate. (B)
- An OGTT may be considered in patients with IFG to better define the risk of diabetes. (E)
- In those identified with prediabetes, identify and, if appropriate, treat other CVD risk factors. (B)

For many illnesses, there is a major distinction between screening and diagnostic testing. However, for diabetes, the same tests would be used for "screening" as for diagnosis. Type 2 diabetes has a long asymptomatic phase and significant clinical risk markers. Diabetes may be identified anywhere along a spectrum of clinical scenarios, ranging from a seemingly low-risk individual who happens to have glucose testing, to a higher-risk individual whom the provider tests because of high suspicion of diabetes, to the symptomatic patient. The discussion herein is primarily framed as testing for diabetes in those without symptoms. Testing for diabetes will also detect individuals with prediabetes.

**Table 3  Criteria for Testing for Prediabetes and Diabetes in Asymptomatic Adult Individuals**

1. Testing should be considered in all adults who are overweight (BMI $\geq$ 25 kg/m$^2$*) and have additional risk factors:
   - physical inactivity
   - first-degree relative with diabetes
   - members of a high-risk ethnic population (e.g. African American, Latino, Native American, Asian American, Pacific Islander)
   - women who delivered a baby weighing > 9 lb or were diagnosed with GDM
   - hypertension ($\geq$ 140/90 mm Hg or on therapy for hypertension)
   - HDL cholesterol level < 35 mg/dl (0.90 mmol/l) and/or a triglyceride level > 250 mg/dl (2.82 mmol/l)
   - women with polycystic ovarian syndrome (PCOS)
   - IGT or IFG on previous testing
   - other clinical conditions associated with insulin resistance (e.g. severe obesity, acanthosis nigricans)
   - history of CVD

2. In the absence of the above criteria, testing for prediabetes and diabetes should begin at age 45 years
3. If results are normal, testing should be repeated at least at 3-year intervals, with consideration of more frequent testing depending on initial results and risk status.

*At-risk BMI may be lower in some ethnic groups.

### 1.2.1. Testing for Prediabetes and Type 2 Diabetes in Adults

Type 2 diabetes is frequently not diagnosed until complications appear, and approximately one-third of all people with diabetes may be undiagnosed. Although the effectiveness of early identification of prediabetes and diabetes through mass testing of asymptomatic individuals has not been definitively proven (and rigorous trials to provide such proof are unlikely to occur), prediabetes and diabetes meet established criteria for conditions in which early detection is appropriate. Both conditions are common, increasing in prevalence, and impose significant public health burdens. There is a long presymptomatic phase before the diagnosis of type 2 diabetes is usually made. Relatively simple tests are available to detect preclinical disease (Engelgau *et al.*, 2007). Additionally, the duration of glycemic burden is a strong predictor of adverse outcomes, and effective interventions exist to prevent progression of prediabetes to diabetes (see Section 1.4) and to reduce the risk of complications of diabetes (see Section 1.6).

Recommendations for testing for prediabetes and diabetes in asymptomatic, undiagnosed adults are listed in Table 3. Testing should be considered in adults of any age with BMI $\geq$ 25 kg/m$^2$ and one or more risk factors for diabetes. Because age is a major risk factor for diabetes, testing of those without other risk factors should begin no later than age 45 years.

Either FPG testing or the 2-h OGTT is appropriate for testing. The 2-h OGTT identifies people with either IFG or IGT, and thus, more prediabetic people at increased risk for the development of diabetes and CVD. It should be noted that the two tests do not necessarily detect the same prediabetic individuals (Gabir *et al.*, 2000). The efficacy of interventions for primary prevention of type 2 diabetes (Knowler *et al.*, 2002; Tuomilehto *et al.*, 2001; Pan *et al.*, 1997; Buchanan *et al.*, 2002; Chiasson *et al.*, 2002; Gerstein, 2006; Ramachandran *et al.*, 2006) has primarily been demonstrated among individuals with IGT, not individuals with IFG (who do not also have IGT). As noted in the diagnosis section (Section 1.1.2), the FPG test is more convenient, more reproducible, less costly, and easier to administer than the 2-h OGTT (Expert Committee on Diagnosis and Classification of Diabetes Mellitus, 1997, 2003). An OGTT may be useful in patients with IFG to better define the risk of diabetes.

The appropriate interval between tests is not known (Johnson *et al.*, 2005). The rationale for the three-year interval is that false-negatives will be repeated before substantial time elapses, and there is little likelihood that an individual will develop significant complications of diabetes within three years of a negative test result.

Because of the need for follow-up and discussion of abnormal results, testing should be carried out within the health care setting. Community screening outside a health care setting is not recommended because people with positive tests may not seek, or have access to, appropriate follow-up testing and care. Conversely, there may be failure to ensure appropriate repeat testing for individuals who test negative. Community screening may also be poorly targeted, i.e. it may fail to reach the groups most at risk and inappropriately test those at low risk (the worried well) or even those already diagnosed (Harris *et al.*, 2003; USPSTF, 2003).

### 1.2.2.  Testing for Type 2 Diabetes in Children

The incidence of type 2 diabetes in adolescents has increased dramatically in the last decade, especially in minority populations (Dabelea *et al.*, 2007), although the disease remains rare in the general adolescent population (Liese *et al.*, 2006). Consistent with recommendations for adults, children and youth at increased risk for the presence or the development of type 2 diabetes, testing should be carried out within the health care setting (American Diabetes Association, 2000). The recommendations of the ADA consensus statement on type 2 diabetes in children and youth, with some modifications, are summarized in Table 4.

### 1.2.3.  Screening for Type 1 Diabetes

Generally, people with type 1 diabetes present with acute symptoms of diabetes and markedly elevated blood glucose levels, and most cases are diagnosed soon after the onset of hyperglycemia. However, evidence from type 1 prevention studies suggests that measurement of islet autoantibodies identifies individuals who are at risk for developing type 1 diabetes. Such testing may be appropriate in high-risk individuals, such as those with prior transient hyperglycemia or those who have relatives with type 1 diabetes, in the context of clinical research studies (see, for example,

**Table 4   Testing for Type 2 Diabetes in Asymptomatic Children**

Criteria:

- Overweight (BMI > 85th percentile for age and sex, weight for height > 85th percentile, or weight > 120% of ideal for height)

Plus any two of the following risk factors:

- Family history of type 2 diabetes in first- or second-degree relative
- Race/ethnicity (Native American, African American, Latino, Asian American, Pacific Islander)
- Signs of insulin resistance or conditions associated with insulin resistance (acanthosis nigricans, hypertension, dyslipidemia, PCOS, or small-for-gestational-age birthweight)
- Maternal history of diabetes or GDM during the child's gestation

Age of initiation: age 10 years or at onset of puberty, if puberty occurs at a younger age

Frequency: every 3 years

Test: FPG preferred

http://www2.diabetestrialnet.org). Widespread clinical testing of asymptomatic low-risk individuals cannot currently be recommended, as it would identify very few individuals in the general population who are at risk. Individuals who screen positive should be counseled about their risk of developing diabetes. Clinical studies are being conducted to test various methods of preventing type 1 diabetes, or reversing early type 1 diabetes, in those with evidence of autoimmunity.

## 1.3.  Detection and Diagnosis of GDM

**Recommendations**

- Screen for GDM using risk factor analysis and, if appropriate, use of an OGTT. (C)
- Women with GDM should be screened for diabetes 6–12 weeks postpartum and should be

followed up with subsequent screening for the development of diabetes or prediabetes. (E)

GDM is defined as any degree of glucose intolerance with onset or first recognition during pregnancy (Expert Committee on Diagnosis and Classification of Diabetes Mellitus, 1997). Although most cases resolve with delivery, the definition applies whether or not the condition persists after pregnancy and does not exclude the possibility that unrecognized glucose intolerance may have antedated or begun concomitantly with the pregnancy. Approximately 7% of all pregnancies (ranging from 1 to 14% depending on the population studied and the diagnostic tests employed) are complicated by GDM, resulting in more than 200,000 cases annually.

Because of the risks of GDM to the mother and neonate, screening and diagnosis are warranted. The screening and diagnostic strategies, based on the 2004 ADA position statement on gestational diabetes mellitus (American Diabetes Association, 2004), are outlined in Table 5.

**Table 5    Screening for and Diagnosis of GDM**

Carry out GDM risk assessment at the first prenatal visit.
Women at very high risk for GDM should be screened for diabetes as soon as possible after the confirmation of pregnancy. Criteria for very high risk are:

- severe obesity
- prior history of GDM or delivery of large-for-gestational-age infant
- presence of glycosuria
- diagnosis of PCOS
- strong family history of type 2 diabetes

Screening/diagnosis at this stage of pregnancy should use standard diagnostic testing (Table 2).
All women of greater than low risk of GDM, including those above not found to have diabetes early in pregnancy, should undergo GDM testing at 24–28 weeks of gestation. Low risk status, which does not require GDM screening, is defined as women with ALL of the following characteristics:

- age < 25 years
- weight normal before pregnancy
- member of an ethnic group with a low prevalence of diabetes
- no known diabetes in first-degree relatives
- no history of abnormal glucose tolerance
- no history of poor obstetrical outcome

Two approaches may be followed for GDM screening at 24–28 weeks:

1. Two-step approach:
   - Perform initial screening by measuring plasma or serum glucose 1 h after a 50-g oral glucose load. A glucose threshold after 50-g load of ≥ 140 mg/dl identifies ~ 80% of women with GDM, while the sensitivity is further increased to ~ 90% by a threshold of ≥ 130 mg/dl.
   - Perform a diagnostic 100-g OGTT on a separate day in women who exceed the chosen threshold on 50-g screening.
2. One-step approach (may be preferred in clinics with high prevalence of GDM): Perform a diagnostic 100-g OGTT in all women to be tested at 24–28 weeks.

The 100-g OGTT should be performed in the morning after an overnight fast of at least 8 h.
To make a diagnosis of GDM, at least two of the following plasma glucose values must be found:

- Fasting: ≥ 95 mg/dl
- 1 h: ≥ 180 mg/dl
- 2 h: ≥ 155 mg/dl
- 3 h: ≥ 140 mg/dl

Results of the Hyperglycemia and Adverse Pregnancy Outcomes study (Metzger *et al.*, 2008), a large-scale (including ~25,000 pregnant women) multinational epidemiologic study, demonstrated that risk of adverse maternal, fetal, and neonatal outcomes increased continuously as a function of maternal glycemia at 24–28 weeks, even within ranges previously considered normal for pregnancy. For most complications, there was no threshold for risk.

These results have led to careful reconsideration of the diagnostic criteria for GDM. An international group representing multiple obstetrical and diabetes organizations, including ADA, is currently working on consensus toward 1) a worldwide standard for which diagnostic test to use for GDM; and 2) rational diagnostic cut points.

Because women with a history of GDM have a greatly increased subsequent risk for diabetes (Kim *et al.*, 2002), they should be screened for diabetes 6–12 weeks postpartum, using nonpregnant OGTT criteria, and should be followed up with subsequent screening for the development of diabetes or prediabetes, as outlined in Section 1.2. For information on the National Diabetes Education Program (NDEP) campaign to prevent type 2 diabetes in women with GDM, go to www.ndep.nih.gov/diabetes/pubs/NeverTooEarly_Tipsheet.pdf.

## 1.4.  Prevention/Delay of Type 2 Diabetes

**Recommendations**

- Patients with IGT (A) or IFG (E) should be referred to an effective ongoing support program for weight loss of 5–10% of body weight and for increasing physical activity to at least 150 min per week of moderate activity such as walking.
- Follow-up counseling appears to be important for success. (B)
- Based on potential cost savings of diabetes prevention, such counseling should be covered by third-party payors. (E)

- In addition to lifestyle counseling, metformin may be considered in those who are at very high risk for developing diabetes (combined IFG and IGT plus other risk factors such as A1C > 6%, hypertension, low HDL cholesterol, elevated triglycerides, or family history of diabetes in a first-degree relative) and who are obese and under 60 years of age. (E)
- Monitoring for the development of diabetes in those with prediabetes should be performed every year. (E)

Randomized controlled trials have shown that individuals at high risk for developing diabetes (those with IFG, IGT, or both) can be given interventions that significantly decrease the rate of onset of diabetes (Knowler *et al.*, 2002; Tuomilehto *et al.*, 2001; Pan *et al.*, 1997; Buchanan *et al.*, 2002; Chiassion *et al.*, 2002; Gerstein *et al.*, 2006; Ramanchandran *et al.*, 2006). These interventions include intensive lifestyle modification programs that have been shown to be very effective ($\geq 58\%$ reduction after three years) and use of the pharmacologic agents metformin, acarbose, orlistat, and thiazolidinediones (TZDs), each of which has been shown to decrease the incident of diabetes by various degrees. A summary of major diabetes prevention trials is shown in Table 6.

Two studies of lifestyle intervention have shown persistent reduction in the rate of conversion to type 2 diabetes with 3 (Lindstrom *et al.*, 2006) to 14 years (Li *et al.*, 2008) of postintervention follow-up.

Based on the results of clinical trials and the known risks of progression of prediabetes to diabetes, an ADA Consensus Development Panel (Nathan *et al.*, 2007) concluded that persons with prediabetes (IGT and/or IFG) should be counseled on lifestyle changes with goals similar to those of the Diabetes Prevention Program (DPP) (5–10% weight loss and moderate physical activity of ~30 min per day). Regarding the more difficult issue of drug therapy for diabetes prevention, the consensus panel felt that metformin should be the only drug considered for use in diabetes prevention. For other drugs, the issues of cost, side effects, and lack of persistence of effect in some studies

**Table 6 Therapies Proven Effective in Diabetes Prevention Trials**

| Study (ref.) | n | Population | Mean Age (years) | Duration (years) | Intervention (daily dose) | Conversion in Control Subjects (%/year) | Relative Risk |
|---|---|---|---|---|---|---|---|
| *Lifestyle* | | | | | | | |
| Finnish DPS (11) | 522 | IGT, BMI $\geq$ 25 kg/m$^2$ | 55 | 3.2 | Individual diet/exercise | 6 | 0.42 (0.30–0.70) |
| DPP (10) | 2161* | IGT, BMI $\geq$ 24 kg/m$^2$, FPG > 5.3 mmol/l | 51 | 3 | Individual diet/exercise | 10 | 0.42 (0.34–0.52) |
| Da Qing (12) | 259* | IGT (randomized groups) | 45 | 6 | Group diet/exercise | 16 | 0.62 (0.44–0.86) |
| Toranomon study (28) | 458 | IGT (men), BMI = 24 kg/m$^2$ | 55 | 4 | Individual diet/exercise | 2 | 0.33 (0.10–1.0)† |
| Indian DPP (16) | 269* | IGT | 46 | 2.5 | Individual diet/exercise | 22 | 0.71 (0.63–0.79) |
| *Medications* | | | | | | | |
| DPP (10) | 2155* | IGT, BMI > 24 kg/m$^2$, FPG > 5.3 mmol/l | 51 | 2.8 | Metformin (1700 mg) | 10 | 0.69 (0.57–0.83) |
| Indian DPP (16) | 269* | IGT | 46 | 2.5 | Metformin (500 mg) | 22 | 0.74 (0.65–0.81) |
| STOP NIDDM (14) | 1419 | IGT, FPG > 5.6 mmol/l | 54 | 3.2 | Acarbose (300 mg) | 13 | 0.75 (0.63–0.90) |
| XENDOS (29) | 3277 | BMI > 30 kg/m$^2$ | 43 | 4 | Orlistat (360 mg) | 2 | 0.63 (0.46–0.86) |
| DREAM (15) | 5269 | IGT or IFG | 55 | 3.0 | Rosiglitazone (8 mg) | 9 | 0.40 (0.35–0.46) |

*Number of participants in the indicated comparisons, not necessarily in the entire study.
†Calculated from information in the article. DPP, Diabetes Prevention Program; DREAM, Diabetes REduction Assessment with ramipril and rosiglitazone Medication; DPS, Diabetes Prevention Study; STOP NIDDM, Study to Prevent Non-Insulin Dependent Diabetes; XENDOS, Xenical in the prevention of Diabetes in Obese Subjects. This table has been reprinted with permission (30) with some modification.

led the panel to not recommend their use for diabetes prevention. Metformin use was recommended only for very-high-risk individuals (those with combined IGT and IFG who are obese and under 60 years of age with at least one other risk factor for diabetes). In addition, the panel highlighted the evidence that in the DPP, metformin was most effective compared to lifestyle in those with BMI of at least 35 kg/m$^2$ and those under age 60 years.

## 1.5. Diabetes Care

### 1.5.1. Initial Evaluation

A complete medical evaluation should be performed to classify the diabetes, detect the presence of diabetes complications, review previous treatment and glycemic control in patients with established diabetes, assist in formulating a management plan, and provide a basis for continuing care. Laboratory tests appropriate to the evaluation of each patient's medical condition should be performed. A focus on the components of comprehensive care (Table 7) will assist the health care team to ensure optimal management of the patient with diabetes.

### 1.5.2. Management

People with diabetes should receive medical care from a physician-coordinated team. Such teams may include, but are not limited to, physicians, nurse practitioners, physician's assistants, nurses, dietitians, pharmacists, and mental health professionals with expertise and a special interest in diabetes. It is essential in this collaborative and integrated team approach that individuals with diabetes assume an active role in their care.

The management plan should be formulated as an individualized therapeutic alliance among the patient and family, the physician, and other members of the health care team. A variety of strategies and techniques should be used to provide adequate education and development of problem-solving skills in the various aspects of diabetes management. Implementation of the management plan requires that each aspect is understood and agreed on by the patient and the care providers and that the goals and treatment plan are reasonable. Any plan should recognize diabetes self-management education (DSME) as an integral component of care. In developing the plan, consideration should be given to the patient's age, school or work schedule and conditions, physical activity, eating patterns, social situation and personality, cultural factors, and presence of complications of diabetes or other medical conditions.

### 1.5.3. Glycemic Control

#### 1.5.3.1. *Assessment of glycemic control*

Two primary techniques are available for health providers and patients to assess the effectiveness of the management plan on glycemic control: Patient self-monitoring of blood glucose (SMBG) or of interstitial glucose and measurement of A1C.

a. *Glucose monitoring*

**Recommendations**

- SMBG should be carried out three or more times daily for patients using multiple insulin injections or insulin pump therapy. (A)
- For patients using less frequent insulin injections, noninsulin therapies, or medical nutrition therapy (MNT) and physical activity alone, SMBG may be useful as a guide to the success of therapy. (E)
- To achieve postprandial glucose targets, postprandial SMBG may be appropriate. (E)
- When prescribing SMBG, ensure that patients receive initial instruction in, and routine follow-up evaluation of, SMBG technique and their ability to use data to adjust therapy. (E)
- Continuous glucose monitoring (CGM) in conjunction with intensive insulin regimens can be a

**Table 7   Components of the Comprehensive Diabetes Evaluation**

Medical history

- age and characteristics of onset of diabetes (e.g. DKA, asymptomatic laboratory finding)
- eating patterns, physical activity habits, nutritional status, and weight history; growth and development in children and adolescents
- diabetes education history
- review of previous treatment regimens and response to therapy (A1C records)
- current treatment of diabetes, including medications, meal plan, physical activity patterns, and results of glucose monitoring and patient's use of data
- DKA frequency, severity, and cause
- hypoglycemic episodes
  - o hypoglycemia awareness
  - o any severe hypoglycemia: frequency and cause
- history of diabetes-related complications
  - o microvascular: retinopathy, nephropathy, neuropathy (sensory, including history of foot lesions; autonomic, including sexual dysfunction and gastroparesis)
  - o macrovascular: CHD, cerebrovascular disease, PAD
  - o other: psychosocial problems,* dental disease*

Physical examination

- height, weight, BMI
- blood pressure determination, including orthostatic measurements when indicated
- fundoscopic examination*

- thyroid palpation
- skin examination (for acanthosis nigricans and insulin injection sites)
- comprehensive foot examination:
  - o inspection
  - o palpation of dorsalis pedis and posterior tibial pulses
  - o presence/absence of patellar and Achilles reflexes
  - o determination of proprioception, vibration, and monofilament sensation

Laboratory evaluation

- A1C, if results not available within past 2–3 months

If not performed/available within past year:

- fasting lipid profile, including total, LDL- and HDL-cholesterol and triglycerides
- liver function tests
- test for urine albumin excretion with spot urine albumin/creatinine ratio
- serum creatinine and calculated GFR
- thyroid-stimulating hormone in type 1 diabetes, dyslipidemia or women over age 50

Referrals

- annual dilated eye exam
- family planning for women of reproductive age
- registered dietitian for MNT
- diabetes self-management education
- dental examination
- mental Health professional, if needed

*See appropriate referrals for these categories.

useful tool to lower A1C in selected adults (age ≥ 25 years) with type 1 diabetes. (A)

- Although the evidence for A1C lowering is less strong in children, teens, and younger adults, CGM may be helpful in these groups. Success correlates with adherence to ongoing use of the device. (C)
- CGM may be a supplemental tool to SMBG in those with hypoglycemia unawareness and/or frequent hypoglycaemic episodes. (E)

The ADA's consensus and position statements on SMBG provide a comprehensive review of the subject

(American Diabetes Association, 1987; 1994). Major clinical trials of insulin-treated patients that demonstrated the benefits of intensive glycemic control on diabetes complications have included SMBG as part of multifactorial interventions, suggesting that SMBG is a component of effective therapy.

SMBG allows patients to evaluate their individual response to therapy and assess whether glycemic targets are being achieved. Results of SMBG can be useful in preventing hypoglycemia and adjusting medications (particularly prandial insulin doses), MNT, and physical activity.

The frequency and timing of SMBG should be dictated by the particular needs and goals of the patients. SMBG is especially important for patients treated with insulin to monitor for and prevent asymptomatic hypoglycemia and hyperglycemia. For most patients with type 1 diabetes and pregnant women taking insulin, SMBG is recommended three or more times daily. For this population, significantly more frequent testing may be required to reach A1C targets safely without hypoglycemia. The optimal frequency and timing of SMBG for patients with type 2 diabetes on noninsulin therapy is unclear. A meta-analysis of SMBG in noninsulin-treated patients with type 2 diabetes concluded that some regimen of SMBG was associated with a reduction in A1C of ≥ 0.4%. However, many of the studies in this analysis also included patient education with diet and exercise counseling and, in some cases, pharmacologic intervention, making it difficult to assess the contribution of SMBG alone to improved control (Welschen *et al.*, 2005). Several recent trials have called into question the clinical utility and cost-effectiveness of routine SMBG in noninsulin-treated patients (Farmer *et al.*, 2007; O'Kane *et al.*, 2007; Simon *et al.*, 2008).

Because the accuracy of SMBG is instrument- and user-dependent (Sacks *et al.*, 2002), it is important to evaluate each patient's monitoring technique, both initially and at regular intervals thereafter. In addition, optimal use of SMBG requires proper interpretation of the data. Patients should be taught how to use the data to adjust food intake, exercise, or pharmacological therapy to achieve specific glycemic goals, and these skills should be reevaluated periodically.

CGM through the measurement of interstitial glucose (which correlates well with plasma glucose) is available. These sensors require calibration with SMBG, and the latter is still recommended for making acute treatment decisions. CGM devices also have alarms for hypo- and hyperglycemic excursions. Small studies in selected patients with type 1 diabetes have suggested that CGM use reduces the time spent in hypo- and hyperglycaemic ranges and may modestly improve glycemic control. A larger 26-week

randomized trial of 322 type 1 patients showed that adults age 25 years and above using intensive insulin therapy and CGM experienced a 0.5% reduction in A1C (from ~7.6 to 7.1%) as compared with usual intensive insulin therapy with SMBG (The Juvenile Diabetes Research Foundation Continuous Glucose Monitoring Study Group, 2008). Sensor use in children, teens, and adults to age 24 years did not result in significant A1C lowering, and there was no significant difference in hypoglycemia in any group. Importantly, the greatest predictor of A1C lowering in this study for all age groups was frequency of sensor use, which was lower in younger age-groups. Although CGM is an evolving technology, emerging data suggest that, in appropriately selected patients who are motivated to wear it most of the time, it may offer benefit. CGM may be particularly useful in those with hypoglycemia unawareness and/or frequent episodes of hypoglycemia, and studies in this area are ongoing.

### b. *A1C*

**Recommendations**

- Perform the A1C test at least twice a year in patients who are meeting treatment goals (and who have stable glycemic control). (E)
- Perform the A1C test quarterly in patients whose therapy has changed or who are not meeting glycemic goals. (E)
- Use of point-of-care testing for A1C allows for timely decisions on therapy changes, when needed. (E)

Because A1C is thought to reflect average glycemia over several months (Sacks *et al.*, 2002), and has strong predictive value for diabetes complications (Knowler *et al.*, 2002; Stratton *et al.*, 2000), A1C testing should be performed routinely in all patients with diabetes at initial assessment and then as part of continuing care. Measurement approximately every three months determines whether a patient's glycemic targets have been reached and maintained. For any individual patient, the frequency of A1C testing should be dependent on the clinical situation, the treatment regimen used, and the judgment of the clinician. Some patients with stable glycemia well within target may do well with testing only twice a year, while unstable or highly intensively managed patients (e.g. pregnant type 1 women) may be tested more frequently than every three months. The availability of the A1C result at the time that the patient is seen (point-of-care testing) has been reported to result in increased intensification of therapy and improvement in glycemic control (Cagliero *et al.*, 1999; Miller *et al.*, 2003).

The A1C test is subject to certain limitations. Conditions that affect erythrocyte turnover (hemolysis, blood loss) and hemoglobin variants must be considered, particularly when the A1C result does not correlate with the patient's clinical situation (Sacks *et al.*, 2002). In addition, A1C does not provide a measure of glycemic variability or hypoglycemia. For patients prone to glycemic variability (especially type 1 patients, or type 2 patients with severe insulin deficiency), glycemic control is best judged by the combination of results of SMBG testing and the A1C. The A1C may also serve as a check on the accuracy of the patient's meter (or the patient's reported SMBG results) and the adequacy of the SMBG testing schedule.

Table 8 contains the correlation between A1C levels and mean plasma glucose levels based on data from the international A1C-Derived Average Glucose (ADAG) trial utilizing frequent SMBG and continuous glucose monitoring in 507 adults (83% Caucasian) with type 1, type 2, and no diabetes (UKPDS, 1998) The ADA and American Association of Clinical Chemists have determined that the correlation ($r = 0.92$) is strong enough to justify reporting both an A1C result and an estimated average glucose (eAG) result when a clinician orders the A1C test. The table in the previous versions of the Standards of Medical Care in Diabetes describing the correlation between A1C and mean glucose was derived from relatively sparse data (one seven-point profile over one day per A1C reading) in the primarily Caucasian type 1 participants in the Diabetes Control and Complications

**Table 8  Correlation of A1C with Average Glucose**

| A1C (%) | Mean Plasma Glucose | |
| --- | --- | --- |
| | mg/dl | mmol/l |
| 6 | 126 | 7.0 |
| 7 | 154 | 8.6 |
| 8 | 183 | 10.2 |
| 9 | 212 | 11.8 |
| 10 | 240 | 13.4 |
| 11 | 269 | 14.9 |
| 12 | 298 | 16.5 |

Estimates based on ADAG data of ~2700 glucose measurements over three months per A1C measurement in 507 adults with type 1, type 2, and no diabetes. Correlation between A1C and average glucose: 0.92 (42). A calculator for converting A1C results into eAG, in either mg/dl or mmol/l, is available at http://professional.diabetes.org/eAG.

Trial (DCCT) (Rohlfing *et al.*, 2002). Clinicians should note that the numbers in the table are now different, as they are based on ~2800 readings per A1C in the ADAG trial. In the ADAG study, there were no significant differences among racial and ethnic groups in the regression lines between A1C and mean glucose, although there was a trend towards a difference between African/African-American and Caucasian participants' regression lines that might have been significant had more African/African-American participants been studied. A recent study comparing A1C to CGM data in 48 type 1 children found a highly statistically significant correlation between A1C and mean blood glucose, although the correlation ($r = 0.7$) was significantly lower than in the ADAG trial (Wilson *et al.*, 2008). Whether there are significant differences in how A1C relates to average glucose in children or in African-American patients is an area for further study. For the time being, the question has not led to different recommendations about testing A1C or to different interpretations of the clinical meaning of given levels of A1C in those populations.

For patients in whom A1C/eAG and measured blood glucose appear discrepant, clinicians should consider the possibilities of hemoglobinopathy or altered red cell turnover and the options of more frequent and/or different timing of SMBG or use of CGM. Other measures of chronic glycemia such as fructosamine are available, but their linkage to average glucose and their prognostic significance are not as clear as is the case for A1C.

### 1.5.3.2. *Glycemic goals in adults*

- Lowering A1C to below or around 7% has been shown to reduce microvascular and neuropathic complications of type 1 and type 2 diabetes. Therefore, for microvascular disease prevention, the A1C goal for nonpregnant adults in general is < 7%. (A)
- In type 1 and type 2 diabetes, randomized controlled trials of intensive versus standard glycemic control have not shown a significant reduction in CVD outcomes during the randomized portion of the trials. Long-term follow-up of the DCCT and UK Prospective Diabetes Study (UKPDS) cohorts suggests that treatment to A1C targets below or around 7% in the years soon after the diagnosis of diabetes is associated with long-term reduction in risk of macrovascular disease. Until more evidence becomes available, the general goal of < 7% appears reasonable for many adults for macrovascular risk reduction. (B)
- Subgroup analyses of clinical trials such as the DCCT and UKPDS and the microvascular evidence from the Action in Diabetes and Vascular Disease: Preterax and Diamicron MR Controlled Evaluation (ADVANCE) trial suggest a small but incremental benefit in microvascular outcomes with A1C values closer to normal. Therefore, for selected individual patients, providers might reasonably suggest even lower A1C goals than the general goal of < 7%, if this can be achieved without significant hypoglycemia or other adverse effects of treatment. Such patients might include those with short duration of diabetes, long life expectancy, and no significant CVD. (B)
- Conversely, less stringent A1C goals than the general goal of < 7% may be appropriate for patients with a history of severe hypoglycemia, limited life expectancy, advanced microvascular or macrovascular complications, extensive comorbid conditions, and those with longstanding diabetes in whom the general goal is difficult to attain despite DSME, appropriate glucose monitoring, and effective doses of multiple glucose-lowering agents including insulin. (C)

Glycemic control is fundamental to the management of diabetes. The DCCT, a prospective, randomized, controlled trial of intensive versus standard glycemic control in patients with relatively recently diagnosed type 1 diabetes, showed definitively that improved glycemic control is associated with significantly decreased rates of microvascular (retinopathy and nephropathy) as well as neuropathic complications (DCCT, 1993). Follow-up of the DCCT cohorts in the Epidemiology of Diabetes Interventions and Complications (EDIC) study has shown persistence of this effect in previously intensively treated subjects, even though their glycemic control has been equivalent to that of previous standard arm subjects during follow-up (DCCT, 2000; Martin *et al.*, 2006).

In type 2 diabetes, the Kumamoto study (Ohkubo *et al.*, 1995) and the UKPDS (UKPDTS, 1998a; UKPDS, 1998b) demonstrated significant reductions in microvascular and neuropathic complications with intensive therapy. Similar to the DCCT-EDIC findings, long-term follow-up of the UKPDS cohort has recently demonstrated a "legacy effect" of early intensive glycemic control on long-term rates of microvascular complications, even with loss of glycemic separation between the intensive and standard cohorts after the end of the randomized controlled (Holman *et al.*, 2008).

In each of these large randomized prospective clinical trials, treatment regimens that reduced average A1C to ≥ 7% (≥ 1% above the upper limits of normal) were associated with fewer long-term microvascular complications; however, intensive control was found to increase the risk of severe hypoglycemia, most notably in the DCCT, and led to weight gain (Stratton *et al.*, 2000; Lawson *et al.*, 1999).

Epidemiological analyses of the DCCT and UKPDS (Stratton *et al.*, 2000; DCCT, 1993) demonstrate a curvilinear relationship between A1C and microvascular complications. Such analyses suggest that, on a population level, the greatest number of complications will be averted if patients are taken from very poor control to fair or good control. These analyses also suggest that further lowering of A1C from 7 to 6% is associated with further reduction in the risk of microvascular complications, albeit the absolute risk reductions become much smaller. Given the substantially increased risk of hypoglycemia (particularly in those with type 1 diabetes) and the relatively much greater effort required to achieve near normoglycemia, the risks of lower targets may outweigh the potential benefits on microvascular complications on a population level. However, selected individual patients, especially those with little comorbidity and long life expectancy (who may reap the benefits of further lowering of glycemia below 7%) may, at patient and provider judgment, adopt glycemic targets as close to normal as possible as long as significant hypoglycemia does not become a barrier.

Whereas many epidemiologic studies and meta-analyses (Selvin *et al.*, 2004; Stettler *et al.*, 2006) have clearly shown a direct relationship between A1C and CVD, the potential of intensive glycemic control to reduce CVD has been less clearly defined. In the DCCT, there was a trend towards lower risk of CVD events with intensive control (risk reduction 41%, 95% CI: 10–68%), but the number of events was small. However, a nine-year post-DCCT follow-up of the cohort has shown that participants previously randomized to the intensive arm had a 42% reduction ($P = 0.02$) in CVD outcomes and a 57% reduction ($P = 0.02$) in the risk of nonfatal myocardial infarction (MI), stroke, or CVD death as compared with those previously in the standard arm (Nathan *et al.*, 2005).

The UKPDS trial of type 2 diabetes observed a 16% reduction in cardiovascular complications (combined fatal or nonfatal MI and sudden death) in the intensive glycemic control arm, although this difference was not statistically significant ($P = 0.052$), and

there was no suggestion of benefit on other CVD outcomes such as stroke. In an epidemiologic analysis of the study cohort, a continuous association was observed, such that for every percentage point lower median onstudy A1C (e.g. 8 to 7%) there was a statistically significant 18% reduction in CVD events, again with no glycemic threshold. A recent report of 10 years of follow-up of the UKPDS cohort describes, for the participants originally randomized to intensive glycemic control as compared with those randomized to conventional glycemic control, long-term reductions in MI (15% with sulfonylurea or insulin as initial pharmacotherapy, 33% with metformin as initial pharmacotherapy, both statistically significant) and in all-cause mortality (13% and 27%, respectively, both statistically significant) (Holman *et al.*, 2008).

Because of ongoing uncertainty regarding whether intensive glycemic control can reduce the increased risk of CVD events in people with type 2 diabetes, several large long-term trials were launched in the past decade to compare the effects of intensive versus standard glycemic control on CVD outcomes in relatively high-risk participants with established type 2 diabetes.

The Action to Control Cardiovascular Risk in Diabetes (ACCORD) study randomized 10,251 participants with either history of a CVD event (ages 40–79 years) or significant CVD risk (ages 55–79) to a strategy of intensive glycemic control (target A1C < 6.0%) or standard glycemic control (A1C target 7.0–7.9%). Investigators used multiple glycemic medications in both arms. ACCORD participants were on average 62-years old and had a mean duration of diabetes of 10 years, with 35% already treated with insulin at baseline. From a baseline median A1C of 8.1%, the intensive arm reached a median A1C of 6.4% within 12 months of randomization, while the standard group reached a median A1C of 7.5%. Other risk factors were treated aggressively and equally in both groups. The intensive glycemic control group had more use of insulin in combination with multiple oral agents, significantly more weight gain, and more episodes of severe hypoglycemia than the standard group.

In February 2008, the glycemic control study of ACCORD was halted on the recommendation of the study's data safety monitoring board due to the finding of an increased rate of mortality in the intensive arm as compared with the standard arm (1.41%/year vs. 1.14%/year; HR 1.22 [95% CI: 1.01–1.46]), with a similar increase in cardiovascular deaths. The primary outcome of ACCORD (MI, stroke, or cardiovascular death) was lower in the intensive glycemic control group due to a reduction in nonfatal MI, although this finding was not statistically significant when the study was terminated (HR 0.90 [95% CI: 0.78–1.04]; $P = 0.16$).

Exploratory analyses of the mortality findings of ACCORD (evaluating variables including weight gain, use of any specific drug or drug combination, and hypoglycemia) were reportedly unable to identify an explanation for the excess mortality in the intensive arm. Prespecified subset analyses showed that participants with no previous CVD event and those who had a baseline A1C < 8% had a statistically significant reduction in the primary CVD outcome.

The ADVANCE study randomized 11,140 participants to a strategy of intensive glycemic control (with primary therapy being the sulfonylurea gliclazide and additional medications as needed to achieve a target A1C of ≤ 6.5%) or to standard therapy (in which any medication but gliclazide could be used and the glycemic target was according to "local guidelines"). ADVANCE participants (who had to be at least 55-year of age with either known vascular disease or at least one other vascular risk factor) were slightly older and of similar high CVD risk as those in ACCORD. However, they had an average duration of diabetes two years shorter, a lower baseline A1C (median 7.2%), and almost no use of insulin at enrollment. The median A1C levels achieved in the intensive and standard arms were 6.3% and 7.0%, respectively, and maximal separation between the arms took several years to achieve. Use of other drugs that favorably impact CVD risk (aspirin, statins, ACE inhibitors) was lower in ADVANCE than in the ACCORD or Veterans Affairs Diabetes Trial (VADT).

The primary outcome of ADVANCE was a combination of microvascular events (nephropathy and retinopathy) and major adverse cardiovascular events (MI, stroke, and cardiovascular death). Intensive glycemic control significantly reduced the primary endpoint (HR 0.90 [95% CI: 0.82–0.98]; $P = 0.01$), although this was due to a significant reduction in the microvascular outcome (0.86 [0.77–0.97], $P = 0.01$), primarily the development of macroalbuminuria, with no significant reduction in the macrovascular outcome (0.94 [0.84–1.06]; $P = 0.32$). There was no difference in the overall or cardiovascular mortality between the intensive and the standard glycemic control arms (Patel *et al.*, 2008).

The VADT randomized 1791 participants with type 2 diabetes uncontrolled on insulin or maximal dose oral agents (median entry A1C 9.4%) to a strategy of intensive glycemic control (goal A1C < 6.0%) or standard glycemic control, with a planned A1C separation of at least 1.5%. Medication treatment algorithms were used to achieve the specified glycemic goals, with a goal of using similar medications in both groups. Median A1C levels of 6.9% and 8.4% were achieved in the intensive and standard arms, respectively, within the first year of the study. Other CVD risk factors were treated aggressively and equally in both groups.

The primary outcome of the VADT was a composite of CVD events (MI, stroke, cardiovascular death, revascularization, hospitalization for heart failure, and amputation for ischemia). During a mean 6-year follow-up period, the cumulative primary outcome was nonsignificantly lower in the intensive arm (HR 0.87 [95% CI: 0.73–1.04]; $P = 0.12$). There were more CVD deaths in the intensive arm than in the standard arm (40 vs. 33; sudden deaths 11 vs. 4), but the difference was not statistically significant. Post hoc subgroup analyses suggested that duration of diabetes interacted with randomization such that participants with duration of diabetes less than about 12 years appeared to have a CVD benefit of intensive glycemic control, while those with longer duration of disease before study entry had a neutral or even adverse effect of intensive glycemic control. Other exploratory analyses suggested that severe hypoglycemia within the past 90 days was a strong predictor of the primary outcome and of CVD mortality (Duckworth, 2008).

The cause of the excess deaths in the intensive glycemic control arm of ACCORD as compared with the standard arm has been difficult to pinpoint. By design of the trial, randomization to the intensive arm was associated with or has led to many downstream effects, such as higher rates of severe hypoglycemia; more frequent use of insulin, TZDs, other drugs, and drug combinations; and greater weight gain. Such factors may be associated statistically with the higher mortality rate in the intensive arm but may not be causative.

It is biologically plausible that severe hypoglycemia could increase the risk of cardiovascular death in participants with high underlying CVD risk. Other plausible mechanisms for the increase in mortality in ACCORD include weight gain, unmeasured drug effects or interactions, or the overall "intensity" of the ACCORD intervention (use of multiple oral glucose-lowering drugs along with multiple doses of insulin, frequent therapy adjustments to push A1C and self-monitored blood glucose to very low targets, and an intense effort to aggressively reduce A1C by ~2% in participants with advanced diabetes and multiple comorbidities entering the trial).

Since the ADVANCE trial did not show any increase in mortality in the intensive glycemic control arm, examining the differences between ADVANCE and ACCORD supports additional hypotheses. ADVANCE participants on average appeared to have earlier or less advanced diabetes, with shorter duration by 2–3 years and a lower A1C at entry despite very little use of insulin at baseline. A1C was also lowered less and more gradually in the ADVANCE trial, and there was no significant weight gain with intensive glycemic therapy. Although severe hypoglycemia was defined somewhat differently in the three trials, it appears that this occurred in fewer than 3% of intensively treated ADVANCE participants for the entire study duration (median 5 years) as compared

with ~16% of intensively treated subjects in ACCORD and 21% in VADT.

It is likely that the increase in mortality in ACCORD was related to the overall treatment strategies for intensifying glycemic control in the population studied, not the achieved A1C *per se*. The ADVANCE study achieved a median A1C in its intensive arm similar to that in the ACCORD study, with no increased mortality hazard. Thus, the ACCORD mortality findings do not imply that patients with type 2 diabetes, who can easily achieve or maintain low A1C levels with lifestyle modifications with or without pharmacotherapy, are at risk and need to "raise" their A1C.

The three trials compared treatments to A1C levels in the "flatter" part of the observational glycemia-CVD risk curves (median A1C of 6.4–6.9% in the intensive arms as compared with 7.0–8.4% in the standard arms). Importantly, their results should not be extrapolated to imply that there would be no cardiovascular benefit of glucose lowering from very poor control (e.g. A1C > 9%) to good control (e.g. A1C < 7%).

All three trials were carried out in participants with established diabetes (mean duration 8–11 years) and either known CVD or multiple risk factors suggesting the presence of established atherosclerosis. Subset analyses of the three trials suggested a significant benefit of intensive glycemic control on CVD in participants with shorter duration of diabetes, lower A1C at entry, and/or or absence of known CVD. The DCCT-EDIC study and the long-term follow-up of the UKPDS cohort both suggest that intensive glycemic control initiated soon after diagnosis of diabetes in patients with a lower level of CVD risk may impart long-term protection from CVD events. As is the case with microvascular complications, it may be that glycemic control plays a greater role before macrovascular disease is well developed and minimal or no role when it is advanced.

The benefits of intensive glycemic control on microvascular and neuropathic complications are well established for both type 1 and type 2 diabetes. The

ADVANCE trial has added to that evidence base by demonstrating a significant reduction in the risk of new or worsening albuminuria when A1C was lowered to 6.3%, as compared with standard glycemic control, achieving an A1C of 7.0%. The lack of significant reduction in CVD events with intensive glycemic control in ACCORD, ADVANCE, and VADT should not lead clinicians to abandon the general target of an A1C < 7.0% and thereby discount the benefit of good control on what are serious and debilitating microvascular complications.

The evidence for a cardiovascular benefit of intensive glycemic control primarily rests on long-term follow-up of study cohorts treated early in the course of type 1 and type 2 diabetes and subset analyses of ACCORD, ADVANCE, and VADT. Conversely, the mortality findings in ACCORD suggest that the potential risks of very intensive glycemic control may outweigh its benefits in some patients, such as those with a very long duration of diabetes, known history of severe hypoglycemia, advanced atherosclerosis, and advanced age/frailty. Certainly, providers should be vigilant in preventing severe hypoglycemia in patients with advanced disease and should not aggressively attempt to achieve near-normal A1C levels in patients in whom such a target cannot be reasonably easily and safely achieved.

Recommended glycemic goals for nonpregnant adults are shown in Table 9. The recommendations are based on those for A1C, with listed blood glucose levels that appear to correlate with achievement of an A1C of < 7%. The issue of pre- versus postprandial SMBG targets is complex (American Diabetes Association, 2001). Elevated postchallenge (2-h OGTT) glucose values have been associated with increased cardiovascular risk independent of FPG in some epidemiological studies. In diabetic subjects, some surrogate measures of vascular pathology, such as endothelial dysfunction, are negatively affected by postprandial hyperglycemia (Ceriello *et al.*, 2002). It is clear that postprandial hyperglycemia, like preprandial hyperglycemia, contributes to elevated A1C levels, with its relative contribution being higher at A1C

**Table 9  Summary of Glycemic Recommendations for Nonpregnant Adults with Diabetes**

| | |
|---|---|
| A1C | < 7.0%* |
| Preprandial capillary plasma glucose | 70–130 mg/dl (3.9–7.2 mmol/l) |
| Peak postprandial capillary plasma glucose | < 180 mg/dl (< 10.0 mmol/l) |

Key concepts in setting glycemic goals:

- A1C is the primary target for glycemic control.
- Goals should be individualized based on:
  - duration of diabetes
  - age/life expectancy
  - comorbid conditions
  - known CVD or advanced microvascular complications
  - hypoglycemia unawareness
  - individual patient considerations
- More or less stringent glycemic goals may be appropriate for individual patients.
- Postprandial glucose may be targeted if A1C goals are not met despite reaching preprandial glucose goals.

*Referenced to a nondiabetic range of 4.0–6.0% using a DCCT-based assay. Postprandial glucose measurements should be made 1–2 h after the beginning of the meal, generally peak levels in patients with diabetes.

levels that are closer to 7%. However, outcome studies have clearly shown A1C to be the primary predictor of complications, and landmark glycemic control trials such as the DCCT and UKPDS relied overwhelmingly on preprandial SMBG. Additionally, a randomized controlled trial presented at the 68th Scientific Sessions of the American Diabetes Association in June 2008 found no CVD benefit of insulin regimens targeting postprandial glucose as compared with those targeting preprandial glucose. A reasonable recommendation for postprandial testing and targets is that for individuals who have premeal glucose values within target but have A1C values above target, monitoring postprandial plasma glucose (PPG) 1–2 h after the start of the meal and treatment aimed at reducing PPG values to < 180 mg/dl may help lower A1C.

As noted above, less stringent treatment goals may be appropriate for adults with limited life expectancies or advanced vascular disease. Severe or frequent hypoglycemia is an absolute indication for the modification of treatment regimens, including setting higher glycemic goals.

Regarding goals for glycemic control for women with GDM, recommendations from the Fifth International Workshop — Conference on Gestational Diabetes Mellitus (Metzger *et al.*, 2007) were to target the following maternal capillary glucose concentrations:

- preprandial: _95 mg/dl (5.3 mmol/l) and either
- 1-h postmeal:_140 mg/dl (7.8 mmol/l) or
- 2-h postmeal:_120 mg/dl (6.7 mmol/l)

For women with preexisting type 1 or type 2 diabetes who become pregnant, a recent consensus statement (Kitzmiller *et al.*, 2008) recommended the following as optimal glycemic goals, if they can be achieved without excessive hypoglycemia:

- premeal, bedtime, and overnight glucose 60–99 mg/dl
- peak postprandial glucose 100–129 mg/dl
- A1C < 6.0%

## 1.6. Prevention and Management of Diabetes Complications

### 1.6.1. CVD

CVD is the major cause of morbidity and mortality for individuals with diabetes and the largest contributor to the direct and indirect costs of diabetes. The common conditions coexisting with type 2 diabetes (e.g. hypertension and dyslipidemia) are clear risk factors for CVD, and diabetes itself confers independent risk. Numerous studies have shown the efficacy of controlling individual cardiovascular risk factors in preventing

or slowing CVD in people with diabetes. Large benefits are seen when multiple risk factors are addressed globally (Gaede *et al.*, 2008). Evidence is summarized in the following sections and reviewed in detail in the ADA technical reviews on hypertension (Arauz-Pacheco, 2002); dyslipidemia (Haffner, 1998); aspirin therapy (Colwell, 1997); and smoking cessation (Haire-Joshu, 1999) and in the American Heart Association (AHA)/ADA scientific statement on prevention of CVD in people with diabetes (Buse *et al.*, 2007).

#### 1.6.1.1. *Hypertension/blood pressure control*
**Recommendations**

*Screening and diagnosis*

- Blood pressure should be measured at every routine diabetes visit. Patients found to have a systolic blood pressure of ≥ 130 mm Hg or a diastolic blood pressure of ≥ 80 mm Hg should have blood pressure confirmed on a separate day. Repeat systolic blood pressure of ≥ 130 mm Hg or diastolic blood pressure of ≥ 80 mm Hg confirms a diagnosis of hypertension. (C)

*Goals*

- Patients with diabetes should be treated to a systolic blood pressure < 130 mm Hg. (C)
- Patients with diabetes should be treated to a diastolic blood pressure < 80 mm Hg. (B)

*Treatment*

- Patients with a systolic blood pressure of 130–139 mm Hg or a diastolic blood pressure of 80–89 mm Hg may be given lifestyle therapy alone for a maximum of three months and then, if targets are not achieved, be treated with the addition of pharmacological agents. (E)
- Patients with more severe hypertension (systolic blood pressure ≥ 140 mm Hg or diastolic blood pressure ≥ 90 mm Hg) at diagnosis or follow-up should receive pharmacologic therapy in addition to lifestyle therapy. (A)

- Pharmacologic therapy for patients with diabetes and hypertension should be with a regimen that includes either an ACE inhibitor or an angiotensin receptor blocker (ARB). If one class is not tolerated, the other should be substituted. If it is necessary to achieve blood pressure targets, a thiazide diuretic should be added for those with an estimated GFR (see below) $\geq$ 30 ml/min per 1.73 $m^2$ and a loop diuretic for those with an estimated GFR < 30 ml/min per 1.73 $m^2$. (C)
- Multiple drug therapy (two or more agents at maximal doses) is generally required to achieve blood pressure targets. (B)
- If ACE inhibitors, ARBs, or diuretics are used, kidney function and serum potassium levels should be closely monitored. (E)
- In pregnant patients with diabetes and chronic hypertension, blood pressure target goals of 110–129/65–79 mm Hg are suggested in the interest of long-term maternal health and minimizing impaired fetal growth. ACE inhibitors and ARBs are contraindicated during pregnancy. (E)

Hypertension is a common comorbidity of diabetes, affecting the majority of patients, with prevalence depending on type of diabetes, age, obesity, and ethnicity. Hypertension is a major risk factor for both CVD and microvascular complications. In type 1 diabetes, hypertension is often the result of underlying nephropathy, while in type 2, it usually coexists with other cardiometabolic risk factors.

### Screening and diagnosis

Measurement of blood pressure in the office should be done by a trained individual and follow the guidelines established for nondiabetic individuals: Measurement in the seated position, with feet on the floor and arm supported at heart level, after 5 min of rest. Cuff size should be appropriate for the upper arm circumference.

Elevated values should be confirmed on a separate day. Because of the clear synergistic risks of hypertension and diabetes, the diagnostic cutoff for a diagnosis of hypertension is lower in people with diabetes (blood pressure $\geq$ 130/80) than in those without diabetes (blood pressure $\geq$ 140/90 mm Hg) (Chobanian *et al.*, 2003).

Home blood pressure self-monitoring and 24-h ambulatory blood pressure monitoring may provide additional evidence of "white coat" and masked hypertension and other discrepancies between office and "true" blood pressure, and studies in nondiabetic populations show that home measurements may better correlate with CVD risk than office measurements (Bobrie *et al.*, 2004; Sega *et al.*, 2005). However, the preponderance of the clear evidence of benefits of treatment of hypertension in people with diabetes is based on office measurements.

### Treatment goals

Randomized clinical trials have demonstrated the benefit (reduction of CHD events, stroke, and nephropathy) of lowering blood pressure to < 140 mm Hg systolic and < 80 mm Hg diastolic in individuals with diabetes (Chobanian *et al.*, 2003, UKPDS; 1998; Hansson *et al.*, 1998; Adler *et al.*, 2000). Epidemiologic analyses show that blood pressure > 115/75 mm Hg is associated with increased cardiovascular event rates and mortality in individuals with diabetes. Therefore, a target blood pressure goal of < 130/80 mm Hg is reasonable if it can be safely achieved. The ongoing ACCORD trial is designed to determine whether blood pressure lowering to systolic blood pressure < 120 mm Hg provides greater cardiovascular protection than a systolic blood pressure level of < 140 mm Hg in patients with type 2 diabetes (www.accord.org).

### Treatment strategies

Although there are no well-controlled studies of diet and exercise in the treatment of hypertension in individuals with diabetes, studies in nondiabetic individuals have shown antihypertensive effects similar to pharmacologic monotherapy of reducing sodium intake and excess body weight; increasing consumption of fruits, vegetables, and low-fat dairy products;

avoiding excessive alcohol consumption; and increasing activity levels (Chobanian *et al.*, 2003; Sacks *et al.*, 2001). These nonpharmacological strategies may also positively affect glycemia and lipid control. Their effects on cardiovascular events have not been established. An initial trial of nonpharmacologic therapy may be reasonable in diabetic individuals with mild hypertension (systolic blood pressure 130–139 mm Hg or diastolic blood pressure 80–89 mm Hg). If the blood pressure is ≥ 140 mm Hg systolic and/or ≥ 90 mm Hg diastolic at the time of diagnosis, pharmacologic therapy should be initiated along with nonpharmacologic therapy (Chobanian *et al.*, 2003).

Lowering of blood pressure with regimens based on a variety of antihypertensive drugs, including ACE inhibitors, ARBs, $\beta$-blockers, diuretics, and calcium channel blockers, has been shown to be effective in reducing cardiovascular events. Several studies have suggested that ACE inhibitors may be superior to dihydropyridine calcium channel blockers in reducing cardiovascular events (Tatti *et al.*, 1998; Estacio *et al.*, 1998; Schrier *et al.*, 2007). However, a variety of other studies have shown no specific advantage to ACE inhibitors as an initial treatment of hypertension in the general hypertensive population, but rather an advantage on cardiovascular outcomes of an initial therapy with low-dose thiazide diuretics (Chobanian *et al.*, 2003; ALLHAT, 2002; Psaty *et al.*, 2002).

In people with diabetes, inhibitors of the renin-angiotensin system (RAS) may have unique advantages for initial or early therapy of hypertension. In a nonhypertension trial of high-risk individuals, including a large subset with diabetes, an ACE inhibitor reduced CVD outcomes (HOPE, 2000). In patients with congestive heart failure (CHF), including diabetic subgroups, ARBs have been shown to reduce major CVD outcomes (Pfeffer *et al.*, 2003; Granger *et al.*, 2003; McMurray *et al.*, 2003, Lindholm *et al.*, 2002), and in type 2 patients with significant nephropathy, ARBs were superior to calcium channel blockers for reducing heart failure (Berl *et al.*, 2003;

Laffel *et al.*, 1995; Bakris *et al.*, 2000). Though evidence for distinct advantages of RAS inhibitors on CVD outcomes in diabetes remains conflicting (UKPDS, 1998; Psaty *et al.*, 1997), the high CVD risks associated with diabetes, and the high prevalence of undiagnosed CVD, may still favor recommendations for their use as a first-line hypertension therapy in people with diabetes (Chobanian *et al.*, 2003). Recently, the blood pressure arm of the ADVANCE trial demonstrated that routine administration of a fixed combination of the ACE inhibitor perindopril and the diuretic indapamide significantly reduced combined microvascular and macrovascular outcomes, as well as CVD and total mortality. The improved outcomes could also have been due to lower achieved blood pressure in the perindopril-indapamide arm (183). The compelling benefits of RAS inhibitors in diabetic patients with albuminuria or renal insufficiency provide additional rationale for use of these agents.

An important caveat is that most patients with hypertension require multidrug therapy to reach treatment goals, especially diabetic patients whose targets are lower. Many patients will require three or more drugs to reach target goals (Chobanian *et al.*, 2003). If blood pressure is refractory to multiple agents, clinicians should consider an evaluation for secondary forms of hypertension.

During pregnancy in diabetic women with chronic hypertension, target blood pressure goals of systolic blood pressure, 110–129 mm Hg and diastolic blood pressure, 65–79 mm Hg are reasonable, as they contribute to long-term maternal health. Lower blood pressure levels may be associated with impaired fetal growth. During pregnancy, treatment with ACE inhibitors and ARBs is contraindicated, since they are likely to cause fetal damage. Antihypertensive drugs known to be effective and safe in pregnancy include methyldopa, labetalol, diltiazem, clonidine, and prazosin. Chronic diuretic use during pregnancy has been associated with restricted maternal plasma volume, which might reduce uteroplacental perfusion (Sibai, 1996).

### 1.6.1.2. *Dyslipidemia/lipid management*

**Recommendations**

*Screening*

- In most adult patients, fasting lipid profile should be measured at least annually. In adults with low-risk lipid values (LDL cholesterol < 100 mg/dl, HDL cholesterol > 50 mg/dl, and triglycerides < 150 mg/dl), lipid assessments may be repeated every two years. (E)

*Treatment recommendations and goals*

- Lifestyle modification focusing on the reduction of saturated fat, *trans* fat, and cholesterol intake; weight loss (if indicated); and increased physical activity should be recommended to improve the lipid profile in patients with diabetes. (A)
- Statin therapy should be added to lifestyle therapy, regardless of baseline lipid levels, for diabetic patients:

  o with overt CVD (A)

  o without CVD who are over the age of 40 and have one or more other CVD risk factors. (A)

- For lower-risk patients than the above (e.g. without overt CVD and under the age of 40), statin therapy should be considered in addition to lifestyle therapy if LDL cholesterol remains above 100 mg/dl or in those with multiple CVD risk factors. (E)
- In individuals without overt CVD, the primary goal is an LDL cholesterol < 100 mg/dl (2.6 mmol/l). (A)
- In individuals with overt CVD, a lower LDL cholesterol goal of < 70 mg/dl (1.8 nmmol/l), using a high dose of a statin, is an option. (B)
- If drug-treated patients do not reach the above targets on maximal tolerated statin therapy, a reduction in LDL cholesterol of ~30–40% from baseline is an alternative therapeutic goal. (A)
- Triglycerides levels < 150 mg/dl (1.7 mmol/l) and HDL cholesterol > 40 mg/dl (1.0 mmol/l) in men and > 50 mg/dl (1.3 mmol/l) in women are desirable. However, LDL cholesterol-targeted statin therapy remains the preferred strategy. (C)

- If targets are not reached on maximally tolerated doses of statins, combination therapy using statins and other lipid lowering agents may be considered to achieve lipid targets but has not been evaluated in outcome studies for either CVD outcomes or safety. (E)
- Statin therapy is contraindicated in pregnancy. (E)

*Evidence for benefits of lipid lowering therapy*

Patients with type 2 diabetes have an increased prevalence of lipid abnormalities, contributing to their high risk of CVD. For the past decade or more, multiple clinical trials demonstrated significant effects of pharmacologic (primarily statin) therapy on CVD outcomes in subjects with CHD and for primary CVD prevention (Baigent, 2005). Subanalyses of diabetic subgroups of larger trials (Pyorala *et al.*, 1997; Heart Protection Study Collaborative Group, 2003; Goldberg *et al.*, 1998; Sheperd *et al.*, 2006; Sever *et al.*, 2005) and trials specifically in subjects with diabetes (Knopp *et al.*, 2006; Sing *et al.*, 2007) showed significant primary and secondary prevention of CVD events ± CHD deaths in diabetic populations. As shown in Table 10, and similar to findings in non-diabetic subjects, reduction in "hard" CVD outcomes (CHD death and nonfatal MI) can be more clearly seen in diabetic subjects with high baseline CVD risk (known CVD and/or very high LDL cholesterol levels), but overall, the benefits of statin therapy in people with diabetes at moderate or high risk for CVD are convincing.

Low levels of HDL cholesterol, often associated with elevated triglyceride levels, are the most prevalent pattern of dyslipidemia in persons with type 2 diabetes. However, the evidence base for drugs that target these lipid fractions is significantly less robust than that for statin therapy (Singh, 2007). Nicotinic acid has been shown to reduce CVD outcomes (Canner, 1986), although the study was done in a non-diabetic cohort. Gemfibrozil has been shown to decrease rates of CVD events in subjects without diabetes (Rubins *et al.*, 1999; Frick *et al.*, 1987) and in the diabetic subgroup in one of the larger trials

**Table 10    Reduction in 10-year Risk of Major CVD End Points (CHD death/non-fatal MI) in Major Statin Trials, or Substudies of Major Trials, in Diabetic Subjects (*n* = 16 032)**

| Study (ref.) | CVD Prevention | Statin Dose and Comparator | Risk Reduction (%) | Relative Risk Reduction (%) | Absolute Risk Reduction (%) | LDL Cholesterol Reduction |
|---|---|---|---|---|---|---|
| 4S-DM (186) | 2° | Simvastatin 20–40 mg vs. placebo | 85.7 to 43.2 | 50 | 42.5 | 186 to 119 mg/dl (36%) |
| ASPEN 2° (191) | 2° | Atorvastatin 10 mg vs. placebo | 39.5 to 24.5 | 34 | 12.7 | 112 to 79 mg/dl (29%) |
| HPS-DM (187) | 2° | Simvastatin 40 mg vs. placebo | 43.8 to 36.3 | 17 | 7.5 | 123 to 84 mg/dl (31%) |
| CARE-DM (188) | 2° | Pravastatin 40 mg vs. placebo | 40.8 to 35.4 | 13 | 5.4 | 136 to 99 mg/dl (27%) |
| TNT-DM (189) | 2° | Atorvastatin 80 mg vs. 10 mg | 26.3 to 21.6 | 18 | 4.7 | 99 to 77 mg/dl (22%) |
| HPS-DM (187) | 1° | Simvastatin 40 mg vs. placebo | 17.5 to 11.5 | 34 | 6.0 | 124 to 86 mg/dl (31%) |
| CARDS (209) | 1° | Atorvastatin 10 mg vs. placebo | 11.5 to 7.5 | 35 | 4 | 118 to 71 mg/dl (40%) |
| ASPEN (191) | 1° | Atorvastatin 10 mg vs. placebo | 9.8 to 7.9 | 19 | 1.9 | 114 to 80 mg/dl (30%) |
| ASCOT-DM (190) | 1° | Atorvastatin 10 mg vs. placebo | 11.1 to 10.2 | 8 | 0.9 | 125 to 82 mg/dl (34%) |

Studies were of differing lengths (3.3–5.4 years) and used somewhat different outcomes, but all reported rates of CVD death and non-fatal MI. In this tabulation, results of the statin on 10-year risk of major CVD end points (CHD death/non-fatal MI) are listed for comparison between studies. Correlation between 10-year CVD risk of the control group and the absolute risk reduction with statin therapy is highly significant (*P* = 0.0007). Analyses provided by Craig Williams, Pharm.D., Oregon Health & Science University, 2007.

(Rubins *et al.*, 1999). However, in a large trial specific to diabetic patients, fenofibrate failed to reduce overall cardiovascular outcomes (Keech *et al.*, 2005).

*Dyslipidemia treatment and target lipid levels*

For most patients with diabetes, the first priority of dyslipidemia therapy (unless severe hypertriglyceridemia is the immediate issue) is to lower LDL cholesterol to a target goal of < 100 mg/dl (2.60 mmol/l) (NCEP, 2001). Lifestyle intervention, including MNT, increased physical activity, weight loss, and smoking cessation, may allow some patients to reach lipid goals. Nutrition intervention should be tailored according to each patient's age, type of diabetes, pharmacological treatment, lipid levels, and other medical conditions and should focus on the reduction of saturated fat, cholesterol, and *trans* unsaturated fat intake. Glycemic control can also beneficially modify plasma lipid levels, particularly in patients with very high triglycerides and poor glycemic control.

In those patients with clinical CVD or over age 40 with other CVD risk factors, pharmacological treatment should be added to lifestyle therapy regardless of baseline lipid levels. Statins are the drugs of choice for LDL cholesterol lowering.

In patients other than those described above, statin treatment should be considered if there is an inadequate LDL cholesterol response to lifestyle modifications and improved glucose control, or if the patient has increased cardiovascular risk (e.g. multiple cardiovascular risk factors or long duration of diabetes). Very little clinical trial evidence exists for type 2 patients under the age of 40, or for type 1 patients of any age. In the Heart Protection Study, the subgroup of 600 patients with type 1 diabetes (lower age limit 40 years) had a proportionately similar reduction in risk as patients with type 2 diabetes, although not statistically significant (Heart Protection Study Collaborative Group, 2003). Although the data are not definitive, consideration should be given to similar lipid-lowering goals in type 1 diabetic patients as those in type 2 diabetic patients, particularly if they have other cardiovascular risk factors.

*Alternative LDL cholesterol goals*

Virtually all trials of statins and CVD outcomes have tested specific doses of statins against placebo, other doses of statin, or other statins, rather than aiming for specific LDL cholesterol goals (Hayward *et al.*, 2006). As can be seen in Table 10, placebo-controlled trials generally achieved LDL cholesterol reductions of 30–40% from baseline.

Hence, LDL cholesterol lowering of this magnitude is an acceptable outcome for patients who cannot reach LDL cholesterol goals due to severe baseline elevations in LDL cholesterol and/or intolerance of maximal, or any, statin doses. Additionally, for those with baseline LDL cholesterol minimally above 100 mg/dl, prescribing statin therapy to lower LDL cholesterol about 30–40% from baseline is probably more effective than prescribing just enough to reduce the LDL cholesterol level to slightly below 100 mg/dl.

Recent clinical trials in high-risk patients, such as those with acute coronary syndromes or previous cardiovascular events (Cannon *et al.*, 2004; de Lemos *et al.*, 2004; Nissen *et al.*, 2004), have demonstrated that more aggressive therapy with high doses of statins to achieve an LDL cholesterol of < 70 mg/dl led to a significant reduction in further events. Therefore, a reduction in LDL cholesterol to a goal of < 70 mg/dl is an option in very-high-risk diabetic patients with overt CVD (Grundy *et al.*, 2004).

In individual patients, LDL cholesterol lowering with statins is highly variable, and this variable response is poorly understood (Chasman, 2004). Reduction of CVD events with statins correlates very closely, with LDL cholesterol lowering (Baigent *et al.*, 2005). When maximally tolerated doses of statins fail to significantly lower LDL cholesterol (< 30% reduction from patients' baseline), the primary aim of combination therapy should be to achieve additional LDL cholesterol lowering. Niacin, fenofibrate, ezetimibe, and bile acid sequestrants all offer additional LDL cholesterol lowering. The evidence that combination therapy provides a significant increment in CVD risk reduction over statin therapy alone is still elusive.

*Treatment of other lipoprotein fractions or targets*

Severe hypertriglyceridemia may warrant immediate therapy of this abnormality with lifestyle and usually pharmacologic therapy (fibric acid derivative or niacin) to reduce the risk of acute pancreatitis. In the absence of severe hypertriglyceridemia, therapy targeting HDL cholesterol or triglycerides has intuitive appeal but lacks the evidence base of statin therapy (Sega *et al.*, 2005). If the HDL cholesterol is < 40 mg/dl and the LDL cholesterol is between 100 and 129 mg/dl, gemfibrozil or niacin might be used, especially if a patient is intolerant to statins. Niacin is the most effective drug for raising HDL cholesterol. It can significantly increase blood glucose at high doses, but recent studies demonstrate that at modest doses (750–2000 mg/day), significant improvements in LDL cholesterol, HDL cholesterol, and triglyceride levels are accompanied by only modest changes in glucose that are generally amenable to adjustment of diabetes therapy (Elam *et al.*, 2000; Grundy *et al.*, 2002).

Combination therapy, with a statin and a fibrate or a statin and niacin, may be efficacious for treatment for all three lipid fractions, but this combination is associated with an increased risk for abnormal transaminase levels, myositis, or rhabdomyolysis. The risk of rhabdomyolysis is higher with higher doses of statins and with renal insufficiency and seems to be lower when statins are combined with fenofibrate than gemfibrozil (Jones and Davidson, 2005). Several ongoing trials may provide much-needed evidence for the effects of combination therapy on cardiovascular outcomes.

In 2008, a consensus panel convened by ADA and the American College of Cardiology recommended a greater focus on non-HDL cholesterol and apolipoprotein B (apo B) in patients who are likely to have small LDL particles, such as people with diabetes (Brunzell *et al.*, 2008). The consensus panel suggested that for statin-treated patients in whom the LDL cholesterol goal would be < 70 mg/dl (non-HDL cholesterol < 100 mg/dl), apo B should be measured and treated to achieve a goal of < 80 mg/dl. For patients on statins with an LDL cholesterol goal of < 100 mg/dl (non-HDL cholesterol < 130 mg/dl), apo B should be measured and treated to below 90 mg/dl.

### 1.6.1.3. *Antiplatelet agents*
**Recommendations**

- Aspirin therapy (75–162 mg/day) should be used as a primary prevention strategy in those with type 1 or type 2 diabetes at increased cardiovascular risk, including those who are > 40 years of age or who have additional risk factors (family history of CVD, hypertension, smoking, dyslipidemia, or albuminuria). (C)
- Aspirin therapy (75–162 mg/day) should be used as a secondary prevention strategy in those with diabetes with a history of CVD. (A)
- For patients with CVD and documented aspirin allergy, clopidogrel (75 mg/day) should be used. (B)
- Combination therapy with ASA (75–162 mg/day) and clopidogrel (75 mg/day) is reasonable for up to a year after an acute coronary syndrome. (B)
- Aspirin therapy is not recommended for people under 30 years of age due to lack of evidence of benefit and is contraindicated in patients under the age of 21 years because of the associated risk of Reye's syndrome. (E)

The use of aspirin in diabetes is reviewed in detail in the ADA technical review (Colwell, 1997) and position statement (American Diabetic Association, 2004) on this topic. Aspirin has been recommended for primary (Hayden *et al.*, 2002; US Preventive Services Task Force, 2002) and secondary (Antithrombotic Trialists Collaboration, 2002) prevention of cardiovascular events in high-risk diabetic and nondiabetic individuals. One large meta-analysis and several clinical trials demonstrate the efficacy of using aspirin as a preventive measure for cardiovascular events, including stroke and myocardial infarction. Many trials have shown a ~30% decrease in myocardial infarction and a 20% decrease in stroke in a wide range of patients, including young and middle-aged patients,

patients with and without a history of CVD, men and women, and patients with hypertension.

Dosages used in most clinical trials ranged from 75 to 325 mg/day. There is little evidence to support any specific dose, but using the lowest possible dosage may help reduce side effects (Campbell *et al.*, 2007). Conversely, a randomized trial of 100 mg of aspirin daily showed less of a primary prevention effect, without statistical significance, in the large diabetic subgroup in contrast to significant benefit in those without diabetes (Sacco *et al.*, 2003), raising the issue of aspirin resistance in those with diabetes.

The systematic review of evidence for the U.S. Preventive Services Task Force (USPSTF) estimated that aspirin reduced the risk for nonfatal and fatal MI (odds ratio 0.72 [95% CI: 0.60–0.87]). The review acknowledged the low numbers of diabetic subjects in most trials but concluded that subset analyses and a single trial in diabetic patients suggested that the estimates extended to those with diabetes (Hayden *et al.*, 2002). The USPSTF stated that the risk to benefit ratio favors aspirin use when a 5-year CHD risk equals or exceeds 3% and suggested aspirin therapy be considered for men > 40 years of age, post-menopausal women, and younger persons with CHD risk factors (including diabetes) (US Preventive Task Force, 2002).

There is no evidence for a specific age at which to start aspirin, but aspirin has not been studied at ages < 30 years. Clopidogrel has been demonstrated to reduce CVD events in diabetic individuals (Bhatt *et al.*, 2002). Adjunctive therapy in the first year after acute coronary syndrome in very-high-risk patients, or as alternative therapy in aspirin-intolerant patients, should be considered.

### 1.6.1.4. *Smoking cessation*

**Recommendations**

- Advice should be given all patients not to smoke. (A)
- Smoking cessation counselling and other forms of treatment should be included as a routine component of diabetes care. (B)

Issues of smoking in diabetes are reviewed in detail in the ADA technical review (Haire-Joshu, 1999) and position statement (American Diabetes Association, 2004) on this topic. A large body of evidence from epidemiological, case-control, and cohort studies provides convincing documentation of the causal link between cigarette smoking and health risks. Cigarette smoking contributes to one of every five deaths in the U.S. and is the most important modifiable cause of premature death. Much of the prior work documenting the impact of smoking on health did not separately discuss results on subsets of individuals with diabetes, suggesting that the identified risks are at least equivalent to those found in the general population. Other studies of individuals with diabetes consistently found a heightened risk of CVD and premature death among smokers. Smoking is also related to the premature development of microvascular complications of diabetes and may have a role in the development of type 2 diabetes.

A number of large randomized clinical trials have demonstrated the efficacy and cost-effectiveness of smoking cessation counseling in changing smoking behavior and reducing tobacco use. The routine and thorough assessment of tobacco use is important as a means of preventing smoking or encouraging cessation. Special considerations should include assessment of level of nicotine dependence, which is associated with difficulty in quitting and relapse (US Preventive Task Force, 2003; Ranney *et al.*, 2006). Free telephone quit lines are available in each state (see www.naquitline.org).

### 1.6.2. Retinopathy Screening and Treatment

**Recommendations**

*General recommendations*

- To reduce the risk or slow the progression of retinopathy, glycemic control should be optimized. (A)
- To reduce the risk or slow the progression of retinopathy, blood pressure control should be optimized. (A)

*Screening*

- Adults and children aged 10 years or older with type 1 diabetes should have an initial dilated and comprehensive eye examination by an ophthalmologist or optometrist within five years after the onset of diabetes. (B)
- Patients with type 2 diabetes should have an initial dilated and comprehensive eye examination by an ophthalmologist or optometrist shortly after the diagnosis of diabetes. (B)
- Subsequent examinations for type 1 and type 2 diabetic patients should be repeated annually by an ophthalmologist or optometrist. Less frequent exams (every 2–3 years) may be considered following one or more normal eye exams. Examinations will be required more frequently if retinopathy is progressing. (B)
- Women with preexisting diabetes who are planning pregnancy or who have become pregnant should have a comprehensive eye examination and be counseled on the risk of development and/or progression of diabetic retinopathy. Eye examination should occur in the first trimester with close follow-up throughout the pregnancy and one year postpartum. (B)

*Treatment*

- Promptly refer patients with any level of macular edema, severe NPDR, or any PDR to an ophthalmologist who is knowledgeable and experienced in the management and treatment of diabetic retinopathy. (A)
- Laser photocoagulation therapy is indicated to reduce the risk of vision loss in patients with high-risk PDR and clinically significant macular edema and in some cases of severe NPDR. (A)
- The presence of retinopathy is not a contraindication to aspirin therapy for cardioprotection, as this therapy does not increase the risk of retinal hemorrhage. (A)

Diabetic retinopathy is a highly specific vascular complication of both type 1 and type 2 diabetes, with prevalence strongly related to the duration of diabetes. Diabetic retinopathy is the most frequent cause of new cases of blindness among adults aged 20–74 years. Glaucoma, cataracts, and other disorders of the eye occur earlier and more frequently in people with diabetes.

In addition to duration of diabetes, other factors that increase the risk of, or are associated with, retinopathy include chronic hyperglycemia (Klein, 1995), the presence of nephropathy (Estacio *et al.*, 1998), and hypertension (Leske *et al.*, 2005). Intensive diabetes management with the goal of achieving near normoglycemia has been shown in large prospective randomized studies to prevent and/or delay the onset and progression of diabetic retinopathy (DCCT, 1993; UKPDS, 1998a; UKPDS, 1998b). Lowering blood pressure has been shown to decrease the progression of retinopathy (UKPDS, 1998) (Table 11). Several case series and a controlled prospective study suggest that pregnancy in type 1 diabetic patients may aggravate retinopathy (Fong *et al.*, 2004; DCCT, 2000); laser photocoagulation surgery can minimize this risk (DCCT, 2000). One of the main motivations for screening for diabetic retinopathy is the established efficacy of laser photocoagulation surgery in preventing vision loss. Two large trials, the Diabetic Retinopathy Study (DRS) and the Early Treatment Diabetic Retinopathy Study (ETDRS), provide the strongest support for the therapeutic benefits of photocoagulation surgery.

The DRS (DRS, 1976) showed that panretinal photocoagulation surgery reduced the risk of severe vision loss from PDR from 15.9% in untreated eyes to 6.4% in treated eyes. The benefit was greatest among patients whose baseline evaluation revealed high-risk characteristics (chiefly disc neovascularization or vitreous hemorrhage). Given the risks of modest loss of visual acuity and contraction of the visual field from panretinal laser surgery, such therapy is primarily recommended for eyes with PDR approaching or having high-risk characteristics.

The ETDRS (ETDRS, 1985) established the benefit of focal laser photocoagulation surgery in

**Table 11   Summary of Recommendations for Glycemic, Blood Pressure, and Lipid Control for Adults with Diabetes**

| | |
|---|---|
| A1C | < 7.0%* |
| Blood pressure | < 130/80 mm Hg |
| Lipids | |
| LDL cholesterol | < 100 mg/dl (< 2.6 mmol/l)‡ |

*Referenced to a nondiabetic range of 4.0–6.0% using a DCCT-based assay.

†In individuals with overt CVD, a lower LDL cholesterol goal of < 70 mg/dl (1.8 mmol/l), using a high dose of a statin, is an option.

eyes with macular edema, particularly those with clinically significant macular edema, with reduction of doubling of the visual angle (e.g. 20/50 to 20/100) from 20% in untreated eyes to 8% in treated eyes. The ETDRS also verified the benefits of panretinal photocoagulation for high-risk PDR, but not for mild or moderate NPDR. In older-onset patients with severe NPDR or less-than-high-risk PDR, the risk of severe vision loss or vitrectomy was reduced ~50% by early laser photocoagulation surgery at these stages.

Laser photocoagulation surgery in both trials was beneficial in reducing the risk of further vision loss, but generally not beneficial in reversing already diminished acuity. This preventive effect and the fact that patients with PDR or macular edema may be asymptomatic provide strong support for a screening program to detect diabetic retinopathy.

As retinopathy is estimated to take at least five years to develop after the onset of hyperglycemia (Klein *et al.*, 1984), patients with type 1 diabetes should have an initial dilated and comprehensive eye examination within five years after the onset of diabetes. Patients with type 2 diabetes, who generally have had years of undiagnosed diabetes (Harris *et al.*, 1992) and who have a significant risk of prevalent diabetic retinopathy at the time of diabetes diagnosis, should have an initial dilated and comprehensive eye examination soon after diagnosis. Examinations should be performed by an ophthalmologist or optometrist who is knowledgeable and experienced in diagnosing the presence of diabetic retinopathy and is aware of its management. Subsequent examinations for type 1 and type 2 diabetic patients are generally repeated annually. Less frequent exams (every 2–3 years) may be cost effective after one or more normal eye exams (Vijan *et al.*, 2000; Klein, 2003; Younis *et al.*, 2003), while examinations will be required more frequently if retinopathy is progressing.

Examinations can also be done with retinal photographs (with or without dilation of the pupil) read by experienced experts. In-person exams are still necessary when the photos are unacceptable and for follow-up of abnormalities detected. This technology has great potential in areas where qualified eye care professionals are not available and may enhance efficiency and reduce costs when the expertise of ophthalmologists can be utilized for more complex examinations and for therapy (Ahmed *et al.*, 2004).

Results of eye examinations should be documented and transmitted to the referring health care professional.

# References

Adler AI, Stratton IM, Neil HA, *et al.* (2000) Association of systolic blood pressure with macrovascular and microvascular complications of type 2 diabetes (UKPDS 36): Prospective observational study. *BMJ* **321**: 412–419.

Ahmed J, Ward TP, Bursell SE, *et al.* (2006) The sensitivity and specificity of nonmydriatic digital stereoscopic retinal imaging in detecting diabetic retinopathy. *Diabetes Care* **29**: 2205–2209.

American Diabetes Association. (1987) Consensus statement on self-monitoring of blood glucose. *Diabetes Care* **10**: 95–99.

American Diabetes Asociation. (1994) Selfmonitoring of blood glucose. *Diabetes Care* **17**: 81–86.

American Diabetes Association. (2000) Type 2 diabetes in children and adolescents (Consensus Statement). *Diabetes Care* **23**: 381–389.

American Diabetes Association. (2001) Postprandial blood glucose (Consensus Statement). *Diabetes Care* **24**: 775–778.

American Diabetes Association. (2003) *Intensive Diabetes Management*. Alexandria, VA, American Diabetes Association.

American Diabetes Association. (2004) Aspirin therapy in diabetes (Position Statement). *Diabetes Care* **27**(1): S72–S73.

American Diabetes Association. (2004) Gestational diabetes mellitus (Position Statement). *Diabetes Care* **27**(1): S88–S90.

American Diabetes Association. (2004) Nephropathy in diabetes (Position Statement). *Diabetes Care* **27**(1): S79–S83.

American Diabetes Association. (2004) Retinopathy in diabetes. *Diabetes Care* **27**(1): S84–S87.

American Diabetes Association. (2004) Smoking and diabetes (Position Statement). *Diabetes Care* **27**(1): S74–S75.

American Diabetes Association. (2008) *Medical Management of Type 1 Diabetes*. 5th ed. Alexandria, VA, American Diabetes Association.

American Diabetes Association. (2008) *Medical Management of Type 2 Diabetes*. 6th ed. Alexandria, VA, American Diabetes Association.

Antithrombotic Trialists Collaboration. (2002) Collaborative meta-analysis of randomised trials of antiplatelet therapy for prevention of death, myocardial infarction, and stroke in high risk patients. *BMJ* **324**: 71–86.

Arauz-Pacheco C, Parrott MA, Raskin P. (2002) The treatment of hypertension in adult patients with diabetes. *Diabetes Care* **25**: 134–147.

Baigent C, Keech A, Kearney PM, *et al*. (2005) Efficacy and safety of cholesterol-lowering treatment: Prospective meta-analysis of data from 90,056 participants in 14 randomised trials of statins. *Lancet* **366**: 1267–1278.

Bakris GL, Siomos M, Richardson DJ, *et al*. (2000) ACE inhibition or angiotensin receptor blockade: Impact on potassium in renal failure: VAL-K Study Group. *Kidney Int* **58**: 2084–2092.

Bakris GL, Williams M, Dworkin L, *et al*. (2000) Preserving renal function in adults with hypertension and diabetes: A consensus approach: National Kidney Foundation Hypertension and Diabetes Executive Committees Working Group. *Am J Kidney Dis* **36**: 646–661.

Berl T, Hunsicker LG, Lewis JB, *et al*. (2003) Cardiovascular outcomes in the Irbesartan Diabetic Nephropathy Trial of patients with type 2 diabetes and overt nephropathy. *Ann Intern Med* **138**: 542–549.

Bhatt DL, Marso SP, Hirsch AT, *et al*. (2002) Amplified benefit of clopidogrel versus aspirin in patients with diabetes mellitus. *Am J Cardiol* **90**: 625–628.

Bobrie G, Chatellier G, Genes N, *et al*. (2004) Cardiovascular prognosis of "masked hypertension" detected by blood pressure self-measurement in elderly treated hypertensive patients. *JAMA* **291**: 1342–1349.

Boden WE, O'Rourke RA, Teo KK, *et al*. (2007) Optimal medical therapy with or without PCI for stable coronary disease. *N Engl J Med* **356**: 1503–1516.

Braunwald E, Domanski MJ, Fowler SE, *et al*. (2004) Angiotensin-converting-enzyme inhibition in stable coronary artery disease. *N Engl J Med* **351**: 2058–2068.

Brenner BM, Cooper ME, de Zeeuw D, *et al*. (2001) Effects of losartan on renal and cardiovascular outcomes in patients with type 2 diabetes and nephropathy. *N Engl J Med* **345**: 861–869.

Brunzell JD, Davidson M, Furberg CD, *et al*. Lipoprotein management in patients with cardiometabolic risk: Consensus statement from the American Diabetes Association and the American.

Buchanan TA, Xiang AH, Peters RK, *et al*. (2002) Preservation of pancreatic-cell function and prevention of type 2 diabetes by pharmacological treatment of insulin resistance in high-risk hispanic women. *Diabetes* **51**: 2796–2803.

Buse JB, Ginsberg HN, Barkis GL, *et al*. (2007) Primary prevention of cardiovascular diseases in people with diabetes mellitus: A scientific statement from the American Heart Association and the American Diabetes Association. *Diabetes Care* **30**: 162–172.

Cagliero E, Levina EV, Nathan DM. (1999) Immediate feedback of HbA1c levels improves glycemic control in type 1 and insulin-treated type 2 diabetic patients. *Diabetes Care* **22**: 1785–1789.

Campbell CL, Smyth S, Montalescot G, *et al*. (2007) Aspirin dose for the prevention of cardiovascular disease: A systematic review. *JAMA* **297**: 2018–2024.

Canner PL, Berge KG, Wenger NK, *et al*. (1986) Fifteen year mortality in Coronary Drug Project patients: Longterm benefit with niacin. *J Am Coll Cardiol* **8**: 1245–1255.

Cannon CP, Braunwald E, McCabe CH, *et al*. (2004) Intensive versus moderate lipid lowering with statins after acute coronary syndromes. *N Engl J Med* **350**: 1495–1504.

Ceriello A, Taboga C, Tonutti L, *et al.* (2002) Evidence for an independent and cumulative effect of postprandial hypertriglyceridemia and hyperglycemia on endothelial dysfunction and oxidative stress generation: Effects of short- and long-term simvastatin treatment. *Circulation* **106**: 1211–1218.

Chasman DI, Posada D, Subrahmanyan L, *et al.* (2004) Pharmacogenetic study of statin therapy and cholesterol reduction. *JAMA* **291**: 2821–2827.

Chiasson JL, Josse RG, Gomis R, *et al.* (2002) Acarbose for prevention of type 2 diabetes mellitus: The STOP-NIDDM randomised trial. *Lancet* **359**: 2072–2077.

Chobanian AV, Bakris GL, Black HR, *et al.* (2003) The Seventh Report of the Joint National Committee on Prevention, Detection, Evaluation, and Treatment of High Blood Pressure: The JNC 7 report. *JAMA* **289**: 2560–2572.

Colhoun HM, Betteridge DJ, Durrington PN, *et al.* (2004) Primary prevention of cardiovascular disease with atorvastatin in type 2 diabetes in the Collaborative Atorvastatin Diabetes Study (CARDS): Multicentre randomised placebo-controlled trial. *Lancet* **364**: 685–696.

College of Cardiology Foundation. (2008) *Diabetes Care* **31**: 811–822.

Colwell JA. (1997) Aspirin therapy in diabetes. *Diabetes Care* **20**: 1767–1771.

Dabelea D, Bell RA, D'Agostino RB Jr, *et al.* (2007) Incidence of diabetes in youth in the United States. *JAMA* **297**: 2716–2724.

Davidson MB, Schriger DL, Peters AL, *et al.* (1999) Relationship between fasting plasma glucose and glycosylated hemoglobin: Potential for false-positive diagnoses of type 2 diabetes using new diagnostic criteria. *JAMA* **281**: 1203–1210.

DCCT. (2000) Effect of pregnancy on microvascular complications in the diabetes control and complications trial: The Diabetes Control and Complications Trial Research Group. *Diabetes Care* **23**: 1084–1091.

de Lemos JA, Blazing MA, Wiviott SD, *et al.* (2004) Early intensive vs a delayed conservative simvastatin strategy in patients with acute coronary syndromes: Phase Z of the A to Z trial. *JAMA* **292**: 1307–1316.

Duckworth W. (2008) VADT results. Presented at the 68th Annual Meeting of the American Diabetes Association, 6–10 June 2008, at the Moscone Convention Center, San Francisco, CA.

Effect of intensive blood-glucose control with metformin on complications in overweight patients with type 2 diabetes (UKPDS 34). (1998) UK Prospective Diabetes Study (UKPDS) Group. *Lancet* **352**: 854–865.

Effect of intensive therapy on the development and progression of diabetic nephropathy in the Diabetes Control and Complications Trial. (1995) The Diabetes Control and Complications (DCCT) Research Group. *Kidney Int* **47**: 1703–1720.

Effects of ramipril on cardiovascular and microvascular outcomes in people with diabetes mellitus. (2000) Results of the HOPE study and MICRO-HOPE substudy: Heart Outcomes Prevention Evaluation Study Investigators. *Lancet* **355**: 253–259.

Effects of the angiotensin-receptor blocker telmisartan on cardiovascular events in high-risk patients intolerant to angiotensin-converting enzyme inhibitors. (2008) A randomised controlled trial. *Lancet* **372**: 1174–1183.

Eknoyan G, Hostetter T, Bakris GL, *et al.* (2003) Proteinuria and other markers of chronic kidney disease: A position statement of the national kidney foundation (NKF) and the national institute of diabetes and digestive and kidney diseases (NIDDK). *Am J Kidney Dis* **42**: 617–622.

Elam MB, Hunninghake DB, Davis KB, *et al.* (2000) Effect of niacin on lipid and lipoprotein levels and glycemic control in patients with diabetes and peripheral arterial disease: the ADMIT study: A randomized trial: Arterial Disease Multiple Intervention Trial. *JAMA* **284**: 1263–1270.

Engelgau MM, Narayan KM, Herman WH. (2000) Screening for type 2 diabetes. *Diabetes Care* **23**: 1563–1580.

Estacio RO, Jeffers BW, Hiatt WR, *et al.* (1998) The effect of nisoldipine as compared with enalapril on cardiovascular outcomes in patients with non-insulin-dependent diabetes and hypertension. *N Engl J Med* **338**: 645–652.

Estacio RO, McFarling E, Biggerstaff S, *et al.* (1998) Overt albuminuria predicts diabetic retinopathy in Hispanics with NIDDM. *Am J Kidney Dis* **31**: 947–953.

Executive Summary of The Third Report of The National Cholesterol Education Program (NCEP). (2001) Expert Panel on Detection, Evaluation, And Treatment of High Blood Cholesterol In Adults (Adult Treatment Panel III). *JAMA* **285**: 2486–2497.

Expert Committee on the Diagnosis and Classification of Diabetes Mellitus. (1997) Report of the Expert Committee on the Diagnosis and Classification of Diabetes Mellitus. *Diabetes Care* **20**: 1183–1197.

Expert Committee on the Diagnosis and Classification of Diabetes Mellitus. (2003) Follow-up report on the diagnosis of diabetes mellitus. *Diabetes Care* **26**: 3160–3167.

Farmer A, Wade A, Goyder E, *et al.* (2007) Impact of self monitoring of blood glucose in the management of patients with non-insulin treated diabetes: Open parallel group randomised trial. *BMJ* **335**: 132.

Fong DS, Aiello LP, Ferris FL III, *et al.* (2004) Diabetic retinopathy. *Diabetes Care* **27**: 2540–2553.

Frick MH, Elo O, Haapa K, *et al.* (1987) Helsinki Heart Study: primary-prevention trial with gemfibrozil in middleaged men with dyslipidemia: Safety of treatment, changes in risk factors, and incidence of coronary heart disease. *N Engl J Med* **317**: 1237–1245.

Gabir MM, Hanson RL, Dabelea D, *et al.* (2000) The 1997 American Diabetes Association and 1999 World Health Organization criteria for hyperglycemia in the diagnosis and prediction of diabetes. *Diabetes Care* **23**: 1108–1112.

Gaede P, Lund-Andersen H, Parving HH, *et al.* (2008) Effect of a multifactorial intervention on mortality in type 2 diabetes. *N Engl J Med* **358**: 580–591.

Gall MA, Hougaard P, Borch-Johnsen K, *et al.* (1997) Risk factors for development of incipient and overt diabetic nephropathy in patients with non-insulin dependent diabetes mellitus: Prospective, observational study. *BMJ* **314**: 783–788.

Garg JP, Bakris GL. (2002) Microalbuminuria: Marker of vascular dysfunction, risk factor for cardiovascular disease. *Vasc Med* **7**: 35–43.

Gerstein HC, Miller ME, Byington RP, *et al.* (2008) Effects of intensive glucose lowering in type 2 diabetes. *N Engl J Med* **358**: 2545–2559.

Gerstein HC, Yusuf S, Bosch J, *et al.* (2006) Effect of rosiglitazone on the frequency of diabetes in patients with impaired glucose tolerance or impaired fasting glucose: A randomised controlled trial. *Lancet* **368**: 1096–1105.

Gerstein HC. (2007) Point: if it is important to prevent type 2 diabetes, it is important to consider all proven therapies within a comprehensive approach. *Diabetes Care* **30**: 432–434.

Goldberg RB, Mellies MJ, Sacks FM, *et al.* (1998) Cardiovascular events and their reduction with pravastatin in diabetic and glucose-intolerant myocardial infarction survivors with average cholesterol levels: Subgroup analyses in the cholesterol and recurrent events (CARE) trial: the Care Investigators. *Circulation* **98**: 2513–2519.

Granger CB, McMurray JJ, Yusuf S, *et al.* (2003) Effects of candesartan in patients with chronic heart failure and reduced left-ventricular systolic function intolerant to angiotensin-converting-enzyme inhibitors: The CHARM-Alternative trial. *Lancet* **362**: 772–776.

Grundy SM, Cleeman JI, Merz CN, *et al.* (2004) Implications of recent clinical trials for the National Cholesterol Education Program Adult Treatment Panel III guidelines. *Circulation* **110**: 227–239.

Grundy SM, Vega GL, McGovern ME, *et al.* (2002) Efficacy, safety, and tolerability of once-daily niacin for the treatment of dyslipidemia associated with type 2 diabetes: Results of the assessment of diabetes control and evaluation of the efficacy of niaspan trial. *Arch Intern Med* **162**: 1568–1576.

Haffner SM. (1998) Management of dyslipidemia in adults with diabetes. *Diabetes Care* **21**: 160–178.

Haire-Joshu D, Glasgow RE, Tibbs TL. (1999) Smoking and diabetes. *Diabetes Care* **22**: 1887–1898.

Hansen HP, Tauber-Lassen E, Jensen BR, *et al.* (2002) Effect of dietary protein restriction on prognosis in patients with diabetic nephropathy. *Kidney Int* **62**: 220–228.

Hansson L, Zanchetti A, Carruthers SG, *et al.* (1998) Effects of intensive blood-pressure lowering and low-dose aspirin in patients with hypertension: Principal results of the Hypertension Optimal Treatment (HOT) randomised trial: HOT Study Group. *Lancet* **351**: 1755–1762.

Harris MI, Klein R, Welborn TA, *et al.* (1992) Onset of NIDDM occurs at least 4–7 yr before clinical diagnosis. *Diabetes Care* **15**: 815–819.

Harris R, Donahue K, Rathore SS, *et al.* (2003) Screening adults for type 2 diabetes: A review of the evidence for the U.S. Preventive Services Task Force. *Ann Intern Med* **138**: 215–229.

Hayden M, Pignone M, Phillips C, *et al.* (2002) Aspirin for the primary prevention of cardiovascular events: A summary of the evidence for the U.S. Preventive Services Task Force. *Ann Intern Med* **136**: 161–172.

Hayward RA, Hofer TP, Vijan S. (2006) Narrative review: lack of evidence for recommended low-density lipoprotein treatment targets: A solvable problem. *Ann Intern Med* **145**: 520–530.

Heart Protection Study Collaborative Group. (2003) MRC/BHF Heart Protection Study of cholesterol-lowering with simvastatin in 5963 people with diabetes: A randomised placebo-controlled trial. *Lancet* **361**: 2005–2016.

Holman RR, Paul SK, Bethel MA, *et al.* (2008) 10-Year follow-up of intensive glucose control in type 2 diabetes. *N Engl J Med* **359**: 1577–1589.

Intensive blood-glucose control with sulphonylureas or insulin compared with conventional treatment and risk of complications in patients with type 2 diabetes (UKPDS 33). (1998) UK Prospective Diabetes Study (UKPDS) Group. *Lancet* **352**: 837–853.

Johnson SL, Tabaei BP, Herman WH. (2005) The efficacy and cost of alternative strategies for systematic screening for type 2 diabetes in the U.S. population 45–74 years of age. *Diabetes Care* **28**: 307–311.

Jones PH, Davidson MH. (2005) Reporting rate of rhabdomyolysis with fenofibrate statin versus gemfibrozil any statin. *Am J Cardiol* **95**: 120–122.

Kasiske BL, Lakatua JD, Ma JZ, *et al.* (1998) A meta-analysis of the effects of dietary protein restriction on the rate of decline in renal function. *Am J Kidney Dis* **31**: 954–961.

Keech A, Simes RJ, Barter P, *et al.* (2005) Effects of long-term fenofibrate therapy on cardiovascular events in 9795 people with type 2 diabetes mellitus (the FIELD study): Randomised controlled trial. *Lancet* **366**: 1849–1861.

Kim C, Newton KM, Knopp RH. (2002) Gestational diabetes and the incidence of type 2 diabetes: A systematic review. *Diabetes Care* **25**: 1862–1868.

Kitzmiller JL, Block JM, Brown FM, *et al.* (2008) Managing preexisting diabetes for pregnancy: Summary of evidence and consensus recommendations for care. *Diabetes Care* **31**: 1060–1079.

Klausen K, Borch-Johnsen K, Feldt-Rasmussen B, *et al.* (2004) Very low levels of microalbuminuria are associated with increased risk of coronary heart disease and death independently of renal function, hypertension, and diabetes. *Circulation* **110**: 32–35.

Klein R, Klein BE, Moss SE, *et al.* (1984) The Wisconsin epidemiologic study of diabetic retinopathy. II. Prevalence and risk of diabetic retinopathy when age at diagnosis is less than 30 years. *Arch Ophthalmol* **102**: 520–526.

Klein R. (1995) Hyperglycemia and microvascular and macrovascular disease in diabetes. *Diabetes Care* **18**: 258–268.

Klein R. (2003) Screening interval for retinopathy in type 2 diabetes. *Lancet* **361**: 190–191.

Knopp RH, d'Emden M, Smilde JG, *et al.* (2006) Efficacy and safety of atorvastatin in the prevention of cardiovascular end points in subjects with type 2 diabetes: The Atorvastatin Study for Prevention of Coronary Heart Disease Endpoints in Non-insulin-dependent diabetes mellitus (ASPEN). *Diabetes Care* **29**: 1478–1485.

Knowler WC, Barrett-Connor E, Fowler SE, *et al.* (2002) Reduction in the incidence of type 2 diabetes with lifestyle intervention or metformin. *N Engl J Med* **346**: 393–403.

Kosaka K, Noda M, Kuzuya T, *et al.* (2005). Prevention of type 2 diabetes by lifestyle intervention: A Japanese trial in IGT males. *Diabetes Res Clin Pract* **67**: 152–162.

Kramer H, Molitch ME. (2005) Screening for kidney disease in adults with diabetes. *Diabetes Care* **28**: 1813–1816.

Kramer HJ, Nguyen QD, Curhan G, *et al.* (2003) Renal insufficiency in the absence of albuminuria and retinopathy among adults with type 2 diabetes mellitus. *JAMA* **289**: 3273–3277.

Laffel LM, McGill JB, Gans DJ. (1995) The beneficial effect of angiotensin-converting enzyme inhibition with captopril on diabetic nephropathy in normotensive IDDM patients with microalbuminuria: North American Microalbuminuria Study Group. *Am J Med* **99**: 497–504.

Lawson ML, Gerstein HC, Tsui E, *et al.* (1999) Effect of intensive therapy on early macrovascular disease in young individuals with type 1 diabetes: A systematic review and meta-analysis. *Diabetes Care* **22**(2): B35–B39.

Leske MC, Wu SY, Hennis A, *et al.* (2005) Hyperglycemia, blood pressure, and the 9-year incidence of diabetic retinopathy: The Barbados Eye Studies. *Ophthalmology* **112**: 799–805.

Levey AS, Bosch JP, Lewis JB, *et al.* (1999) A more accurate method to estimate glomerular filtration rate from serum creatinine: a new prediction equation: Modification of

Diet in Renal Disease Study Group. *Ann Intern Med* **130**: 461–470.

Levey AS, Coresh J, Balk E, *et al.* (2003) National Kidney Foundation practice guidelines for chronic kidney disease: evaluation, classification, and stratification. *Ann Intern Med* **139**: 137–147.

Levinsky NG. (2002) Specialist evaluation in chronic kidney disease: Too little, too late. *Ann Intern Med* **137**: 542–543.

Lewington S, Clarke R, Qizilbash N, *et al.* (2002) Age-specific relevance of usual blood pressure to vascular mortality: A meta-analysis of individual data for one million adults in 61 prospective studies. *Lancet* **360**: 1903–1913.

Lewis EJ, Hunsicker LG, Bain RP, *et al.* (1993) The effect of angiotensin-converting-enzyme inhibition on diabetic nephropathy: The Collaborative Study Group. *N Engl J Med* **329**: 1456–1462.

Lewis EJ, Hunsicker LG, Clarke WR, *et al.* (2001) Renoprotective effect of the angiotensin-receptor antagonist irbesartan in patients with nephropathy due to type 2 diabetes. *N Engl J Med* **345**: 851–860.

Li G, Zhang P, Wang J, *et al.* (2008) The long-term effect of lifestyle interventions to prevent diabetes in the China Da Qing Diabetes Prevention Study: A 20-year follow-up study. *Lancet* **371**: 1783–1789.

Liese AD, D'Agostino RB Jr, Hamman RF, *et al.* (2006) The burden of diabetes mellitus among US youth: Prevalence estimates from the SEARCH for Diabetes in Youth Study. *Pediatrics* **118**: 1510–1518.

Lindholm LH, Ibsen H, Dahlof B, *et al.* (2002) Cardiovascular morbidity and mortality in patients with diabetes in the Losartan Intervention For Endpoint reduction in hypertension study (LIFE): A randomised trial against atenolol. *Lancet* **359**: 1004–1010.

Lindstrom J, Ilanne-Parikka P, Peltonen M, *et al.* (2006) Sustained reduction in the incidence of type 2 diabetes by lifestyle intervention: Follow-up of the Finnish Diabetes Prevention Study. *Lancet* **368**: 1673–1679.

Major outcomes in high-risk hypertensive patients randomized to angiotensin-converting enzyme inhibitor or calcium channel blocker vs diuretic. (2002) the Antihypertensive and Lipid-Lowering Treatment to Prevent Heart Attack Trial (ALLHAT). *JAMA* **288**: 2981–2997.

Martin CL, Albers J, Herman WH, *et al.* (2006) Neuropathy among the diabetes control and complications trial cohort 8 years after trial completion. *Diabetes Care* **29**: 340–344.

McMurray JJ, Ostergren J, Swedberg K, *et al.* (2003) Effects of candesartan in patients with chronic heart failure and reduced left-ventricular systolic function taking angiotensinconverting- enzyme inhibitors: The CHARM-Added trial. *Lancet* **362**: 767–771.

Metzger BE, Buchanan TA, Coustan DR, *et al.* (2007) Summary and recommendations of the Fifth International Workshop-Conference on Gestational Diabetes Mellitus. *Diabetes Care* **30**(2): S251–S260.

Metzger BE, Lowe LP, Dyer AR, *et al.* (2008) Hyperglycemia and adverse pregnancy outcomes. *N Engl J Med* **358**: 1991–2002.

Miller CD, Barnes CS, Phillips LS, *et al.* (2003) Rapid A1c availability improves clinical decision-making in an urban primary care clinic. *Diabetes Care* **26**: 1158–1163.

Mogensen CE, Neldam S, Tikkanen I, *et al.* (2000) Randomised controlled trial of dual blockade of renin-angiotensin system in patients with hypertension, microalbuminuria, and non-insulin dependent diabetes: The candesartan and lisinopril microalbuminuria (CALM) study. *BMJ* **321**: 1440–1444.

Nathan DM, Cleary PA, Backlund JY, *et al.* (2005) Intensive diabetes treatment and cardiovascular disease in patients with type 1 diabetes. *N Engl J Med* **353**: 2643–2653.

Nathan DM, Davidson MB, DeFronzo RA, *et al.* (2007) Impaired fasting glucose and impaired glucose tolerance: Implications for care. *Diabetes Care* **30**: 753–759.

Nathan DM, Kuenen J, Borg R, *et al.* (2008) Translating the A1C assay into estimated average glucose values. *Diabetes Care* **31**: 1473–1478.

Nissen SE, Tuzcu EM, Schoenhagen P, *et al.* (2004) Effect of intensive compared with moderate lipid-lowering therapy on progression of coronary atherosclerosis: A randomized controlled trial. *JAMA* **291**: 1071–1080.

O'Kane MJ, Bunting B, Copeland M, *et al.* (2008) Efficacy of self monitoring of blood glucose in patients with newly diagnosed type 2 diabetes (ESMON study): Randomised controlled trial. *BMJ* **336**: 1174–1177.

Ohkubo Y, Kishikawa H, Araki E, *et al.* (1995) Intensive insulin therapy prevents the progression of diabetic microvascular complications in Japanese patients with non-insulindependent diabetes mellitus: A randomized prospective 6-year study. *Diabetes Res Clin Pract* **28**: 103–117.

Pan XR, Li GW, Hu YH, *et al*. (1997) Effects of diet and exercise in preventing NIDDM in people with impaired glucose tolerance: The Da Qing IGT and Diabetes Study. *Diabetes Care* **20**: 537–544.

Parving HH, Lehnert H, Brochner-Mortensen J, *et al*. (2001) The effect of irbesartan on the development of diabetic nephropathy in patients with type 2 diabetes. *N Engl J Med* **345**: 870–878.

Parving HH, Persson F, Lewis JB, *et al*. (2008) Aliskiren combined with losartan in type 2 diabetes and nephropathy. *N Engl J Med* **358**: 2433–2446.

Patel A, MacMahon S, Chalmers J, *et al*. (2008) Intensive blood glucose control and vascular outcomes in patients with type 2 diabetes. *N Engl J Med* **358**: 2560–2572.

Patel A, MacMahon S, Chalmers J, *et al*. (2007) Effects of a fixed combination of perindopril and indapamide on macrovascular and microvascular outcomes in patients with type 2 diabetes mellitus (the ADVANCE trial): A randomised controlled trial. *Lancet* **370**: 829–840.

Pedrini MT, Levey AS, Lau J, *et al*. (1996) The effect of dietary protein restriction on the progression of diabetic and nondiabetic renal diseases: A meta-analysis. *Ann Intern Med* **124**: 627–632.

Pepine CJ, Handberg EM, Cooper-De-Hoff RM, *et al*. (2003) A calcium antagonist vs a non-calcium antagonist hypertension treatment strategy for patients with coronary artery disease: The International Verapamil-Trandolapril study (INVEST): a randomized controlled trial. *JAMA* **290**: 2805–2816.

Pfeffer MA, Swedberg K, Granger CB, *et al*. (2003) Effects of candesartan on mortality and morbidity in patients with chronic heart failure: The CHARM-Overall programme. *Lancet* **362**: 759–766.

Photocoagulation for diabetic macular edema. (1985) Early Treatment Diabetic Retinopathy Study report number 1: Early Treatment Diabetic Retinopathy Study Research Group. *Arch Ophthalmol* **103**: 1796–1806.

Pijls LT, de Vries H, Donker AJ, *et al*. (1999) The effect of protein restriction on albuminuria in patients with type 2 diabetes mellitus: A randomized trial. *Nephrol Dial Transplant* **14**: 1445–1453.

Psaty BM, Lumley T, Furberg CD, *et al*. (2003) Health outcomes associated with various antihypertensive therapies used as first-line agents: A network metaanalysis. *JAMA* **289**: 2534–2544.

Psaty BM, Smith NL, Siscovick DS, *et al*. (1997) Health outcomes associated with antihypertensive therapies used as first-line agents: A systematic review and meta-analysis. *JAMA* **277**: 739–745.

Pyorala K, Pedersen TR, Kjekshus J, *et al*. (1997) Cholesterol lowering with simvastatin improves prognosis of diabetic patients with coronary heart disease: A subgroup analysis of the Scandinavian Simvastatin Survival Study (4S). *Diabetes Care* **20**: 614–620.

Ramachandran A, Snehalatha C, Mary S, *et al*. (2006) The Indian Diabetes Prevention Programme shows that lifestyle modification and metformin prevent type 2 diabetes in Asian Indian subjects with impaired glucose tolerance (IDPP-1). *Diabetologia* **49**: 289–297.

Ranney L, Melvin C, Lux L, *et al*. (2006) Systematic review: smoking cessation intervention strategies for adults and adults in special populations. *Ann Intern Med* **145**: 845–856.

Ravid M, Lang R, Rachmani R, *et al*. (1996) Long-term renoprotective effect of angiotensin-converting enzyme inhibition in non-insulin-dependent diabetes mellitus: A 7-year follow-up study. *Arch Intern Med* **156**: 286–289.

Reichard P, Nilsson BY, Rosenqvist U. (1993) The effect of long-term intensified insulin treatment on the development of microvascular complications of diabetes mellitus. *N Engl J Med* **329**: 304–309.

Remuzzi G, Macia M, Ruggenenti P. (2006) Prevention and treatment of diabetic renal disease in type 2 diabetes: The BENEDICT study. *J Am Soc Nephrol* **17**: S90–S97.

Retinopathy and nephropathy in patients with type 1 diabetes four years after a trial of intensive therapy. (2000) The Diabetes Control and Complications Trial/Epidemiology of Diabetes Interventions and Complications Research Group. *N Engl J Med* **342**: 381–389.

Rohlfing CL, Wiedmeyer HM, Little RR, *et al*. (2002) Defining the relationship between plasma glucose and HbA(1c): Analysis of glucose profiles and HbA(1c) in the Diabetes Control and Complications Trial. *Diabetes Care* **25**: 275–278.

Rubins HB, Robins SJ, Collins D, *et al*. (1999) Gemfibrozil for the secondary prevention of coronary heart disease in men with low levels of high-density lipoprotein cholesterol: Veterans Affairs High-Density Lipoprotein Cholesterol Intervention Trial Study Group. *N Engl J Med* **341**: 410–418.

Sacco M, Pellegrini F, Roncaglioni MC, *et al.* (2003) Primary prevention of cardiovascular events with low-dose aspirin and vitamin E in type 2 diabetic patients: Results of the Primary Prevention Project (PPP) trial. *Diabetes Care* **26**: 3264–3272.

Sacks DB, Bruns DE, Goldstein DE, *et al.* (2002) Guidelines and recommendations for laboratory analysis in the diagnosis and management of diabetes mellitus. *Clin Chem* **48**: 436–472.

Sacks FM, Svetkey LP, Vollmer WM, *et al.* (2001) Effects on blood pressure of reduced dietary sodium and the Dietary Approaches to Stop Hypertension (DASH) diet: DASH-Sodium Collaborative Research Group. *N Engl J Med* **344**: 3–10.

Schjoedt KJ, Jacobsen P, Rossing K, *et al.* (2005) Dual blockade of the renin-angiotensin-aldosterone system in diabetic nephropathy: The role of aldosterone. *Horm Metab Res* **37**(1): 4–8.

Schjoedt KJ, Rossing K, Juhl TR, *et al.* (2005) Beneficial impact of spironolactone in diabetic nephropathy. *Kidney Int* **68**: 2829–2836.

Schrier RW, Estacio RO, Mehler PS, *et al.* (2007) Appropriate blood pressure control in hypertensive and normotensive type 2 diabetes mellitus: A summary of the ABCD trial. *Nat Clin Pract Nephrol* **3**: 428–438.

Scognamiglio R, Negut C, Ramondo A, *et al.* (2006) Detection of coronary artery disease in asymptomatic patients with type 2 diabetes mellitus. *J Am Coll Cardiol* **47**: 65–71.

Sega R, Facchetti R, Bombelli M, *et al.* (2005) Prognostic value of ambulatory and home blood pressures compared with office blood pressure in the general population: follow-up results from the Pressioni Arteriose Monitorate e Loro Associazioni (PAMELA) study. *Circulation* **111**: 1777–1783.

Selvin E, Marinopoulos S, Berkenblit G, *et al.* (2004) Meta-analysis: glycosylated haemoglobin and cardiovascular disease in diabetes mellitus. *Ann Intern Med* **141**: 421–431.

Sever PS, Poulter NR, Dahlof B, *et al.* (2005) Reduction in cardiovascular events with atorvastatin in 2,532 patients with type 2 diabetes: Anglo-Scandinavian Cardiac Outcomes Trial–Lipid-Lowering Arm (ASCOT-LLA). *Diabetes Care* **28**: 1151–1157.

Shepherd J, Barter P, Carmena R, *et al.* (2006) Effect of lowering LDL cholesterol substantially below currently recommended levels in patients with coronary heart disease and diabetes: The Treating to New Targets (TNT) study. *Diabetes Care* **29**: 1220–1226.

Sibai BM. (1996) Treatment of hypertension in pregnant women. *N Engl J Med* **335**: 257–265.

Simon J, Gray A, Clarke P, *et al.* (2008) Cost effectiveness of self monitoring of blood glucose in patients with non-insulin treated type 2 diabetes: Economic evaluation of data from the Di-GEM trial. *BMJ* **336**: 1177–1180.

Singh IM, Shishehbor MH, Ansell BJ. (2007) High-density lipoprotein as a therapeutic target: A systematic review. *JAMA* **298**: 786–798.

Singh IM, Shishehbor MH, Ansell BJ. (2007) High-density lipoprotein as a therapeutic target: A systematic review. *JAMA* **298**: 786–798.

Smith SC Jr, Allen J, Blair SN, *et al.* (2006) AHA/ACC guidelines for secondary prevention for patients with coronary and other atherosclerotic vascular disease: 2006 update: Endorsed by the National Heart, Lung, and Blood Institute. *Circulation* **113**: 2363–2372.

Stamler J, Vaccaro O, Neaton JD, *et al.* (1993) Diabetes, other risk factors, and 12-yr cardiovascular mortality for men screened in the Multiple Risk Factor Intervention Trial. *Diabetes Care* **16**: 434–444.

Stettler C, Allemann S, Juni P, *et al.* (2006) Glycemic control and macrovascular disease in types 1 and 2 diabetes mellitus: Meta-analysis of randomized trials. *Am Heart J* **152**: 27–38.

Stratton IM, Adler AI, Neil HA, *et al.* (2000) Association of glycaemia with macrovascular and microvascular complications of type 2 diabetes (UKPDS 35): Prospective observational study. *BMJ* **321**: 405–412.

Tatti P, Pahor M, Byington RP, *et al.* (1998) Outcome results of the Fosinopril Versus Amlodipine Cardiovascular Events Randomized Trial (FACET) in patients with hypertension and NIDDM. *Diabetes Care* **21**: 597–603.

The Diabetic Retinopathy Study (DRS) Research Group. (1976) Preliminary report on the effects of photocoagulation therapy: DRS Report #1. *Am J Ophthalmol* **81**: 383–396.

The effect of intensive treatment of diabetes on the development and progression of long-term complications in insulin-dependent diabetes mellitus. (1993) The Diabetes Control and Complications Trial Research Group. *N Engl J Med* **329**: 977–986.

The Juvenile Diabetes Research Foundation Continuous Glucose Monitoring Study Group. (2008) Continuous glucose monitoring and intensive treatment of type 1 diabetes. *N Engl J Med* **359**: 1464–1476.

Tight blood pressure control and risk of macrovascular and microvascular complications in type 2 diabetes. (1998) UKPDS 38: UK Prospective Diabetes Study Group. *BMJ* **317**: 703–713.

Torgerson JS, Hauptman J, Boldrin MN, *et al.* (2004) XENical in the prevention of diabetes in obese subjects (XENDOS) study: A randomized study of orlistat as an adjunct to lifestyle changes for the prevention of type 2 diabetes in obese patients. *Diabetes Care* **27**: 155–161.

Tsalamandris C, Allen TJ, Gilbert RE, *et al.* (1994) Progressive decline in renal function in diabetic patients with and without albuminuria. *Diabetes* **43**: 649–655.

Tuomilehto J, Lindstrom J, Eriksson JG, *et al.* (2001) Prevention of type 2 diabetes mellitus by changes in lifestyle among subjects with impaired glucose tolerance. *N Engl J Med* **344**: 1343–1350.

US Preventive Services Task Force. (2002) Aspirin for the primary prevention of cardiovascular events: Recommendation and rationale. *Ann Intern Med* **136**: 157–160.

US Preventive Services Task Force. (2003) Counseling to prevent tobacco use and tobacco-related diseases: Recommendation statement. Rockville, MD, Agency for Healthcare Research and Quality.

USPSTF. (2003) Screening for type 2 diabetes mellitus in adults: Recommendations and rationale. *Ann Intern Med* **138**: 212–214.

Vijan S, Hofer TP, Hayward RA. (2000) Costutility analysis of screening intervals for diabetic retinopathy in patients with type 2 diabetes mellitus. *JAMA* **283**: 889–896.

Wackers FJ, Chyun DA, Young LH, *et al.* (2007) Resolution of asymptomatic myocardial ischemia in patients with type 2 diabetes in the Detection of Ischemia in Asymptomatic Diabetics (DIAD) study. *Diabetes Care* **30**: 2892–2898.

Welschen LM, Bloemendal E, Nijpels G, *et al.* (2005) Self-monitoring of blood glucose in patients with type 2 diabetes who are not using insulin: A systematic review. *Diabetes Care* **28**: 1510–1517.

Wilson DM, Kollman C. (2008) Relationship of A1C to glucose concentrations in children with type 1 diabetes: Assessments by high-frequency glucose determinations by sensors. *Diabetes Care* **31**: 381–385.

Younis N, Broadbent DM, Vora JP, *et al.* (2003) Incidence of sight-threatening retinopathy in patients with type 2 diabetes in the Liverpool Diabetic Eye Study: A cohort study. *Lancet* **361**: 195–200.

# Chapter 2

# Clinical Presentation of Retinopathy

## José Cunha-Vaz

Diabetic Retinopathy is composed of a characteristic group of lesions found in the retina of individuals having diabetes, generally for several years.

It has serious significance for the affected eye in that the ocular sequellae may progress to blindness.

Medical intervention can decrease some of the risk to vision caused by diabetic retinopathy, i.e. the control of glycemia decreases the risk of incidence and progression of retinopathy, but diabetic retinopathy may still in many cases progress to the loss of vision in well–controlled patients.

Klein and Klein (2003) stated that though maintaining normal blood glucose levels from the onset would be ideal, any improvement in glycemic control at virtually any stage in the course of retinopathy seems to be associated with a decreased risk of progression. This question is still a matter of controversy and there is much information indicating that good metabolic control is not effective when the retinopathy has progressed to a point of no return. In this situation rigorous control may even worsen the retinopathy (Lauritzen *et al.*, 1983; Canny *et al.*, 1985). They state also that the abnormalities that characterize diabetic retinopathy occur in predictable progression with minor variations in the order of their appearance. This is clearly not the case and there is much variation in the rate of progression of the retinopathy between different individuals, even when they have been submitted to similar levels of glycemic control (Ribeiro *et al.*, 2002). The different steps of the Early Treatment Diabetic Retinopathy Study (ETDRS) classification do not necessarily follow in an orderly fashion and it is possible to find different

evolutions of the retinopathy, such as, regression from moderate to mild nonproliferative or rapid progression from mild to preproliferative retinopathy. The only clear and regular evolutive pattern to be observed in diabetic retinopathy is the progression from the preproliferative stage to the proliferative stage if there is no intervention.

The evolution of diabetic retinopathy has been considered to progress in stages, based on two landmarks: presence of alterations on ophthalmoscopic examination and the development of retinal neovascularization, a late development, which appears to be fundamentally independent of the diabetic metabolic disease.

I prefer to consider non-proliferative retinopathy as the retinal disease resulting from diabetes mellitus. As it progresses it may, then, develop two major complications, each one dependent on different mechanisms of disease, macular edema and proliferative retinopathy.

The involvement of retina in diabetes may, therefore, be divided into:

1. Preclinical stage
2. Nonproliferative retinopathy
3. Complications of Diabetic Retinopathy
   3.1. Diabetic macular edema
   3.2. Preproliferative and proliferative retinopathy

It is to be realized that considering all individuals suffering from diabetes the natural history of diabetic retinopathy does not follow a rigid timetable, on the contrary, it has a rather variable course. Factors that influence the evolution of the disease and its staging are numerous but the ones considered most important are the type of diabetes and level of metabolic control, duration of diabetes, increased blood pressure and genetic susceptibility.

## 2.1. Preclinical Stage

This stage is characterized by the absence of lesions on ophthalmoscopic examination. However, alterations preceding ophthalmoscopic changes have been demonstrated by a variety of other more sensitive methods of examination and by histological examination.

Basically a microangiopathy, the initial pathologic findings are characterized by endothelial proliferation in the capillaries and venules and endothelial swelling and degeneration on the smallest arteriolar branchings (Fig. 2.1). Pericyte damage is also widespread and has been considered to be characteristic of diabetic retinal disease but its distribution is irregular and is only made more apparent by an accumulation of eosinophilic material. The apparent predominance of pericytic lesions when compared to the alteration of the endothelial cells may be explained by the different

anatomical location of these cells, encased in basement membrane.

The damaged pericytes remain in place for longer periods of time becoming, therefore, more conspicuous (Cunha-Vaz, 1978).

Microaneurysms occur preferentially in the posterior pole and on the venous side of the circulation in association with endothelial proliferation (Cunha-Vaz, 1967). As the disease spreads the endothelial swelling and degeneration on the arterial side leads to areas of vascular cell loss and capillary closure, increasing progressively until they reach sizes that become visible on fluorescein angiography.

The initial changes in the diabetic retina are, therefore, endothelial proliferation and microaneurysm formation on the venous side and endothelial cell loss and capillary closure on the arterial side (Cunha-Vaz, 1972). It appears to be initially a posterior pole disease, primarily affecting the cells of the small retinal vessels (Fig. 2.2). The topographical distribution of its lesions differs markedly from the hematological disorders (e.g. macroglobulinemia and sickle-cell disease) which manifest characteristically peripheral changes, and hypertensive retinopathy, which demonstrates preferential involvement of the arterial side.

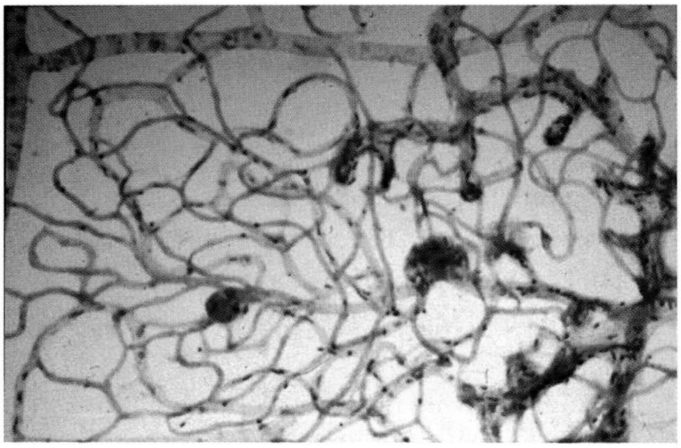

**Fig. 2.1.** Diabetic retinopathy. Retinal digest showing endothelial proliferation and microaneurysm formation preferentially on the venous side with cell loss on the arteriolar side.

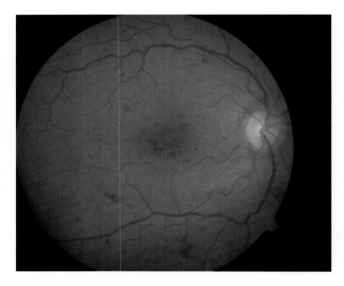

**Fig. 2.2.** Diabetic retinopathy. Fundus photography of the posterior pole showing typical alterations, predominantly microaneurysms and hemorrhages.

Diabetic retinopathy, however, can be compared with radiation retinopathy, in which endothelial cell damage predominates.

Fluorescein angiography confirmed the histopathological findings of diabetic retinal disease in a dynamic manner. It was the first technique to document the abnormal leakage of fluorescein through the walls of the retinal vessels (Fig. 2.3) that was demonstrated to be due to breakdown of the blood-retinal barrier (Cunha-Vaz and Maurice, 1967). Fluorescein angiography also reinforced the importance of capillary closure as a reliable indicator of the progression of ischemia, one of its most characteristic changes.

Increased capillary visibility on fluorescein angiography is also a characteristic feature of early diabetic retinopathy. Retinal blood vessels do not have autonomic systemic innervation. They attempt to maintain constant blood flow through a mechanism called autoregulation. Thus, under hypoxic conditions, they dilate to provide a better blood supply. Under hyperoxic conditions, they constrict. The loss of the supporting pericytes from the capillary walls may also contribute to permanent loss of this tonic control, resulting in chronic diffuse distention of the vessel

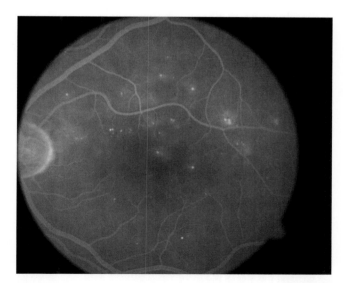

**Fig. 2.3.** Diabetic retinopathy. Fluorescein angiography showing fluorescent dots (microaneurysms) and diffusion of fluorescein around the lesions (fluorescein leakage).

walls. Hyperglycemia by itself impairs autoregulation. Furthermore, as the retinopathy worsens, there is evidence that autoregulation deteriorates (Sinclair et al., 1982).

Ashton (1950) was the first to demonstrate areas of capillary closure in diabetic patients. Since that time it has become recognized that areas of retinal capillary closure or capillary nonperfusion, as demonstrated by fluorescein angiography, are a hallmark feature of diabetic retinopathy. It is one of the two fundamental alterations occurring in the retina. As some capillaries are occluded, the blood is diverted to other vessels that dilate and function as shunt vessels. Progressive capillary occlusion actually causes an increase in the speed of flow in large retinal vessels, apparently due to this shunting mechanism. It is this shunting mechanism that appears to be responsible for the multiple vascular abnormalities that progressively develop in the retina.

More recently, vitreous fluorophotometry has been used to quantify the alteration of the blood-retinal barrier (Cunha-Vaz et al., 1975). This sensitive method has confirmed that alteration of the blood-retinal barrier (fluorescein leakage) is one of the earliest changes to occur in the diabetic retina, again suggesting the importance of the retinal endothelial damage.

The alteration of the blood-retinal barrier is detected by vitreous fluorophotometry, with values higher than 2 SD above the normal in approximately 30–40% of the eyes that did not show any ophthalmoscopical changes, in comparison with fluorescein angiography, which detects microaneurysms, leakage or capillary nonperfusion in approximately 18% of the eyes that appear to be normal on ophthalmoscopic examination (Cunha-Vaz et al., 1979).

Vitreous fluorophotometry, which was introduced for clinical use in 1975, is the only commercially available method that can quantify, in a reproducible manner, the breakdown of the blood-retinal barrier. Fluorophotometry shows a distinct separation between normal control eyes and diabetic eyes with retinopathy. Diabetic eyes with no visible retinopathy may be distributed almost equally into the three groups: one showing fluorophotometric values within the normal range, another demonstrating borderline leakage and a third showing clearly abnormal leakage. There is evidence that this increased leakage may be of prognostic value, indicating the eyes that are at risk for more rapidly progressing to severe retinopathy. Krupin and Waltman (1985) in the first long term study of diabetic patients using vitreous fluorophotometry showed that high vitreous fluorescein values were harbingers of the development or progression of retinopathy. The vascular changes involving the small retinal vessels are, therefore, the initial alterations occurring in the diabetic retina. There is some evidence of early neural tissue damage from other methods of examination but this evidence has been scanty and neuroglial damage does not appear to be an initial feature of the preretinopathy stage.

One of the early symptoms of diabetic retinopathy is poor night vision and poor recovery from bright light. Testing with the Goldmann dark adaptometer and with the nyctometer shows that they deteriorate in advanced stages of retinopathy (Frost-Larsen *et al.*, 1981). Dark adaptation may indeed be affected by decreased oxygen levels and hypoglycemia, (McFarland *et al.*, 1946) but in diabetics dark adaptation usually is normal until clinical retinopathy develops. Similarly, color vision tends to deteriorate as diabetic retinopathy advances, involving blue-yellow discrimination (Roy *et al.*, 1984).

Visual fields are usually within normal limits and when changes are present they correlate with areas of capillary nonperfusion demonstrated by fluorescein angiography, (Bell and Feldon, 1984) again showing that the retinal neural tissue involvement appears to be secondary to the vascular alterations.

Finally, the same conclusions can be drawn from the electrophysiological abnormalities detected in the diabetic retina. The most significant and earliest electrophysiologic abnormality seen in patients with diabetic retinopathy is a diminution of the amplitude of the oscillatory potentials of the electroretinogram. It is noteworthy that here again the alterations in oscillatory potentials appear clearly linked to capillary

nonperfusion and ischemia and this evaluation appears particularly useful to predict overall ischemia and evolution to the preproliferative stage (Bresnick *et al.*, 1984).

## 2.2. Nonproliferative Diabetic Retinopathy

Nonproliferative diabetic retinopathy is said to be present when alterations of the fundus are detected by ophthalmoscopy.

On ophthalmoscopic examination, the characteristic features of nonproliferative diabetic retinopathy are: microaneurysms, intrarretinal hemorrhages, hard exudates and some degree of retinal edema.

Retinal microaneurysms are usually the first ophthalmoscopic sign of diabetic retinopathy. They are located predominantly within the inner nuclear layer and in the deep retinal capillary network (Asthon, 1958). On ophthalmoscopy, fresh microaneurysms appear as small red dots (Figs. 2.4 and 2.5). Microaneurysms may later become yellowish due to increased thickening of basement membrane due to the associated leakage. Finally, they occlude. Microaneurysms fill during the early venous phase of fluorescein angiography

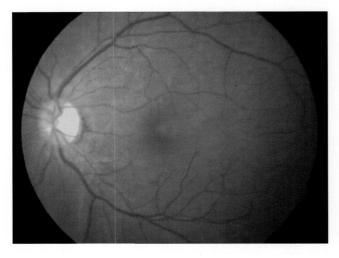

**Fig. 2.4.**   Diabetic retinopathy. Isolated microaneurysms in the posterior pole.

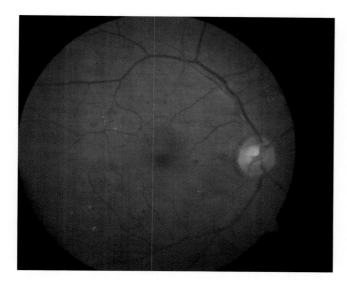

**Fig. 2.5.** Diabetic retinopathy. Microaneurysms and small hemorrhages in posterior pole with isolated hard exudates.

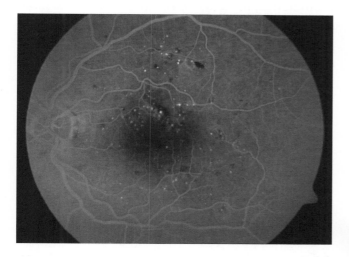

**Fig. 2.6.** Diabetic retinopathy. Fluorescein angiography showing multiple microaneurysms and a few areas of capillary closure.

indicating their characteristic origin in the venous side of the circulation.

Fluorescein angiography demonstrates the microaneurysms particularly well as they become hyperfluorescent and leak profusely (Fig. 2.6). However, later in the disease process, as they become occluded, fluorescein angiography is not able to identify them. Microaneurysm counts on fluorescein angiography

are, therefore, only reliable as an indicator of diabetic retinal disease in the initial stages of diabetic retinopathy.

Intraretinal hemorrhages are another predominant ophthalmoscopical feature of nonproliferative diabetic retinopathy and result from ruptured microaneurysms, capillaries and venules, and are mostly located within the outer plexiform and inner nuclear layers.

In the diabetic eye, retinal intraretinal hemorrhages are characteristically most numerous in the posterior pole. Numerous peripheral hemorrhages should lead one to suspect of another concomitant systemic disease process.

Hard exudates are another ophthalmoscopic feature of background diabetic retinopathy. They are extracellular accumulations of lipoproteins derived from leakage from abnormal vessels. Clinically, these yellowish deposits vary in size from small dots to a confluent arrangement that may even cover most of the posterior pole (Fig. 2.7).

Finally, retinal edema leads to the development of central macular edema, which is the most frequent cause of vision loss in diabetes. It is clinically defined as thickening of the macula and is due to accumulation of fluid in the central macular area. Subclinical macular edema is detected frequently in diabetic eyes using the new methods to measure retinal thickness,

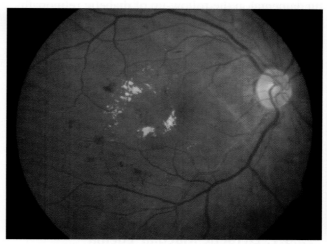

**Fig. 2.7.** Diabetic retinopathy. Hard exudates in a circiunrate pattern in the posterior pole.

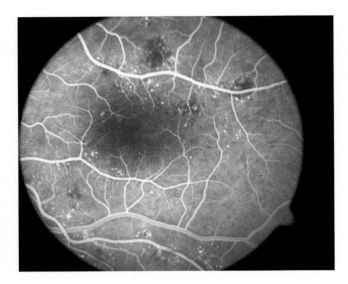

**Fig. 2.8.** Diabetic retinopathy. Fluorescein angiography showing numerous microaneuryms and areas of capillary closure.

optical coherence is apparently due to the associated alteration of the blood-retinal barrier, well demonstrated by fluorescein leakage. Leakage is, with capillary closure, the two fundamental alterations occurring in the diabetic retina (Fig. 2.8). It is this leakage due to the alteration of the blood-retinal barrier that ultimately leads to clinically significant macular edema. The role of fluorescein angiography and vitreous fluorophotometry in detecting and measuring the alteration of the blood-retinal barrier is, therefore, fundamental in the follow-up of diabetic retinopathy.

The need to document leakage (alteration of the blood-retinal barrier) and capillary closure demonstrate clearly that ophthalmoscopic examination and its documentation by fundus photography alone has limited value for characterization of diabetic retinopathy.

## 2.3. Complications of Diabetic Retinal Disease

### 2.3.1. Diabetic Macular Edema

Diabetic macular edema is the largest cause of visual acuity reduction in patients with diabetes (Aiello *et al.*, 1998). It affects central vision from the early stages of retinopathy and is extremely frequent, particularly in older type 2 diabetic patients. Its role in the process of vision loss in diabetic patients and its occurrence in the evolution of the retinopathy is being increasingly recognized.

Diabetic macular edema, also frequently denominated diabetic maculopathy leads to distortion of visual images and may cause a significantly decreased visual acuity despite possible absence of severe retinopathy.

Macular edema, while a frequent and characteristic complication of diabetic retinopathy and showing a clear association with the systemic metabolic alterations of diabetes, does not fit necessarily into the regular course of progression of diabetic retinopathy, as it may occur at any stage of DR, nonproliferative, moderate or severe or even at the more advanced stages of the retinopathy (Klein and Klein, 2003).

These facts are particularly important regarding the relevance of diabetic macular edema in the natural history of diabetic retinopathy.

First, the retinopathy in diabetes frequently progresses for many years without visual loss, making particularly difficult to consider and accept outcomes to signal retinopathy progression and need for treatment that do not include vision loss. Diabetic macular edema is particularly frequent in diabetes type 2 and is often the first alteration occurring in the retina that causes vision loss.

Second, diabetic macular edema does not fit clearly in the presently accepted ETDRS classification of diabetic retinopathy. This is a clear indication that this classification has major shortcomings and needs to be revised as we progress in our understanding of the natural history of diabetic retinopathy. The ETDRS classification of diabetic retinopathy was constructed in order to be prognostic of progressive ischemia resulting in the development neovascularization and proliferative retinopathy. This was, indeed, an acceptable orientation when treatment of proliferative retinopathy remained the main priority. Improved understanding of the evolution of retinal disease and the development of new therapies that offer the possibility for early treatment of diabetic retinopathy have shifted the focus towards the initial stages of diabetic retinal disease. It is now clear that management of diabetic retinopathy has to address the initial stages of retinal disease when the pathology is still reversible, there is retinal edema where there is any increase of water in the retinal tissue resulting in an increase in its volume, i.e. thickness.

This increase in water content of the retinal tissue may be initially intracellular or extracellular.

In the retina there is a specialized structure, the Blood-Retinal Barrier, that regulates the fluid movements in and out of the retinal tissue. The BRB is essentially formed by two major components: the inner BRB and the outer BRB (Cunha-Vaz, 1976). The inner BRB is formed by the endothelial membrane of the retinal vessels, whereas the outer BRB is structurally organized around the retinal pigment epithelium. In diabetes, the inner BRB becomes dysfunctional and does not fulfil its prospective role. When that occurs the barrier opens resulting in increased movements of fluids and molecules into the retina.

In diabetes, in the initial stages of diabetic retinal disease, we may be dealing with two different situations: a situation of intact BRB and an open BRB (Cunha-Vaz and Travassos, 1984; Lobo *et al.*, 1999).

Intracellular edema, in the retina in diabetes, may occur when there is a situation of intact BRB and the retinal cells are swollen due to an alteration of the cellular ionic changes resulting in excessive accumulation of $Na^+$ inside the cells. This is a situation of cytotoxic edema. It may be induced by accumulation of excitatory transmitters, such as glutamate and excessive accumulation of lactic acid and may be the immediate result of ischemia, trauma or toxic cell damage.

Extracellular edema is directly associated with a situation of open BRB, i.e. results from a breakdown of the inner BRB, one of the earliest alterations occurring in the diabetic retina. The increase in tissue volume is due to an increase in the retinal extracellular space and the breakdown of the BRB is well identified by fluorescein leakage, which can be detected in a clinical environment by fluorescein angiography or

vitreous fluorometry measurements. Extracellular edema can also be called vasogenic edema because of its direct association with vascular changes, namely, in this case, the endothelial membrane of the retinal vessels. This type of edema is characterized by its reversibility, if addressed in its initial stages, and due to an open BRB situation when the Starling law governing the movements of fluids applies. With an open BRB, any loss of equilibrium between hydrostatic, oncotic and osmotic pressure gradients across the retinal vessels contribute to further water movements and may result in increased edema formation.

In this situation, the "force" driving water across the capillary wall is represented by the result of a hydrostatic pressure $\Delta P$ and an effective osmotic pressure difference $\Delta \pi \sigma$. The equation regulating movements across the BRB is, therefore:

(driving force)
$$= L_p \left[ (P_{\text{plasma}} - P_{\text{tissue}}) - \sigma (\pi_{\text{plasma}} - \pi_{\text{tissue}}) \right],$$

where $L_p$ is the hydraulic conductivity or membrane permeability of the BRB and $\sigma$, an osmotic reflection coefficient, $P_{\text{plasma}}$, the blood pressure, $P$ tissue, the retinal tissue pressure, $\pi$ plasma, blood omostic pressure and $\pi$ tissue, the tissue osmotic pressure.

An increase in $\Delta P$, contributing to increased movements of fluids into the retinal tissue and retinal extracellular edema, may be due to an increase in $P_{\text{plasma}}$ or a decrease in $P_{\text{tissue}}$ or both. An increase in $P_{\text{plasma}}$ due to increased systemic blood pressure does contribute to retinal edema formation only after loss of autoregulation of retinal blood flow and breakdown of the BRB, as mentioned before.

A decrease in $P_{\text{tissue}}$ is also an important component that has not been given sufficient attention. Any alteration in the cohesion of the retinal tissue due to pathologies, such as localized cell loss, cyst formation and vitreous traction with pulling on the inner limiting membrane of the retina will lead to a decrease in $P_{\text{tissue}}$, thus facilitating fluid accumulation in the retina and an increase in retinal thickness, i.e. retinal edema.

Similarly, a decrease in $\Delta \pi_+$ contributes to retinal edema due to protein accumulation in the retina associated with the breakdown of the BRB. Extravasation of proteins and lipoproteins, such as in hard exudates, increase the osmotic pressure in the retinal tissue and draw more water into the retinal extracellular space contributing to edema formation and maintenance. This is the main factor associated with oncotic-driven fluid movements in the retina, as reduction in plasma osmolarity high enough to contribute to edema formation is an extremely rare event.

When there is a breakdown of the BRB there is formation of extracellular edema and the progression of the edema depends directly on the gradient induced by differences between blood pressure, tissue pressure and the oncotic gradient induced by protein accumulation in the retina.

The clinical evaluation of macular edema has been characterized by its difficulty and subjectivity. Direct and indirect ophthalmoscopy may only show an alteration of the focal reflexes. Stereoscopic fundus photography and slit-lamp microscopy have played an important role demonstrating changes in retinal volume in the macular area, but they are dependent on the observer experience and the results do not offer a reproducible measurement of the volume change. In a study by Gonzalez *et al.*, 1995, the results from stereofundus photography and slit-lamp examination by experienced observers were compared and an agreement of only 45% was found, supporting the unreliability of the clinical methods to document macular edema objectively.

This ETDRS, made an effort to establish some guidelines to define "clinically significant macular edema" in order to establish an outcome when designing clinical trials to test the efficacy of treatment for diabetic macular edema. They paid special attention to the involvement of the center of the macula taking into the consideration the associated visual loss, with its clinical significance.

Their definition of clinically significant macular edema is as follows:

1. Thickening of the retina (as seen either by slitlamp biomicroscopy or by stereofundus photography) at or within 500 microns of the center of the macular.
2. Hard exudates at or within 500 microns of the center of the macular associated into the thickening of the adjacent retina (but not residual exudates remaining after disappearance of retinal thickening);
3. A zone, or zones, of retinal thickening one disc area or larger size, any part of which is within one disc diameter of the center of the macula.

The problems associated with these guidelines are self-evident, taking into account the subjectivity of the evaluation regarding "abnormal" thickening, the presence of "hard exudates," which are not "residual" and the relative involvement of the central 500 microns circle of the macula.

Recently, two methodologies capable of meaning objectively changes in retinal thickness became available, Optical Coherence Tomography (OCT) and the Retinal Thickness Analyzer (RTA) (Zeimer *et al.*, 1984; Puliafito *et al.*, 1995). The advent of these techniques are changing our understanding of the incidence dramatically, evolution and rates of progression of diabetic macular edema. They will be described at length in the Section dedicated to Clinical Evaluation of Diabetic Retinopathy.

We are now able to measure changes in retinal thickness and identify macular edema, using non-invasive instrumentation in a clinical setting. Diabetic macular edema now needs to be identified regarding its type, distribution, evolution, pathophysiology and degree of involvement of the central macular area, central 500 microns circle of the retina (Figs. 2.9–2.12).

It is, therefore, necessary to consider:

1. the distribution of the edema in the macula;
2. the evolution of the edema and its the response to laser treatment;
3. the presence or absence of a situation of "open-barrier";
4. the degree of involvement of the central fovea;

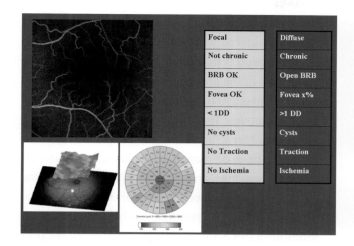

**Fig. 2.9.**   Focal edema with intact BRB. Indication for tighter metabolic control.

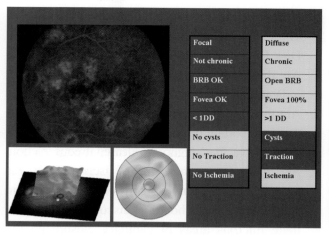

**Fig. 2.11.**   Diffuse edema with open BRB and ischemia. Need for close follow-up and progressive tightening of metabolic control.

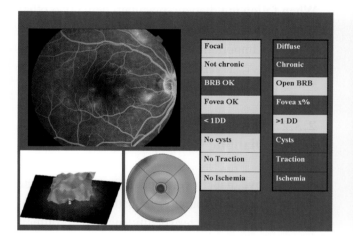

**Fig. 2.10.**   Focal edema with open BRB. Indication for focal laser treatment.

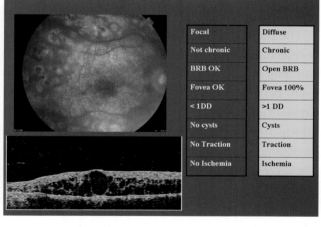

**Fig. 2.12.**   Diffuse macular edema with vitreous traction. Indication for vitrectomy.

5. the extent of the macular edema;
6. the presence or absence of cysts in the retina demonstrating decreased retinal tissue pressure;
7. the presence or absence of vitreous traction and finally;
8. the presence of signs of ischemia, such as loss of continuity of the capillary net surrounding the Foveal Avascular Zone or extensive areas of capillary closure.

We should, therefore, consider when characterizing a situation of diabetic macular edema, the following alternatives:

1. Is the edema focal or difuse.
2. Is the edema recently developed or has already been treated by laser without responding to treatment (chronic).
3. Is there a situation of "intact-barrier" or "open-barrier."

4. Is the fovea involved (central 300 $\mu$m)? How much?
5. The extent of the edema. More or less than one Disk Diameter (1500 $\mu$m).
6. Are there large cysts visible on OCT examination indicating decreased tissue pressure?
7. Are there signs of vitreous traction? This information is important because the edema will only probably resolve after surgery to release vitreous traction.
8. Are there important signs of ischemia? Is the retinal capillary network surrounding the Foveal Avascular Zone showing discontinuities? Are there microns areas of capillary closure on the fluorescein angiography?

The classification according to evolution into acute and chronic is dependent on the its evolution over a six-month period looking for its reversibility, with treatment.

The classification into open barrier or intact barrier is dependent on documentation of fluorescein leakage and may be achieved by fluorescein angiography or, even better, by vitreous fluorometry or with the Retinal Leakage Analyzer (Lobo *et al.*, 1999). Indirect information on Blood-Retinal Barrier breakdown may be obtained through the OCT (Bernardes *et al.*, 2009). The three main mechanisms of macular edema formation must also be identified in order to choose the best therapeutical option. All these three mechanisms of edema formation may be present simultaneously but it is fundamental to evaluate which one predominates and is probably responsible for the increased macular thickness. A predominance of the hemodynamic component must be considered when the signs of open barrier identified by abnormal fluorescein leakage dominate the fundus picture with minimal or absent signs of vitreous traction and moderate evidence of capillary dropout. In this situation control of blood pressure is particularly relevant.

A predominance of the tractional component should be considered when there is clear evidence of vitreous traction associated with a situation of open barrier predominantly in the central macular over signs of ischemia, demonstrated by capillary dropout.

Finally, a predominance of the ischemic component must be considered when capillary dropout predominates in the central macular area.

The extent of the area of increased thickness and the percentage coverage of the central macular area of 500 microns is another fundamental feature that must be registered in order to achieve a good characterization of a particular case of diabetic macular edema and its prognosis regarding potential loss of vision in the immediate future. A specific case of diabetic macular edema should then be classified, as shown in Table 2.1.

Multiple combinations of these alternatives are possible defining different types of diabetic macular edema. Four clinical cases are presented to illustrate the proposed classification. The indicated therapeutic option is given in the caption of each figure.

When following diabetic macular edema two other parameters must be considered in the analysis and are particularly important for management. These are Hemoglobin $A_{1C}$ levels and blood pressure values.

### 2.3.2. Preproliferative and Proliferative Diabetic Retinopathy

Preproliferative diabetic retinopathy is an intermediate stage between background retinopathy and proliferative retinopathy. Characteristically, in the preproliferative stage, signs of retinal ischemia increase. These

**Table 2.1**

| Diabetic Macular Edema – characterization | | |
|---|---|---|
| 1. Thickness Measurement | >300 μm | <500 μm |
| 2. Visual Acuity <3/10> | >3/10 | <3/10 |
| 3. Focal vs recurring | Focal | Recurring |
| 4. Foveal involvement | No Fovea | Fovea |
| 5. BRB Open | Normal BRB | BRB Open |
| 6. "Cystoid" spaces | No cystoid | Cystoid |
| 7. Traction | No Traction | Traction |
| 8. Ischemia | No Ischemia | Ischemia |
| 9. HgA$_{1C}$ | HgA$_{1C}$< 8 % | HgA$_{1C}$≥ 8% |
| 10. Blood Pressure | BP≤ 130/80 mmHg | BP> 130/80 mmHg |

include soft exudates, venous beading and loops, intraretinal microvascular abnormalities (IRMA) and widespread areas of capillary nonperfusion (Benson *et al.*, 1988).

Soft exudates are also called nerve fiber layer infractions or cotton-wool spots. They are due to obstruction of terminal retinal arterioles. On ophthalmoscopic examination they appear as superficial, whitish, fluff-like patches. A large number of soft exudates (greater than five) often indicates a rapidly progressing retinopathy with high risk of development of neovascularization within 12 to 24 months (Kohner and Dollery, 1975).

Severe venous dilatation with beading is an important indicator of preproliferative retinopathy because it indicates severe and diffuse hypoxia and a poor visual prognosis. Late venous changes include a line degeneration and diffuse thickening of the vessel wall. These changes account for the venous thickening that contributes to progressive circulatory stasis and blood sluggishness in the retina (Fig. 2.13).

Widespread and increasing capillary closure is another fundamental feature of the preproliferative retinopathy stage.

In preproliferative diabetic retinopathy it is no more the isolated area of capillary nonperfusion that predominates, but large areas of the retina become completely closed to the blood circulation (Fig. 2.14).

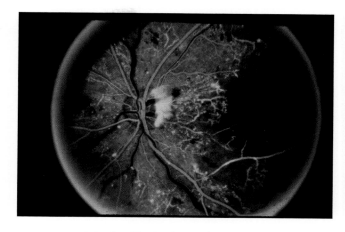

**Fig. 2.14.** Proliferative diabetic retinopathy. Fluorescein angiography showing extensive vascular closure and neovascularization at the optic disk.

Retinal nonperfusion may be suspected on ophthalmoscopic examination but can only be well demonstrated by fluorescein angiography. In some eyes this increase in nonperfused areas is better seen in the foveal avascular zone (FAZ), which becomes enlarged due to progressive closure of the perifoveal capillaries. Automated image analysis of the FAZ is one of the most promising ways of quantifying areas of retinal nonperfusion and ischemia. Preliminary results have shown it to be a reproducible method, particularly useful regarding follow-up of retinopathy progression and as indicator of prognosis and future neovascularization (Leite *et al.*, 1989).

IRMAs are dilated and often telangiectatic capillaries that result from their role as shunts between arterioles and venules in areas of increasing capillary closure. They leak fluorescein although not as profusely as does preretinal neovascularization.

The exact cause of new vessel formation is not known. It is, however, always secondary to the presence of large areas of capillary nonperfusion, usually associated with nonperfusion of arterioles and venules. It is, therefore, not specific to diabetic retinopathy, but occurs in a number of other retinal vascular diseases characterized by marked ischemia, such as sickle cell disease and retinal vein occlusion (Valone *et al.*, 1981; Cunha-Vaz, 1986).

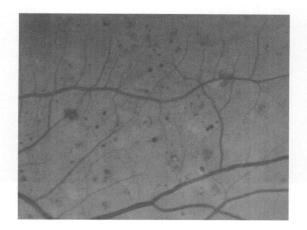

**Fig. 2.13.** Preproliferative diabetic retinopathy. Dilated venules and hemorrhages dominate the picture.

In diabetic patients it is usually preceded by a stage of preproliferative retinopathy characterized by progressive signs of widespread ischemia, such as multiple cotton-wool spots, intraretinal vascular abnormalities and a variety of venous abnormalities, such as leading loop formation and reduplication, clusters of relatively large blot hemorrhages and occluded vessels.

New vessels arise from the optic disk or from the retina periphery (Figs. 2.15 and 2.16a, b). Their origin is usually a venule, but they may occasionally arise from arterioles. New Vessels on the Disc (NVD) sometimes arise from the choroidal circulation. Peripheral new vessels lie initially in the plane of the retina but soon pierce the internal limiting membrane and are preretinal, forming adhesions with the overlying vitreous. While the vitreous is attached to the retina the new vessels are symptomless. However the presence of the new vessels leads to retraction of the vitreous. It is this pulling effect that leads to the progressive complications associated with retinal neovascularization, such as vitreous hemorrhage and progressive visual distortion.

As the neovascularization progresses fibrous tissue grows and follows it. When the fibrovascular meshwork becomes extensive and adherent to the posterior hyaloid face, vitreous contracture, apparently due to leakage and marked alterations of the blood-retinal barrier lead to tractional and marked alterations of the blood-retinal barrier lead to tractional retinal detachment.

Characteristically, retinal neovascularization leaks fluorescein profusely demonstrating an absent or very abnormal blood-retinal barrier (Fig. 2.16b). Eyes with

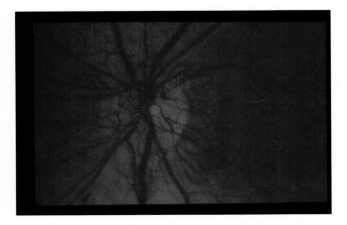

**Fig. 2.15.** Proliferative diabetic retinopathy. Neovascularization in the optic disk.

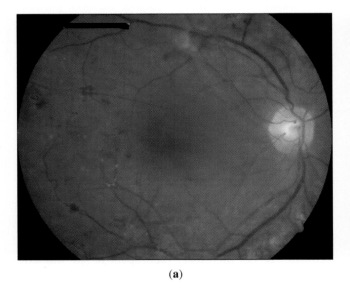

(a)

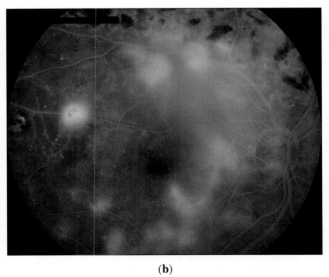

(b)

**Fig. 2.16.** (a) Diabetic Retinopathy. Fundus photography showing hemorrhages and sites of suspected retinal neovascularization. (b) Diabetic Retinopathy. Fluorescein angiography of the same eye identified the sites of retinal neovascularization (NVE).

NVD have always been generalized and widespread capillary nonperfusion, again confirming that retinal neovascularization is a direct consequence of generalized ischemia as in other non-diabetic retinal vascular diseases. Proliferative diabetic retinopathy is usually a bilateral disease. Approximately 90% of patients who present with proliferative diabetic retinopathy have it in both eyes at the time of initial examination (Valone *et al.*, 1981).

Neovascularization elsewhere in the retina (NVE), originates from the remaining perfused vessels, almost exclusively venules, next to areas of capillary nonperfusion. NVE in diabetic patients involves the posterior pole and midperiphery in contrast to other systemic diseases that cause peripheral NVE.

As the vitreous shrinks, possibly due to the abnormal leakage associated with the new vessels, it gradually pulls the neovascular fronds, causing preretinal and intravitreal bleeding, a frequent cause of acute vision loss in diabetic patients. The vitreous alterations associated with fibrovascular tissue contraction and cellular proliferation lead sooner or later to localized or generalized detachment. The vision prognosis for eyes with new vessels is poor.

This is particularly so, when there are "high risk" characteristics present, as described in the Diabetic Retinopathy Study. These are disc new vessels of more than minimal degree of severity, disc new vessels with present or previous hemorrhage and peripheral new vessels associated with hemorrhage.

Proliferative retinopathy responds well to photocoagulation, but it is essential that it is treated early and adequately, at a time when it is symptomless, before tractional complications have developed.

# References

Aiello LP, Gardner TW, King GL, *et al.* (1998) Diabetic Retinopathy. *Diabetes Care* **21**: 143–156.

Ashton N. (1950) The pathology of retinal microaneurysms. *Acta XVI Concilium Ophthalmologicum* **1**: 411–421.

Ashton N. (1958) Diabetic microaniopathy. *Adv Ophthalmol* **8**: 1–84.

Bell JA, Feldon SG. (1984) Retinal microangiopathy. Correlation of OCTOPUS perimetry with fluorescein angiography. *Arch Ophthalmol* **102**: 1294–1298.

Benson WE, Brown GC, Tasman W. (1988) *Diabetes and Its Ocular Complications*. WR Saubders Company, Philadelphia.

Bernardes R, Santos T, Horne M, Cunha-Vaz J. (2009) Non-invasive Assessment of Blood-retinal Barrier Changes by Cirrus HD-OCT. Arvo Annual Meeting, **A268**.

Bresnick GH, Korth K, Groo A, *et al.* (1984) Electroretinographic oscillatory potentials predict progression of diabetic retinopathy. Preliminary report. *Arch Ophthalmol* **102**: 1307–1311.

Canny CLB, Kohner EM, Traultman J, *et al.* (1985) Comparison of stereofundus photographs in patients with insulin-dependent diabetes during conventional insulin treatment or continuous subcutaneous insulin infusion. *Diabetes* **34**(Suppl. 3): 50–55.

Cunha-Vaz JG. (1972) Diabetic retinopathy. Human and experimental studies. *Trans Ophthalmol Soc UK* **92**: 111–124.

Cunha-Vaz JG, Abreu JRF, Campos AJ, Figo G. (1975). Early breakdown of the blood-retinal barrier in diabetes. *Br J Ophthalmol* **59**: 649–656.

Cunha-Vaz JG. (1976). The Blood-Retinal Barrier. *Doc Ophthalmol* **41**: 287–327.

Cunha-Vaz JG. (1978) Pathophysiology of diabetic retinopathy. *Br J Ophthalmol* **62**: 351–355.

Cunha-Vaz JG. (1986) Diabetic retinopathy. In: Crepaldi G, Cunha-Vaz JG, Fedele D, Morgensen C, Ward S (eds.), *Microvascular and Neurological Complications of Diabetes*. Padova Liviana Press, Springer Verlag, p. 3.

Cunha-Vaz JG, Faria de Abreu JR, Campos AJ, *et al.* (1975). Novos métodos de estudo da circulação retiniana. *O Médico* **70**: 195–197.

Cunha-Vaz JG, Goldberg MF, Vygantas C, Noth J. (1979) Early detection of retinal involvement in diabetes by vitreous fluorophotometry. *Ophthalmology* **86**: 264–275.

Cunha-Vaz JG, Maurice DM. (1967) Fluorescein transport by retinal vessels. Proc. 20 Internat. Congr. Ophthalmol. (*Excerpta Medica International Congress Series*) **146**: 187–188.

Cunha-Vaz JG, Travassos A. (1984) Breakdown of the blood-retinal barriers and cystoid macular edema. *Surv Ophthalmol* **28**(Suppl.) 465–492.

Early Treatment Diabetic Retinopathy Study Research Group. (1987) Treatment techniques and clinical guidelines for photocoagulation of diabetic macular edema. ETDRS report no 2. *Ophthalmology* **94**: 761–774.

Frost-Larsen K, Larsen HW, Simonsen SE. (1981) The value of dark-adaptation as a prognostic tool in diabetic retinopathy. *Metab Pediatr Ophthalmol* **5**(1): 39–44.

Gonzalez ME, Gonzalez C, Stern MP, *et al.* (1995) Concordance in diagnosis of diabetic retinopathy by fundus photography between retina specialists and standardized reading center. Mexico City Diabetes Study Retinopathy Group. *Arch Med Res* **26**: 127–130.

Klein BEK, Klein R. (2003) *Diabetic Retinopathy*. In: Johnson GJ, Minassian DC, Weale RA, West SK. (eds.), *The Epidemiology of Eye Disease*, 2nd ed, Oxford University Press, Chap. 20, pp. 341–355.

Kohner E, Dollery CT. (1975) Diabetic Retinopathy. In: Keen H, Jarret, M. (eds.), *Complications of Diabetes*, London, Edward Arnold, pp. 1–98.

Krupin T, Waltman SR. (1985) Fluorophotometry in juvenile-onset diabetes: Long-term follow-up. *Jpn J Ophthalmol* **29**(2): 139–145.

Lauritzen T, Frost-Larsen K, Larsen HW, Deckert T and the Steno Study Group. (1983) Effect of one year near normal blood glucose levels on retinopathy in insulin-dependent diabetics. *Lancet* **1**: 200–204.

Leite E, Mota MC, Faria de Abreu JR, Murta JN, Oliveira MA, Sousa Peeara A. Cunha-vaz JG. (1989) Quantification of the foveolar zone in normal and diabetic patients. *J Fr Ophthalmol* **12**(10): 665–668.

Lobo C, Bernardes R, Faria de Abreu JR, Cunha-Vaz JG. (1999) Novel imaging techniques for diabetic macular edema. *Doc Ophthalmol* **97**: 341–347.

McFarland RA, Halperin MH, Niven JI. (1946) Visual Thresholds as an index of physiological imbalance during insulin hypoglycemia. *Am J Physiol* **145**: 299–313.

Puliafito CA, Hee MR, Lin CP, *et al.* (1995) Imaging of macular disease with optical coherence tomography. *Ophthalmology* **102**: 217–229.

Ribeiro ML, Lobo CL, Figueira JP, *et al.* (2003). Correlation between Progression of Retinopathy and Metabolic Control in a Two-year Follow-up Study of Mild Nonproliferative Retinopathy in Subjects with Type 2 Diabetes. *Invest Ophthalmol Vis Sci* **44**: E-Abstract 3980.

Roy MS, McCulloch C, Hanna HK, *et al.* (1984) Colour vision long-standing diabetes mellitus. *Br J Ophthalmol* **68**: 215–217.

Sinclair SH, Grunwald JE, Riva CE, *et al.* (1982) Retinal vascular autoregulation in diabetes mellitus. *Ophthalmology* **89**(7): 748–750.

Valone JA, McNeel JW, Franks EP. (1981) Unilateral proliferative diabetic retinopathy. I. Initial Findings. *Arch Ophthalmol* **99**: 1357–1361.

Zeimer R, Mori MT, Khoobebi B. (1989) Feasibility test of a new method to measure retinal thickness noninvasively. *Invest Ophthalmol Vis Sci* **30**: 2099–2105.

# Chapter 3

# Clinical Diagnostic Methodologies

The early diagnosis of diabetic retinopathy, before the development of fundus lesions that are invisible on ophthalmoscopy or slit-lamp examination, should be a major priority for any one interested in this retinal disease and its management. It is fundamental to follow the initial stages of the retinopathy, when the retinal alterations are still reversible and may, therefore, be controlled by medical therapy and adequate metabolic control.

The development of drugs for DR and the evaluation of their efficacy will only be possible when the initial changes, occurring in the retina, can be identified and their evolution and natural history understood.

The major problem associated with early detection of diabetic retinal disease and development of new drugs for DR is the fact that vision loss is a relatively late development in the disease. Fundus photography, the accepted method for following the evolution of the retinal changes, detects changes that have, in general, reached an irreversible stage.

The predominant cause of vision loss in DR is advanced macular edema and proliferative diabetic retinopathy, both late stages of the evolution of the retinopathy.

Visual acuity examination is, therefore, not an appropriate method to follow the initial stages of DR, and must be kept in mind that vision loss due to DR is a sure indication that the retinopathy has already reached a stage of no return and at present, the only option of the treating doctor is to stabilize and delay the disease progression.

## 3.1. Fundus Photography and Fluorescein Angiography

### Lilianne Duarte and José Cunha-Vaz

Ophthalmoscopy and fundus imaging are used for screening DR. However, direct ophthalmoscopy, even in the hands of an experienced ophthalmologist, has a sensivity as low as 65% for the detection of sight-threatening disease (Harding *et al.*, 1995).

### Fundus Photography

Color fundus photography is the tool most frequently used to document retinal disease and its evolution in diabetic patients. It is used for tracking disease progression and is still accepted as the best screening method for DR.

Fundus photographs allow to identify small red dots in the fundus, corresponding to microaneurysms and hemorrhages as the initial lesions of DR. They show the development of hard and soft exudates and, finally, show well the major changes occurring in the retinal venules and arterioles as the disease progresses (Klein *et al.*, 1985). Fundus photographs or fundus digital images must be produced in a consistent manner following well defined protocols, in order to allow comparisons between different examinations performed on different occasions.

Color fundus photographs or maps may be obtained in either stereoscopic or nonstereoscopic fashion. They can be performed in the standards 30° (or 35°) or 45°–50° field of view or in the wide-angle 60° field. Higher field size is allows in a single image to record widespread retinal pathology, but the higher the field size, the lower is the magnification of detail. Therefore, the angle must be chosen according to the purpose: for a quick screening/evaluation method of widespread disease with peripheral ischemia and proliferative retinopathy the 60° field is one of the first choices. Because much retinal pathology occurs around the disk and macula, a standard for photographic composition has evolved, with a 30° field that includes the entire macula, the entire optic disk, and the major vascular arcades recorded in one view.

Seven standard fields of 30° were described as the Arlie House Classification and were used on the Diabetic Retinopathy Study Protocol. This was slightly modified for the ETDRS to the Modified 7-standard field protocol and became the standard protocol in fundus photography for diabetic retinopathy (Fig. 3.1).

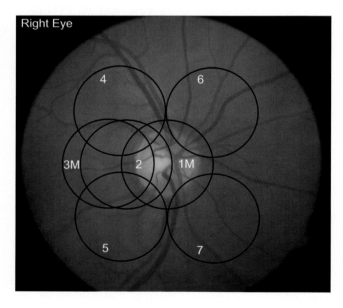

**Fig. 3.1.** Seven standard field protocol (ETDRS).

Traditional 35-mm color film fundus photography is still the standard technique, but digital photography is being progressively adopted in the screening and follow-up of diabetic retinopathy. Problems related to reliable image resolution and file size for digital images are being supplanted with the evolution of informatic systems.

### Microaneurysms earmarking

In order to allow earmarking microaneurysms on digital images, software was developed that allows graders to pinpoint microaneurysms by mouse point-and-clicking over the fundus images.

To make all images to be digitally available and normalized for their appearance to the grader, all of them were digitally processed. Color slide films were taken using a Kowa FX-500S fundus camera and a SX-type Polaroid pach type 600/779 film (100 ASA) and were digitalized at 1200 dpi resolution into 4032 × 2688 pixels images using a Minolta SC-100 scanner. Digital color fundus photographs, on the other hand, were taken using a Zeiss fundus camera FF-450 model, with a Sony DXL-390P 3CCD camera to produce 768 × 576 pixel images. Both sets are of field two (centered on the macula) and of 50° field-of-view. To best match both image sources, digitized images were reduced in size to a resolution similar to the digital ones, while preserving the proportion ratio, therefore, resulting on 1008 × 672 pixels images.

Digital images are composed of a black background plus the eye fundus, the latter constituting the region of interest (ROI), while fundus images on color slide films have an extra rectangular area on the image to hold patient identification. So to further process images to facilitate microaneurysm earmarking by graders, the ROI of each image has to be considered independently of the rest of the image and, therefore, image masks were created for each individual image. While for original digital images the ROI is always at the same place within the image, images from scanned slide films depend on the film holder thus showing translations, rotations or both. To overcome this added difficulty, an automated procedure was developed that identifies the ROI for each of the scanned images, being it a circular area delimited by two approximately parallel lines, which are detected through a generalized and through a modified Hough transform, respectively.

The quality of the images are sometimes lower than expected. To normalize image appearance to the grader in terms of color and intensity, another procedure was developed that corrects non-uniform illumination conditions (prior to any color processing) and generates three different digital versions of each: one that corrects intensity of the RGB color channels altogether; one that corrects intensity of each RGB color channels independently and one last image composed only of the green channel, respectively options A, B and C.

Non-uniform illumination condition correction is achieved by low-pass filtering images using a 2D Gaussian kernel of $31 \times 31$ pixels in size and standard variation ($\sigma$) of 10 pixels, while color correction is achieved by linearly increasing its dynamic range.

The grader can, at any moment during the grading process, decide which version to use (options A, B and C) plus the original unprocessed image.

By using this software, the grader has to pinpoint every microaneurysms seen at each visit image (Fig. 3.2). Some of the software facilities include zooming in and out (shown at their natural scale — 1:1 scale — by default), switching between any of the image versions and undo some or all earmarked microaneurysm for the image at hand. An off-line procedure allows user-assisted image registration, that is to say, to bring images into alignment so the same pixel coordinates always refer to the same retinal location along the follow-up. In this way, earmarked microaneurysm can be checked for their existence at different visits.

Using this facility each microaneurysm is identified as a single entity, thus making possible to track each one individually along the follow-up study and hence computing a set of parameters for the study as the number of microaneurysms at each visit, number

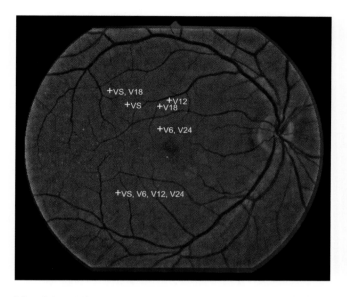

**Fig. 3.2.** Microaneurysm identification by location in the macular in a two-year period of follow-up at the initial visit (VS), 6 (V6), 12 (V12), 18 (V18) and 24 (V24) month.

of new, as well as missing ones, from the previous visit, rates of formation/disappearance, etc.

### Fluorescein angiography

Since 1961, when Novotny and Alvis introduced the technique of fluorescein angiography, its routine use has contributed significantly to the present understanding of diabetic retinal disease, buying to the clinical area concepts that were previously only perceived in the research laboratory.

Sodium fluorescein, which is approximately 80% protein-bound to albumin, is the dye used in fluorescein angiography. Fluorescein, because it is a small molecule that remains unbound in 10–20% of the amount injected, diffuses freely through the choriocapillaries, Bruch's membrane, optic nerve and sclera. However, it does not diffuse through the tight junctions of the retinal endothelial cells and of the retinal pigment epithelium which are the inner and outer blood-retinal barriers. A physiologic inner blood-retinal barrier exists at the level of the retinal vessels due to the zonula occludens that unite firmly and tightly neighboring retinal endothelial cells (Shakib and Cunha-Vaz, 1966). If there is a disruption of the blood-retinal barrier, dye leakage occurs. The tight junctions (zonula occludens) between the retinal pigment epithelial cells constitute the outer blood-retinal barrier, which under normal physiological conditions, does not allow visible leakage of fluorescein from the choroid into the retina.

Understanding the outer and inner retinal vascular barriers is the key to understanding and interpreting a fluorescein angiogram (Cunha-Vaz, 1976).

Another fundamental contribution of fluorescein angiography to our understanding of DR is the identification of areas of capillary closure or capillary drop-out (Fig. 3.3). The normal regular distribution of the capillary network appears interrupted by areas which are not perfused by the dye, identifying well areas outlined by perfused capillaries. Capillary closure and fluorescein leakage were identified clinically, for the first time, using fluorescein angiography and they are still accepted today as the determinant alterations occurring in the diabetic retina that better identify retinopathy progression (Kohner and Henkind, 1970).

Fluorescein angiography quality, however, depends on technique, filters, film, ocular media and patient cooperation. Finally, the information obtained is not quantitative depending on all these variables.

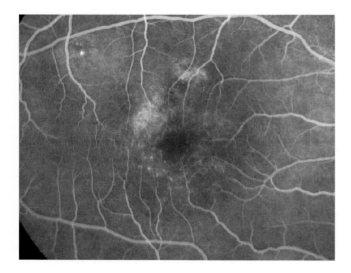

**Fig. 3.3.** Fluorescein angiography showing microaneurysms, leakage and damage of the fovea avascular zone contour.

Fluorescein angiography, because of the need for intravenous injection of fluorescein, is used much less frequently than fundus photography. Although sodium fluorescein is generally safe and is used in the daily routine of every ophthalmological care centre, severe anaphylactic reactions may occur sporadically (1 in 200.000) — (Yannuzzi *et al.*, 1986).

### 3.1.1. Mild Nonproliferative Retinopathy

The earliest lesions detected in the diabetic retina by fundus photography and fluorescein angiography are isolated microaneurysms or small blot hemorrhages. They occur in the presence of normal vision. Fluorescein angiography also identifies the presence of sites of fluorescein leakage demonstrating the presence of localized alterations of the inner blood-retinal barrier.

Although fluorescein angiography may show more microaneurysms than are detected by fundus photography and may also identify the microaneurysms that have closed, contributing to a much better evaluation of disease progression, it is not considered to be necessary for management or evaluating severity of retinopathy (DCCT, 1987). Fluorescein angiography has been reported to have greater sensivity than color stereoscopic fundus photographs for the detection of microaneurysms (Nielsen, 1980).

Hyalinised microaneurysms, i.e. closed microaneurysms, are not identifiable in fundus photographs because of lack of contrast (Bresnick *et al.*, 1977). One report documented that four times more microaneurysms were detected with fluorescein angiography than with color or red-free photographs (Helstedt, Vesti and Immonen, 1996).

There is a clear disagreement between different authors, so much so that Shah and Brown (2000) in their chapter in *Diabetes and Ocular Disease*, monograph of the American Academy of Ophthalmology, suggest that microaneurysms detected with fluorescein angiography and photographs "may reflect different structural alterations in the retina." It is recognized that small microaneurysms in color fundus photographs represent also hemorrhages and not only microaneurysms.

Several types of microaneurysms have been identified on histological examinations (Cunha-Vaz, 1972). The main types are:

1. endothelium lined microaneurysms containing blood cells.
2. microaneurysms devoid of endothelium and in the process of thrombosis.
3. occluded microaneurysms containing cell debris.
4. sclerotic, picnotic, hyalinised remnants of microaneurysms.

From histological examinations it is clear that microaneurysms are localized dilatations or outpouchings of retinal capillaries that will ultimately close, probably by thrombosis. It is therefore, likely that two stages of microaneurysms may occur in the diabetic retina, perfused and non-perfused microaneurysms, the last ones being the end-stage of the disease process. It is not expected, except in extremely rare circumstances, to have reperfused microaneurysms. The information obtained from the appearance of these initial lesions is of major importance to follow progression of diabetic retinal disease.

Microaneurysms on fundus images have the potential to become the reference lesion in the initial stages of DR (Fig. 3.2), when the retinopathy is still reversible. The development of new drugs targeted at the initial stages of the retinal disease pinpoints the need for improved follow-up of these lesions.

Red dot counting on fundus images may become an easily accessible and non-invasive tool to follow progression of DR. The red dot formation rate has been proposed recently by our group as a good way to characterize vascular disease progression and remodeling, whereas red dot disappearance rate was proposed as an appropriate indicator of microvascular thrombosis and development of capillary closure (Torrent-Solans *et al.*, 2004). Validation of these methodologies is urgently needed.

In summary, in the initial stages of diabetic retinal disease the use of fundus photography has been clearly preferred to fluorescein angiography because of its non-invasive nature. It is also to be kept in mind that no therapies have been available that could interfere with retinopathy progression in these initial stages of DR.

Now, that new therapies are being tested, better characterization of microaneurysms on fundus photography and their correspondence with fluorescein angiography images, becomes an urgent need. The development of new techniques for microaneurysm counting on fundus color images will be described again in the last chapter of this report.

It is also of importance to keep in mind that when following the initial stages of DR and microaneurysm changes, the examiner must focus on the area of greatest interest and yield, i.e. in the posterior pole. Diabetic retinopathy initiates in the posterior pole, in the macula and around the fovea.

### 3.1.2. Moderate Nonproliferative Retinopathy Without Macular Edema

This stage is characterized, basically, by an increase in number and size of the retinal hemorrhages, hard exudates and the development of changes in the retinal arterioles and venules. Again, because of lack of useful treatments for this stage of DR fluorescein angiography has not been considered necessary, follow-up being generally restricted to color fundus photography performed at regular intervals.

### 3.1.3. Nonproliferative Retinopathy with Clinically Significant Macular Edema

Clinically significant macular edema is a definition proposed by the Early Treatment Diabetic Retinopathy

Study (ETDRS, 1987a, b) in order to have a clear outcome that could be used to test the need for laser photocoagulation and its value.

The diagnosis of clinically significant macular edema is a clinical one and is not based on fluorescein angiography. It may be made by ophthalmoscopy or slit-lamp examination and documented by stereo fundus photography. It is also based in the detection of hard exudates close to the fovea and hard exudates are considered to be equivalent to retinal edema, past or present. Fluorescein angiography may be helpful in guiding treatment by identifying sites of leakage or by defining areas of capillary nonperfusion. These alterations are fundamental to our understanding of the specific situation of macular edema that we are dealing with. Is it a situation associated with increased leakage and marked breakdown of the inner blood-retinal barrier? In this situation, management of the blood pressure, improvement of metabolic control and prompt laser treatment are likely to contribute and effectively reduce the retinal edema. When the macular edema is associated with extensive capillary closure, identified on fluorescein angiography, the chances of improvement in visual acuity are minimal, and the improvement to be obtained may be restricted to improved fundus appearance with any improvement in visual acuity.

Measurements of retinal thickness using the Retinal Thickness Analyzer and the OCT are changing some of these concepts by objectively quantifying and mapping macular edema.

### 3.1.4. Severe Nonproliferative Retinopathy

The risk of progression from very severe nonproliferative diabetic retinopathy to high-risk proliferative diabetic retinopathy (PDR) is approximately 50% within a year (ETDRS Report #9, 1991). Fluorescein angiographic features demonstrate better the defining fundus lesions, such as, venous abnormalities and intraretinal vascular abnormalities (IRMAs). Fluorescein angiography also demonstrates the extension of widespread capillary closure, which is the direct indicator of ischemia, the factor that is behind the development of retinal neovascularization. However, because of the real benefit-to-risk ratio associated with the fact that the fundus color images are reasonably informative and are obtained by a non-invasive procedure fluorescein angiography is not considered necessary to perform an appropriate evaluation of severe nonproliferative diabetic retinopathy (ETDRS, 1991c).

### 3.1.5. Diabetic Retinopathy Screening

Screening for retinopathy in diabetic patients is one of the first and more important ways to prevent vision loss.

Retinopathy screening recommendations were established by the American Academy of Ophthalmology (AAO) and the American Diabetes Association (ADA).

— Adults with type 1 diabetes should have an initial dilated and comprehensive eye examination by an ophthalmologist or optometrist within five years after the onset of diabetes (AAO and ADA).
— Patients with type 2 diabetes should have an initial and comprehensive eye examination by an ophthalmologist or optometrist at the time of diagnosis of diabetes (AAO and ADA).
— Subsequent examinations for type one and type two patients should be repeated annually by an ophthalmologist or optometrist who is knowledgeable and experienced in diagnosing the presence of diabetic retinopathy and is aware of its management. Less frequent exams (every 2–3 years) may be considered with the advice of an eye care professional in the setting of a normal eye exam. Examinations will be required more frequently if retinopathy is progressing (ADA).
— When planning pregnancy, women with preexisting diabetes should have a comprehensive eye examination and should be counseled on the risk

of development and/or progression of diabetic retinopathy. Women with diabetes who become pregnant should have a comprehensive eye examination in the first trimester and close follow-up throughout pregnancy and for one-year post-partum. This guideline does not apply to women who developed gestational diabetes, because such individuals are not at increased risk for diabetic retinopathy (AAO and ADA).

Ideally, screening of diabetic retinopathy should be performed with a complete and midriatic eye fundus examination by an ophthalmologist.

However, to perform a diabetic retinopathy screening to a larger population of diabetic patients, several programs in several countries were developed using nonmydriatics color fundus photography. This screening method, which can be performed by technicians, nurses or optometrist, enables to track signs of early stages of diabetic retinopathy and direct those patients for ophthalmological follow-up and treatment.

Methods for screening diabetic retinopathy vary in type of camera, fields and type of images. Some screening programs uses cameras with a field angle of 45°, with a single image for each eye. Other use non-mydriatic cameras, which allows faster screening but the quality of images sometimes is not very good. The gold standard of fundus photography is a 30° or 35° seven-fields, as described on the ETDRS. This method provides good quality and detailed information of almost all retina area. It must be performed with midriatic pupils and takes longer than the other methods, making it inappropriate to use for screening.

Software needs to be created to establish automated methods to detect retinopathy. Automated detection of diabetic retinopathy with digital analysis to fundus photography has, however, still some limitations. The interest of this technology is to replace current procedures that depend on manual labor and visual inspection.

With the evolution and improvement of informatics, the future in fundus photography will progressively shift to digital imaging and, certainly, automated screening for diabetic retinopathy.

### 3.1.6. Grading Diabetic Retinopathy from Stereoscopic Color Fundus Photographs-an Extension of the Modified Airlie House Classification. ETDRS Report Number 10

The modified Airlie House classification of diabetic retinopathy has been extended for use in the Early Treatment Diabetic Retinopathy Study (ETDRS, 1991b). The revised classification provides additional steps in the grading scale for some characteristics, separates other characteristics previously combined, expands the section on macular edema and adds several characteristics not previously graded. The classification is described and illustrated and its reproducibility between graders is assessed by calculating percentages of agreement and kappa statistics for duplicate gradings of baseline color nonsimultaneous stereoscopic fundus photographs. For retinal hemorrhages and/or microaneurysms, hard exudates, new vessels, fibrous proliferations and macular edema, agreement was substantial (weighted kappa, 0.61 to 0.80). For soft exudates, intraretinal microvascular abnormalities and venous beading, agreement was moderate (weighted kappa, 0.41 to 0.60). A double grading system, with adjudication of disagreements of two or more steps between duplicate gradings, led to some improvement in reproducibility for most characteristics (Tables 3.1, 3.2 and 3.3).

### *Limitations of fundus photography gradings to follow early diabetic retinopathy*

Fundus photography has been the method of choice to follow diabetic retinopathy (DR), because 1) it is non-invasive, technically easy and well accepted by patients and 2) its usefulness has been demonstrated in a large-scale randomized clinical trial, the Diabetic Retinopathy Study (DRS), which showed the benefits of photocoagulation in the treatment of proliferative DR.

Fundus photography is very useful in addressing the specific problem of new vessel formation.

**Table 3.1    ETDRS Final Retinopathy Severity Scale (for Individual Eyes)**

| Level | Severity | Definition |
|---|---|---|
| 10 | **DR absent** | Microaneurysms and other characteristics absent |
| 14* | DR questionable | 14 A HE definite; microaneurysms absent<br>14 B SE definite; microaneurysms absent<br>14 C IRMA definite; microaneurysms absent |
| 15* | DR questionable | Hemorrhage(s) definite; microaneurysms absent |
| 20 | **Microaneurysms only** | Microaneurysms definite, other characteristics absent |
| 35† | **Mild NPDR** | 35 A Venous loops $\geq$ D/1;<br>35 B SE, IRMA, or VB = Q;<br>35 C Retinal hemorrhages present;<br>35 D HE $\geq$ D/1<br>35 E HE $\geq$ M/1<br>35 F SE $\geq$ D/1 |
| 43 | **Moderate NPDR** | 43 A H/Ma = M/4–5 – S/1<br>43 B IRMA = D1–3 |
| 47 | **Moderately severe NPDR** | 47 A Both L43 characteristics<br>47 B IRMA = D4–5<br>47 C H/Ma = S/2–3<br>47 D VB = D/1 |
| 53 | **Severe NPDR†** | 53 A $\geq$ 2 of the 3 L47 characteristics;<br>53 B H/Ma $\geq$ S/4-5<br>53 C IRMA $\geq$ M/1<br>53 D VB $\geq$ D/2-3 |
| 53 E | Very severe NPDR | $\geq$ 2 of 53B, 53C and 53D |
| 61 | **Mild NPDR** | 61 A FPD and/or FPE only (regressed PDR)<br>61 B NVE < 1/4 DA in $\geq$ 1 field (borderline PDR)<br>61 C NVE $\geq$ 1/4 but < 1/2 DA in $\geq$ 1 field |
| 65 | **Moderate PDR** | 65 A NVE $\geq$ M/1 $\geq$ 1/2 but < 1/2 DA in $\geq$ 1 field<br>65 B NVD = D; and VH and PRH = A or Q<br>65 C VH or PRH = D and NVE < M/1 and NVD absent |
| 71 | **High-risk PDR** | 71 A VH or PHR $\geq$ M/1 (M = about 1 DA)<br>71 B NVE $\geq$ M/1 and VH or PRH $\geq$ D/1<br>71 C NVD = D and VH or PRH $\geq$ D/1<br>71 D NVD $\geq$ M |
| 75 | **High risk PDR** | NVD $\geq$ M and VH or PRH $\geq$ D/1 |
| 81 | Advanced PDR: fundus partially obscured, center of macula attached | NVD = cannot grade, or NVD < D and NVE = cannot grade in $\geq$ 1 field and absent in all others; and retinal detachment at center of macula < D |
| 85 | Advanced PDR: posterior fundus obscured, or center of macula detached | 85 A VH = VS in fields 1 or 2<br>85 B Retinal detachment at center of macula = D |

*(Continued)*

**Table 3.1**  (*Continued*)

| Level | Severity | Definition |
|---|---|---|
| 90 | Cannot grade, even sufficiently for level 81 or 85 | |

DR = diabetic retinopathy; NPDR = nonproliferative DR; PDR = proliferative DR; HE = hard exudates; SE = soft exudates; IRMA = intraretinal microvascular abnormalities; VB = venous bleedings; H/Ma = hemorrhages/microaneurysms; NVE = new vessels elsewhere; NVD = new vessels on or adjacent to optic disc; VH = vitreous hemorrhage; PRH = preretinal hemorrhage.
Severity categories: absent (A), questionable (Q), definitely present (D); moderate (M), severe (S), or very severe (VS). Extent is the number of photographic fields at that severity level, example, M/2-3 means there are two or three fields from fields 3 to 7 with moderate severity and none higher severity.
*Levels 14 and 15 are not considered separate steps in the scale, but are pooled with level 10 or 20 (or excluded).
†NPDR levels 35 and above all require presence of microaneurysms.

**Table 3.2   Major Levels, with Subcategories for Diabetic Macular Edema Disease Severity Scale**

| Proposed Disease Severity Level | Findings Observable Upon Dilated Ophthalmoscopy |
|---|---|
| Diabetic Macular Edema Apparently Absent | • No retinal thickening or hard exudates in posterior pole |
| Diabetic Macular Edema Apparently Absent | • Some retinal thickening or hard exudates in posterior pole |

If diabetic macular edema is present, it can be categorized as follows:

| Proposed Disease Severity Level | Findings Observable Upon Dilated Ophthalmoscopy |
|---|---|
| Diabetic Macular Edema Present | • Mild Diabetic Macular Edema Some retinal thickening or hard exudates in posterior pole but distant from the center of the macula |
| | • Moderate Diabetic Macular Edema Retinal thickening or hard exudates approaching the center of the macula but not involving the center |
| | • Severe Diabetic Macular Edema Retinal thickening or hard exudates involving the center of the macula |

Following the success of the DRS, another large-scale trial, the Early Treatment Diabetic Retinopathy Study (ETDRS), examined early photocoagulation treatment for macular edema and eyes at high risk for proliferative DR Again, fundus photography was demonstrated to be useful for well-defined alterations (macular edema and new vessel formation) in advanced stages of DR.

Fundus photography was, therefore, chosen to monitor retinopathy in the Diabetes Control and Complications Trial in the U.S. and United Kingdom Prospective Diabetes Study Trial. Elaborate fundus

**Table 3.3 Initial Stages of Nonproliferative Diabetic Retinopathy (Scale for Individual Eyes)**

| Level | Severity | Definition |
|---|---|---|
| 10 | DR absent | MA absent |
| 20 | MA only | MA definite, other characteristics absent |
| 35b | Mild NPDR | Venous loops ≥ D/1 + one of the following: SE/IRMA/H/HE/SE |
| 43 | Moderate NPDR | H/MA – M/4–5 or S/1; IRMA – D/1 – 3 |
| 47 | Moderately severe NPDR | Both level 43 characteristics + IRMA – D/4–5; H/MA – S/2-#; VB-D/1 |

photography gradings were developed from the original Airlie House Diabetic Retinopathy Classification to document progression and delineate the natural history of retinal disease, from the earliest visible alterations to more advanced stages, e.g. maculopathy and high-risk proliferative DR.

These gradings consist of only five steps for the early stage (Table 3.1) and many problems and limitations are associated with their use, particularly for obtaining information on the initial stages. Microaneurysms (MAs) appear in the second step of the scale #20. Although they are an important and frequent alteration in the retinal circulation in diabetes, they are not counted. Furthermore, MA formation and disappearance is a dynamic process. During a two-year follow-up of 24 type 1 diabetics with mild background DR using fluorescein angiography, Hellsted *et al.* observed 395 new MAs and the disappearance of 258 previously identified MAs. MAs need to be counted to assess progression of retinopathy and new MAs should always be added to those previously identified in the same retina (Torrent Solans *et al.*, 2003). It must be realized that the disappearance of an MA is not a reversible process, but indicates vessel closure and progressive vascular damage.

Other major alterations in the initial stages of DR that may affect disease progression are capillary closure and the blood-retinal barrier (BRB) alteration. Capillary closure is the first sign of ischemia and BRB alteration indicates development of macular edema; neither is identified by fundus photography or included in the fundus photography grading or classifications.

Many important fundus photography studies have been performed on the advanced stages of DR. The future now lies in the examination of its initial reversible stages, where metabolic control and drugs are expected to play a major role, and a case must be made to use markers for DR disease progression other than from fundus photography. Number of MAs, retinal leakage (BRB alteration) and capillary closure (blood-flow changes) must be measured in studies of the development and progression of the initial stages of DR.

Fluorescein angiography and quantitative methods, such as retinal leakage analysis, retinal thickness analysis and capillary blood flow measurements should be added to fundus photography for improved understanding, management and prevention of DR.

# References

American Academy of Ophthalmology (AAO). (2003) Preferred Practice Patterns™ diabetic retinopathy. Approved 2003 Sep.

American Diabetes Association (ADA). (2005) Standards of medical care in diabetes. Revised 2004 Oct. *Diabetes Care* **28**(1): S4–S36.

Bresnick GH, Davis MD, Myers FL, de Venecia G. (1977) Clinicopathologic correlations in diabetic retinopathy, II: Clinical and histologic appearances of retinal capillary microaneurysms. *Arch Ophthalmol* **95**: 1215–1220.

Cunha-Vaz JG. (1972) Diabetic retinopathy. Human and Experimental studies. *Trans Ophthalmol Soc UK* **92**: 111–124.

Cunha-Vaz JG. (1976) The blood-retinal barriers. *Doc Ophthalmol* **41**: 287–327.

Diabetes Control and Complications Trial Research Group. (1987) Color photography versus fluorescein angiography in the detection of diabetic retinopathy in the Diabetes Control Complications Trial. *Arch Ophthalmol* **105**: 1344–1351.

Early Treatment Diabetic Retinopathy Study Research Group. (1987a) Treatment techniques and clinical guidelines for photocoagulation of diabetic macular edema. Early Treatment Diabetic Retinopathy Study Report Number 2. *Ophthalmology* **94**(7): 761–774.

Early Treatment Diabetic Retinopathy Study Research Group. (1987b) Photocoagulation for diabetic macular edema. ETDRS Report Number 4. *Int Ophthalmol Clin* **27**: 265–272.

Early Treatment Diabetic Retinopathy Study Research Group. (1991a) Early photocoagulation for diabetic retinopathy. ETDRS Report Number 9. *Ophthalmology* **98**: 766–785.

Early Treatment Diabetic Retinopathy Study Research Group. (1991b) Grading diabetic retinopathy from stereoscopic color fundus photography: An extension of the modified Airlie House classification. ETDRS Number 10. *Ophthalmology* **98** (Suppl. 5): 786–806.

Early Treatment Diabetic Retinopathy Study Research Group. (1991c) Fundus photographic risk factors for progression of diabetic retinopathy. ETDRS Report Number 12. *Ophthalmology* **98**: 823–833.

Harding SP, Boradbent DM, Neoh C, *et al.* (1995) Sensitivity and specificity of photograph and direct ophthalmoscopy in screening for sight threatening eye disease: The Liverpool Diabetic Eye Study. *Br Med J* **311**: 1131–1135.

Hellstedt T, Vesti E, Immonen I. (1996) Identification of individual microaneurysms: A comparison between fluorescein angiograms and red-free and colour photographs. *Graefes Arch Clin Exp Ophthalmol* **234** (Suppl. 1): S13–S17.

Klein R, Klein BE, Neider MW, *et al.* (1985) Diabetic retinopathy as detected using ophthalmology, A nonmydriatic and a standard fundus camera. *Ophthalmology* **92**: 485–491.

Kohner EM, Henkind P. (1970) Correlation of fluorescein angiogram and retinal digest in diabetic retinopathy. *Am J Ophthalmol* **69**: 403–414.

Nielsen NV. (1980) Fluorescein angiography in persons with slightly abnormal glucose tolerances. *Acta Endocrinol* **238** (Suppl.): 77–84.

Novotny HR, Alvis DL. (1961) A method of photographing fluorescein in the human retina. *Circulation* **24**: 72–77.

Shah GK, Brown GC. (2000) Photography, angiography and ultrasonography in diabetic retinopathy. In: Flynn HW, Smiddy WE (eds), *Diabetes and Ocular Disease*. The foundation of the American Academy of Ophthalmology, pp. 101–113.

Shakib M, Cunha-Vaz JG. (1966) Studies on the permeability of the blood-retinal barrier. IV. Junctional complexes of the retinal vessels and their role on their permeability. *Exp Eye Res* **5**: 229–234.

Torrent-Solans T, Duarte L, Monteiro R, *et al.* (2004) Microaneurysms counting on digitalized fundus images of mild nonproliferative retinopathy in Diabetes type 2. *Invest Ophthalmol Vis Sci* **45**: E-Abstract 2985.

Yannuzzi LA, Rohrer KT, Tindel LJ, *et al.* (1986) Fluorescein angiography complication survey. *Ophthalmology* **93**: 611–617.

## 3.2. Measurements of Retinal Thickness

### João Figueira, Rui Bernardes and José Cunha-Vaz

Macular edema is a frequent alteration in type 2 diabetes and is the most frequent cause of vision loss (Aiello *et al.*, 1998). Clinically significant macular edema, as defined by the ETDRS, is the presence of one or more of the following criteria: a) thickening of the retina located less than 500 $\mu$m from the center of the macula; b) hard exudates (with thickening of the adjacent retina) located less than 500 $\mu$m from the center of the macula; and c) a zone of retinal thickening one disk area or larger in size, located within one disk diameter from the center of the macula (ETDRS, 1987). Current diagnostic methods for its detection and evaluation are slit-lamp biomicroscopy and stereo fundus photography, providing a subjective evaluation of retinal thickness.

Detection of retinal thickening by means of slit-lamp examination or stereo fundus photography however, appears, to be associated with relatively low sensitivity. A report by Shahidi *et al.*, (1994) using the Retinal Thickness Analyzer (RTA-Talia Technology, Ltd, Mevaseret, Zion, Israel), shows that slit-lamp examination and stereo fundus photography may only detect increases in thickness when they show values of more than 60% over the reference population and may, therefore, be unable to identify mild or localized macular thickening.

Improved detection of macular edema is expected to offer new perspectives for treatment of diabetic retinopathy. The ETDRS, which is based on slit-lamp biomicroscopy and stereo fundus photography has demonstrated that photocoagulation for clinically significant macular edema (CSME) only reduces the risk of moderate visual loss by approximately 50%.

Optical imaging instruments, like the RTA and Optical Coherence Tomography (OCT-Humphrey Instruments, CA, USA), have been proposed as powerful tools for the objective assessment of macular edema. It appears desirable to test these methods when minimal changes in retinal thickness may be present, a stage where other methods cannot identify changes and when visual acuity is not affected. Both techniques, which are able to measure retinal thickness and rapidly generate thickness maps at the posterior pole, (Shahidi *et al.*, 1994; Hee *et al.*, 1995) are noninvasive and non-contact procedures.

## 3.2.1. Retinal Thickness Analyzer (RTA)

The RTA is a quantitative and reproducible method to evaluate retinal thickness (Shahidi *et al.*, 1994).

The principle of the RTA is based on projecting a thin He-Ne laser (543 nm) slit obliquely on the retina and viewing it at an angle in a manner similar to slit-lamp biomicroscopy. The separation between the reflections (and scatter) from the vitreoretinal interface and the chorioretinal interface is a measure of the retinal thickness. The reflected image of the intersection of the laser slit with the retina — optical cross section — is recorded by a video camera and digitized. Nine scans are obtained covering the central 20° area around the fovea in the posterior pole. Each one of these scans is composed of 10 optical cross sections of the retina, separated by 200 $\mu$m, measuring an area of 2000 $\mu$m × 2000 $\mu$m within 200 ms. The total area scanned with the RTA is 6000 $\mu$m × 6000 $\mu$m with each "thixel" representing an area of 200 $\mu$m × 200 $\mu$m.

The whole set of scans is processed, and the output may be displayed as 10 adjacent cross sections of the retina, as color-coded topographic map in two or three dimensions or as a numeric report.

Optimal depth precision of the RTA is 5 to 10 $\mu$m and its optimal depth resolution is 50 $\mu$m.

Newly available RTAII version performs four scans with a fifth overlapping them in the central area. The principle and generated data remains the same.

## 3.2.2. Optical Coherence Tomography (OCT)

Time domain optical coherence tomography is an imaging diagnostic technique that provides cross sectional tomograms (B-scan) of retinal structure, *in vivo*, in which optical interferometry is used to resolve the distances of reflective structures within the eye (Hee *et al.*, 1995). It is analogous to ultrasound but with superior resolution.

The OCT system uses a +78 dioptre lens to visualize the eye fundus and deliver the probe beam onto the retina. It has an infrared video camera to show the position of the OCT scan on the retina on a computer monitor and to record the position of each tomogram on the retina.

Low coherence light from a superluminescent diode source, operating at 840 nm (infrared light), is split into two beams: one incident on the retina and the other incident on a translating mirror. The two reflected beams, one on the mirror and the other on retinal structures, are recombined and optical interference detected by a photodiode.

The OCT image closely approximates the histological appearance of the retina. The top of the image corresponds to the vitreous cavity. In healthy eyes, this will be optically silent, or may show the posterior hyaloidal face in an eye with a posterior vitreous detachment. The posterior vitreous face appears as a thin horizontal or oblique line above or inserting into retina. The anterior surface of the retina demonstrates high reflectivity, and in the fovea of normal eyes, demonstrates the central foveal depression. The horizontally aligned nerve fiber layer (NFL) demonstrates higher tissue signal strength and is thicker closer to the optic nerve. The internal structure of the retina consists of heterogeneous reflections, corresponding to the ultrastructural anatomy. The axially aligned cellular layers of the retina (inner nuclear, outer nuclear and ganglion cells layers) demonstrate less backscattering and back-reflection of incident OCT light, and thus appear with a lower tissue signal (darker), compared to horizontally aligned structures (internal limiting membrane, Henle's layer, and NFL) that appear brighter. The retinal pigment epithelium, Bruch's membrane, and choriocapillaris complex collectively comprise the highly reflective external band. Just anterior to this band is another highly reflective line representing the junction between the photoreceptors' inner and outer segments. Reproducible patterns of retinal morphology seen by OCT have been shown to correspond to the location of retinal layers seen on light microscopic overlays in both normal and pathologic retinas.[1]

Fourier or spectral-domain technology delivers almost a 100-fold improvement in acquisition speed over time-domain OCT because no physical movement of the reference mirror is required, and data is therefore acquired at a much faster rate. Furthermore, this technique is able to simultaneous detect reflexions from a broad range of depths, whereas time-domain OCT acquires signals from various depths sequentially. This improves the signal-to-noise ratio by a factor proportional to the number of detector elements in the spectrometer (typically 1024 or 2048). With increased imaging speed and greater signal to noise ratio, the Fourier-domain OCT scanners produce more detailed and brighter images.

Fourier-domain OCT of the macula has been shown to provide greater detail than previously available time-domain OCT systems image in a shorter period of time. This dramatically decreases motion artefact. The faster scanning time allows also a larger area to be scanned and offers more precise registration. It is also possible to acquire three-dimensional OCT data that achieve comprehensive retinal coverage and allow correlation between OCT images and clinical fundus features.

### 3.2.3. Retinal Thickness Measurements

We have used RTA and OCT to measure retinal thickness in eyes of healthy volunteers and diabetic patients with minimal nonproliferative diabetic retinopathy in order to compare both methods. (Pires *et al.*, 2002).

A series of diabetic patients, with an established diagnosis of type 2 diabetes mellitus, were recruited to participate in this study. The diabetes in this group of patients was reasonably well controlled and the blood pressure within the normal range.

Fundus examination was performed by slit-lamp using a +90 diopter lens or Goldmann contact lens and seven-field stereo fundus photography obtained and classified according to the criteria of the ETDRS protocol. Stereoscopic pairs of fields were obtained using a 30° fundus camera. Thirty-six percent of the eyes were classified as level 10 (DR absent), while the remaining 64% were classified as levels 20 and 35 (microaneurysms only and mild nonproliferative DR, respectively). Only one eye of each patient was studied.

Retinal thickness was assessed by performing RTA and OCT in a single session.

Two normal populations volunteered to participate as control age matched groups for RTA (N = 14; mean age 48 years; range 42–55 years) and OCT (N = 10; mean age 56 years; range 43–68). Retinal thickness was measured in only one eye with both methods and reference maps were computed using the mean + 2SD.

OCT scans were performed in the control and diabetic eye, using the six radial line pattern, each of 3.45 mm in length passing through the center of fixation, following the protocol proposed by Hee *et al.*, 1998.

Each one of the six tomograms (B-scans) was oriented along a line intersecting the central fovea and containing 100 equally spaced axial profiles (A-scans) of optical reflectivity.

In a study performed with the RTA and OCT, five measurements of retinal thickness were considered. These five values were automatically obtained in five retinal locations, within a circle: a central disc area of 1 mm in diameter, centered on the patient's fixation, which was assumed to correspond to the central fovea and in a peripheral ring area, 1–3 mm in diameter in four retinal quadrants — papilomacular, superior, temporal and inferior.

In order to make possible the comparison of RTA and OCT areas of retinal thickness, a new thickness map of the RTA was computed taking into account the values that best fit the locations covered by the OCT map as shown in Fig. 3.4.

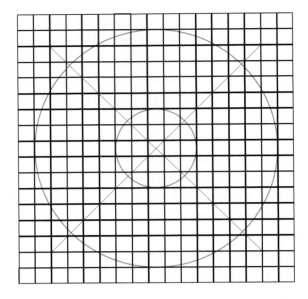

**Fig. 3.4.** The figure shows the best-fit overlapping areas by the RTA and OCT measurements to allow the comparison on the measures performed with both methods. Each square represents a single RTA measure covering an area of 200 $\mu$m × 200 $\mu$m. The two-concentric circles overlapped on the grid, as well as the 45 and 135 degrees lines, show the limits of the 5 locations measured by the OCT (foveal area; papilomacular and temporal areas; and superior and inferior areas). The circles are of 1000 and 3000 $\mu$m radii, centered in the fovea.

RTA detected abnormal increases in most diabetic eyes, with increases ranging from 0.3% to 73.5%. RTA increased values were frequently noted in more than one location in the eyes with increased retinal thickness.

OCT detected retinal thickness increases in only 11% of the same series of eyes, with percentages of increase above reference ranging from 0.3% to 4.8%, always located on the foveal area.

This study showed that there are localized areas of retinal edema, i.e. abnormal increases in retinal thickness, occurring in the macula in the early stages of diabetic retinal disease. These localized areas of increased retinal thickness were identified in 86% of the eyes examined when using the RTA but only in 11% when using the OCT.

From this study the RTA appears, to be able to detect abnormal increases in retinal thickness in the diabetic retina well before OCT.

Furthermore, the results obtained with the RTA showed that localized retinal edema is one of the earliest alterations occurring in the macula in type 2 diabetes.

The highest increase found with the RTA in eyes with Wisconsin grading 10 was 19.2%, whereas larger increases reaching values of 56.5% and 73.5% were detected in eyes graded as 20 and 35. Although our results indicate that increases in retinal thickness are a very early finding in diabetic retinas, they also show that progression of retinal microvascular alterations are associated with larger increases in retinal thickness. It is also clear from this study that the development of localized areas of retinal edema is not a constant finding, as a number of eyes, 14%, with gradings 10, 20 and 35 remained edema-free.

In our clinical experience with the RTA and OCT another advantage of the RTA is its short acquisition time. The 200 ms required for the scanning procedure with the RTA are associated with less discomfort to the patient, because of less prolonged light exposures, easier to maintain steadily ocular fixation and less problems associated with blinking. On the other hand, in more advanced stages of the retinopathy, the RTA results may be affected by irregular reflections from hard exudates accumulated in the retina and the interference of media opacities, such as severe cataract or vitreous opacities.

Comparing the two techniques to measure retinal thickness, the RTA appears to be particularly appropriate in measuring changes in retinal thickness when these changes are minimal and localized, particularly in the initial stages of diabetic retinal disease. We consider it to be an extremely promising tool in quantitatively evaluating the changes in retinal thickness before the development of clinical macular edema, and when an early therapeutical intervention may be more effective. OCT, in our experience, is particularly

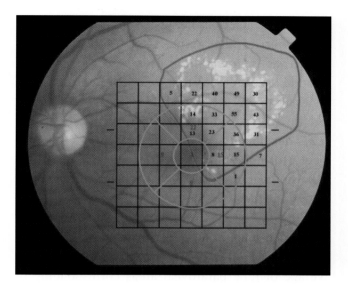

**Fig. 3.5.** Agreement for retinal edema seen by stereo fundus photography (hand delimited area in red), by retinal thickness analyzer (squared grid showing the percentage of increased retinal thickness) and optical coherence tomography (circular grid with number indicating the percentage of increased retinal thickness).

informative when there are changes in the retinal architecture, namely through the formation of cysts or localized fluid detachments. None of these situations are found, however, in the initial stages of diabetic retinal disease.

In conclusion, localized areas of increased retinal thickness, i.e. edema, occur in the retina in type 2 diabetes in the initial stages of the retinopathy. These areas of localized retinal edema may be identified and quantified by the RTA and OCT, offering a unique opportunity to study the effects of early intervention in the evolution of diabetic retinal edema in order to prevent its progression to advanced stages of macular edema (Fig. 3.5).

### 3.2.4. Macular Edema

Image processing software can quantify retinal thickness from the OCT tomograms as the distance between the anterior and posterior highly reflective boundaries of the retina. A software algorithm known as segmentation uses the processes of smoothing, edge detection, and error correction to facilitate this process. Retinal thickness can therefore be determined at any transverse location. Hee et al.[2] developed a standardized mapping OCT protocol (for time domain OCT), consisting of six radial tomograms, each 6 mm in length, in a spoke pattern centered on the fovea. Retinal thickness is then displayed in two different manners: first as a two-dimensional color-coded map of retinal thickness in the posterior pole; and secondly as a numeric average of nine parafoveal areas corresponding to the ETDRS subfields. Additionally acquisition algorithms include the fast macular mapping protocol, which allows six radial scans to be performed in a single session of 1.92s; and the high-density scan protocol consisting of six separate 6-mm radial lines, acquired in 7.32s. Over the last decade, the development of OCT has progressed rapidly. The first and second generations of commercial OCT instruments had an axial resolution of 10-15 $\mu$m. Third generation OCT (OCT Stratus; Carl Zeiss Meditec, Dublin, California, USA) provides an axial resolution of 8-10 $\mu$m.

OCT retinal thickness measurements have been shown in a number of studies to be highly reproducible.

Thus, changes in central retinal thickness greater than 10% are likely to be due to true changes in retinal thickness rather than inconsistencies in the OCT measurements.

Changes in macular thickness may be reported in absolute values before and after treatment or in percentage change. However no uniform method currently exists for reporting changes in macular thickness.

## Morphologic Patterns of Macular Edema

At least five different morphologic patterns of macular edema can be seen on OCT (Otani *et al.*, 1999; Alkuraya *et al.*, 2005).

Diffuse retinal thickening appears as increased sponge-like retinal thickness greater than 200 $\mu$m with reduced intraretinal reflectivity, particularly in the outer retinal layers (Fig. 3.6). Cystoid macular edema appears as small, round or oval, hyporeflective lacunae with highly reflective septae bridging the retinal layers and separating the cystoid-like cavities (Fig. 3.7). The cystoid spaces are located primarily in the outer retinal layers, leaving a thin, outer layer in the fovea. Some morphological differences exist between newly developed and long-standing cystoid macular edema. In early cystoid

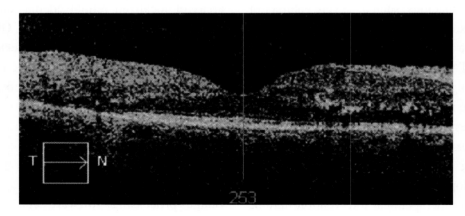

**Fig. 3.6.** OCT scan of difuse macular edema appearing as increased sponge-like retinal thickening with reduced intraretinal reflectivity, particularly in the outer retinal layers.

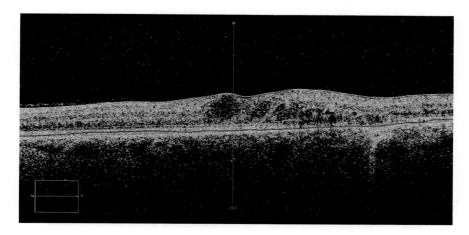

**Fig. 3.7.** OCT scan of cystoid macular edema appearing as round or oval, hyporeflective cystoid-like intraretinal spaces with septae bridging the retinal layers and separating the cavities. The cystoid spaces are located primarily in the outer retinal layers.

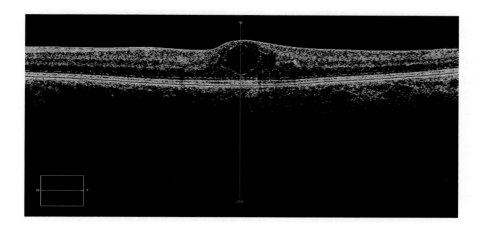

**Fig. 3.8.** OCT scan of chronic cystoid macular edema showing a large intraretinal cystoid cavity with loss of septae.

macular edema, cystoid spaces are primarily located in the outer retinal layers, and the inner retinal layers are relatively preserved. In chronic cystoid macular edema, the septa of each cystoid space disappear, forming confluent large cystoid cavities (Fig. 3.8). Large cystoid spaces may involve the entire retinal layer. Posterior hyaloidal traction is defined as a highly reflective signal arising from the inner retinal surface and extending toward the optic nerve or peripherally (Fig. 3.9).

Subretinal fluid or serous retinal detachment appears as a shallow elevation of the retina resembling a dome, with an optically clear space between the retina and the RPE, and a distinct outer boarder of the detached retina (Fig. 3.10). The identification of the highly reflective posterior border of detached retina distinguishes subretinal from intraretinal fluid. Finally, tractional retinal detachment is defined as a peak-shaped detachment of the retina with an area of low signal underlying the highly reflective border of the neurosensory retina, and it is accompanied by posterior hyaloidal traction.

Although diffuse retinal thickening is often found as a single pattern of diabetic macular edema, the remaining OCT patterns usually do not appear alone.

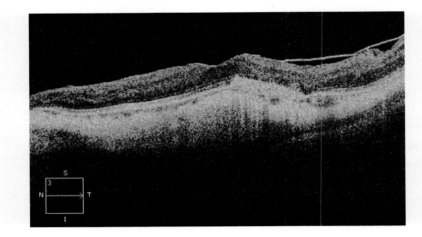

**Fig. 3.9.** OCT scan of epiretinal membrane appearing as highly reflective horizontal signal on the inner surface of the retina, with irregularities of the retinal surface beneath.

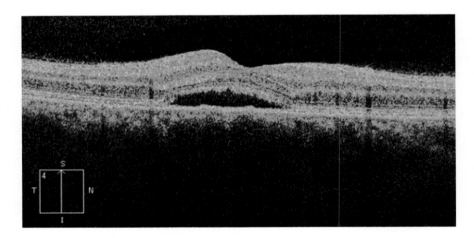

**Fig. 3.10.** OCT scan of subretinal fluid apprearing as a shallow elevation of the retina with an optically clear space between the retina and the RPE.

A number of studies have compared the use of OCT with slit-lamp biomicroscopy and stereo fundus photography in the detection of macular thickening. OCT was found to be sensitive to small changes in retinal thickness despite normal findings by slit-lamp biomicroscopy. Brown *et al.* reported good agreement between OCT and contact lens examination for the presence or absence of foveal edema when OCT thickness was considered normal ($\leq 200$ $\mu$m) or significantly increased ($>300$ $\mu$m) (Brown *et al.*, 2004). However, when OCT foveal thickness was mildly increased (201–300 $\mu$m), slit-lamp biomicroscopy was sensitive in only 14% of cases.

## References

Aiello LP, Gardner TW, King GL, *et al.* (1998) Diabetic retinopathy. *Diabetes Care* **21**: 143–156.

Alkuraya H, Kangave D, Abu El-Asrar AM. (2005) The correlation between optical coherence tomography features and severity of retinopathy, macular thickness and visual acuity in diabetic macular edema. *Int Ophthalmol* **26**(3): 93–99.

Bernardes RC, Nunes S, Duarte LG, Cunha-Vaz JG. (2005) Comparison between retinal edema by color fundus photography and retinal thickness maps. *Invest Ophthalmol Vis Sci* **46**: E-Abstract 1587.

Brown JC, Solomon SD, Bressler SB *et al.* (2004) Detection of diabetic foveal edema: Contact lens biomicroscopy compared with optical coherence tomography. *Arch Ophthalmol* **122**(3): 330–335.

Early Treatment Diabetic Retinopathy Study Research Group. (1987) Photocoagulation for diabetic macular edema. Early treatment Diabetic Retinopathy Study Report Number 4. *Int Ophthalmol Clin* **27**: 265–272.

Hee MR, Puliafito CA, Wong C, *et al.* (1995) Quantitative assessment of macular edema with optical coherence tomography. *Arch Ophthalmol* **113**: 1019–1029.

Hee MR, Puliafito CA, Duker JS, *et al.* (1998) Topography of diabetic macular edema with optical coherence tomography. *Ophthalmology* **105**: 360–370.

Margolis R, Kaiser K. (2008) Diagnostic Modalities in Diabetic Retinopathy; In Due E: Diabetic Retinopathy. Humana Press: 109–133.

Otani T, Kishi SH, Maryuama Y. (1999) Patterns of diabetic macular edema with optical coherence tomography. *Am J Ophthalmol* **127**: 688–693.

Pires I, Bernardes R, Lobo C, *et al.* (2002) Retinal thickness in eyes with mild nonproliferative retinopathy in subjects with type 2 diabetes. Comparison of measurements obtained with RTA and OCT. *Arch Ophthalmol* **120**: 1301–1306.

Shahidi M, Ogura Y, Blair NP, Zeimer R. (1994) Retinal thickness changes after focal laser treatment of diabetic macular edema. *Br J Ophthalmol* **78**: 827–830.

## 3.3.  Vitreous Fluorometry and Retinal Leakage Measurements

### José Cunha-Vaz and Conceição Lobo

In the early 1960s, two research groups contributed significantly to our understanding of the pathological picture of diabetic retinopathy: Ashton and his group, in London (1963), and Cogan and his co-workers in Boston (1963, 1965). Injection and digestion techniques allowed the observation and characterization of the initial vascular changes occurring in diabetic retinal disease. The first changes are limited to the cellular constituents of the retinal vessels, involving both the endothelial cells and pericytes. Microaneurysms appear associated with endothelial proliferation, being localized predominantly on the venous side of retinal circulation. With progression of the disease the capillaries on the arterial side show increased cell loss and capillary closure.

From these observations the endothelial cells were seen to be affected from the earlier stages of diabetic retinopathy. When the Blood-Retinal Barrier was found to be located primarily at the level of the endothelial membrane of retinal vessels it was only natural to assume that an alteration of the endothelial cells could play a major role in diabetic retinal disease. Asthon, in his 1965 Bowman Lecture, stated that early lesions of diabetic retinopathy are "focal breakdowns of the BRB."

The advent of fluorescein angiography confirmed most of what was known about the initial pathological picture of diabetic retinopathy and showed in the initial stages of the disease focal leaks of fluorescein, demonstrating well, in a clinical setting, the existence of focal breakdowns of the BRB.

In 1975, vitreous fluorometry, a clinical quantitative method for the study of the BRB, was introduced by our group, showing that an alteration of the BRB could be detected and measured in diabetic eyes apparently normal fundi. The disturbance of the BRB, as evidenced by vitreous fluorometry, appeared before microaneurysms or capillary closure could be demonstrated by fluorescein angiography. These results were soon confirmed by Waltman *et al.* (1978).

Thereafter, many experimental and clinical studies have examined the alteration of the BRB in diabetes with conflicting results at times, but showing in general that an alteration of the BRB is present in the diabetic retina and may have an important role in its development and progression.

The barrier system that separates the intraocular structures and fluids from the blood can be viewed as formed by two different boundaries (Cunha-Vaz and Maurice, 1965).

One, regulating exchanges between the blood and the aqueous humor is called the Blood-Aqueous Barrier (BAB). Here, inward movement from the blood into the eye predominates.

The other barrier, particularly tight, is the BRB. It is responsible for the microenvironment of the retina. It regulates the exchanges between the blood and the extravascular space of the retina. From there, substances diffuse and exchange with the vitreous humor. There is evidence of an intimate relationship between the alteration of this BRB and almost every retinal disease, particularly the vascular retinopathies and diseases involving the retinal pigment epithelium. Retinal edema, a very common alteration causing vision loss, results at least from BRB breakdown.

The development of a quantitative method capable of detecting minimal alterations in the barrier and monitoring their progress has obvious clinical interest.

Vitreous fluorometry was developed as a method that should be appropriate for clinical application. Principal reason for its success is the tracer chosen (fluorescein). This allowed the development of a very sensitive method, which is basically non-invasive.

Fluorescein is a non-toxic molecule of only 5.5 Å radius. When mixed with blood, a high proportion (about 20%) remains free. It does not form a firm bond to vital tissues, is excreted rapidly by the kidney and liver and minimal concentrations ($10^{-9}$ g/ml) can be detected in the intraocular fluids by measuring its fluorescence intensity.

Initial experimental studies using a fluorophotometric slit lamp showed that it was possible to quantify the distribution of fluorescein within the axial regions of the vitreous in the living animal and estimate the movement of fluorescein across the retinal surface by measuring the concentration gradients of the dye in the vitreous body. These experimental

measurements where made not only *in vivo*, but also on frozen sections of enucleated eyes. This allowed a complete mapping of the distribution of fluorescein in the eye and made it possible to correlate the patterns of distribution with the concentration contours obtained *in vivo* in the axial region of the vitreous (Cunha-Vaz and Maurice, 1965). These experimental studies were the foundation of Vitreous Fluorometry studies. Clinical studies were initiated later and published for the first time by Cunha-Vaz *et al.* in 1975.

In Vitreous Fluorometry fluorescein, the tracer, is introduced into the blood circulation (first compartment) and from there it will cross the blood-ocular barriers in variable amounts, and penetrate into the intraocular fluids (second compartment). The concentration gradients between the fluorescein present in the blood and the fluorescein that penetrated into the eye namely into the vitreous and aqueous, will allow quantification of the permeability of the boundaries separating the blood from the intraocular fluids, the blood-ocular barriers (Cunha-Vaz, 1985).

Finally, after fluorescein has reached maximum levels in the vitreous, it is eliminated anteriorly through the main aqueous drainage pathway and posteriorly transported by the BRB. The rate of loss of fluorescein from the vitreous will give information on the transport mechanism for organic anions of the blood-retinal barrier, providing a good index of the cellular function of the BRB.

### 3.3.1. Basic Principles of Ocular Fluorometry

#### 3.3.1.1. *Quantitative Measurement of Fluorescein*

By measuring the fluorescence emitted by fluorescein in a solution, one cannot only detect its presence, but also obtain quantitative measurements of its concentration. Hence, the name of the technique stems from the dependence of the number of emitted fluorescent photons on the number of fluorescein molecules being irradiated. There is a wide range of fluorescein concentrations for which this relation is linear (proportional) with the concentration. However, in order to perform reliable fluorophotometric measurements, one has to realize that there are situations in which the relation between fluorescence intensity and concentrations is not linear. Moreover, the linearity constant may be influenced by different factors. The factors that are relevant to the clinical application of ocular fluorometry include light absorption by the ocular structures, spectrum shift in the eye and chemical quenching of fluorescence (Cunha-Vaz, 1985).

### 3.3.1.2. *Instrumentation and Measurement*

In the original ocular fluorometer light emitted by a light source is filtered by an excitation that transmits efficiently only wavelengths in the excitation bandwidth. This light is then focused in the eye by the optics of delivery. Some of the fluorescence emitted in the eye enters the pick up optics, which are designed to gather only light originating from the focal plan of the illuminating beam. This intersection of the delivery and pick up optical paths defines a

volume inside the eye from which fluorescence is detected by the photodetector. The photodetector outputs a signal that is proportional to the number of photons detected and this signal is, in turn, registered by the data processor. The volume, in which the fluorophotometric measurement is performed, is defined by the intersection of the illuminating beam and the pick up path.

Having realized that we are scanning across the eye with a probing volume of finite axial length, it is important to understand distribution of the fluorescein in the eye, in the vitreous fluorometry recording (Fig. 3.11).

### 3.3.1.3. *Evaluation of Blood-retinal Barrier Permeability*

The inward permeability across the BRB can, therefore, be estimated by calculating the mass of fluorescein that has penetrated posteriorly into the vitreous and the integral over time of the free plasma fluorescein concentration.

$$P_{in} = \int Cv(r) \times dv \, / \int Cp(t) \times dt \qquad (1)$$

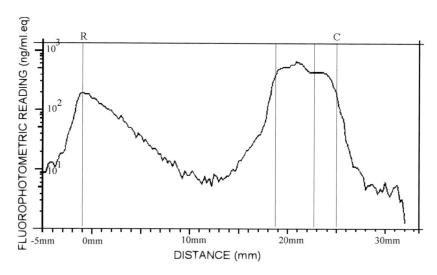

**Fig. 3.11.** Vitreous fluorophotometry recording from an eye with nonproliferative retinopathy from a patient with diabetes type 2 obtained one hour after intravenous fluorescein injection. Note the fluorescence curve in the vitreous across an altered blood-retinal barrier. Reference landmarks: R-retina; C-cornea.

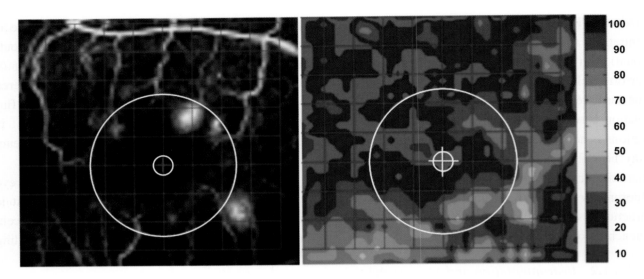

**Fig. 3.12.** Macula from a patient with diabetes type 2. *Left*: fluorescein angiography obtained by scanning laser ophthalmoscope. *Right*: Retinal Leakage Analyzer blood-retinal barrier permeability map (RLmap) in a false color-code map. Two-concentric circles of 100 $\mu$m and 750 $\mu$m radii centered on the fovea are shown on the figure. Note that not all hyperfluorescent areas in the *left* picture correspond to sites of increased fluorescein leakage into the vitreous, well depicted in the *right*.

Where $P_{in}$ is the inward permeability; $Cv(r)$ is the concentration in the vitreous at location $r$; $dv$ is a volume element; $Cp(t)$ is the free fluorescein in the plasma as a function of time; $dt$ the time element.

This equation (1) demonstrates the importance of evaluating the course of the plasma concentration and of basing the evaluation on more than one point in the vitreous. The role of outward transport may be ignored if we consider the movements of fluorescein in the period following injection of fluorescein, typically one hour (Zeimer, Blair and Cunha-Vaz, 1983; Cunha-Vaz *et al.*, 1993).

### 3.3.2. Retinal Leakage Analyzer

One major limitation of the available commercial instrumentation for Vitreous Fluorometry was associated with the fact that the permeability of the BRB is measured as an average over the macular area. Accurate mapping of localized changes in the permeability of the BRB would be beneficial for early diagnosis, to explain the natural history of retinal disease and to predict its effect on visual acuity.

We have recently developed a new method of retinal leakage mapping, the Retinal Leakage Analyzer (RLA), that is capable of measuring localized changes in fluorescein leakage across the BRB while simultaneously imaging the retina (Fig. 3.12). The instrument is based on a prototype Zeiss confocal scanning laser ophthalmoscope that was modified into a confocal scanning laser fluorometer (Lobo *et al.*, 1999).

Retinal and vitreous fluorescence is measured within the first five minutes after the intravenous injection of 14 mg/kg of 20% sodium fluorescein and at 30 minutes after the injection. Blood is sampled for plasma fluorescein estimation. The RLA acquires an entire image of the retina with real three-dimensional information. With use of appropriate software, it is possible to select an arbitrary sized ROI over an image as small as 75 mm $\times$ 75 $\mu$m or the total area and to build the corresponding fluorescence axial graphic.

Axial graphics of the fluorescence measurements obtained from the vitreous representing a volume of 75 $\mu$m $\times$ 75 $\mu$m $\times$ 2550 $\mu$m are converted into RLmaps (Fig. 3.12).

The permeability index of the BRB at 30 minutes in a series of normal eyes showed values ranging from a mean $13 \pm 4 \times 10^{-7}$ cm/s over vessels in retina, with a mean of $1.9 \pm 0.4 \times 10^{-7}$ cm/sec for the central macular area (3150 $\mu$m × 2700 $\mu$m).

We have also examined and followed eyes with mild diabetic retinopathy (Lobo *et al.*, 2000; 2002).

The vascular lesions included dilated retinal capillaries and microaneurysms showing different degrees of leakage both on fluorescein angiography and RLA imaging. Increased BRB permeability was measured in sites of morphological vascular abnormalities and also in areas where no retinal pathology could be identified (Fig. 3.13).

The multiple measurements of retinal leakage using the RLA may be graphically assembled in RLmaps, representing the distribution of the localized alterations in the BRB in any chosen area of the total 3150 $\mu$m × 2700 $\mu$m of the posterior pole under examination.

The method described allows localized measurements of BRB permeability discriminating leaking sites of approximately 75 $\mu$m to 100 $\mu$m size. This capability offers unique opportunities to examine the focal alteration of the BRB that occurs in a variety of retinal diseases. Simultaneous imaging of the retina is another important feature of the RLA. It is now possible to measure BRB permeability in specific locations of the fundus where there are retinal abnormalities and to follow the changes in retinal pathology together with modifications in the BRB.

The Retinal Leakage Analyzer, by performing quantitative mapping of retinal fluorescein leakage and simultaneous imaging of the retina offers, therefore, a novel approach to examine the role of BRB breakdown in the development and progression of retinal pathology.

### 3.3.3. Experimental Studies

An alteration of the BRB has been frequently reported in experimental diabetes. These studies, initiated by Waltman and co-workers (1978), showed an alteration of the BRB in rats with streptozotocin-induced diabetes. That was well demonstrated by vitreous fluorometry, soon after induction of chronic

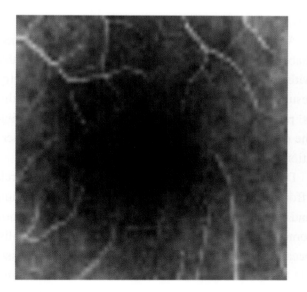
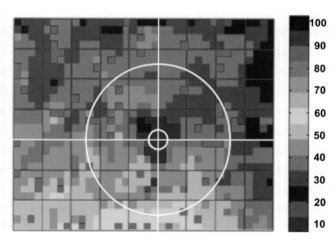

**Fig. 3.13.** Retinal leakage map. Color-coded blood-retinal barrier function. Index values of permeability can be deciphered with the aid of the color bar on the right. Units are × $10^{-7}$ cm.s$^{-1}$. Red squares represent leaking sites, defined as central sites of fluorescein diffusion. They are, therefore, identified as the sites showing permeability values higher than their immediate neighborhood. The red circles are centered on the fovea with 100- and 750-$\mu$m radii.

hyperglycemia. Furthermore, this alteration of the BRB was reversed by the administration of insulin and regularization of the glycemia.

Other studies have confirmed the alteration of the BRB in the rat in streptozotocin-induced diabetes only one week after the administration of streptozotocin. There were, however, contradicting observations regarding the site of the RBR breakdown. Studies using horseradish peroxidase as a tracer for electron microscopic investigation, pointed to the retinal pigmented epithelium as the main structure affected. However, studies using histochemical localization of naturally occurring albumin, performed by Murta *et al.* (1993) and Vinores *et al.* (1990), have clearly shown that the main site of increased permeability of the BRB is located at the level of the inner BRB involving the retinal vessels. More recently, our group in Coimbra have demonstrated using confocal microscopy that the breakdown of the BRB occurring in rats one week after onset of streptozotocin-induced diabetes is localized preferentially in the inner BRB (Carmo *et al.*, 1998).

In alloxan-induced diabetes, Engerman (1976) was able to demonstrate in the dog the development of a retinopathy presenting many of the features seen in man. Ultrastructural studies, using horseradish peroxidase, a relatively large protein, demonstrated the breakdown of the BRB preferentially in vessels showing signs of endothelial proliferation (Tso *et al.*, 1980).

An alteration of the transport of glucose has also been demonstrated in the retinal vessels of rabbits with alloxan-induced diabetes, using a model of microperfusion (Murta, Serra and Cunha-Vaz, 1994; 1996). These studies may offer an explanation for the differences in retinal and brain involvement in diabetes. In the alloxan-diabetic rabbit, the transport of glucose increases significantly increasing its Tm and promoting increased access of glucose to the retina, in contrast to the brain where the transport of glucose has been shown to be decreased, maintaining a low Tm in diabetic animals.

### 3.3.4. Clinical Studies

Our clinical studies on the application of vitreous fluorophotometry to diabetes were reported for the first time in 1975. The examination of a series of predominantly adult-onset diabetics with apparently normal fundi revealed the presence of a significant alteration of the BRB. The disturbance of the BRB appeared before microaneurysms or capillary closure could be demonstrated by fundus fluorescein angiography. The fluorescein concentration curves in the vitreous in the diabetic patients followed a typical pattern, the gradient indicating penetration of fluorescein across the BRB.

Our results were confirmed by Waltman and co-workers in St Louis (1978), who reported on the vitreous fluorometry examination of a series of juvenile-onset, insulin-dependent diabetics.

Initial studies suggested a direct association between an increase in vitreous fluorometry values and development of the retinal lesions. Higher fluorescein concentrations in the vitreous were observed in eyes showing more pathology. Another aspect of much interest was the observation of a relation between breakdown of the BRB, as shown by vitreous fluorometry, and metabolic control (Cunha-Vaz *et al.*, 1978; 1979).

A series of subsequent studies have examined diabetic patients with different degrees of retinopathy with conflicting results. Increased vitreous fluorometry results have generally been observed when retinopathy is present, but there is still controversy regarding the percentage of diabetic patients who show an alteration of the BRB without visible retinopathy.

During the following years many of the research efforts were directed at improving the instrumentation and standardization of the method. An ocular fluorometer described by Zeimer *et al.* (1983) finally became available commercially, thus making it possible to repeat studies at different centers and avoiding much of the variability in instrumentations that characterized some of the earlier studies.

More recently, in 1997, the results of a European multicentre study by Van Schaik *et al.* (1997) involving six different research groups showed that vitreous fluorometry, performed using the Fluorotron Master and following a well-defined protocol is a highly sensitive and reliable method for measuring the permeability of the BRB. An alteration of the BRB appear to be common after development of ophthalmoscopically visible retinopathy and is sometimes present even before the development of clinically visible retinopathy. This breakdown of the BRB increases with duration of the disease and is associated with poor metabolic control.

## 3.3.5. Prognostic Value of Leakage Measurements

Waltman (1984) published for the first time a five-year follow-up study involving 59 type 1 diabetic patients, examining the correlation between vitreous fluorometry values and the deterioration of the retinopathy. He found that increasing vitreous fluorometry values were harbingers of more rapid progression of diabetic retinopathy.

We have published a seven-year prospective follow-up study of 40 patients with adult-onset diabetes mellitus, with retinopathy no greater than level three of the modified Airlie House Classification of diabetic retinopathy at the commencement of the study (Cunha-Vaz *et al.*, 1998). They were examined by fundus photography, fluorescein angiography and vitreous fluorometry, at entry into the study and one, four, five and seven years of follow-up and a total of 22 of the 40 eyes had received photocoagulation. The eyes that needed photocoagulation were those that had higher vitreous fluorometry values at entry to the study and showed higher rates of deterioration. The eyes that did not need photocoagulation during the seven years follow-up showed stable vitreous fluorometry readings. Abnormally higher vitreous fluorometry values and their rapid increase over time were shown to be good indicators of progression and worsening of retinopathy in diabetes type 2.

Similar findings have been reported by Engler *et al.* (1991) in an eight-year follow-up study of 50 type 1

diabetic patients. Initially, the patients were submitted to fundus photography and vitreous fluorometry for determination of the BRB permeability. After eight years the patients were re-examined. A positive correlation between a higher initial permeability value and an unfavorable clinical course, using photocoagulation as the outcome parameter, was found. In summary, in patients showing the same retinal morphology, higher permeability of the BRB indicates an unfavorable disease course.

It appears, therefore, that the alteration of the BRB, measured by vitreous fluorometry, is an early finding in diabetic retinal disease and correlates well with progression and worsening of the retinopathy, both in type 1 and in type 2 diabetics. The quantitative nature of vitreous fluorometry and the demonstration of its clinical significance makes it the preferred outcome variable when evaluating drug therapy directed at the earliest stages of diabetic retinopathy.

Randomized studies using fundus photography as the main outcome have consistently produced negative results, particularly when studying initial stages of the retinopathy. Clinical studies using the alteration of the BRB as the outcome variable have shown that the progressive deterioration of the BRB that occurs in the diabetic patients may be decreased and possibly stabilized by drug administration. A favorable effect on the BRB has been observed in pilot studies using aldose reductase inhibitors, such as sorbinil, sulindac and calcium dobesilate antioxidants and antihistamine drugs (Cunha-Vaz, 1992).

Permeability of the BRB, measured by vitreous fluorometry, appears to be particularly valuable in the early stages of retinal disease as a quantifiable outcome variable of clinical significance.

The development of a retinal leakage analyzer, with the ability to map retinal fluorescein leakage while simultaneously imaging the retina, is expected to improve in the near future our understanding of the role breakdown of the BRB in diabetic retinal disease. It is now possible to follow the natural history of the main morphological changes occurring in the diabetic retina, such as microaneurysms, capillary closure and retinal oedema, and study their association with localized alterations of the BRB identified and measured by the retinal leakage analyzer.

More recently, the Retinal Leakage Analyzer, a modified scanning laser ophthalmoscope for fluorometry measurements, has been introduced. This novel instrumentation allows localized measurement of the alterations of the BRB and mapping of these alterations in the initial steps of diabetic retinal disease.

# References

Ashton N. (1963) Studies of retinal capillaries in relation to diabetic and other retinopathies. *Br J Ophthalmol* **47**: 521–538.

Ashton N. (1965) The blood-retinal barrier and vasoglial relationships in retinal disease. *Trans Ophthalmol Soc UK* **85**: 199–229.

Carmo A, Ramos P, Reis A, *et al.* (1998) Breakdown of the inner and outer blood-retinal barriers in streptozotocin-induced diabetes. *Exp Eye Res* **67**: 569–575.

Cogan DG, Kwabara T. (1963) Capillary shunts in the pathogenesis of diabetic retinopathy. *Diabetes* **12**: 293–300.

Cunha-Vaz JG, Abreu JR, Campos AJ, Figo G. (1975) Early breakdown of the blood-retinal barrier in diabetes. *Br Ophthalmol* **59**: 649–656.

Cunha-Vaz JG, Fonseca JR, Faria de Abreu JR, Ruas MA. (1978) A follow-up study by vitreous fluorometry of early retinal involvement in diabetes. *Am J Ophthalmol* **86**: 467–473.

Cunha-Vaz JG, Goldberg MF, Vygantas C, Noth J. (1979) Early detection of retinal involvement in diabetes by vitreous fluorophotometry. *Ophthalmology* **86**: 264–275.

Cunha-Vaz JG, Leite E, Ramos C. (1993) Manual of Ocular Fluorometry. Protocols approved within the framework of a Concerted Action of the European Community Biomedical Programme on Ocular Fluorometry. pp. 1–16, Coimbra.

Cunha-Vaz JG, Lobo C, Castro Sousa JP, *et al.* (1998) Progression of retinopathy and alteration of the blood-retinal barrier in patients with type 2 diabetes: A 7-year prospective follow-up study. *Graefes Arch Clin Exp Ophthalmol* **236**: 264–268.

Cunha-Vaz JG, Maurice DM. (1965) Fluorescein transport by retinal vessels. *J Physiol* **183**: 42–43.

Cunha-Vaz JG. (1985) Vitreous Fluorometry. *Prog Retinal Res* **4**: 89–114.

Cunha-Vaz JG. (1992) Prespectives in the treatment of diabetic retinopathy. *Diabetes Metab Rev* **8**: 105–116.

Engerman RL. (1976) Animal models of diabetic retinopathy. *Trans Am Acad Ophthalmol Otolaryngon* **81**: 710–715.

Engler C, Krogssa B, Lund-Andersen H. (1991) Blood-retinal barrier permeability and its relation to the progression of diabetic retinopathy in type 1 diabetes. *Graefes Arch Clin Exp Ophthalmol* **229**: 442–446.

Lobo C, Bernardes R, Cunha-Vaz JG. (2000) Alterations of the blood-retinal barrier and retinal thickness in preclinical retinopathy in subjects with type 2 diabetes. *Arch Ophthalmol* **118**: 1364–1369.

Lobo C, Bernardes R, Faria de Abreu JR, Cunha-Vaz JG. (2002) One year follow-up of blood-retinal barrier and retinal thickness alterations in patients with type 2 diabetes mellitus and mild nonproliferative retinopathy. *Arch Ophthalmol* **119**: 1469–1474.

Lobo C, Bernardes R, Santos F, Cunha-Vaz JG. (1999) Mapping retinal fluorescein leakage with confocal scanning laser fluorometry of the human vitreous. *Arch Ophthalmol* **117**: 631–637.

Murta JN, Serra A, Cunha-Vaz JG. (1994) Organic anion transport and reabsorptive fluid flux in diabetic retinal vessels: a microperfusion study. *Exp Eye Res* **58**: 567–572.

Murta JN, Serra A, Cunha-Vaz JG. (1996) Characterization of D-glucose transport across diabetic retinal vessels. *Invest Ophthalmol* **38**: 979.

Murta T, Ishibashi T, Inomata H. (1993) Immunohistochemical detection of blood-retinal barrier breakdown in streptozotocin-diabetic rats. *Graefes Arch Clin Exp Ophthalmol* **231**: 175–177.

Tso MOM, Cunha-Vaz JG, Shih CY, *et al.* (1980) Clinical pathologic study of blood-retinal barrier in experimental diabetes mellitus. *Arch Ophthalmol* **98**: 2032–2040.

Van Schaik HJ, Heintz B, Larsen M, *et al.* (1997) Permeability of the blood-retinal barrier in healthy humans. *Graefes Arch Clin Exp Ophthalmol* **235**: 639–646.

Vinores SA, McGree RO, Lee A, *et al.* (1990) Ultrastructural localization of blood-retinal barrier breakdown in diabetic and galactosemic rats. *J Histochem Cytochem* **38**: 1341–1352.

Waltman SR, Oestrich C, Krupin T, *et al.* (1978) Quantitative vitreous fluorometry: A sensitive technique for measuring early breakdown of the blood-retinal barrier in young diabetic patients. *Diabetes* **27**: 85–87.

Waltman SR, Krupin T, Hanish S. (1978) Alterations of the blood-retinal barrier in experimental diabetes mellitus. *Arch Ophthalmol* **96**: 878–879.

Waltman SR. (1984) Sequential vitreous fluorometry in diabetes mellitus. A five-year prospective study. *Trans Am Ophthalmol* **82**: 827–842.

Zeimer R, Blair N, Cunha-Vaz JG. (1983) Pharmacokinetic interpretation of vitreous fluorophotometry. *Invest Ophthalmol Vis Sc* **24**: 1374–1381.

Zeimer RC, Blair NP, Cunha-Vaz JG. (1983) Vitreous fluorophotometry for clinical research. II Methodology of data acquisition and processing. *Arch Ophthalmol* **11**: 1757–1761.

## 3.4.  Blood Flow

### José Cunha-Vaz

The nutritional and waste removal needs of the retina are met by two separate sources. The central retinal artery (CRA) supplies approximately the inner two-thirds of the retina. The deeper outer layers, including photoreceptors and bipolar cells, are nourished by the uveal system, specifically the choriocapillaries. The retinal pigment epithelial layer which separates the retina from the choroid, actively transports metabolites and waste to and from the deep layers of the retina to the choroid.

The CRA typically branches into four major trunks, each of which supplies a quadrant of the retina. The retinal arteries and veins lie within the nerve fiber layer of the superficial retina.

The retinal capillaries run parallel to the nerve fiber layer. In the posterior pole, the retinal capillaries form several layers are higher in number than in the more peripheral retina. The peripapillary retina has a superficial layer of fine capillaries. In approximately 30% of all people a cilioretinal artery may be present and supply a variably sized region of the retina, temporal to the optic nerve.

Retinal venous drainage occurs via the central retinal vein, which exits the eye through the optic nerve and parallels the CRA. The central retinal vein drains into the superior ophthalmic veins or, rarely, directly into the cavernous sinus.

Normally, retinal blood flow remains relatively constant over a substantial range of intraocular pressure and systemic blood pressure. Compared with the choroidal circulation (a high-flow, variable-rate system) the retinal circulation is a lower flow, constant-rate system supplying a highly metabolic active tissue. The choroid receives 85% of the ocular circulation, as compared to 15% to the retinal circulation. The autonomic nervous system controls vascular resistance in the choroid. The autonomic nervous system contributes to retrobulbar and choroidal circulatory regulation, but it ends at the lamina cribosa, so the retinal and anterior optic nerve head (ONH) vasculature do not possess direct innervation (Malmfors, 1965). Although retinal and optic nerve head vessels have alpha-adrenergic, beta-adrenergic and cholinergic receptors, the role of these receptors in vascular control remains unclear. Consequently, retinal blood flow is autoregulated locally in response mainly to variable oxygen content.

### 3.4.1.  General Hemodynamic Principles

In general, the physical laws formulated to describe steady laminar flow of uniform fluids through nondistensible tubes are also helpful in understanding *in vivo* retinal vascular hemodynamics (Traytsman, 1983). Ohm's law predicts that flow (Q) is proportional to the pressure gradient between inflow and outflow ($\Delta P$) divided by the resistance to flow ($R$):

$$Q = \frac{\Delta P}{R}.$$

Analogously in the retina, retinal perfusion pressure, the difference between arterial inflow and downstream outflow pressure ($\Delta P$), is used as the relevant driving pressure ($Q$) for retinal blood flow (RBF). Retinal perfusion pressure is the difference between intraarterial pressure and the pressure in the thin walled veins.

Venous pressure changes in parallel with intraocular pressure (IOP) and is normally 2–5 mm Hg higher than IOP. Therefore, the driving pressure is calculated as the difference between mean arterial blood pressure (MAP) and retinal venous pressure or IOP, whichever is higher. Resistance is determined principally by vessel radius and can be calculated to estimate retinal vascular resistance (RVR). Poiseuille's law shows that the major determinants of RBF are perfusion pressure ($\Delta P$), blood viscosity ($\eta$) and vessel radius ($r$). Vessel length ($L$) is generally not a measurable parameter in physiological conditions and is assumed to be non manipulable:

$$Q = (\pi r 4 \Delta P/(8\eta L)).$$

Poiseuille's law demonstrates that all factors except radius are linearly related to flow. It bears emphasis that blood flow is related to the fourth power of vessel radius, thus, even small changes in luminal diameter have significant effects on RBF. It is by this mechanism that RVR can change rapidly and dramatically alter regional or global RBF during normal or pathophysiological conditions. Autoregulation is achieved via fine tuning of vessel diameter in response to fluctuations in perfusion pressure.

Retinal blood flow should be distinguished, as either a volume rate (ml per min), a volume flow rate for a specific tissue weight (ml per min per 100 g) or a velocity (cm per sec). With steady flow, blood flow can be expressed as the product of velocity (cm/sec) and cross-sectional area (cm$^2$): $Q = V\pi r^2$ (Wise *et al.*, 1971).

### 3.4.2. Pressure-Volume Relationships

The vascular network of the retina is contained within the eye relatively rigid structure maintained by the sclera. Therefore, extravascular pressure is critically important in retinal vascular dynamics because

arterial transmural pressure (difference between intrasterial and extra vascular pressures) is equivalent to IOP.

### 3.4.3. Retinal Blood Volume

Retinal blood volume (RBV) is determined by two factors, retinal blood flow and capacitance vessel diameter (i.e. small veins and venules). Retinal blood volume increases with vasodilatation and decreases with vasoconstriction. Although RBF frequently changes in the same direction as retinal blood volume, these variables are inversely related in some normal situations (e.g. autoregulation) or in pathological situations.

### 3.4.4. Pressure-Flow Relationships

One of the characteristic aspects of both, retinal and cerebral circulations, is its diameter responses to changes in perfusion pressure. In healthy brain, for instance, arterial diameter increases or decreases over 30 sec to 2 min in order to actively control central blood flow and maintain constant flow over a range of cerebral perfusion pressures (approximately between 60 and 160 mmHg). It is this vascular phenomenon which comprises autoregulation. Within the autoregulatory range RBF remains constant via vasoconstriction when perfusion pressure increases and blood volume decreases. Below the autoregulatory range, a decrease in perfusion pressure results in decreased RBF and RBV.

In conclusion, application of general hemodynamics principles offers an initial understanding of RBF, mechanical control of the retinal circulation and the basis for understanding blood flow in retinal vascular disease.

### 3.4.5. Biophysical Factors Affecting Retinal Capillary Flow

The flow of red blood cells through retinal capillaries is modulated by intravascular and extravascular factors. The intravascular pressure gradient between the precapillary arteriole and the postcapillary venule is the most important regulator of capillary flow. This pressure gradient is influenced by the systemic arterial pressure; the pressure drop across the retinal resistance vessels and the venous outflow pressure. Despite the presence of retinal blood flow (RBF) autoregulation, rapid changes in arterial pressure are transmitted to the microcirculation and result in transient changes in capillary flow velocity. Dilatation of resistance arterioles and venules, which are responsible for a major component of retinal vascular resistance, increases the microvascular pressure gradient, and, therefore, increases capillary flow velocity. On the other hand, an increase in capillaries diameter, in the absence of a change in arteriolar diameter, has a relatively small effect on the pressure gradient and, therefore, results in a decrease in capillary flow velocity.

The flow of red cells in capillaries is also modulated by the flow of leukocytes. Leukocytes are believed to navigate selected flow pathways with high red blood cell and plasma flow in the microvascular network. Under conditions of low perfusion, leukocytes may stop in these capillaries. Very slow perfusion also contributes to erythrocyte and platelet aggregation, reducing blood fluidity, which becomes significant under pathological conditions.

### 3.4.6. Velocity and Intermittence of Retinal Capillary Flow

One the most striking characteristics of the retinal capillary circulation like in the brain circulation are the irregular, tortuous course of its capillaries and the remarkably high velocity of red blood cells (Keith *et al.*, 1967; Hudetz *et al.*, 1995). Under resting conditions there is a significant heterogeneity in flow velocity within each microvascular network. This heterogeneity is important because it may influence the effectiveness of oxygen transport to tissue. The direction of flow and the average rate of red blood cell perfusion in each capillary are stable. A fundamental question is whether perfusion heterogeneity is determined by network architecture or by vascular tone and capillary diameter.

Under normal physiological conditions, almost all capillaries are perfused by both plasma and red blood cells. Despite the heterogeneity of flow among neighboring capillaries, some degree of red blood cell perfusion is present in every capillary segment.

It has been suggested that the capillaries with high resting flow and absent autoregulation represent functional thoroughfare channels, while the capillaries with slow resting flow represent the true "exchange" capillaries. The significance of this specialization is that thoroughfare channels would provide a physiological reserve of flow, which could be recruited when retinal blood supply is challenged. A decrease in retinal perfusion pressure may initiate redistribution of flow from the thoroughfare channels to the exchange capillaries. This may help to maintain balanced perfusion and transcapillary exchange. In addition, the maintenance of flow velocity in the slower capillaries may protect the microcirculation from perfusion failure. Red cells fail to enter capillaries with slow flow (plasma skimming) and slow flow capillaries are more prone to plugging by leukocytes.

Moderate hypoxia increases retinal blood flow and increases the velocity of flow in retinal capillaries. In the brain, when the inspired $O_2$ is lowered to 15%, red blood cell velocity in individual capillaries increases by about 40%. This increase in velocity is somewhat less than the corresponding increase in cortical central blood flow at 58% (Berecki *et al.*, 1993) and, therefore, suggests that a small increase in the number of perfused capillaries or in capillary diameter may have also occurred. Moderate distension of capillaries due to an upstream vasodilatation or opening of capillary shunts may be an alterative explanation. Nevertheless, the major mechanism, by which central blood flow increases in hypoxia, appears to be an increase in capillary flow velocity.

### 3.4.7. Regulation of Retinal Capillary Blood Flow

Changes in the arterioles, alone cannot explain the autoregulatory responses of retinal and brain capillary blood flow.

It is, therefore, postulated that cerebral and retinal capillary flow distribution is regulated by contractile cells of the microvascular bed. Smooth muscle cells with potential regulatory functions exist in precapillary areas of terminal arterioles and may regulate red cell entry into capillaries. Endothelial or pericyte contraction and relaxation may also be involved. Actin and myosin are present in retinal and brain capillaries and endothelial cells contract in response to mechanical, electrical and pharmacological stimulation. Retinal pericytes have been shown to contract or relax in response to a number of hormones and endothelial derived mediators, such as angiotensin II, endothelin, serotonin, thromboxan A, prostaglandin and NO (Haefliger *et al.*, 1994).

Physiological regulation also requires an adequate sensing mechanism of capillary flow. Changes in red blood cells flow in capillaries may be detected by endothelial shear receptors. Signals generated by a change in capillary flow velocity may then be communicated to the terminal arterioles or pericytes by cell to cell communication within the vessel wall or via perivascular nerves or astrocytic networks. Capillary cells may integrate information about flow velocity with those representing functional/metabolic status of the retinal cells ($K^+$, $H^+$, adenosine, glutamate, NO) and communicate these signals to the contractile elements where capillary flow may be regulated.

When perfusion pressure and flow are severely reduced, the intermittency in capillary perfusion becomes more apparent. Transient plugging of capillaries by leukocytes at the capillary orifices becomes frequent and the periods of flow stagnation increase with a decrease in perfusion pressure (Yamakawa *et al.*, 1987). In severe ischemia, capillary obstruction may be aggravated by endothelial swelling and formation of microvilli, platelet aggregation and external compression of capillaries due to edema or perivascular astrocyte swelling. A varying combination of these factors may be involved in capillary perfusion failure.

The maintenance of flow velocity of erythrocytes in retinal capillaries has regulatory importance to maintain optimum capillary exchange and for protecting the microcirculation from perfusion failure. The main mechanism of a change in blood flow in cerebral capillaries is a change in linear velocity with a minor role for capillary recruitment, change in capillary diameter or flow shunting. In hypoxia, red cell velocity increases in the capillaries. Decreased perfusion pressure, on the other hand, involves a decrease in the heterogeneity of capillary flow, in which redistribution of red cell flow between thoroughfare channels and exchange capillaries may play an important role.

### 3.4.8. Autoregulation of Retinal Blood Flow

In summary autoregulation of blood flow in the retina and brain is a regulatory mechanism that allows blood flow to remain relatively constant during variations of arterial pressure in order to keep an extremely high degree of homeostasis with respect to a balance of tissue nutrients and fluids. Retinal resistance arterioles dilate during reductions in retinal perfusion pressure (mean arterial pressure) and constrict during increases. As a result, retinal blood flow remains relatively constant over a fairly broad range of arterial pressure defined as the autoregulatory plateau. When retinal perfusion pressure exceeds the limits of the autoregulatory plateau, resistance arterioles respond passively to further changes in pressure. Thus, once the limits of autoregulation are reached, retinal blood flow increases or decreases passively with increases or reductions in perfusion pressure.

Breakthrough of the upper limit of retinal autoregulation is also accompanied, like in the brain, by damage to the retinal endothelium and disruption in the Blood-Retinal Barrier (BRB). Disruption of the BRB results in extravasation of plasma proteins into the retina, neuronal dysfunction and development of edema. Finally, retinal blood flow may decrease further as a result of the edema and constriction due to vasoconstrictor hormones that gain access to vascular smooth muscle or pericytes after disruption of the BRB and development of signs of ischemia.

The mechanisms responsible for blood flow autoregulation are not yet clearly understood but three major hypothesis remain viable. One involves a myogenic response and is based on the concept that resistance arteries respond directly to alterations in perfusion pressure by contraction during increases in pressure and relaxation during reductions. Most evidence favoring this hypothesis has been obtained *in vitro*, whereas *in vivo* data does not support the myogenic hypothesis (Busija and Heistad, 1984). The second is the metabolic hypothesis and it states that reductions in retinal and cerebral blood flow stimulate the release of vasoactive substances from the tissue that in turn stimulate the dilatation of resistance arterioles. Finally, the third hypothesis considers endothelial factors as the most relevant (Iadecola *et al.*, 1994). In this concept, endothelium may react to changes in transmural pressure or shear stress by a decreased liberation of endothelium derived relaxing factor or bed an increase in liberation of an endothelium derived contracting factor.

### 3.4.9. Measurement of Blood Flow

From the most basic standpoint, the eye offers a unique opportunity to study hemodynamics. It is the only location in the body where capillary blood flow may be observed noninvasively in humans. However, the technical complexities involved in obtaining accurate measurements of retinal blood flow have been, up to now, insurmountable. Only one commercially available technique can provide volumetric blood flow measurements in absolute units and it is limited to measurements of flow in large retinal vessels. At this time volumetric flow measurements in absolute units from retinal tissue are unobtainable.

The techniques that can be used for measuring retinal blood flow include pulsability measurement devices and laser devices (the Canon laser blood

flowmeter, fluorescein angiographic methods using scanning laser optical systems and laser Doppler flowmetry). For a complete review of the different techniques the work of Harris *et al.* (2003) should be read.

All these techniques have shown major limitations. The results that have been published using the different techniques available have, however, given some useful indications on the behavior of retinal blood flow in diabetes.

### 3.4.10. Retinal Blood Flow in Diabetes

Blood flow parameters are altered as a result of acute and subacute changes in blood glucose levels. In one report, patients with insulin-dependent diabetes and no clinical evidence of retinopathy when subjected to acute elevation of glucose levels in the blood for periods as short as one hour responded by a decrease in retinal blood flow when compared to nondiabetics (Bursell, *et al.*, 1996). Ludovico *et al.* (2003), however, have shown that not all eyes of diabetic patients, even before the development of clinical retinopathy, have similar retinal blood flow values. They showed that some eyes show decreased retinal blood flow values in contrast with other eyes that have significantly increased values of retinal blood flow. This observation may explain the many contradictory reports existing in the literature.

It is becoming clear that not all patients with diabetes will develop retinopathy at the same rate of progression or with the same severity. In their lifetime only a few diabetic patients, particularly in type 2 diabetes, will ever develop proliferative retinopathy.

There is, however, some agreement that when nonproliferative diabetic retinopathy is present there is initially some degree of increase in retinal blood flow (Blair *et al.*, 1982; Cunha-Vaz *et al.*, 1978; Kohner *et al.*, 1975; Yoshida *et al.*, 1983). These results have been confirmed in studies using both laser Doppler flowmetry and fluorescein angiography dye-dilution techniques (Grunwald *et al.*, 1986 and 1993). Later in the disease, with increasing ischemia and development of neovascularization, the results available indicate a widespread decrease in retinal blood flow, but at this stage of the retinal disease the results obtained with the available techniques are even more difficult to interpret.

It is accepted that there is an alteration of retinal blood autoregulation in diabetes that may play a fundamental role in the development and progress of the retinal lesions.

In patients with diabetes, the inability of the retinal vessels to constrict in response to increased arterial blood oxygen content is one of several pieces of evidence showing that the diseased retina lacks normal autoregulatory responsiveness. Diabetics suffer, apparently, from retinal autoregulatory incapacity in proportion to disease severity. For example, when intravenous tyramine administration is used to elevate mean arterial pressure, a 35% pressure rise is required to increase bulk retinal blood flow in healthy persons (Rassam *et al.*, 1995). In normoglycemic diabetics, a 25% pressure elevation increased was needed to retinal blood flow, whereas only a 15% rise in pressure was required to increase blood flow in hyperglycemic diabetic patients.

Furthermore, using the blue light entoptic phenomenon, investigators have demonstrated faulty retinal capillary autoregulation in response to both isocapnic hypoxia and to intraocular pressure elevation (Sinclair *et al.*, 1982; Fallon, Maxwell and Kohner, 1987).

# References

Berecki D, Wei L, Otsuka T, *et al.* (1993) Hypoxia increases velocity or blood flow through parenclymal microvascular systems in rat brain. *J Cereb Blow Metabol* **13**: 475–486.

Blair NP, Feke GT, Moralles-Stopeelo J, *et al.* (1982) Prolongation of the retinal mean circulation time in diabetes. *Arch Ophthalmol* **100**: 764–768.

Bursell S, Clermont A, Kinsley BT, *et al.* (1996) Retinal blood flow changes in patients with insulin-dependent diabetes mellitus and no diabetic retinopathy. *Invest Opthalmol Vis Sci* **37**: 886–897.

Busija DW, Heistad DD. (1984) Factors involved in the physiologic regulation of the cerebral circulation. *Rec Physiol Biochem Pharmacol* **101**: 161–211.

Cunha-Vaz JG, Fonseca JR, Faria de Abreu JR. (1978) Vitreous fluorophotometry and retinal blood flow studies in proliferative retinopathy. *Albrecht Graefe's Arch Klin Exp Ophthalmol* **207**: 71–76.

Fallon TJ, Maxwell, DL, Kohner EM. (1987) Autoregulation of retinal blood flow in diabetic retinopathy measured by blue-light entoptic technique. *Ophthalmology* **94**: 1410–1415.

Grunwald JE, Brucker CE, Grunwald SE, Riva CE. (1993) Retinal hemodynamics in proliferative diabetic retinopathy. *Invest Ophthalmol Vis Sci* **34**: 66–71.

Grunwald JE, Riva LE, Sinclair SH, *et al.* (1986) Laser Doppler velocimetry study of retinal circulation in diabetes mellitus. *Arch Ophthalmol* **104**: 991–996.

Haefliger IO, Zschauer A, Anderson DA. (1994) Relaxation of retinal pericyte contractile tone through the nitric-oxide-cyclic guanosine nonphosphate pathway. *Invest Ophthalmol Vis Sci* **35**: 991–997.

Harris A, Jonescu-Cuypers CP, Kageman L, *et al.* (2003) *Atlas of Ocular Blood Flow.* Butterworth, Heinemann.

Hudetz AG, Fcher G, Weigle CG, *et al.* (1995) Viedomicroscopy of cerebral cortical capillary flow: Response to hypotension and intracranial hypertension. *Am J Physiol* **268**: H2202–H2210.

Iadecola C, Pelligrino DA, Moskowitz MA, Lassen NA. (1994) Nitric oxide synthase inhibition and cerebrovascular regulation. *J Cereb Blood Flow Metab* **14**: 175–192.

Keith CG, Cunha-Vaz JG, Shakib M. (1967) Studies on the effect of osmotically active substances on the retina. I Observations *in vivo. Invest Ophthalmol Vis Sci* **6**: 192–197.

Kohner EM, Hamilton AM, Saunders SJ, *et al.* (1975) The retinal blood flow in diabetes. *Diabetologia* **27**: 48–52.

Ludovico J, Bernardes R, Pires I, *et al.* (2003) Alterations of retinal capillary blood flow in preclinical retinopathy in subjects with type 2 diabetes. *Graefe's Arch Clin Exp Ophthalmol* **41**: 181–186.

Mamlfors T. (1965) The adrenergic innervation of the eye as demonstrated by fluorescence microscopy. *Acta Physiol Scand* **65**: 259–267.

Rassam SMB, Patel V, Kohner EM. (1995) The effect of experimental hypertension on retinal vascular autoregulation in humans: A mechanism for the progression of diabetic retinopathy. *Exp Physiol* **80**: 53–68.

Sinclair SH, Grunwald JE, Riva CE, *et al.* (1982) Retinal vascular autoregulation in diabetes mellitus. *Ophthalmology* **89**: 748–750.

Traystman RM. (1983) Microcirculation in the brain. In: Mortillaro N (ed.), *The Physiology and Pharmacology of the Microcirculation*, Vol. 1, Academic Press, San Diego, pp. 237–298.

Wise G, Dollery CT, Henkind P. (1971) *The Retinal Circulation*. Harper and Row, New York, pp. 87–115.

Yamakawa T, Yaniguchi S, Nimi H, Sugiyama I. (1987) White blood cell plugging and blood flow mal distribution in the capillary network of cat cerebral cortex in acute hemorrhagic hypotension: An intravital microscopic study. *Circ Shock* **22**: 323–332.

Yoshida A, Feke GT, Morales-Stopello J, *et al.* (1983) Retinal blood flow alterations during progression of diabetic retinopathy. *Arch Ophthalmol* **101**: 225–227.

## 3.5. Retinal Neural Impairment

### Miguel Castelo-Branco

Current trends in the study of retinal neural impairment in diabetic retinopathy focus on functional assays that can specifically examine a given pathway or layer within the retinal network. This rationale is well demonstrated by studies that have aimed to show a large rod contribution to retinal deficits in diabetes, by means of measurement of dark adaptation curves (Amemiya, 1977; Henson and North, 1979; Greenstein *et al.*, 1993). This significant rod contribution to overall impairment may be related to the fact that these cells require larger amounts of oxygen than cones, which might lead to outer retinal hypoxia in the dark-adapted state (Arden, *et al.*, 1998).

Retinal capillaries within the inner nuclear layer (close to cell bodies of amacrine and bipolar cells) seem to be affected in the early stages of diabetic retinopathy (Chakrabarti *et al.*, 2000, Ciulla *et al.*, 2003), which renders techniques that measure this part of the retinal network also useful.

It is important to recognize that when evaluating topographic structural and functional impairment in diabetic retinas, one should consider that even in normal subjects, performance of retinal networks is asymmetrical in space. Accordingly, Miyake *et al.* (1989) have demonstrated an asymmetry of the focal ERG in the human macular region. It is known for a long time that there is a higher density of photoreceptors in the upper retinal areas, (Oesterberg, 1935) and the standing potential, which reflects the function of the retinal pigment epithelium, is also larger in the upper retina (Skrandies and Baier, 1986).

Recently, high-resolution mfERG in which a large number of retinal locations were functionally mapped with an array of 509 elements, have further suggested that some of the observed variations are a clear consequence of inhomogeneities in retinal anatomy and physiology (Poloschek and Sutter, 2002). In fact, these differences can be sufficiently strong to become visible even in the analysis of cortical responses. Indeed, consistent latency differences do exist between the nasal and temporal mfVEP responses. Responses to visual field peripheral nasal stimuli are faster than that to peripheral temporal stimuli (Hood and Zhang, 2000).

Accordingly, Curcio *et al.* (1993) found the highest rod density 4 – 5 mm above the fovea in healthy eyes. Interestingly, multifocal electrophysiology of oscillatory potentials has shown topographic asymmetries in retinal quadrants for the second-order kernel, which is more dependent on rod activity than the first order kernel (Kurtenbach *et al.*, 2000). These waveforms were larger from the temporal retina as compared with those from the nasal retina, and were larger in the upper retina than in the lower retina. This pronounced nasal-temporal difference in amplitude had been observed previously for focal OPs and mfOPs (Wu and Sutter, 1995; Hood *et al.*, 1997; Bearse *et al.*, 2000; Rangaswamy *et al.*, 2000).

Other forms of mfERG, such as the slow flash mfERG, evoke temporal response waveforms, are slightly larger and contain relatively more high-frequency wavelets at corresponding eccentricities (Onozu and Yamamoto, 2003; Bearse *et al.*, 2000, 2004).

We do believe that these asymmetries may have a retinal ganglion cell origin. Indeed, in a human glaucoma, which is a model of ganglion cell death, an oscillatory component is lost in the temporal retina (Fortune *et al.*, 2002) and, in monkey, high-frequency and oscillatory components of the mfERG are reduced by experimental glaucoma (Frishman *et al.*, 2000), tetrodotoxin (TTX) treatment (Hood *et al.*, 1999), and induced nerve fiber layer defects (Fortune *et al.*, 2003). Nevertheless, some authors do still argue that prolonged latencies in mfOP recordings observed in patients with diabetes without retinopathy, indicate an alteration in inner retinal sensitivity that can be explained by impaired rod–cone interactions (Wu and Sutter, 1995; Kurtenbach *et al.*, 2000). These methods based on isolation of oscillatory potentials may not be best suited to investigate foveal function because density plots show a more marked absence of activity in the central 6° to 7° of the retina (Kurtenbach *et al.*, 2000). This is consistent with strong rod and magnocellular (with small foveal populations) contributions to these responses.

There is more consensus that the primary generators of the flash mfERG, are located in the region that contains the cell bodies of the bipolar cells (Han *et al.* 2002, Hare *et al.*, 2002). Since flash diabetic retinopathy is largely caused by defects of retinal capillaries in the inner nuclear layer, the flash mfERG seems to be also a valuable testing procedure in this context. Interestingly, both first- and second-order kernel responses are significantly altered in type 1 diabetes without retinopathy, between 5° and 22° eccentricity, for the nasal retina.

It is believed that ERG changes in diabetes have a microvascular origin (Scholl and Zrenner, 2000), although direct retinal dysfunction has also been hypothesized (Tzekov and Arden, 1999). In any case, permeability changes and small vessel closure, leading to ischemia and cell death, seem to be pivotal in the nonproliferative stage of diabetic retinopathy.

Despite the widely described psychophysical and electrophysiological methods that have often been used to document diabetic retinopathy, a consensus on the ideal tool to detect retinal dysfunction before the appearance of diabetic retinopathy is still missing. It is indeed important to identify individuals and retinal locations at risk so that it becomes possible to assess new preventive therapies.

Vascular damage is a central issue in diabetic retinopathy, but it is also important to know whether any concomitant independent neural damage occurs. It could be argued that methods that can directly assess perfusion would be more appropriate and that psychophysical/electrophysiological methods would be mainly appropriate for the later type of damage. It is, however, still an open question whether primary neural damage occurs early in the natural history of diabetic retinopathy.

The vascular vs. neural damage discussion is also pertinent to other fields of research, such as glaucoma (Castelo-Branco *et al.*, 2004). Here, a central question is whether the high pressure in the eye directly attacks the fibers of the ganglion cell or alternatively, damages the blood vessels that nourish such fibers.

### 3.5.1. New Psychophysical Techniques to Assess Retinal Neural Impairment in Diabetic Retinopathy

It is important to study retinal function in the early stages and in particular to study macular function, since diabetic maculopathy is the most frequent sight-threatening complication of diabetes. In this respect, assessment of standard visual acuity is not very rewarding since acuity remains stationary until ~50% of the neuroretinal pathways are affected (Frisèn, 1976), and the foveal avascular zone is frequently enlarged in diabetic patients without any sign of change in visual acuity (Arend *et al.*, 1995). This suggests that psychophysical techniques should aim to assess separately distinct functional channels (Bresnick *et al.*, 1985; Green *et al.*, 1985). Evidence for predominant early involvement of the parvocellular pathway suggests that the physiology of the perifoveal area should be under scrutiny in future studies, since changes in the microvasculature in this region may be predictive of visual outcome.

Short-wavelength automated perimetry is probably more valuable in detecting early damage in diabetic retinopathy than conventional perimetric methods. Accordingly, the presence of perifoveal ischemia is related to a subtle deterioration of visual function as measured by SWAP (Remky *et al.*, 2000). These authors suggested further that in patients without clinically significant macular edema and with normal visual acuity, SWAP could be a clinical adjunct for further identifying early ischemic diabetic maculopathy. The rationale behind this strategy lies in the fact that short wavelength sensitive cones have been shown to be particularly sensitive to ischemic and phototoxic damage.

We are currently evaluating alternative psychophysical strategies to study chromatic function in retinal disorders in a specific manner (Fig. 3.14). Luminance

and size noise in the stimulus ensure that only chromatic signals are being used in the task. If chromatic contrast is modulated only along three main confusion lines, then the test can be applied in a few minutes, and it can still isolate L, M and S cone responses (Castelo-Branco *et al.*, 2004; Campos *et al.*, 2004). A longer version of the test allows the determination of "areas of color confusion" (discrimination ellipses), which allows evaluation damage along areas of impairment instead of axes of damage. This strategy has been applied successfully in early glaucoma and might show good promise in diabetes even in pre-retinopathy stages. Figure 3.15 shows a four-fold enlarged chromatic discrimination ellipse in a patient with diabetes but no apparent signs of diabetic retinopathy.

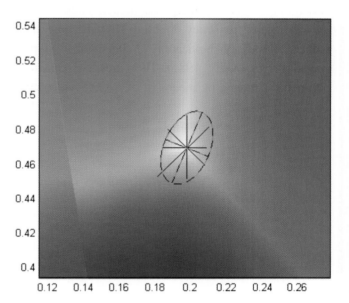

**Fig. 3.15.** Chromatic discrimination ellipse (raw discrimination vectors and fitted ellipses) taken from a subject with diabetes in a pre-retinopathy stage. The large ellipse corresponds to increased color "confusion area" and impaired performance. Black solid lines: measured color axes. Curved solid line: fitted ellipse. Green dotted lines: fitted ellipse axes. Color rendering (which is only approximate in the printed version) is based on the IEC1996 2.1 standard, with the white point set to the white point of the test and the monitor gamut set to the gamut of our SONY GDM-F520 monitor equipped with Trinitron phosphors. Parameters extracted from fitted ellipse were as follows: Length, 0.0443; Axis ratio, 1.716; Angle, 67.7°. Trivector (P, D and T) results: 0.019, 0.010, 0.021, which were all abnormal.

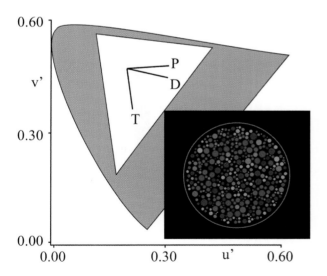

**Fig. 3.14.** *Right* inset: Schematic illustration of the luminance noise stimulus. The Landolt C shape is visible due to the presence of high chromatic contrast in this image. *Left graph* depicts axes (confusion lines in CIE 1976 u′ v′ color space) along which color contrast is modulated, in order to study cone function human subjects. P: protan; D: Deutan and T: Tritan axes (corresponding to L, M and S cones).

We are currently also assessing achromatic contrast discrimination within the magnocellular system using a perimetric strategy. Retinal damage is assessed using frequency-doubling (FD) stimuli that preferentially activate a subset of neurons within the magnocellular dorsal pathway. These FD stimuli are used as detection targets in contrast sensitivity (CS) measurements performed in multiple locations in visual space. We have recently generated a database FD-CS thresholds using a custom-based approach that is comparable to commercially available 30-2 and N-30-F frequency-doubling perimetry.

In our both custom-based approach and N-30-F perimetric strategy, inducing stimuli are patches of 0.25 cyc/deg vertically oriented sinusoidal gratings, undergoing 25 Hz counterphase flicker. These stimuli are labeled as frequency-doubling (FD) because they induce an illusory duplication of the number of perceived stripes (Kelly, 1981). They are generated in a perimetric strategy, by means of a VSG2/5 video card (Cambridge Research Systems, Rochester, UK) and displayed on a gamma-corrected 21 inch Trinitron Sony GDM-F520 color monitor (frame rate 100 Hz). Figure 3.16 shows the results for a normal control subject. Figure 3.17 shows the results of such a FD strategy for the same patient that showed impaired chromatic discrimination illustrated in Fig. 3.15. Figures 3.17–3.22 show that diabetic patients often have significantly changed contrast thresholds in many visual field locations, even in the absence of retinopathy. These preliminary findings suggest strong early involvement of the magnocellular pathway in diabetes, which may occur concomitantly to damage of chromatic pathways.

## 3.5.2. Classical Electrophysiological Findings in Diabetic Retinopathy

Diabetic retinopathy is often focal in its nature, which renders standard electrophysiological methods that

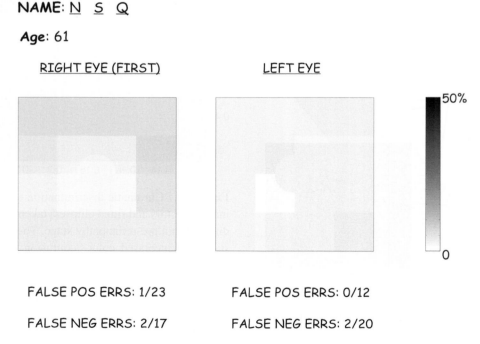

**Fig. 3.16.** Perimetric assessment of achromatic contrast sensitivity of a control subject with normal ophthalmological examination, using a frequency doubling strategy (FDT) that determined % threshold contrast in different regions of the visual field. Darker regions in gray scale plots correspond to higher contrast thresholds. Stimuli were patches of 0.25 cyc/deg vertically oriented sinusoidal gratings, undergoing 25 Hz counterphase flicker. These stimuli are labeled as frequency-doubling (FD) because they induce an illusory duplication of the number of perceived stripes.

NAME: J C P

Age: 74

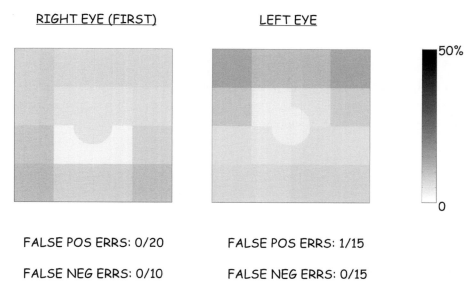

RIGHT EYE (FIRST)    LEFT EYE

FALSE POS ERRS: 0/20     FALSE POS ERRS: 1/15

FALSE NEG ERRS: 0/10     FALSE NEG ERRS: 0/15

**Figs. 3.17–3.23.** Perimetric assessment of achromatic contrast sensitivity in patients with diabetes. All patients were in pre-retinopathy stage, except the one whose performance is depicted in Fig. 3.21 (with nonproliferative diabetic retinopathy).

NAME: A J J O

Age: 46

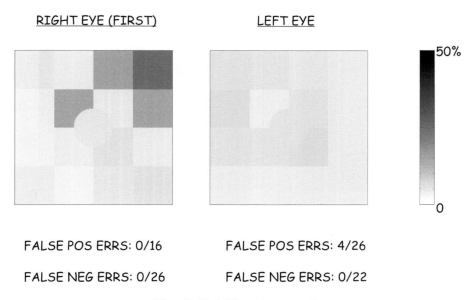

RIGHT EYE (FIRST)    LEFT EYE

FALSE POS ERRS: 0/16     FALSE POS ERRS: 4/26

FALSE NEG ERRS: 0/26     FALSE NEG ERRS: 0/22

**Figs. 3.17–3.23.** *(Continued)*

**NAME:** <u>M</u> <u>A</u> <u>G</u> C

**Age:** 69

RIGHT EYE          LEFT EYE (FIRST)

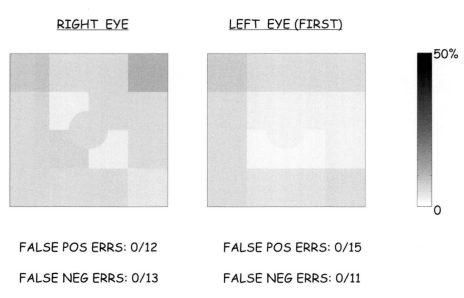

FALSE POS ERRS: 0/12          FALSE POS ERRS: 0/15

FALSE NEG ERRS: 0/13          FALSE NEG ERRS: 0/11

**Figs. 3.17–3.23.** (*Continued*)

**NAME:** <u>S</u> <u>L</u>

**Age:** 22

RIGHT EYE (FIRST)          LEFT EYE

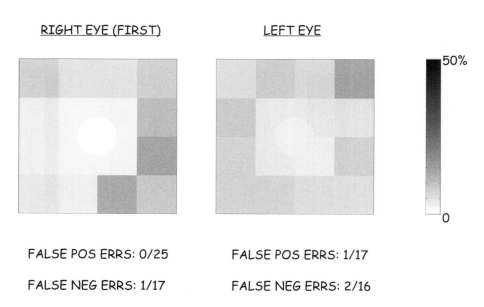

FALSE POS ERRS: 0/25          FALSE POS ERRS: 1/17

FALSE NEG ERRS: 1/17          FALSE NEG ERRS: 2/16

**Figs. 3.17–3.23.** (*Continued*)

NAME: J  S  B

Age: 64

RIGHT EYE (FIRST)              LEFT EYE

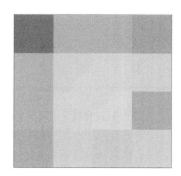 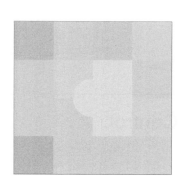 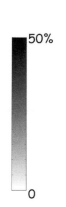

FALSE POS ERRS: 0/25          FALSE POS ERRS: 1/17

FALSE NEG ERRS: 1/17          FALSE NEG ERRS: 2/16

**Figs. 3.17–3.23.**    (*Continued*)

NAME: I  A  L

Age: 60

RIGHT EYE (FIRST)              LEFT EYE

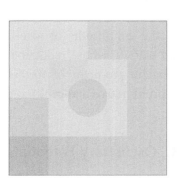 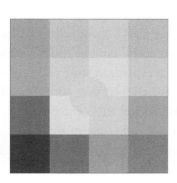 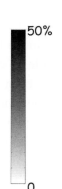

FALSE POS ERRS: 1/13          FALSE POS ERRS: 0/13

FALSE NEG ERRS: 0/21          FALSE NEG ERRS: 0/16

**Figs. 3.17–3.23.**    (*Continued*)

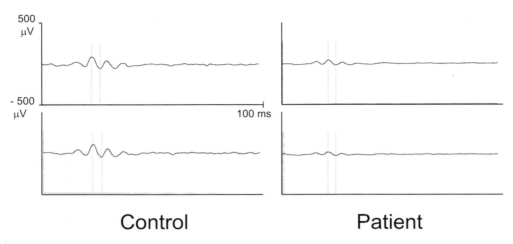

Figs. 3.17–3.23. (*Continued*)

measure the global response of retinal photoreceptors, such as the flash electroretinogram (ERG), rather unpromising approaches. For these reason, conflicting reports have emerged in the literature, some describing significant differences (Juen and Kieselbach, 1990; Bresnick, 1991; Holopigian *et al.*, 1992) and others not (Jenkins and Cartwright, 1990). The reduction of the b wave of the conventional ERG is often reported only for advanced cases, and more sensitive results can only be obtained with the calculation of intensity-response functions, which are of limited clinical applicability. Variations of these methods, such as the relation between photopic and scotopic b waves in the adapto-electroretinogram or changes in response latencies in 30 Hz flicker ERG, have been suggested as capable of detecting early damage, but they have so far not been widely accepted. In spite of the limitations as mentioned, it is believed that both the amplitude and timing of 30 Hz flicker ERG waveforms are good indicators of the ischemic state of the retina, flicker ERG being abnormal in up to 85% of the patients with proliferative retinopathy (Bresnick and Palta, 1987).

There is an ongoing search of measures capable of detecting earlier dysfunction. Recent candidates concerning parametric evaluation have included amplitude and delay of oscillatory potentials, pattern-ERG, scotopic threshold response (STR), and more recently, the multifocal ERG. The STR (Sieving *et al.*, 1986) is a near absolute psychophysical threshold response that may therefore represent responses solely from the rod pathway. This response has a likely postsynaptic origin between the inner plexiform layer and the ganglion cell layer (Frishman *et al.*, 1988).

In summary, despite the mentioned difficulties, it has been shown that even standard ERG methods are often capable of detecting electrophysiological damage well before the detection of any sign of vascular damage. Furthermore, the evolution of electrophysiological markers has shown good correlation with fundoscopic and angiographic criteria of severity of the retinopathy. This has been the case, in particular the case for the amplitude of oscillatory potentials (discussed below), whose reduction has proved to be an independent predictor of further deterioration of both non-proliferative and proliferative retinopathy.

### 3.5.3. Oscillatory Potentials (OPs)

These are high frequency responses (100–160 Hz) which are superimposed on the ascending limb of the bwave (Yonemura, 1962; Wachtmeister and Dowling, 1978), and seem to be changed by early retinal dysfunction in diabetes. They are a signature of the involvement of the inner retinal layers, since they are thought to originate in the inner plexiform layer, namely from inhibitory circuits connecting amacrine and ganglion cells.

OPs are usually taken as good indicators of the extent of retinal ischemia and may be reduced at all stages of diabetic retinopathy, with a good correlation with severity, especially during the proliferative stages (Fig. 3.23). A reduced amplitude of OPs implies a several-fold risk of evolution to retinopathy. Simonsen *et al.* (1975) conducted a long-term follow-up study of OP amplitudes in a population of diabetic patients with nonproliferative diabetic retinopathy, and could show that of the 129 eyes with normal OP amplitudes at the start of the study, five developed proliferative diabetic retinopathy, in striking contrast with the 38 out of 51 eyes with reduced OP amplitudes which developed proliferative diabetic retinopathy.

Bresnick and colleagues (1984, 1985, 1987) confirmed and extended these results, by showing that OP amplitude predicts progression (independently from predictors taken from fundus photography and fluorescein angiography) of eyes with nonproliferative diabetic retinopathy or mild proliferative diabetic retinopathy to severe proliferative diabetic retinopathy. Eyes with abnormal OP amplitudes had a steady rate of progression to severe proliferation (28% after one year, and 52% after two years). Eyes with normal OPs had a much lower rate of progression (0 and 7%, respectively).

Other authors have, however (e.g. Wanger and Persson, 1985), questioned these changes, probably due to the high intra- and interindividual variability of OP measurements.

Peak latencies of OPs may represent a better marker of damage than amplitudes, since they are changed earlier (Shirao and Kawasaki, 1998). This has been well documented in rats with streptozotocin-induced diabetes, with changes of the latency of the second peak of OPs occurring as early as two weeks after induction, which suggests that direct neuropathy may occur, concomitantly to the angiopathy (Shirao and Kawasaki, 1998).

### 3.5.4. Pattern ERG

Pattern ERG is a useful method to assess the function of retinal ganglion cells, which explains its wide use in the assessment of glaucoma and other optic neuropathies. In diabetes, it has been suggested that PERG produces less variable measurements than OPs (Arden *et al.*, 1986), which might render this strategy more clinically useful, given that amplitudes were changed under the presence of cotton-wool spots and ischemia as documented by angiography (for opposite results, see Jenkins and Cartwright, 1990 and Wanger and Persson, 1985).

### 3.5.5. Multifocal Electrophysiology

Multifocal electroretinography (mfERG; Sutter and Tran, 1992) provides functional topographic detail that overcomes the disadvantages of conventional electrophysiology. Objective measurement of retinal dysfunction simultaneously at multiple locations, by means of this technique, is now being increasingly used in diabetes research. Sutter and Tran pioneered this field and have also introduced new methods for response amplitude estimation such as the scalar product method. In this method, a template for the response waveform is normalized to a root-mean-square amplitude of one. The amplitude of a local response waveform is estimated by multiplying it, data point by corresponding data point, with the matching template and summing of all the products. The matching template consists of the average of traces that contain approximately the same response waveform.

Electrophysiological local amplitude changes and delays have been found in the retinas of diabetic patients with or without retinopathy, both in regional and local averages (Palmowski *et al.*, 1997; Fortune *et al.*, 1999; Scholl and Zrenner, 2000; Bearse *et al.*, 2004.) This promising technique is, however, still largely exploratory. It is believed that second-order responses of mERG should be more useful in diabetes since they are better related with responses of the inner-retina (Palmowski, 1997), but first-order responses have also been shown to be useful in detecting early diabetic retinopathy (Fortune *et al.*, 1999). New variants of the mfERG, such as the slow-flash technique (Bearse, 1994), have also been tested as a potential clinical tool in the future.

Multiple prospective analyses of local mfERGs should now confirm functional abnormalities in eyes with diabetic retinopathy, both in retinal regions corresponding to retinopathy and in areas without signs of it (Fortune *et al.*, 1999; Bearse *et al.*, 2004). Along the same line, it has been found that mfERG implicit time delays are associated with retinal locations in which new nonproliferative diabetic retinopathy (NPDR) will develop one year later (Han *et al.*, 2004). All these promising results suggest that mfERG will become a pivotal technique for the study of neural impairment in the diabetic retina.

### 3.5.6. Future Directions

Current electrophysiological and psychophysical methods should probably be combined in the future with current electrophysiological approaches to study cone function and color vision. Given the abovementioned solid evidence supporting early and substantial damage of the blue-cone pathway in diabetes (see also Roth and Lanthony, 1999; Grange, 1995; Weiner *et al.*, 1997), some groups have attempted electrophysiological characterization of chromatic responses in diabetic retinopathy. (Yamamoto *et al.*, 1996; Greenstein *et al.*, 1989) It was found that even in diabetes without retinopathy, S-cone amplitudes may be significantly reduced. Given that cone function is predominant in the macula, extending this approach in the future may be helpful in improving the assessment of macular damage in diabetes.

It is still unclear what the neural pathways more commonly impaired in diabetic retinopathy are, how early they are affected, and how specific patterns of functional deficits evolve during disease progression.

Newly developed psychophysical and electrophysiological methods have the advantage that they can provide improved isolation of different pathways. These sensitive tools will allow the documentation of retinal impairment, including optimal detection of dysfunction before the appearance of clinically evident retinopathy.

The value of techniques that attempt to assess separately distinct functional channels has been emphasized by studies that have shown substantial contrast sensitivity deficits for high spatial frequencies, which suggests involvement of the parvocellular pathway. We have extended these findings into the magnocellular domain, by showing strongly reduced contrast sensitivity within the magnocellular stream, both in the macula and visual periphery, even in the pre-retinopathy stage. It is an open question whether these neurosensory deficits are primary, although the prevailing view for parvocelullar deficits is that they might be related to changes in the macular microvasculature. (Remky *et al.*, 2000)

Color vision quantitative assessment methods can detect visual dysfunction in diabetic patients with good acuity in the presence of maculopathy. Our own studies have confirmed that substantial chromatic discrimination impairment may be found in diabetic patients even in the absence of retinopathy.

It will become important in the future to better understand the physiology of the perifoveal area, since changes in the microvasculature in this region may be predictive of visual outcome. Accordingly, an enlarged foveal avascular zone occurs even in the absence of overt macular edema and in the presence of normal visual acuity. Later on, in advanced diabetic disease, reduction of capillary density is correlated with decreased acuity. Functional psychophysical losses should be correlated with measures of the disruption of the blood-retinal barrier. This philosophy of correlating independent structural and measures may help improve strategies that aim to assess early damage. Short-wavelength automated perimetry may show some promise in detecting early damage in diabetic retinopathy due to the particular susceptibility of short-wavelength sensitive cones to ischemic and phototoxic damage.

Psychophysical strategies must be compared with flash and pattern ERG measurements as well as with the objective measurement of retinal dysfunction simultaneously at multiple locations, by means of flash multifocal electroretinography (mfERG). This technique has shown some promise in detecting amplitude changes and delays in the retinas of diabetic patients with or without retinopathy. Multifocal electrophysiology of oscillatory potentials may also provide a promising avenue to investigate neural function of the retinal circuitry in the context of diabetic retinopathy.

# References

Amemiya T. (1977) Dark adaptation in diabetics. *Ophthalmologica* **174**: 322–326.

Arden GB, Hamilton AM, Wilson-Holt J, *et al.* (1986) Pattern electroretinograms become abnormal when background diabetic retinopathy deteriorates to a pre-proliferative stage: Possible use as a screening test. *Br J Ophthalmol* **70**: 330–335.

Arden GB, Wolf JE, Tsang Y. (1998) Does dark adaptation exacerbate diabetic retinopathy? Evidence and a linking hypothesis. *Vision Res* **38**: 1723–1729.

Arend O, Wolf S, Harris A, Reim M. (1995) The relationship of macular microcirculation to visual acuity in diabetic patients. *Arch. Ophthalmol.* **75**: 610–614.

Bearse, MA, Schneck ME, Adams AJ. (2004) Retinal function in normal and diabetic eyes mapped with the slow flash multifocal electroretinogram. *Inv Ophthalmol Vis Science* **45**(1): 296–304.

Bearse MA, Shimada Y, Sutter EE. (2000) Distribution of oscillatory components in the central retina. *Doc Ophthalmol* **100**: 185–205.

Bresnick GH. (1991) Diabetic Retinopathy, in Heckenlively JR, Arden GB (eds): Principles and Practice of Clinical Electrophysiologyof Vision. *St Louis Mosby Year Book*, pp. 619–635.

Bresnick GH, Condit RS, Palta M, *et al.* (1985) Association of hue discrimination loss and diabetic retinopathy. *Arch Ophthalmol* **103**: 1317–1324.

Bresnick GH, Korth K, Groo A, Palta M. (1984) Electroretinographic oscillatory potentials predict progression of diabetic retinopathy. *Arch Ophthalmol* **102**: 1307–1311.

Bresnick GH, Palta M. (1987a) Temporal aspects of the electroretinogram in diabetic retinopathy. *Arch Ophthalmol* **105**: 660–664.

Bresnick GH, Palta M. (1987b) Predicting progression to severe proliferative diabetic retinopathy. *Arch Ophthalmol* **105**: 810–814.

Castelo-Branco M, Faria P, Forjaz V, *et al.* (2004) Early and late damage of parvo and koniocellular function in ocular hypertension and glaucoma. *Inv Ophtalmol Vis Sci* 499–504.

Campos SH, Forjaz V, Kozak LR, *et al.* (2004) Chromatic dysfunction in Best's macular dystrophy: New quantitative strategies for improval of clinical staging. *Arch Ophthalmol.* In Press

Chakrabarti S, Cukiernik M, Hileeto D, *et al.* (2000) Role of vasoactive factors in the pathogenesis of early changes in diabetic retinopathy. *Diabetes Metab Res Ver* **16**: 393–407.

Ciulla TA, Amador AG, Zinman B. (2003) Diabetic retinopathy and diabetic macular edema. Pathophysiology, screening and novel therapies. *Diabetes Care* **26**: 2653–2664.

Curcio C, Millican L, Allen K, Kalina R. (1993) Aging of the human photoreceptor mosaic: Evidence for selective vulnerability of rods in central retina. *Invest Ophthalmol Vis Sci* **34**: 3278–3296.

Fortune B, Schneck ME, Adams AJ. (1999) Multifocal electroretinogram delays reveal local retinal dysfunction in early diabetic retinopathy. *Invest Ophthalmol Vis Sci* **40**(11): 2638–2651.

Fortune B, Wang L, Bui BV, *et al.* (2003) Local ganglion cell contributions to the macaque electroretinogram revealed by experimental nerve fiber layer bundle defect. *Invest Ophthalmol Vis Sci* **44**: 4567–4579.

Fortune B, Bearse MA, Cioffi GA, Johnson CA. (2002) Selective loss of an oscillatory component from temporal retinal multifocal ERG responses in glaucoma. *Invest Ophthalmol Vis Sci* **43**: 2638–2647.

Frisen FM. (1976) A simple relationship between the probability distribution of visual acuity and the density of retinal output channels. *Acta Ophthalmol* **54**: 437–444.

Frishman L, Sieving PA, Steinberg RH. (1988) Contributions to the electroretinogram of currents originating in proximal retina. *Vis Neurosci* **1**: 307–315.

Frishman LJ, Saszik S, Harwerth RS, *et al.* (2000) Effects of experimental glaucoma in macaques on the multifocal ERG: Multifocal ERG in laser-induced glaucoma. *Doc Ophthalmol* **100**: 231–251.

Grange JD. (1995) La Rétinopathie Diabétique, In: Grange JD (ed.), Masson, Paris of Vision, Mosby Year Book, *St Louis* 1991, pp. 643–645.

Green FD, Ghafour IM, Allan D, *et al.* (1985) Color vision of diabetics. *Br J Ophthalmol* **69**: 533–536.

Greenstein VC, Hood DC, Ritch R, *et al.* (1989) S (blue) cone pathway vulnerability in retinitis pigmentosa, diabetes and glaucoma. *Invest Ophthalmol Vis Sci* **30**: 1732–1737.

Greenstein VC, Holopigian K, Hood DC, *et al.* (2000) The nature and extent of retinal dysfunction associated with diabetic macular edema. *Invest Ophthalmol Vis Sci* **41**: 3643–3654.

Greenstein VC, Thomas SR, Blaustein H, *et al.* (1993) Effects of early diabetic retinopathy on rod system sensitivity. *Optom Vis Sci* **37**: 1140–1148.

Han Y, Bearse MA, Schneck ME, *et al.* (2004) Multifocal electroretinogram delays predict sites of subsequent diabetic retinopathy. *Invest Ophthalmol Vis Sci* **45**: 948–954.

Hare WA, Ton H. (2002) Effects of APB, PDA, and TTX on ERG responses recorded using both multifocal and conventional methods in monkey: Effects of APB, PDA, and TTX on monkey ERG responses. *Doc Ophthalmol* **105**: 189–222.

Henson DB, North R. (1979) Dark adaptation in diabetes mellitus. *Br J Ophthalmol* **63**: 539–541.

Holopigian K, Seiple W, Lorenzo M, Carr R. (1992) A comparison of photopic and scotopic electroretinographic changes in early diabetic retinopathy. *Invest Ophthalmol Vis Sci* **33**: 2773–2780.

Hood DC, Seiple W, Holopigian K, Greenstein V. (1997) A comparison of the components of the multifocal and full-field ERGs. *Vis Neurosci* **14**: 533–544.

Hood DC, Frishman LJ, Viswanathan S, *et al.* (1999) Evidence for a ganglion cell contribution to the primate electroretinogram (ERG): Effects of TTX on the multifocal ERG in macaque. *Vis Neurosci* **16**: 411–416.

Hood DC, Frishman LJ, Saszik S, Viswanathan S. (2002) Retinal origins of the primate multifocal ERG: Implications for the human response. *Invest Ophthalmol Vis Sci* **43**: 1673–1685.

Hood DC, Zhang X. (2000) Multifocal ERG and VEP responses and visual fields: Comparing disease-related changes. *Doc Ophthalmol* **100**(2–3): 115–137.

Kurtenbach A, Langrova E, Zrenner E. (2000) Multifocal oscillatory potentials in type 1 diabetes without retinopathy. *Invest Ophthalmol Vis Sci* **41**(10): 3234–3241.

Jenkins TC, Cartwright JP. (1990) The electroretinogram in minimal diabetic retinopathy. *Br J Ophthalmol* **74**: 681–684.

Juen S, Kieselbach GF. (1990) Electrophysiological changes in juvenile diabetics without retinopathy. *Arch Ophthalmol* **108**: 372–375.

Miyake Y, Shiroyama N, Horiguchi M, Ota I. (1989) Asymmetry of focal ERG in human macular region. *Invest Ophthalmol Vis Sci* **30**: 1743–1749.

Onozu H, Yamamoto S. (2003) Oscillatory components of multifocal electroretinogram in diabetic retinopathy. *Doc Ophthalmol* **106**: 327–332.

Osterberg G. (1935) Topography of the layer of rods and cones in the human retina. *Acta Ophthalmol* **6**(suppl): 1–102.

Palmowski AM, Sutter EE, Bearse MA, Fung W. (1997) Mapping of retinal function in diabetic retinopathy using the multifocal electroretinogram. *Invest Ophthalmol Vis Sci* **38**: 2586–2596.

Poloschek CM, Sutter EE. (2002) The fine structure of multifocal ERG topographies. *J Vis* **2**(8): 577–587.

Rangaswamy NV, Hood DC, Frishman LJ. (2003) Regional variations in local contributions to the primate photopic flash ERG: Revealed using the slow-sequence mfERG. *Invest Ophthalmol Vis Sci* **44**: 3233–3247.

Regan D, Neima D. (1984) Low-contrast letter charts in early diabetic retinopathy, ocular hypertension, glaucoma, and Parkinson's disease. *Br J Ophthalmol* **68**: 885–889.

Remky A, Arend O, Hendricks S. (2000) Short-wavelength automated perimetry and capillary density in early diabetic maculopathy. *Invest Ophthalmol Vis Sci* **41**(1): 274–281.

Roth A, Lanthony P. (1999) Vision des couleurs. In: Risse JF (ed.), *Exploration de la Fonction Visuelle*, Masson, Paris, pp. 129–151.

Scholl H, Zrenner E. (2000) Electrophysiology in the investigation of acquired retinal disorders. *Surv Ophthalmol* **45**(1): 29–47.

Skrandies W, Baier M. (1986) The standing potential of the human retina. *Vision Res* **26**: 577–581.

Simonsen SE. (1975) Prognostic value of ERG (oscillatory potential) in juvenile diabetics. *Acta Ophthalmol* **123**: 223–224.

Sokol S, Moskowitz A, Skarf B, Evans R, *et al.* (1985) Contrast sensitivity in diabetics with and without background retinopathy. *Arch Ophthalmol* **103**: 51–54.

Sperling HG. (1991) Vulnerability of the blue-sensitive mechanism. In: Foster D (ed.), *Inherited and Acquired Colour Vision Deficiencies: Fundamental Aspects on Clinical Studies.* Macmillan, London, 72–87.

Sieving PA, Frishman LJ, Steinberg RH. (1986) Scotopic threshold response of proximal retina in cat. *J Neurophysiol* **56**: 1049–1061.

Shirao Y, Kawasaki K. (1998) Electrical responses from diabetic retina. *Prog Ret Eye Res* **17**: 59–76.

Sutter EE, Tran D. (1992) The field topography of ERG components in man-I. The photopic luminance response. *Vision Res* **32**: 433–446.

Tzekov R, Arden GB. (1999) The electroretinogram in diabetic retinopathy. *Surv Ophthalmol* **44**: 53–60.

Wachtmeister L, Dowling JE. (1978) The oscillatory potentials of the mudpuppy retina. *Invest Ophthalmol Vis Sci* **17**: 1176–1188.

Wanger P, Persson HE. (1985) Early diagnosis of retinal changes in diabetes: A comparison between electroretinography and retinal biomicroscopy. *Acta Ophthalmol (Copenh)* **63**: 716–20.

Weiner A, Christopoulos VA, Gussler CH, Adams DH, *et al.* (1997) Foveal cone function in nonproliferative diabetic retinopathy and macular edema. *Invest Ophthalmol Vis Sci* **38**: 1443–1449.

Wu S, Sutter EE. (1995) A topographic study of oscillatory potentials in man. *Vis Neurosci* **12**: 1013–1025.

Yonemura D. (1962) The oscillatory potential of the electroretinogram. *Acta Soc Ophthalmol* Jpn **66**: 1566–1584.

Yamamoto S, Kamiyama M, Nitta K. *et al.* (1996) Selective reduction of the S cone electroretinogram in diabetes. *Br J Ophthalmol* **80**: 973–975.

## Abbreviations

| | |
|---|---|
| OPs | oscillatory potentials; |
| mfVEP | multifocal visual evoked potentials; |
| mfERG | multifocal electroretinogram; |
| SWAP | short-wavelength perimetry; |
| FDT | frequency-doubling perimetry. |

## 3.6. Multimodal Macula Mapping

### Rui Bernardes, Conceição Lobo and José Cunha-Vaz

There is currently a variety of diagnostic tools and techniques to examine the macular region and to obtain information on its structure and function. The different methods available offer different perspectives and fragmentary information. Multimodal Macula Mapping aims to combine different methodologies and to obtain maps of the alterations occurring in the macular region in health and in different stages of disease, and therefore to establish correlation between the fragmentary pieces of information and so to build the complete puzzle (Bernardes *et al.*, 2002).

Digital imaging, fluorescence measurement and new optical devices, are just a few of the possible data sources that can be integrated into a map of the macula. The treatment of this complex information requires additional instrumentation beyond that of the detector. The volume of data that can be acquired, the speed at which it is analyzed and the treatment of the signals needed for interpretation, depend on the computer. The complexity of the registration for the large number of modalities, as well as their differences in the imaging acquisition systems, sensors included, presents a quite large and complex number of questions to be addressed.

The use of color, contours, and other visual signals to differentiate differences in thickness, visual function, capillary density, alteration in vascular permeability, and other attributes of structures or function should produce holistic views of the retina.

Available maps of the macula, obtained either from digital imaging, fluorescence measurements, electrophysiological potentials, or using a variety of other optical devices, have different degrees of spatial resolution. Generally, spatial resolution has been determined by the kind of detector used to collect the data.

Increasing the field of view typically results in lower spatial resolution. Similarly, increasing the temporal resolution, by decreasing the acquisition time, results in loss of image quality due to eye movements. Spatial resolution is clearly fundamental for a useful map of the macula.

Maps that present correlative, multimodality or otherwise derived data can greatly extend the map usefulness beyond that available from the individual sources alone and therefore possess a tremendous potential.

### 3.6.1. Imaging Systems

From the wealth of imaging systems, the one most used is the photography modality. Although being probably the simplest of the medical image modalities, it can be of color or gray scale type, thus conveying different information. A digital image may be defined as a sampled and quantized function in two dimensions, sampled in equally spaced grid (most common) and uniformly quantized (most common).

Nevertheless, images can be functions of higher order dimensions and produced by different means, containing and conveying different information and being sampled in different coordinating systems. Images represent in this away the imaged object, although typically conveying less information than represented by the original imaged object.

Digital images are composed of individual elements, pixels for 2D images and voxels for volumes.

Each picture's element, either pixel or voxel is represented by a value measured or computed by the acquisition system.

In medical imaging systems, the pixel/voxel values do not represent structural information but a measure that indicates the behavior of some function, e.g. using a confocal scanning laser ophthalmoscope, which primarily acquires the fluorescence level for a set of confocal planes, performing a set of computing steps, it is possible to compute the permeability of the blood-retinal barrier, i.e. it is possible to compute the function image that indicates a function of a particular structure and not the structure itself.

### 3.6.2. Multimodal Macula Mapping. Integration of Information and Representation

A map improves our representation of an object and helps to place in the right location additional information contributing to a progressive reconstruction of the same object. It is a way of organizing data, representing it, and communicating results.

The challenge of mapping in general lies in the need for appropriate presentation strategies to convey the pertinent information without obscuring other data, reference systems suitable for equating the map with the real object, and a product that is compatible with its intended use.

### 3.6.3. Multimodal Macula Mapping

Detection devices for obtaining information for macula mapping are numerous and varied, often complementing one another with differing degrees of invasiveness, accuracy and object of measurement. Some chart anatomy, whereas others measure an aspect of physiology. Together, they can combine structure and function. Our research group has been developing methods to combine and integrate data from fundus photography, angiographic images (scanning laser ophthalmoscope — fluorescein angiography), maps of fluorescein leakage into the vitreous (scanning laser ophthalmoscopy — retinal leakage analyzer), maps of retinal thickness and maps of visual function (automated perimetry — Humphrey Field Analyzer HFA II 750) of the macular area to achieve multimodal macula mapping (Lobo *et al.*, 1999; Lobo *et al.*, 2000; Bernardes *et al.*, 2002). Scanning laser ophthalmoscopy (SLO) produces high-resolution images using much less light for illumination of the fundus than that used for conventional photography. High contrast images of the foveal and perifoveal structures are produced with this technique using directly reflected light. In confocal scanning laser ophthalmoscopy, a laser beam illuminates an area of the eyes fundus. A confocal stop placed in front of the detector rejects most the light coming from both the

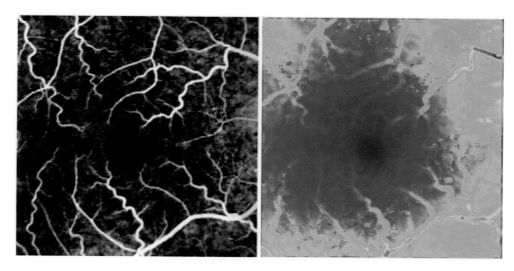

**Fig. 3.24.** Macula from a patient with diabetes type 2. *Left*: fluorescein angiography obtained by a scanning laser ophthalmoscope. *Right*: Retinal Leakage Analyzer blood-retinal barrier permeability map (RLmap) in a false color-code map.

anterior and posterior planes. A set of moving mirrors allows the scanning of an area of interest. In SLO imaging, a laser beam illuminates an area of the ocular fundus, forming a rectangular pattern (raster) on the retina. The light reflected from each retinal point is captured by the detector. Thus, a point-by-point video image is constructed, with each retinal point corresponding to a point on the monitor screen. SLO, because of its monochromatic wavelength emission, minimizes scattering and chromatic aberration. This feature of SLO increases contrast and improves visibility as compared with slit-lamp biomiscrocopy and fundus photography.

SLO can also be used to perform high-resolution fluorescein angiographies. The contrast of the images allows acquisition of high-quality morphological information on the retinal vasculature. A system combining SLO with Doppler flowmetry provides non-invasive evaluation of regional blood flow. We have been able to develop the Retinal Leakage Analyzer (RLA), for measuring and mapping the permeability of the BRB based on a SLO system (Lobo *et al.*, 1999; Bernardes *et al.*, 2005). The combination of two data sets, angiographic and permeability mapping, obtained simultaneously using the same instrumentation, provided a set of landmark references of the macula, giving simultaneously functional and morphological information (Fig. 3.24), and was in this

way an important step in the development of multi-modal mapping.

To integrate the information from the above sources, a common reference has to be established. The reference fundus image may be given by the RLA or by fundus digital images.

We have been able to combine in multimodal macula mapping, information on structure and function by integrating data from fluorescein angiography, retinal leakage analysis, retinal thickness analysis and visual perimetry (Fig. 3.25). Other available detection devices that may be used for macula mapping include laser Doppler retinal flowmetry using the Heidelberg Retina Flowmeter, indocyanine green angiography (ICG), electrophysiology (ERG), autofluorescence mapping and Optical Coherence Tomography. Each one of these methods adds more information and appears as potentially valuable tools for evaluating the structure and function of the retinal macula.

More recently we were able to integrate color fundus photography, leakage analysis and mfERG using deformable models to correct for deformations due to saccadics during data acquisition (Fig. 3.26).

When examining diabetic macular edema, OCT and HRF methodologies become particularly interesting especially when diabetic macular edema is associated with some degree of vision loss. The HRF

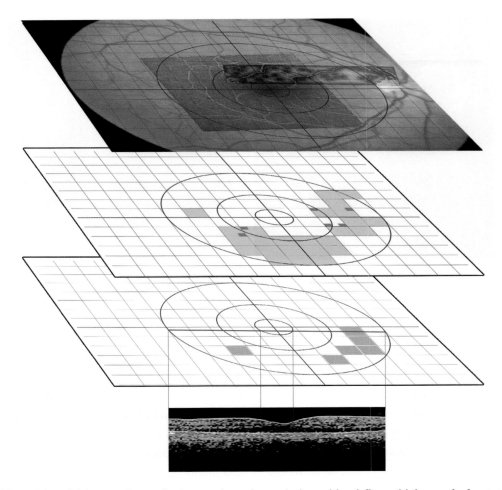

**Fig. 3.25.** This multimodal image shows the integration of morphology, blood flow, thickness, leakage, visual function and OCT cross-section image as a stack of images. The top image contains information on morphology (color fundus photograph plus SLO fluorescein angiography) and flow measurements. The second shows thickness changes (yellow areas) and identifies leaking sites (green spots). The third represents visual field changes (shaded areas). Finally, in the bottom, the OCT cross-sectional image.

appears to be particularly useful and reliable for following changes in capillary perfusion in the macular area and we are examining its value to indicate progression of ischemia.

### 3.6.4. Contribution to the Evaluation of Diabetic Retinopathy

A key issue when dealing with medical images and for medical purposes consists of extracting more information than the one provided by the traditional approaches in a particular field or gain access to the same information in a faster and/or reliable way. Multimodal macula mapping fits in the first category, i.e. it allows for the extraction of more information than the one provided by each modality when seen independently. The clinical interest and usability of such a technique of correlating different imaging modalities is evident in different studies performed involving diabetic patients.

One example is the application of multimodal macula mapping to study diabetic eyes with preclinical retinopathy, looking for changes that may be present before overt ophthalmoscopic retinopathy develops (Lobo *et al.*, 2000). Abnormal increases in fluorescein

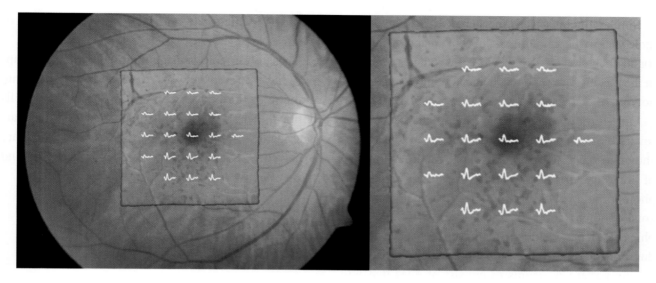

**Fig. 3.26.**  Deformable image registration between color fundus photograph (background image), leakage analysis (retinal leakage analyzer) (central squared area) and multifocal electroretinogram (mfERG) (curve responses in white). Global (*left*) and zoomed (*right*) view for details. Please note the deformation on the leakage map, which is due to saccadics during the scanning laser acquisition for leakage analysis. Although not visible, mfERG is also corrected for this intrinsic deformation.

leakage were present at some time during the follow-up in 90% of examined eyes and abnormal increases in retinal thickness were found in 70% of the eyes examined, even though no other abnormalities were visible in the retina or detected by ophthalmoscopy or 7-field stereofundus photography. These findings have clear clinical value, since increased retinal fluorescein leakage identifies an alteration of the BRB and increased retinal thickness characterizes the presence of retinal edema. Retinal edema, the major cause of visual loss in people with type 2 diabetes, has often been associated in the retina with an alteration of the BRB. This study indicates that in the initial stages of diabetic retinal disease, breakdown of the BRB and retinal tissue thickening may occur simultaneously, either with each other or independently. The BRB damage may modulate and play a role in the development of retinal tissue thickening, but the opposite is also a possibility.

Another study involving diabetic patients with type 2 diabetes mellitus and mild nonproliferative retinopathy followed during one year showed the interest of the use of multimodal macula mapping technique (Lobo *et al.*, 2001). It allows correlations to be established between fundus lesions, localized alterations of the BRB identified by mapping fluorescein leakage into the vitreous, and changes in retinal thickness.

The most frequent alterations observed were, in decreasing order of frequency, RLA-leaking sites, areas of increased retinal thickness, microaneurysms, and drusen. A particularly interesting observation in this study is the widespread presence of increased retinal thickness, i.e. retinal edema. Our findings offer some insight into the mechanisms of the development of retinal edema in the initial stages of diabetic retinopathy. The location of RLA-leaking sites appears to be predictive of the later development in the same location of areas of increased retinal thickness. An alteration of the BRB appears, therefore, to be associated with the development of diabetic retinal edema, at least at this stage of retinopathy.

It was suggested that the dominant alterations in the retina of patients with type 2 diabetes mellitus and mild nonproliferative retinopathy is the presence of RLA-leaking sites, indicating spotty retinal vascular damage characterized by alteration of the BRB. The spotty retinal vascular damage appears to be reversible and directly associated with variation in metabolic glicemic control.

Similar findings were registered in a follow-up of three years, where multimodal macula mapping allowed for an integrated view of the different changes occurring in the macular area and made apparent three major phenotypes of diabetic retinopathy, (Lobo *et al.*, 2004).

One group of patients included eyes with reversible and little abnormal fluorescein leakage, as shown in successive retinal leakage maps, a slow rate of microaneurysm formation identified on fundus photograph images and a normal foveal avascular zone contour demonstrated on fluorescein angiographies. Patients included in this group had a longer duration of their diabetes. This group designated as having pattern A, seems to consist of eyes that will progress slowly and may never develop clinically significant macular edema or proliferative diabetic retinopathy.

A second group included eyes with persistently high leakage values, well demonstrated by the Retinal Leakage Analyzer images, high rates of microaneurysm formation on successive fundus images and a normal foveal avascular zone contour identified on fluorescein angiography images. The duration of diabetes in this group of patients was relatively short. All these combined features suggest a "wet" form of diabetic retinopathy that has rapid progression. This group was designated as having pattern B.

The third group included eyes with reversible retinal leakage and progressive abnormalities of the contours of the foveal avascular zone. The presence of progressive capillary closure from the initial stages of the retinal disease suggests a different evolutionary,

pattern C, which may represent an ischemic form of the disease.

These observations using multimodal macula mapping have offered new perspectives for phenotyping diabetic retinopathy. The identification of well-defined phenotypes is a fundamental step in the characterization of genotype-phenotype studies which are expected to offer new opportunities for specific and more effective therapies of diabetic retinopathy.

# References

Bernardes R, Lobo C, Cunha-Vaz JG. (2002) Multimodal macula mapping. A new approach to study diseases of the macula. *Surv Ophthalmol* **47**: 580–589.

Bernardes R, Dias J, Cunha-Vaz JG. (2005) Mapping the human blood-retinal barrier function. *IEEE TBE* **52**(1): 106–116.

Lobo C, Bernardes R, Cunha-Vaz JG. (1999) Mapping retinal fluorescein leakage with confocal scanning laser fluorometry of the human vitreous. *Arch Ophthalmol* **117**: 631–637.

Lobo C, Bernardes R, Cunha-Vaz J. (2000) Alterations of the blood-retinal barrier and retinal thickness in preclinical retinopathy in subjects with type 2 diabetes. *Arch Ophthalmol* **118**: 1364–1369.

Lobo C, Bernardes R, Faria de Abreu J, Cunha-Vaz J. (2001) One-year follow-up of blood-retinal barrier and retinal thickness alterations in patients with type 2 diabetes mellitus and mild nonproliferative retinopathy. *Arch Ophthalmol* **119**: 1469–1474.

# Chapter 4

# Pathogenesis

## 4.1. Molecular Mechanisms

**Paulo Pereira**

Diabetic retinopathy is the leading cause of blindness in developed countries (Stratton *et al.*, 2000). After 20 years of diabetes, virtually all type 1 patients will have at least some retinopathy (Klein *et al.*, 1989). As described elsewhere in this book in detail, the sight-threatening stages of this disease are characterized by progressive retinal vessel loss, increasing retinal ischemia, development of pathologic retinal neovascularization and increased vascular permeability (Cunha-Vaz, 1978; Engerman, 1989; Stratton *et al.*, 2000). Subsequent bleeding, fibrosis and tissue edema frequently results in vision loss.

Apparently hyperglycemia is sufficient to initiate development of diabetic retinopathy as revealed by development of retinopathy in animals experimentally made hyperglycemic (Engerman and Kern, 1984; Kador *et al.*, 1990; Kern and Engerman, 1996; Robison *et al.*, 1990). Consistently, a number of studies have shown that intensive therapy sufficient to minimize hyperglycemia inhibits the development of retinopathy (Engerman *et al.*, 1977; 1993). Excessive transport or concentration of glucose within cells of the retina is a common thread underlying most of the biochemical and molecular mechanisms that have been postulated to play a role in the pathogenesis of diabetic retinopathy.

The observation that not all patients with poor metabolic control develop advanced stages of diabetic retinopathy suggests that other factors, such as genetic predispositions, are likely to determine individual susceptibility to the disease.

The retina consists of three major types of cells: neurons, glial cells and blood vessels and most, if not all, of these cell types are affected to some degree in diabetic retinopathy. As described in previous chapters the retina is primarily a neuronal tissue. Indeed, neurons and glial cells comprise about 95% of the retinal mass. The glial cells of the retina, Muller cells and astrocytes serve as support cells for the neurons and blood vessels. High sensitivity tests have demonstrated subtle defects in neurosensory retinal function of diabetic patients before any obvious visual symptoms and before signs of retinal damage are visible (Daley *et al.*, 1987; Della Sala *et al.*, 1985; Sokol *et al.*, 1985). These and other observations indicate that dysfunction of the inner retina may affect retinal neurons before any obvious signs of vascular lesions. Neuronal damage in early stages of diabetic retinopathy is further confirmed by animal models of diabetes, where neuronal damage is observed before major vascular lesions are visible (Barber *et al.*, 1998). Glial cells also appear to be affected and implicated in early stages of diabetic retinopathy. For example, accumulation of glutamate in the retinas of diabetic patients and animal models of diabetes suggests a dysfunction of glial cells, since these cells are responsible for glutamate metabolism (Lieth *et al.*, 1998; Mizutani *et al.*, 1998). Accumulation of glutamate is known to cause neuronal cell death through mechanisms of excitotoxicity (Lipton and Rosenberg, 1994; Vorwerk *et al.*, 1996). Diabetic retinopathy is also associated with pericyte loss presumably through apoptosis (Mizutani *et al.*, 1996). It has further been suggested that pericytes are lost more rapidly than endothelial cells. However, it still remains a matter of controversy whether or not pericytes are lost preferentially on diabetic retinopathy and if so, to which extent pericyte loss contributes to diabetic retinopathy (de Oliveira, 1966).

Despite virtually all retinal cells and tissues being potentially affected in diabetic retinopathy, an overwhelming amount of experimental data suggests that vascular cells are dramatically affected during progression of diabetic retinopathy. Moreover, it has been suggested by some authors that endothelial cell dysfunction may be the initial event leading to the progression of diabetic retinopathy ending up by producing injury to many different cell types. Indeed, impaired vascular autoregulation appears to be an early feature in development and progression of diabetic retinopathy. For example, increased blood-retinal barrier permeability appears to occur very early in diabetic patients and in animal models of diabetes, significantly before major signs or retinal damage or symptoms of vision loss occur (Cunha-Vaz *et al.*, 1975, Bursell *et al.*, 1995; Enea *et al.*, 1989; Grunwald *et al.*, 1996; Krogsaa *et al.*, 1987).

As described in greater detail elsewhere in this book, the retinal circulation consists of a progressive circuit of vessels that includes conduits in and out of the retina and microvessels. The microcirculation includes precapillary arterioles, capillaries and postcapillary venules. Arterioles possess smooth muscle that allows regulation of local delivery of blood to retina. The venules are primarily passive conducting tubes that drain blood out of the retina.

Autoregulation is a general feature of blood vessels of central nervous system that is also present in the retina. The main feature of autoregulation is to ensure appropriate supply of blood to neuronal tissues despite alterations in systemic arterial pressure. The retinal arterial vessels possess smooth muscle, while capillaries, arterioles and venules possess pericytes, which may function as modified smooth muscle cells. These features allow the retinal circulation to autoregulate in response to systemic and local metabolic demands. Diabetes creates the conditions that favor

endothelial vascular damage. In early stages of diabetic retinopathy, vascular changes include delayed leukocyte migration in the perifoveal capillaries, increased blood flow and increased permeability of BRB (Krogsaa *et al.*, 1987; Sander *et al.*, 1994). As the disease progresses vascular lesions become more obvious and include microaneurysms, intraretinal hemorrhages and vasodilatation. At later stages, capillary closure occurs and results subsequently in retinal ischemia. Parallel to capillary closure and presumably in an attempt to compensate retinal ischemia, there is a remarkable increase in proliferation of endothelial cells resulting in neovascularization of the optic disk, retina and iris.

Some of the above observations suggest that diabetic retinopathy is primarily a vascular disorder. However, the molecular mechanism that underlies tissue and cell damage associated with diabetic retinopathy in humans are still largely unknown. Despite the variety of hypothesis that have been suggested to contribute to the development and progression of diabetic retinopathy, it remains relatively undisputed that the main feature of diabetic retinopathy, as of other diabetes-related diseases, is hyperglycemia. Moreover, if diabetic retinopathy involves primarily a vascular dysfunction, then it is conceivable that excessive entry of glucose into endothelial cells is the triggering event leading to the endothelial cell lesion and subsequent development of major relevant features of diabetic retinopathy.

This chapter will initially focus on the mechanisms of glucose transport into endothelial cells and will subsequently review some of the major hypothesis and molecular mechanisms that have proposed to explain glucose toxicity associated with diabetic retinopathy.

### 4.1.1. Glucose Transport in the Retina

Oxygen consumption and metabolic activity in the retina is one of the highest in the body. The neuroretina is nourished by transport of glucose across the endothelial cells of the capillaries of the inner BRB and from the choroidal vessels across the retinal pigment epithelium of the outer BRB (Kumagai, 1999). A number of *in vivo* studies confirmed the presence in the retina of saturable, stereospecific, facilitative glucose transporters identical to glucose transporter type 1 (GLUT1) of human red blood cells (Birnbaum *et al.*, 1986). A number of biochemical and physiological studies were further undertaken in isolated microvessels to characterize the blood-retina barrier glucose transporter. It is now clearly established that glucose is transported to the retina mainly through GLUT1 transporter. In addition to erythrocytes, GLUT1 is characteristically expressed in tissues with blood barrier properties, such as blood-brain barrier (BBB) and the blood-ocular barriers (Harik *et al.*, 1990; Takata *et al.*, 1997; Takata *et al.*, 1990). Other isoforms of glucose transporters, such as GLUT2 and GLUT3, are also present in the retina, mainly at the level of the Muller and neuronal cells, respectively (Mantych *et al.*, 1993; Watanabe *et al.*, 1994). Studies of immunohystochemistry and of western blot analysis revealed that the GLUT4 and

GLUT5 glucose transporters isoforms are not expressed in the eye tissues (Mantych *et al.*, 1993).

In the human eye, as in most mammals, GLUT1 is expressed in a variety of tissues, such as capillary endothelial cells, retinal pigmented epithelium, ciliary body, endothelium of the canal of Schlemm and capillaries and pigmented epithelium of the iris (Harik *et al.*, 1990; Kumagai, 1999; Kumagai *et al.*, 1994; Mantych *et al.*, 1993).

Analysis of the GLUT1 sequence together with the secondary structure predictions that the protein is predominantly in $\alpha$-helice (Alvarez *et al.*, 1987; Cairns *et al.*, 1987; Chin *et al.*, 1986), enabled to propose a model for the two-dimensional orientation of the GLUT1 protein in the plasma membrane (Mueckler *et al.*, 1985) (Fig. 4.1). The model predicts that the protein traverses the membrane 12 times. The N- and C-terminal regions of the protein (residues 1-12 and 451-492), and a large hydrophylic region (residues 207-271), linking proposed transmembrane helices 6 and 7, are predicted to lie at the cytoplasmic face of the membrane (Cairns *et al.*, 1987; Davies *et al.*, 1987; Haspel *et al.*, 1988; Mueckler *et al.*, 1985).

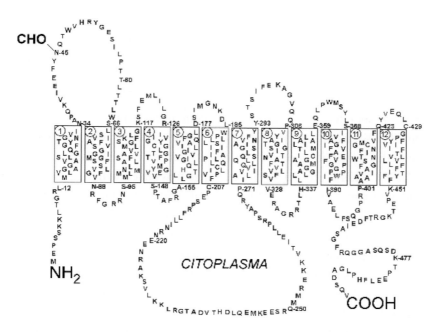

**Fig. 4.1.** Simplified schematic representation of GLUT1 orientation in the cell plasma membrane. The transmembrane segments are signed between 1 and 12. The potential glycosylation site is found in the extracellular loop 1. (Adapted from Hruz and Mueckler, 2001.)

Glucose enters the cytoplasm of endothelial cells of the inner BRB by transport across the endothelial lumenal membrane via GLUT1. GLUT1 also mediates subsequent transport across the ablumenal membrane into the neuroretina (Kumagai, 1999). As in the brain, retina endothelial cells express GLUT1 both in luminal and abluminal membranes (Kumagai *et al.*, 1996; Takata *et al.*, 1992) and a significant portion of the transporter (about 40%) is present in intracellular pools (Kumagai *et al.*, 1996). Only GLUT1 present at plasma membrane is available for glucose transport across endothelial cells. Cytosolic stores of GLUT1 can be translocated to the plasma membrane in response to stimuli, such as growth factors (Kumagai, 1999; Mandarino *et al.*, 1994; Takagi *et al.*, 1998). As in other tissues GLUT1 expression is modulated by hypoxia, growth factors and glucose (Mandarino *et al.*, 1994; Takagi *et al.*, 1998).

Another important aspect of GLUT1, that is relevant to diabetes, is related to its kinetic properties. Indeed for normal concentrations of blood glucose, GLUT1-mediated transport operates at near saturation levels (Mueckler, 1994). Thus, even in conditions where blood glucose concentration increases, such as diabetes, the amount of glucose that is transported into retinal endothelial cells is only marginally affected (Kumagai, 1999). Because GLUT1 is the only glucose transporter present in retinal endothelial cells, the increase in intracellular glucose available to trigger the cytotoxic processes associated with diabetic retinopathy, is likely to be associated with alteration on the expression, subcellular distribution or stability of GLUT1 (Kumagai, 1999). Alterations on absolute amount and/or subcellular distribution of GLUT1 in retinal endothelial cells are likely to be of critical importance in the development of diabetic retinopathy. However, information on the amount of GLUT1 present in retinal endothelial cells of human diabetic patients or in animal models of diabetes has produced some unclear and apparently conflicting results. For example, in galactosemic rats (which develop retinal lesions similar to those seen in diabetic patients) there appears to be an upregulation of total retinal GLUT1

mRNA (Roy, 1996). On the other hand in retinas of streptozotocin-induced diabetic rats the abundance of GLUT1 mRNA does not change significantly (Poulsom *et al.*, 1990). Moreover, while some studies showed that GLUT1 is upregulated in membranes from retinal microvessels of diabetic patients (Kumagai *et al.*, 1996), other studies have shown a decrease in the total amount of GLUT1 in retinas of animal models of diabetes (Fernandes *et al.*, 2004). Moreover, it appears that the decrease in GLUT1 is related to an increased degradation of the protein under high glucose, presumably by the ubiquitin-proteasome pathway.

The distribution of GLUT1 between luminal and abluminal membranes of endothelial cells is critical for the accumulation of intracellular pools of glucose and was shown to be altered in diabetic retinas (Kumagai *et al.*, 1996).

As in the endothelial cells of the brain, glucose uptake by retinal endothelial cells occurs in excess of metabolic rates. The intracellular level of glucose in endothelial cells is approximately 16 times higher than the amount of glucose that can be metabolized by hexokinase (Berkowitz *et al.*, 1995). This leads to the existence of a large pool of intracellular glucose in endothelial cells. The concept of intracellular hyperglycemia is critical in the conceptualization of many molecular mechanisms associated with glucose cytotoxicity contributing to the pathophysiology of diabetic retinopathy.

There is chronic exposure of the retina to high levels of glucose is the upstream event leading to cell damage associated with diabetes. Two major lines of clinical evidence support this hypothesis. The severity of retinopathy is correlated with poor metabolic control (Klein, 1995) and conversely near-normalization of blood glucose levels delay the progression of diabetic retinopathy in patients with type 1 diabetes (Klein *et al.*, 1993; Kumagai, 1999). Glucose can, indeed, be cytotoxic and over the years various mechanisms were suggested to account for glucose toxicity to the retina as well as to other tissues affected in diabetes.

## 4.1.2. Aldose Reductase and Polyol Pathway

In the context of diabetes the "polyol pathway" refers to the enzymatic reduction of glucose to an acyclic polyol, such as sorbitol, which in some cases is reoxidized to another carbohydrate, such as fructose. Although the polyol pathway is common in microorganisms, the mammalian polyol pathway was recognized only about forty years ago in association with early studies in experimental diabetes.

Aldose reductase (AR) is the first enzyme of the polyol pathway that catalyses the NADPH-dependent reduction of a wide variety of carbonyl compound, including glucose. Aldose reductase is characterized by high enzymatic capacity but low affinity with respect to glucose, therefore, at the normal glucose concentration the amount of glucose that is metabolized by the AR is virtually negligible. However, for higher glucose concentrations, the enzyme can be activated resulting in an intracellular accumulation of sorbitol, with a concomitant decrease in NADPH. Opposite to AR, sorbitol dehydrogenase has a high affinity but a low enzymatic capacity for sorbitol, so that sorbitol oxidation to fructose is relatively independent of sorbitol concentration within the physiological range. Therefore, sorbitol accumulates in response to hyperglycemia in tissues that contain high titres of polyol pathway enzymes and in which glucose entry is not rate limiting for glycolysis or mediated by insulin.

Flux through the polyol pathway in hyperglycemia varies from 33% of total glucose in rabbit lenses to 11% in human erythrocytes. Activation of AR in hyperglycemia and the resulting production of sorbitol can have a number of detrimental effects to the affected cells, including sorbitol-induced osmotic stress, decreased $Na^+K^+$-ATPase activity, an increase in cytosolic $NADH/NAD^+$ and a decrease in cytosolic NADPH. However, the amount of sorbitol detected *in vivo* in most tissues is, by far, insufficient to cause osmotic damage. The $Na^+K^+$-ATPase activity was indeed shown to decrease in diabetes in various

studies and in different experimental conditions of hyperglycemia. Although some early studies suggested that activation of AR could account for this reduced activity, more recent data demonstrated that the decrease in $Na^+K^+$-ATPase activity is due to activation of PKC (as described elsewhere in this chapter) (Brownlee, 2001).

Oxidation of sorbitol by sorbitol dehydrogenase reduces $NAD^+$ to NADH so that the ratio $NADH/NAD^+$ increases. This increase could inhibit the activity of the enzyme glyceraldehyde-3-phosphate dehydrogenase, thus leading to an accumulation of triose phosphate (Williamson *et al.*, 1993). Increased levels of triose phosphate may increase formation of methylglyoxal (MGX) and diacylglycerol (DAG). Both MGX and DAG may induce cell damage characteristic of diabetes although through different pathways. As discussed before, DAG is an endogenous activator of PKC, whereas MGX is a precursor of advanced glycation products (AGE). Despite accumulation of MGX and DAG being consistently reported in cells or tissues on diabetes, this appears to have very little to do with activation of AR. In fact, the increase in the ratio $NADH:NAD^+$ that is reported in endothelial cells on hyperglycemia, appears to be the result of a decrease in absolute levels of $NAD^+$ as a result of the activation of poly (ADP-ribose) polymerase (Williamson *et al.*, 1993) in response to hyperglycemia and not related to an increase in the ratio $NADH:NAD^+$ (Brownlee, 2001).

An alternative mechanism has been proposed to explain how AR activation could induce cell damage associated with diabetes. It has been suggested that the initial reduction of glucose to sorbitol by AR would consume NADPH, thus contributing to deplete intracellular reducing potential leading to accumulation of oxidized glutathione and a reduction of reduced GSH. Although a decrease in the levels of GSH has been observed in the lens of transgenic mice over expressing the enzyme AR (Lee and Chung, 1999), it is not obvious that a similar decrease in the levels of GSH is consistently observed in the tissues of diabetic patients. Moreover, the specific vascular abnormalities typical of diabetic retinopathy, such as breakdown of BRB, cannot be explained by this hypothesis. Studies with aldose reductase inhibitors in animal models, including diabetic dogs and rats, have produced conflicting results (Engerman and Kern, 1993; McCaleb *et al.*, 1991). The above observations together with some inconsistent results from clinical trials on beneficial effects of inhibitors of AR makes it rather unlikely that activation of AR can significantly account for cell damage associated with diabetes.

### 4.1.3. Protein Glycation

Glucose has long been known to cause damage to proteins *in vivo*. The food chemists in the early 20th century identified a mechanism through which glucose and other sugars could damage proteins. The chemistry of this reaction came to be known as the Maillard reaction and has since then been shown to occur *in vivo* in various cells and tissues, presumably accounting for the post-translational modification of long-lived proteins. Glucose can react spontaneously with amino groups of a wide range of proteins to form Schiff bases, which through multiple rearrangements are transformed into irreversibly bound, chemically reactive adducts. Indeed, the chemical and conformational modifications that follow glucose binding to proteins appear to be sufficient to expose SH groups. Oxidation of SH residues could then lead to protein cross-linking and aggregation, as well as, to inactivation of various enzymes (Stevens *et al.*, 1978; Swamy and Abraham, 1987). Subsequent reactions following glucose binding to amino groups in proteins result in the formation of the Amadori product. The Amadori product can also be oxidized and undergo further reactions to produce alpha-cetoaldehydes, such as 1 and 3-deoxyglucosones. These products are usually more reactive than the initial monosaccharide and can further react with proteins yielding a heterogeneous mixture of fluorescent and colored compounds that

can crosslink proteins (Brownlee *et al.*, 1984). These compounds were originally known as Maillard products and subsequently by the broader and the more inspired designation of Advanced Glycation End products (AGEs) (Monnier, 1989).

Over the years a wide range of evidence confirmed that AGE form and accumulate *in vivo* and mostly on diabetes. For example, the levels of glycated hemoglobin became a widely accepted marker of metabolic control in diabetic patients (Kennedy and Baynes, 1984). A wide variety of results further suggested that many modifications observed in a number of biomolecules in diabetic patients are consistent with the occurrence of protein glycation *in vivo*. For example, lenses extracted from diabetic patients present higher levels of glycated proteins as compared with healthy individuals (Rao and Cotlier, 1986). Although the hypothesis that protein glycation contribute to the pathophysiology of diabetes has been popular for a long time, there are a few unresolved issues that persisted over the years. Although increased in diabetes, the total amount of glycated proteins present in tissues of diabetic patients (even with poor metabolic control) was too low to account for the extent of cell damage observed. For example, the total amount of amino groups that is glycated in the hemoglobin of diabetic patients after three months is less than 2.5% (Shapiro *et al.*, 1980). On the other hand, although the accumulation of glycated proteins and AGE-modified proteins can be relevant for tissues with long-lived proteins, such as the lens, where a protein will remain exposed to glucose for many years, it is not clear that the same happens for organs with faster protein turnover, such as the retina. It, thus, appears that *per se* direct modification of proteins by glucose would produce only limited damage to most cells. Moreover, it was later realized that the rate of AGE-formation from glucose is orders of magnitude slower than the rate of formation of AGEs from glucose-derived dicarbonyls formed inside the cells (Degenhardt *et al.*, 1998). It, thus, appears that intracellular hyperglycemia is the primary initiating event in the formation of AGEs. AGEs can originate from a number of pathways including auto-oxidation of glucose to glyoxal, decomposition of the Amadori product to 3-deoxyglucosone and fragmentation of glyceraldehyde-3-phosphate and dihydroxyacetone phosphate to methylglyoxal (Thornalley, 1990). These highly reactive dicarbonyl precursors then react with amino-groups of proteins to form AGEs. Methylglyoxal (MG), for example, reacts with arginine residues to form imidazolone adducts and also with lysine residues in proteins to form N (epsilon)-(carboxymethyl) lysine (Degenhardt *et al.*, 1998). Despite its cytotoxic potential, MG is detoxified by the glyoxalase system producing D-lactate via the intermediate S-D-lactoylgluthathione (Thornalley, 1990). Moreover, the above described dicarbonyl precursors are also metabolized by other reductases (Suzuki *et al.*, 1998).

AGEs formed from dicarbonyls, such as MG, were shown to the accumulate in cells and tissues from diabetic patients or in animal models of diabetes (McLellan *et al.*, 1994; Oya *et al.*, 1999; Phillips *et al.*, 1993). Indeed, in endothelial cells cultured under high glucose, it was demonstrated that MG is the major precursor of AGEs (Shinohara *et al.*, 1998). MG irreversibly modifies a variety of proteins under physiological conditions and at physiologically relevant concentrations of MG (Thornalley, 1990). Modification of proteins by MG is closely associated with cell toxicity. MG selectively inhibits mitochondrial respiration and glycolysis as well as inactivates a number of other enzymes, such as membrane ATPases and glyceraldehydes-3-phosphate dehydrogenase (Biswas *et al.*, 1997; Halder *et al.*, 1993). Adducts of MGX to proteins may also target the protein for proteasome dependent degradation (Bulteau *et al.*, 2001) or interfere with other key enzymes of the ubiquitin proteasome pathway. In addition to direct modification of protein and enzymes AGE-precursors may induce further damage to cells by other mechanisms, such as by disrupting interaction between extracellular matrix components and integrins or by binding to AGE receptors in endothelial cells inducing receptor mediated production of reactive oxygen species and activation of NF-kB with the consequent alteration in gene expression. Proteins involved in the macromolecular endocytosis are also modified by AGEs (Shinohara *et al.*, 1998). AGEs formation on extracellular matrix also interferes with matrix-matrix interactions, as well as, with cell-matrix interaction, which can result in decreased endothelial cell adhesion (Haitoglou *et al.*, 1992).

AGEs were also shown to contribute to the vascular damage characteristic of diabetic retinopathy, such as disruption of blood-retinal barrier (BRB) (Leto *et al.*, 2001; Stitt *et al.*, 2000). AGEs are further known to accumulate in the neuronal retina and vascular cells of diabetic animals (Hammes *et al.*, 1999; Stitt *et al.*, 1997) where they appear to initiate pathophysiological changes in retinal microvascular function (Stitt *et al.*, 2000). Although the mechanisms whereby AGEs increase permeability of retinal vessels is still not clear, it has been suggested that VEGF is involved in this process. For example, it has been shown that AGEs enhance VEGF expression in retinal cells (Hirata *et al.*, 1997; Hoffmann *et al.*, 2002; Lu *et al.*, 1998; Mamputu and Renier, 2002). VEGF then leads to neovascularization of endothelial cells and increased permeability of retinal microvessels.

The major piece of evidence in favor of a role for AGEs in the pathophysiology of diabetes, including, diabetic retinopathy, resulted from the study of inhibitors of protein glycation. Indeed, in animal models, inhibitors of glycation, such as aminoguanidine, appear to prevent part of the functional and structural manifestations of diabetic retinopathy, as well as, other microvascular diseases associated with diabetes (Hammes *et al.*, 1999; Nakamura *et al.*, 1997; Soulis-Liparota *et al.*, 1991). More importantly, some clinical trials indicate that aminoguanidine slows the progression of diabetic retinopathy (Bolton *et al.*, 2004).

### 4.1.4. VEGF and Angiogenesis

Aberrant neovascularization of the retina is a hallmark of proliferative diabetic retinopathy and is closely associated with loss of vision associated with diabetes. Formation of new capillaries from preexisting vessels is a complex process and is regulated by a number of different stimuli including the action of growth factors, such as VEGF, interaction between endothelial cells and support cells, such as pericytes and interaction of endothelial cells with extracellular matrix. Ultimately, new vessels are formed when there is an imbalance that favors proangiogenic factors over antiagiogenic factors occurs (Chavakis and Dimmeler, 2002). Apparently, angiogenesis is closely associated with an inhibition of endothelial cell apoptosis (Chavakis and Dimmeler, 2002). Increased production of VEGF has been considered a major factor contributing to retinopathy on diabetes. VEGF is produced primarily, but not exclusively, by non-vascular retinal cells, including pericytes, ganglion cells, Muller cells and retinal pigment epithelial cells (Lutty *et al.*, 1996). VEGF, a key regulator of angiogenesis, acts by preventing apoptosis of endothelial cells (Alon *et al.*, 1995). In fact, VEGF was shown to induce the expression of the antiapoptotic proteins Bcl-2, A1, survinin and XIAP (Gerber *et al.*, 1998a; Nor *et al.*, 1999; Tran *et al.*, 1999). Furthermore, VEGF was shown to promote endothelial cell survival by activation of the phosphatidylinositol 3-kinase (PI3K)/Akt pathway (Fujio and Walsh, 1999; Gerber *et al.*, 1998b). The downstream effector pathways mediating the antiapoptotic VEGF effect include Akt-dependent activation of the endothelial nitric oxide synthase (NOS) resulting in an enhanced synthesis of NO by endothelial cells. NO, in turn, promotes endothelial cell survival (Dimmeler *et al.*, 1999; Dimmeler *et al.*, 1997; Fulton *et al.*, 1999; Hoffmann *et al.*, 2001). Alternatively, the PI3K/Akt pathway also activates the transcription of survinin and can inhibit the p38 mitogen-activated protein kinase (MAPK) (Gratton *et al.*, 2001; Papapetropoulos *et al.*, 2000). On the other hand it was also demonstrated that the antiaptotic effect of VEGF is also associated with activation of the MAPK/extracellular signal-regulated kinase (ERK) pathway and with inhibition of the

stress-activated protein kinase /c-Jun amino-terminal kinase pathway (Gupta *et al.*, 1999).

VEGFs are a family of peptides produced by a single gene by alternative splicing. VEGF stimulate proliferation of endothelial cells and significantly increase permeability at blood-tissue barriers. VEGF binds with high affinity to the vascular endothelium via two receptors: fms-like tyrosine kinase 1 (VEGF-R1) and fetal liver kinase 1 (VEGF-R2). VEGF-R1 is expressed both in endothelial and non-endothelial cells, whereas VEGF-R2 is expressed only in endothelial cells and mostly in the retinal microcirculation (Jakeman *et al.*, 1992). In addition to activating anti-apoptotic pathways, stimulating endothelial cell proliferation, VEGF also triggers phosphoinositol hydrolysis and release of DAG, which then leads to activation of PKC-a, b and d (Xia *et al.*, 1996). *In vitro* studies have shown that VEGF induces endothelial fenestrations that presumably lead to increased vascular permeability (Esser *et al.*, 1998).

Production of VEGF is induced by a number of stimuli with one of the best known being hypoxia. VEGF expression is increased about 30 fold by hypoxia (Wise, 1956). However, it is still not clear whether hypoxia is the stimulus that leads to production of VEGF in diabetic retinopathy. The mechanism for VEGF overexpression appears to be dependent on selective activation of various PKC isoforms, however PKC-beta seems to be especially important in VEGF signaling (Suzuma *et al.*, 2002). In fact transcription of VEGF gene in response to hypoxia and/or hyperglycemia is dependent on activation of such specific kinases. The mechanisms through which hypoxia leads to increased production of VEGF and by consequence to neovascularization have been extensively studied over the last few years.

VEGF can be produced in response to a variety of stimuli, one of the best known involves activation of Hypoxia Inducible Factor (HIF). HIF-1 is an oxygen-dependent transcriptional activator, which plays crucial roles in the agiogenesis. HIF-1 induces the expression of more than 60 proteins including VEGF. HIF-1 consists of a constitutively expressed HIF-1$\beta$

subunit and one of three inducible expressed subunits: HIF-1$\alpha$, HIF-2$\alpha$, HIF-3$\alpha$. The stability of HIF-1$\alpha$ is regulated in various ways.

Under non-hypoxic (normoxia) conditions, HIF-1$\alpha$ is subject to oxygen dependent prolyl hydroxylation (Ivan *et al.*, 2001; Jaakkola *et al.*, 2001), which is required for binding of the von Hippel-Lindau tumor supressor protein (VHL), the recognition component of an ubiquitin-protein ligase, which targets HIF-1$\alpha$ for ubiquitin-dependent proteasomal degradation (Maxwell *et al.*, 1999). HIF-1$\alpha$ contains two sites for hydroxylation, Pro402 and Pro564 within the oxygen-dependent degradation (ODD) domain and each site contains a conserved LXXLAP motif (Masson *et al.*, 2001).

Under hypoxic conditions oxygen becomes limiting for prolyl hydroxylase activity (Epstein *et al.*, 2001) and ubiquitination of HIF-1$\alpha$ is inhibited (Sutter *et al.*, 2000). As a result, HIF-1$\alpha$ accumulates, dimerizes with HIF-1$\beta$ and activates transcription of target genes, including VEGF.

Ubiquitination of HIF-1$\alpha$, as of most proteins, requires primarily formation of a polyubiquitin chain through lysine 48 of ubiquitin. Subsequently, the polyubiquitinated HIF-1$\alpha$ needs to be translocated for the 26S proteasome for degradation.

In further support of the hypothesis that increased production of VEGF is associated with diabetic retinopathy is the observation that increased levels of VEGF are present in the eyes of persons with diabetes even before the onset of detectable retinopathy.

Moreover, levels of VEGF correlate with new vessel formation in patients with diabetes (Aiello *et al.*, 1994) and were further shown to be increased in the vitreous of eyes with neovascularization and diminish after panretinal photocoagulation (Aiello *et al.*, 1994).

In animal models local injection of VEGF causes neovascularization of the retina (Tolentino *et al.*, 2002). Conversely strategies to block VEGF, such as those, using antibodies that can bind to VEGF before it can activate its receptors or antisense oligonecleotides that inhibit VEGF mRNA appear to prevent retinal neovascularization (Robinson *et al.*, 1996; Tolentino *et al.*, 2002).

Despite its important role in angiogenesis, VEGF is probably not the only player that leads to neovascularization in diabetic retinopathy. Indeed, the switch from quiescent to active vessels involves not only an increase in inducers of neovascularization but also a decrease in concentration of negative regulators of angiogenesis, such as pigment epithelium-derived factor (PEDF) (Dawson *et al.*, 1999; Stellmach *et al.*, 2001). PEDF is also responsible for the anti-angiogenic activity of human vitreous and for excluding vessels from cornea (Chader, 2001; Dawson *et al.*, 1999). PEDF is regulated by oxygen concentration and behaves in a manner opposite to VEGF, falling in concentration when oxygen is limited and rising when it is in good supply (Becerra, 1997; Dawson *et al.*, 1999; Gao *et al.*, 2001). It, thus, appears that the balance between the levels of VEGF and PEDF may be critical in preventing neovascularization. A number of agents that block VEGF or stimulate PEDF are currently being tested, including on clinical trials. For example gene therapy may prove useful in increasing the levels of PEDF in the eye (Frank, 2004; Rasmussen *et al.*, 2001).

## 4.1.5. Activation of Protein Kinase C

As described before, glucose enters retinal endothelial cells via glucose transporters (GLUTs) mostly GLUT1. Under hyperglycemia GLUT1 will transport more glucose inside endothelial cells. Accumulation of intracellular glucose stimulates glycolysis leading to accumulation of glycolitic intermediates, including glyceraldehydes-3-phosphate (G-3-P). Accumulation of G-3-P stimulates synthesis of diacylglycerol (DAG), which in turn activates one or more isoforms of protein kinase C (PKC). Through a variety of direct and indirect mechanisms activation of PKC contribute to the pathophysiology of diabetic retinopathy (Donnelly *et al.*, 2004).

Protein kinase C consists of a family of about 13 members of structurally and functionally related proteins derived both from multiple genes and from alternative splicing of single mRNA transcripts. All PKC members consist of serine/threonine kinases that are activated by a number of different mechanisms, including receptor tyrosine kinases, non-receptor tyrosine kinases and G protein coupled receptors. The classic or conventional PKC isoforms require an endogenous activator, diacylglycerol (DAG), calcium and phosphatidylserine for their activation. The novel isoforms do not require calcium, whereas the atypical isoforms require only phosphatidylserine. PKC is recruited to cellular membranes by binding to either DAG/phorbol ester or to anionic lipids, but both DAG/phorbol ester and phosphatidylserine binding must occur to release the substrate from the active site (Newton and Johnson, 1998). DAG binding and membrane attachment induces unfolding of a domain (pseudo-substrate) to reveal the catalytic site. The active site binds ATP and the substrate protein resulting in phosphorylation of serine and threonine residues in the target proteins. PKC activity is mainly regulated by its phosphorylation state. Upon ligand binding and recruitment to the membrane, PKC becomes a substrate for kinases, mainly phosphoinositide-dependent kinase 1 (PDK-1), resulting in autophosphorylation (at three sites on the catalytic domain) and enhanced catalytic activity (Parekh *et al.*, 2000). In diabetic retinopathy, PKC mediated changes in endothelial permeability, blood flow and the response to angiogenic growth factors, contribute to retinal leakage, ischemia and neovascularization (Huang and Yuan, 1997; Park *et al.*, 2000b; Williams *et al.*, 1997).

In animal models it was shown that both PKC activity and DAG expression are increased in rat retinas early in experimental diabetes and in endothelial cells cultured in high glucose conditions (Shiba *et al.*, 1993). Significantly, chronic activation of PKC may play a critical role in the activation of the signaling pathways that promote increased vascular permeability associated with diabetes (Harhaj and Antonetti, 2004). For example, PKCb isoform has

been implicated as a regulator of VEGF induced increased permeability *in vivo* (Aiello *et al.*, 1997). Consistently, PKC agonists are sufficient to increase permeability in many cell models (Lynch *et al.*, 1990; Marano *et al.*, 2001). A number of other studies involving expression of PKC mutants in cell culture models further support the notion that PKC signaling pathway lead to increased permeability.

The mechanisms that lead to activation of PKC under hyperglycemia, as well as, the downstream pathways that lead to cell damage are not yet fully understood. However, it has, for example, been demonstrated that DAG (an endogenous activator of PKC) is increased in vascular endothelial cells in high glucose, as are the levels of DAG in tissues from diabetic animals, including retina (Shiba *et al.*, 1993). It seems likely that different species of DAG, selectively activate specific PKC isoforms in different tissues (Inoguchi *et al.*, 1992). Moreover, the importance of PKC in human diabetic patients is further emphasized by the observation of a correlation between PKC activity in monocytes and plasma glucose (Ceolotto *et al.*, 1999).

In addition, hyperglycemia induced PKC activation augments biochemical responses triggered by other pathophysiological mechanisms, including hypoxia, shear stress and raised capillary pressure (Aiello *et al.*, 1995; Liao *et al.*, 1997).

There are also a number of indirect mechanisms that involve activation of PKC and that may result in deleterious effects to retina cells. For example, transcription of VEGF gene is, in part, induced by PKC activation (Aiello *et al.*, 1995; Williams *et al.*, 1997). PKC activation is, in part, responsible for reduction of activity of membrane transporters, such as $Na^+K^+$-ATPase and $Ca^{2+}$-ATPase in response to high glucose (Kowluru *et al.*, 1998; Xia *et al.*, 1995). Activation of PKC increases cytosolic phospholipase A2 activity, which increases the production of two inhibitors of $Na^+K^+$-ATPase, arachidonate and PGE2 (Xia *et al.*, 1995). PKC activation is also involved in leukocyte adhesion to retinal endothelial cells (Park *et al.*, 2000a), which is a characteristic pathophysiological event, associated with diabetic retinopathy leading to capillary occlusion and microthrombosis.

Given that PKC activation is involved in a wide variety of pathophysiological events associated with diabetes, a considerable interest has been raised in finding inhibitors of different isoforms of PKC. On the other hand PKC pays a crucial role in signal transduction and other vital signaling pathways in various tissues, therefore, general PKC inhibitors are of very limited use. About 10 years ago a selective and reversible inhibitor of isoforms PKC-bI and PKC-bII, ruboxistaurin, was characterized and reported to be effective at very low concentrations (5 nM) (Ishii *et al.*, 1996). In animal models of diabetes, ruboxistaurin was shown to decrease retinal PKC activity and to restore $Na^+$-$K^+$-ATPase activity (Jirousek *et al.*, 1996). Moreover, in other animal models ruboxistaurin reduces VEGF induced retinal permeability and attenuates new vessel formation on the retina and optic nerve (Aiello *et al.*, 1997; Danis *et al.*, 1998). Clinical studies have further shown a favorable effect of ruboxistaurin on normalizing retinal blood flow in patients with type 1 and type 2 diabetes. A number of PKC inhibitors are now being tested.

A puzzling question has been the apparent absence of downregulation of PKC in diabetes. Indeed, whereas, the vast majority of *in vitro* studies show that PKCs, activated in response to phorbol esters, downregulate after a period typically of a few minutes. Although not all isoforms downregulate in the same way or the same cell types the general and overall response is still a downregulation. This, however, does not happen or at least is not obvious in diabetes. The resistance to downregulation can presumably be explained by a number of factors: the synthesis of PKCs could be increased, the activity of the enzymes responsible for the downregulation could be impaired on diabetes or DAGs, for example, are produced in such a way that they compensate for downregulation of PKC (Curtis and Scholfield, 2004).

Another interesting, and presumably more complex, hypothesis is that degradation of PKCs is impaired on diabetes. In fact, the ubiquitin proteasome pathway degrades PKCs and this appears to be a major mechanism for downregulation of PKC following activation by phorbol esters. However, recent data suggests that the UPP itself is altered in diabetes (White, 2002). The major effect of insulin on protein metabolism is to suppress protein degradation (Gelfand and Barrett, 1987). It has been demonstrated that in diabetes the ubiquitin-proteasome pathway is upregulated as revealed by the increase in content of mRNA encoding components of the pathway (Mitch *et al.*, 1999; Price *et al.*, 1996).

### 4.1.6.   Oxidative Stress

For many years oxidative stress has been proposed to contribute in a significant manner to the pathophysiology of diabetes and diabetes-related complications. Oxidative stress may induce cell and tissue damage through a variety of different mechanisms.

Indeed, it has been shown that sustained generation of reactive oxygen species (ROS) at the levels shown in endothelial cells exposed to high glucose may contribute significantly to the endothelial cell dysfunction associated with diabetic retinopathy. The contribution of free radicals to endothelial cell dysfunction is further supported by the observation that both *in vitro* and *in vivo* the acute effects of hyperglycemia can be contrabalanced by antioxidants (Beckman *et al.*, 2001; Diederich *et al.*, 1994; Marfella *et al.*, 1995; Tesfamariam and Cohen, 1992).

There are a number of mechanisms through which high glucose may induce oxidative stress to various biomolecules. These mechanisms are briefly summarized and then major player and most recent developments are described in greater detail:

(a) The increased availability of glucose appears to increase mitochondria activity resulting in an increased production of superoxide anions (Nishikawa *et al.*, 2000a);

(b) A number of chemical and enzymatic antioxidant defenses were shown to be decreased on diabetes, thus, favoring cell damage associated with production of ROS (Chen *et al.*, 1983; Karpen *et al.*, 1985; Nourooz-Zadeh and Pereira, 1999). Consistently, markers for oxidative damage are increased in tissues of diabetics, including retina where products of lipid oxidation were shown to accumulate (Nourooz-Zadeh and Pereira, 1999);

(c) Glucose itself, as other dicarbonyls, can undergo autoxidation in the presence of transition metals yielding reactive oxygen species;

(d) An early step in protein glycation consists in the formation of a so-called Amadori product. The Amadori product can autoxidise producing dycarbonyls and hydroxyl radicals (Baynes and Thorpe, 1999; Wolff and Dean, 1987);

(e) AGE can bind to membrane receptors triggering a cascade of events that lead to production of reactive oxygen species;

(f) Nitric oxide is critical in modulating endothelial function. The inducible form of NO synthase (iNOS) is expressed in response to hyperglycemia (Spitaler and Graier, 2002). Through activation of NFkB, hyperglycemia favors increased expression of iNOS, which in turn leads to increased production of NO (Spitaler and Graier, 2002). Accumulation of NO together with overproduction of superoxide favors formation of the strong oxidant peroxynitrite (Beckman and Koppenol, 1996), which in turn can oxidize iNOS cofactors leading to further production of superoxide (Brodsky *et al.*, 2002; Cosentino *et al.*, 1997).

The oxidative stress hypothesis is not inconsistent with other downstream events that are likely to participate in the pathogenesis of diabetic retinopathy. It rather appears that production of ROS in response to high glucose is the upstream event that may trigger other cellular events. Indeed, the oxidative insult hypothesis has recently emerged as a "unifying hypothesis" to explain many pathogenic pathways initially proposed to explain retinal degeneration in response to hyperglycemia (Brownlee, 2001).

Excessive production of reactive oxygen species (ROS) and specifically the superoxide anion in respiratory chain, in the retina may by itself provide an explanation for pathways, such as activation of PKC, activation of polyol pathway, alterations in redox potential and formation of advanced glycation end products (AGE) (Brownlee, 2001).

## 4.1.7. Hyperglycemia and Oxidative Damage: A Unifying Hypothesis

Some of the major mechanisms described above to explain toxicity of glucose in diabetes: activation of protein kinase C (PKC), activation of aldose reductase, formation of AGE and the hexosamine pathway appear to account significantly for the pathophysiology of diabetic retinopathy. Moreover, inhibitors of some of these pathways or enzymes were shown to ameliorate, although at times only marginally, many of the modifications associated with diabetes both in cell culture and animal models (for a review: (Brownlee, 2001)). For many years all of these mechanisms were considered to explain modifications associated with pathogenesis of diabetic retinopathy independently.

More recently, however, it was realized that a common thread might exist that could account for the hyperglycemia-induced damage in diabetes. Indeed, over the past four years it has consistently been shown that hyperglycemia induces overproduction of superoxide by the mitochondrial electron transport chain (Brownlee, 2001; Du *et al.*, 2000; Nishikawa *et al.*, 2000b) and that this excess production of reactive oxygen species (ROS) can be the upstream event leading to other mechanisms implicated in endothelial cell damage associated with diabetes. The use of endothelial cell lines as a model system to assess the effects of high glucose on production of ROS and other molecular events associated with diabetes is most useful not only because vascular endothelial cells are shown to be major sites of damage in diabetes-associated diseases, such as retinopathy, but also because, as discussed before, glucose transport into endothelial cells is mediated by the insulin-independent transporter GLUT1. Transport through GLUT1 facilitates the diffusion of high levels of glucose when endothelial cells are exposed to physiologically relevant glucose concentrations.

## 4.1.8. Hyperglycemia and Production of Superoxide

The mechanism whereby hyperglycemia induces increased production of superoxide by mitochondria appears to be related to the excessive production of oxygen donors from trycarboxylic acid cycle (TCA). Glucose oxidation inside the cells begins with glycolisis in cytosol, which generates NADH and pyruvate. The intracellular pool of pyruvate that is not reduced to lactate is then transported into the mitochondria where it is oxidized producing water, carbon dioxide and reducing potential in the form of NADH and FADH2. Mitochondrial NADH and FADH2 enter the electron-transport chain producing energy in the form of ATP through oxidative phosphorylation. ATP is produced in complex V (ATP synthase), but it is the electron transport through complexes I, III and IV that generates the proton gradient that drives ATP synthase. For every four electrons fed into the cytochrome oxidase complex, a molecule of oxygen is reduced to two molecules of water. Cytochrome oxidase releases no detectable oxygen radicals into free solution. Unlike cytochrome oxidase, some other components of the electron transport chain do "leak" a few electrons while passing the great bulk of them on to the next component in the chain. There are two main sites of electron "leakage" in inner mitochondrial membrane and, therefore, two major sites where superoxide is likely to form: NADH dehydrogenase at complex I and the interface between ubiquinone and complex III (Kwong and Sohal, 1998; Wallace, 1992). When the electrochemical potential difference, generated by the proton gradient in inner mitochondrial

membrane is high the half-life of intermediates in electron transport is also higher. Some of these intermediates, such as ubisemiquinone, are then more likely to transfer an electron to oxygen producing superoxide (Brownlee, 2001). Hyperglycemia appears to increase the proton gradient resulting in a significant increase in the production of superoxide as a result of excessive production of electron donors by the TCA cycle (Du *et al*., 2001). It has consistently been shown in endothelial cells, that flux through the TCA cycle increases about 2.2 fold in response to high glucose (Nishikawa *et al*., 2000b). Conversely, inhibition of glycolysis derived pyruvate transport into mitochondria completely inhibited hyperglycemia-induced ROS production (Nishikawa *et al*., 2000b). These data indicate that the TCA cycle is the source of increased ROS-generating substrate induced by hyperglycemia. All together the increased production of glycolysis intermediates increase flux through TCA cycle and an increased electrochemical potential difference in inner mitochondrial membrane cause a marked increase in the production of superoxide by endothelial cells.

A number of experimental data appear to support this hypothesis. For example, overexpression of manganese superoxide dismutase (MnSOD), the mitochondrial enzyme that dismutates superoxide abolishes the signal generated by reactive oxygen species under physiologically relevant hyperglycemia (Nishikawa *et al*., 2000b). Overexpression of the uncoupling protein-1 (UCP-1), a specific protein uncoupler of oxidative phosphorylation collapsed the proton gradient and prevented hyperglycemia-induced overproduction of superoxide (Nishikawa *et al*., 2000b). Consistently, antisense complementary DNA in the same gene transfer vector did not produce any effect. A number of pharmacological inhibitors of different complexes in mitochondrial electron transport chain have shown that inhibitor of complex II and uncouplers of oxidative phosphorylation are the only inhibitors that completely prevented effects of hyperglycemia in production of ROS (Nishikawa *et al*., 2000b). Thus the main site of production of superoxide in mitochondria of endothelial cells following exposure to high glucose is the mitochondrial complex II (succinate:ubiquinone oxidoreductase).

This unifying hypothesis is consistent with the four pathways suggested to be involved in the development of diabetic complications (activation of aldose reductase, increased formation of AGEs, activation of protein kinase C and increased hexosamine pathway flux). This hypothesis further accounts for the relevance of increased production of reactive oxygen species in diabetes and also provides a unifying hypothesis regarding the effects of hyperglycemia on cellular dysfunction (Brownlee, 2001; Nishikawa *et al.*, 2000b).

Furthermore, the activation of the transcription factor NF-kB by superoxide (Nishikawa *et al.*, 2000b) provides an extra link between hyperglycemia and the expression of multiple genes related to vascular stress response (Collins, 1993). Significantly, hyperglycemia-induced activation of NF-kB is also prevented by inhibiting mitochondrial superoxide overproduction (Nishikawa *et al.*, 2000b).

### 4.1.9. Activation of Hexosamine Pathway

A few years ago it was demonstrated that hyperglycemia-induced mitochondrial superoxide overproduction inhibits glyceraldehyde-3-phosphate dehydrogenase (GAPDH) activity and activates the hexosamine pathway by diverting the upstream metabolite fructose-6-phosphate from glycolysis to glucosamine formation (Du *et al.*, 2000). Hyperglycemia-induced mitochondrial superoxide dismutase overproduction consistently leads to a 2.5 fold increase in the activity of hexosamine pathway (Du *et al.*, 2000).

Activation of the hexosamine pathway increases O-GlcNAcylation and decreases serine/threonine phosphorylation of the transcription factor SP1. This leads to SP1 transactivation and increased SP1 dependent expression of both TGFb1 and PAI-1.

This hypothesis has been confirmed by a number of independent and consistent reports. For example, it was shown that activity of GAPDH is reversibly inhibited by reactive oxygen species (Fig. 4.2) (Knight *et al.*, 1996). Moreover inhibition of mito-

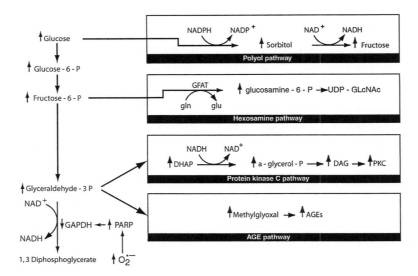

**Fig. 4.2.** Hyperglycaemia increases the proton gradient through the electron transport chain resulting in a significant increase in the production of superoxide in the mitochondria. Superoxide can activate the hexosamine pathway by inhibiting the activity of the enzyme GAPDH and diverting fructose-6-phosphate into the hexosamine pathway leading to an increase in Udp-GLCnac. This increase can, in turn, lead to increased transactivation of SP1 with the resulting Sp1-dependent gene expression. Adapted from Brownlee M. *Nature* **414**: 813–820, 2001.

chondrial superoxide overproduction by inhibitors of complex II, uncouplers of oxidative phosphorylation or superoxide dismutase mimetic completely prevented the reduction of GAPDH activity induced by hyperglycemia (Du *et al.*, 2000). Overexpression of UCP-1 or MnSOD also prevented inactivation of GAPDH (Du *et al.*, 2000).

Hyperglycemia further induces an increase in TGFbeta1 and PAI-1 promoter activity and both are prevented by inhibiting mitochondrial superoxide production and by inhibiting the hexosamine pathway. The glutamine-rich transactivating domain of Sp1 contains a dominant O-GlcNAc epitope and this modification was found to block Sp1 protein interactions (Roos *et al.*, 1997). It appears that hyperglycemia-induced increases in GlcNAc modification of Sp1 activate transcription by blocking Sp1 interaction with repressor proteins, such as p. 74 and p. 107 (a retinoblastoma related protein) (Datta *et al.*, 1995; Murata *et al.*, 1994).

### 4.1.10.  Activation of PKC

As previously discussed there is significant evidence that activation of PKC is relevant in the development of diabetic complications in endothelial cells. Hyperglycemia activates PKC by increasing the synthesis of its endogenous activator DAG (Koya and King, 1998), thus the effect of hyperglycemia on PKC activation probably reflects increased dihydroxyacetone phosphate levels resulting from inhibition of GAPDH by superoxide (Du *et al.*, 2000).

Moreover, chemical inhibitors of mitochondrial electron transport chain, overexpression of uncoupler protein 1 (UCP-1) or overexpression of manganese superoxide dismutase, all inhibited PKC activation in response to hyperglycemia (Nishikawa *et al.*, 2000b). Furthermore, GAPDH antisense oligonucleotides cause activation of PKC in the presence of physiological concentrations of glucose (Brownlee, 2001). All together these and other results indicate that it is superoxide produced in mitochondria as a result of

hyperglycemia that leads to inhibition of GAPDH that subsequently activates PKC.

### 4.1.11.  Formation of AGEs

Protein modification by AGE on diabetes or under condition of hyperglycemia can also be explained by overproduction of superoxide by the mitochondria. In fact, methylglyoxal, a major AGE-precursor is produced by fragmentation of triose phosphates. As discussed before, overproduction of superoxide leads to inhibition of GAPDH, which in turn may increase intracellular levels of triose phosphate available to form methylglyoxal or other AGE precursors (Du *et al.*, 2000). This hypothesis is further supported by the experimental observation that in the absence of hyperglycemia GAPDH antisense causes an increase in the intracellular levels of AGE comparable to that observed upon cell exposure to high glucose (Brownlee, 2001) (Fig. 4.3).

### 4.1.12.  Production of Nitric Oxide

Increased production of superoxide may further interfere with NO function in the retina and, as mentioned before, may even result in an increased production of superoxide by a mechanism that does not involve the mitochondria, thus amplifying the production of reactive oxygen species. NO is generated from the metabolism of L-arginine by the enzyme nitric oxide synthase (NOS). There are three known isoforms of the enzyme: the constitutive brain (bNOS); endothelial (eNOS) isoforms and an inducible isoform (iNOS). A number of stimuli were shown to induce iNOS, including hyperglycemia (Baek *et al.*, 1993). Overproduction of superoxide may interfere with NO function at different stages. For example, superoxide may quench NO, thus, reducing its vasodilator properties and disrupting the general homeostasis of the vasculature (Benz *et al.*, 2002). On the other hand, induction of iNOS in

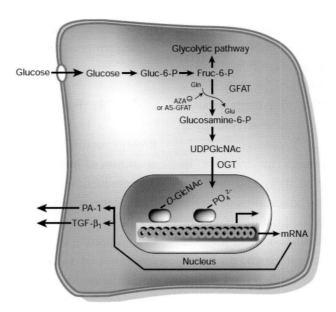

**Fig. 4.3.** A unifying mechanism for glucose-induced tissue damage in diabetes. The increased availability of glucose inside the cells leads to an increased flow of electrons through the electron transport chain resulting in increased production of superoxide anion. Excessive production of superoxide by mitochodria can lead to inhibition of GAPDH, activating four of the major pathways involved in the pathophysiology of diabetes, including polyol pathway, hexosamine pathway, activation of Protein Kinase C and the AGE pathway. Adapted from Brownlee M. (2001), *Nature* **41**: 4813–4820.

response to hyperglycemia and the resulting accumulation of NO may, in the presence of superoxide, lead to formation of peroxynitrite (Beckman and Koppenol, 1996). Peroxynitrite may then oxidize tetrahydrobiopterin, an iNOS cofactor (Beckman and Koppenol, 1996) rendering iNOS to an uncoupled state, which results in electrons being diverted from the original path iNOS reductase domain — oxidase domain, to molecular oxygen leading to formation of more superoxide rather then NO (Brodsky *et al.*, 2002; Cosentino *et al.*, 1997).

inhibition of prostacyclin synthetase and prevents inhibition of eNOS induced by hyperglycemia (Du *et al.*, 2001). Transgenic animals overexpressing human $Cu^{2+}/Zn^{2+}$ SOD and in which diabetes is induced chemically showed a considerable attenuation in markers associated with progression of diabetic disease as compared to wild-type animals. These markers included albuminuria, glomerular hypertrophy and glomerular content of TGF-beta and collagen type IV (Craven *et al.*, 2001).

### 4.1.14. Genetic Factors

### 4.1.13. Animal Models

Finally it has been consistently shown that overexpression of UCP-1 or MnSOD is able to correct a variety of phenotypes in cells that are generally affected in diabetes (for a review: (Brownlee, 2001)). For example, overexpression of either UCP-1 or MnSOD in aortic endothelial cells blocks the hyperglycemia induced monocyte adhesion and hyperglycemia-induced

Over the past few years it has become widely accepted that high glucose is the critical event in the development of diabetic retinopathy. Although the current rise in prevalence of diabetes is most certainly driven by life-style changes, individual differences in susceptibility to the complications associated with diabetes can, at least in part, be attributed to genetic differences in susceptibility to the disease. It is conceivable both that some genes expressed in certain groups of individuals make them less prone to retinopathy and, on the other hand, that specific genes are differentially induced in response to hyperglycemia (Engerman and Kern, 1987). There appears to be genetic determinants in the susceptibility to micro and macrovascular complications associated with diabetes. This is supported by familial clustering of diabetic retinopathy and nephropathy (Quinn *et al.*, 1996). The DCCT reported familial clustering of diabetic retinopathy with an odds ratio of 5.4 for the risk of severe retinopathy in diabetic relatives of retinopathy-positive subjects from the conventional treatment group compared with subjects with no retinopathy (DCCT, 1997).

The study of a number of monogenic disorders has also provided a new insight in genetic determinants of diabetes. Indeed a number of monogenic disorders were already identified that have diabetes as a main phenotypic feature. Molecular characterization of some of these diseases has reveled that molecules involved are primarily associated with insulin signal transduction cascade or with lipodystrophy (O'Rahilly, 2002; O'Rahilly *et al.*, 2005). If major mutations in some of these critical molecules result in severe human diabetes, then it is conceivable that more subtle mutations may alter genetic susceptibility to type 2 diabetes (O'Rahilly *et al.*, 2005). For example, a common missense variant (Pro12Ala) of the $\gamma2$ isoform of peroxisome proliferator-activated receptor gamma (PPARg) was shown to be associated with an increased risk for diabetes of about 25% (Altshuler *et al.*, 2000). A common variant (Glu23Lys) in the gene encoding the inwardly rectifying potassium channel KIR 6.2 also seems to increase diabetes risk by about 25%. Again, major mutations in this gene lead to an inherited form of severe diabetes or hypoglycemia (O'Rahilly *et al.*, 2005).

Despite recent developments and information gathered from monogenic diseases and animal models, there is still a major lack and a great need for gene-mapping studies designed to identify genes that predispose to complications of diabetes. It should, however, be noted that no single approach to study the determinants and susceptibility to diabetes-related complications is likely to be successful. Indeed, a number of factors from lifestyle to diet, from glycemia control to genetics background, are likely to contribute to development of diabetes. Thus, an optimal strategy will involve a variety of different approaches including the use of appropriate animal models. A major goal will be to examine the relationship between genetic polymorphisms and responses to different therapies and preventive strategies. Perhaps in the future the description of individual genetic profiles or, in the nearer future, the relationship between the presence of particular genetic variants in an individual and its response to particular therapies (pharmacogenomics) is a promising avenue to address treatment of diabetes and its complications, such as diabetic retinopathy.

# References

The Diabetes Control and Complications Trial Research Group. (1993) The effect of intensive treatment of diabetes on the development and progression of long-term complications in insulin-dependent diabetes mellitus. *N Engl J Med* **329**: 977–986.

The Diabetes Control and Complications Trial Research Group. (1997) Clustering of long-term complications in families with diabetes in the diabetes control and complications trial. *Diabetes* **46**: 1829–1839.

UK Prospective Diabetes Study (UKPDS) Group. (1998) Intensive blood-glucose control with sulphonylureas or insulin compared with conventional treatment and risk of complications in patients with type 2 diabetes (UKPDS 33). *Lancet* **352**: 837–853.

The Diabetes Control and Complications Trial/Epidemiology of Diabetes Interventions and Complications Research Group. (2000): Retinopathy and nephropathy in patients with type 1 diabetes four years after a trial of intensive therapy. *N Engl J Med* **342**: 381–389.

Aiello LP, Avery RL, Arrigg PG, *et al.* (1994) Vascular endothelial growth factor in ocular fluid of patients with diabetic retinopathy and other retinal disorders. *N Engl J Med* **331**: 1480–1487.

Aiello LP, Bursell SE, Clermont A, *et al.* (1997) Vascular endothelial growth factor-induced retinal permeability is mediated by protein kinase C *in vivo* and suppressed by an orally effective betaisoform-selective inhibitor. *Diabetes* **46**: 1473–1480.

Aiello LP, Northrup JM, Keyt BA, *et al.* (1995) Hypoxic regulation of vascular endothelial growth factor in retinal cells. *Arch Ophthalmol* **113**: 1538–1544.

Alon T, Hemo I, Itin A, *et al.* (1995) Vascular endothelial growth factor acts as a survival factor for newly formed retinal vessels and has implications for retinopathy of prematurity. *Nat Med* **1**: 1024–1028.

Altshuler D, Hirschhorn JN, Klannemark M, *et al.* (2000) The common PPARgamma Pro12Ala polymorphism is associated with decreased risk of type 2 diabetes. *Nat Genet* **26**: 76–80.

Alvarez J, Lee DC, Baldwin SA, Chapman D. (1987) Fourier transform infrared spectroscopic study of the structure and conformational changes of the human erythrocyte glucose transporter. *J Biol Chem* **262**: 3502–3509.

Baek KJ, Thiel BA, Lucas S, Stuehr DJ. (1993) Macrophage nitric oxide synthase subunits. Purification, characterization, and role of prosthetic groups and substrate in regulating their association into a dimeric enzyme. *J Biol Chem* **268**: 21120–21129.

Barber AJ, Lieth E, Khin SA, *et al.* (1998) Neural apoptosis in the retina during experimental and human diabetes. Early onset and effect of insulin. *J Clin Invest* **102**: 783–791.

Baynes JW, Thorpe SR. (1999) Role of oxidative stress in diabetic complications: A new perspective on an old paradigm. *Diabetes* **48**: 1–9.

Becerra SP. (1997) Structure-function studies on PEDF. A noninhibitory serpin with neurotrophic activity. *Adv Exp Med Biol* **425**: 223–237.

Beckman JA, Goldfine AB, Gordon MB, Creager MA. (2001) Ascorbate restores endothelium-dependent vasodilation impaired by acute hyperglycemia in humans. *Circulation* **103**: 1618–1623.

Beckman JS, Koppenol WH. (1996) Nitric oxide, superoxide, and peroxynitrite: The good, the bad, and ugly. *Am J Physiol* **271**: C1424–1437.

Benz D, Cadet P, Mantione K, *et al.* (2002) Tonal nitric oxide and health — a free radical and a scavenger of free radicals. *Med Sci Monit* **8**: RA1–4.

Berkowitz BA, Garner MH, Wilson CA, Corbett R.J. (1995) Nondestructive measurement of retinal glucose transport and consumption *in vivo* using NMR spectroscopy. *J Neurochem* **64**: 2325–2331.

Birnbaum MJ, Haspel HC, Rosen OM. (1986) Cloning and characterization of a cDNA encoding the rat brain glucose-transporter protein. *Proc Natl Acad Sci USA* **83**: 5784–5788.

Biswas S, Ray M, Misra S, *et al.* (1997) Selective inhibition of mitochondrial respiration and glycolysis in human leukaemic leucocytes by methylglyoxal. *Biochem J* **323**(Pt 2): 343–348.

Bolton WK, Cattran DC, Williams ME, *et al.* (2004) Randomized trial of an inhibitor of formation of advanced glycation end products in diabetic nephropathy. *Am J Nephrol* **24**: 32–40.

Brodsky SV, Gao S, Li H, Goligorsky MS. (2002) Hyperglycemic switch from mitochondrial nitric oxide to superoxide production in endothelial cells. *Am J Physiol Heart Circ Physiol* **283**: H2130–2139.

Brownlee M. (2001) Biochemistry and molecular cell biology of diabetic complications. *Nature* **414**: 813–820.

Brownlee M, Vlassara H, Cerami A. (1984) Nonenzymatic glycosylation and the pathogenesis of diabetic complications. *Ann Intern Med* **101**: 527–537.

Bulteau AL, Verbeke P, Petropoulos I, *et al.* (2001) Proteasome inhibition in glyoxal-treated fibroblasts and resistance of glycated glucose-6-phosphate dehydrogenase to 20 S proteasome degradation *in vitro*. *J Biol Chem* **276**: 45662–45668.

Bursell SE, Clermont AC, Oren B, King GL. (1995) The in vivo effect of endothelins on retinal circulation in nondiabetic and diabetic rats. *Invest Ophthalmol Vis Sci* **36**: 596–607.

Cairns MT, Alvarez J, Panico M, *et al.* (1987) Investigation of the structure and function of the human erythrocyte glucose transporter by proteolytic dissection. *Biochim Biophys Acta* **905**: 295–310.

Ceolotto G, Gallo A, Miola M, *et al.* (1999) Protein kinase C activity is acutely regulated by plasma glucose concentration in human monocytes *in vivo*. *Diabetes* **48**: 1316–1322.

Chader GJ. (2001) PEDF: Raising both hopes and questions in controlling angiogenesis. *Proc Natl Acad Sci USA* **98**: 2122–2124.

Chavakis E, Dimmeler S. (2002) Regulation of endothelial cell survival and apoptosis during angiogenesis. *Arterioscler Thromb Vasc Biol* **22**: 887–893.

Chen MS, Hutchinson, ML, Pecoraro RE, *et al.* (1983) Hyperglycemia-induced intracellular depletion of ascorbic acid in human mononuclear leukocytes. *Diabetes* **32**: 1078–1081.

Chin JJ, Jung EK, Jung CY. (1986) Structural basis of human erythrocyte glucose transporter function in reconstituted vesicles. *J Biol Chem* **261**: 7101–7104.

Collins T. (1993) Endothelial nuclear factor-kappa B and the initiation of the atherosclerotic lesion. *Lab Invest* **68**: 499–508.

Cosentino F, Hishikawa K, Katusic ZS, Luscher TF. (1997) High glucose increases nitric oxide synthase expression and superoxide anion generation in human aortic endothelial cells. *Circulation* **96**: 25–28.

Craven PA, Melhem MF, Phillips SL, DeRubertis FR. (2001) Overexpression of $Cu^{2+}/Zn^{2+}$ superoxide dismutase protects against early diabetic glomerular injury in transgenic mice. *Diabetes* **50**: 2114–2125.

Cunha-Vaz J. (1975) Early breakdown of the blood-retinal barrier in diabetes. *Br J Ophthalmol* **59**(11): 649–656.

Cunha-Vaz J. (1978) Pathophysiology of diabetic retinopathy. *Br J Ophthalmol* **62**(6): 351–355.

Curtis TM, Scholfield CN. (2004) The role of lipids and protein kinase Cs in the pathogenesis of diabetic retinopathy. *Diabetes Metab Res Rev* **20**: 28–43.

Daley ML, Watzke RC, Riddle MC. (1987) Early loss of blue-sensitive color vision in patients with type I diabetes. *Diabetes Care* **10**: 777–781.

Danis RP, Bingaman DP, Jirousek M, Yang Y. (1998) Inhibition of intraocular neovascularization caused by retinal ischemia in pigs by PKCbeta inhibition with LY333531. *Invest Ophthalmol Vis Sci* **39**: 171–179.

Datta PK, Raychaudhuri P, Bagchi S. (1995) Association of p107 with Sp1: Genetically separable regions of p107 are involved in regulation of E2F- and Sp1-dependent transcription. *Mol Cell Biol* **15**: 5444–5452.

Davies A, Meeran K, Cairns MT, Baldwin SA. (1987) Peptide-specific antibodies as probes of the orientation of the glucose transporter in the human erythrocyte membrane. *J Biol Chem* **262**: 9347–9352.

Dawson DW, Volpert OV, Gillis P, *et al.* (1999) Pigment epithelium-derived factor: A potent inhibitor of angiogenesis. *Science* **285**: 245–248.

DCCT — The Diabetes Control of Complications Trial Research Group. (1997). Clustering of long-term complications in families trial. *Diabetes* **46**(11): 1829–1839.

de Oliveira F. (1966) Pericytes in diabetic retinopathy. *Br J Ophthalmol* **50**: 134–143.

Degenhardt TP, Thorpe SR, Baynes JW. (1998) Chemical modification of proteins by methylglyoxal. *Cell Mol Biol* (Noisy-le-grand) **44**: 1139–1145.

Della Sala S, Bertoni G, Somazzi L, *et al.* (1985) Impaired contrast sensitivity in diabetic patients with and without retinopathy: A new technique for rapid assessment. *Br J Ophthalmol* **69**: 136–142.

Diederich D, Skopec J, Diederich A, Dai FX. (1994) Endothelial dysfunction in mesenteric resistance arteries of diabetic rats: Role of free radicals. *Am J Physiol* **266**: H1153–1161.

Dimmeler S, Fleming I, Fisslthaler B, *et al.* (1999) Activation of nitric oxide synthase in endothelial cells by Akt-dependent phosphorylation. *Nature* **399**: 601–605.

Dimmeler S, Haendeler J, Nehls M, Zeiher AM. (1997) Suppression of apoptosis by nitric oxide via inhibition of interleukin-1beta-converting enzyme (ICE)-like and cysteine protease protein (CPP)-32-like proteases. *J Exp Med* **185**: 601–607.

Donnelly R, Idris I, Forrester JV. (2004) Protein kinase C inhibition and diabetic retinopathy: A shot in the dark at translational research. *Br J Ophthalmol* **88**: 145–151.

Du XL, Edelstein D, Dimmeler S, *et al.* (2001) Hyperglycemia inhibits endothelial nitric oxide synthase activity by posttranslational modification at the Akt site. *J Clin Invest* **108**: 1341–1348.

Du XL, Edelstein D, Rossetti L, *et al.* (2000) Hyperglycemia-induced mitochondrial superoxide overproduction activates the hexosamine pathway and induces plasminogen activator inhibitor-1 expression by increasing Sp1 glycosylation. *Proc Natl Acad Sci USA* **97**: 12222–12226.

Enea NA, Hollis TM, Kern JA, Gardner TW. (1989) Histamine H1 receptors mediate increased blood-retinal barrier permeability in experimental diabetes. *Arch Ophthalmol* **107**: 270–274.

Engerman R, Bloodworth JM Jr., Nelson S. (1977) Relationship of microvascular disease in diabetes to metabolic control. *Diabetes* **26**: 760–769.

Engerman RL. (1989) Pathogenesis of diabetic retinopathy. *Diabetes* **38**: 1203–1206.

Engerman RL, Kern TS. (1984) Experimental galactosemia produces diabetic-like retinopathy. *Diabetes* **33**: 97–100.

Engerman RL, Kern TS. (1987) Progression of incipient diabetic retinopathy during good glycemic control. *Diabetes* **36**: 808–812.

Engerman RL, Kern TS. (1993) Aldose reductase inhibition fails to prevent retinopathy in diabetic and galactosemic dogs. *Diabetes* **42**: 820–825.

Epstein AC, Gleadle JM, McNeill LA, *et al.* (2001) C. elegans EGL-9 and mammalian homologs define a family of dioxygenases that regulate HIF by prolyl hydroxylation. *Cell* **107**: 43–54.

Esser S, Wolburg K, Wolburg H, Breier G. (1998) Vascular endothelial growth factor induces endothelial fenestrations in vitro. *J Cell Biol* **140**: 947–959.

Fernandes R, Carvalho AL, Kumagai A, Seica R. (2004) Downregulation of retinal GLUT1 in diabetes by ubiquitinylation. *Mol Vis* **10**: 618–628.

Frank RN. (2004) Diabetic retinopathy. *N Engl J Med* **350**: 48–58.

Fujio Y, Walsh K. (1999) Akt mediates cytoprotection of endothelial cells by vascular endothelial growth factor in an anchorage-dependent manner. *J Biol Chem* **274**: 16349–16354.

Fulton D, Gratton JP, McCabe TJ, *et al.* (1999) Regulation of endothelium-derived nitric oxide production by the protein kinase Akt. *Nature* **399**: 597–601.

Gao G, Li Y, Zhang D, *et al.* (2001) Unbalanced expression of VEGF and PEDF in ischemia-induced retinal neovascularization. *FEBS Lett* **489**: 270–276.

Gelfand RA, Barrett EJ. (1987) Effect of physiologic hyperinsulinemia on skeletal muscle protein synthesis and breakdown in man. *J Clin Invest* **80**: 1–6.

Gerber HP, Dixit V, Ferrara N. (1998a) Vascular endothelial growth factor induces expression of the antiapoptotic proteins Bcl-2 and A1 in vascular endothelial cells. *J Biol Chem* **273**: 13313–13316.

Gerber HP, McMurtrey A, Kowalski J, *et al.* (1998b) Vascular endothelial growth factor regulates endothelial cell survival through the phosphatidylinositol 3′-kinase/Akt signal transduction pathway. Requirement for Flk-1/KDR activation. *J Biol Chem* **273**: 30336–30343.

Gratton JP, Morales-Ruiz M, Kureishi Y, *et al.* (2001) Akt down-regulation of p38 signaling provides a novel mechanism of vascular endothelial growth factor-mediated cytoprotection in endothelial cells. *J Biol Chem* **276**: 30359–30365.

Grunwald JE, DuPont J, Riva CE. (1996) Retinal haemodynamics in patients with early diabetes mellitus. *Br J Ophthalmol* **80**: 327–331.

Gupta K, Kshirsagar S, Li W, *et al.* (1999) VEGF prevents apoptosis of human microvascular endothelial cells via opposing effects on MAPK/ERK and SAPK/JNK signaling. *Exp Cell Res* **247**: 495–504.

Haitoglou CS, Tsilibary EC, Brownlee M, Charonis AS. (1992) Altered cellular interactions between endothelial cells and nonenzymatically glucosylated laminin/type IV collagen. *J Biol Chem* **267**: 12404–12407.

Halder J, Ray M, Ray S. (1993) Inhibition of glycolysis and mitochondrial respiration of Ehrlich ascites carcinoma cells by methylglyoxal. *Int J Cancer* **54**: 443–449.

Hammes HP, Alt A, Niwa T, *et al.* (1999) Differential accumulation of advanced glycation end products in the course of diabetic retinopathy. *Diabetologia* **42**: 728–736.

Harhaj NS, Antonetti DA. (2004) Regulation of tight junctions and loss of barrier function in pathophysiology. *Int J Biochem Cell Biol* **36**: 1206–1237.

Harik SI, Kalaria RN, Whitney PM, *et al.* (1990) Glucose transporters are abundant in cells with "occluding" junctions at the blood-eye barriers. *Proc Natl Acad Sci USA* **87**: 4261–4264.

Haspel HC, Rosenfeld MG, Rosen OM. (1988) Characterization of antisera to a synthetic carboxyl-terminal peptide of the glucose transporter protein. *J Biol Chem* **263**: 398–403.

Hirata C, Nakano K, Nakamura N, *et al.* (1997) Advanced glycation end products induce expression of vascular endothelial growth factor by retinal Muller cells. *Biochem Biophys Res Commun* **236**: 712–715.

Hoffmann J, Haendeler J, Aicher A, *et al.* (2001) Aging enhances the sensitivity of endothelial cells toward apoptotic stimuli: Important role of nitric oxide. *Circ Res* **89**: 709–715.

Hoffmann S, Friedrichs U, Eichler W, *et al.* (2002) Advanced glycation end products induce choroidal endothelial cell proliferation, matrix metalloproteinase-2 and VEGF upregulation *in vitro*. *Graefes Arch Clin Exp Ophthalmol* **240**: 996–1002.

Hruz PW, Mueckler MM. (2001) Structural analysis of the GLUT1 facilitative glucose transporter (review). *Mol Membr Biol* **18**: 183–193.

Huang Q, Yuan Y. (1997) Interaction of PKC and NOS in signal transduction of microvascular hypermeability. *Am J Physiol* **273**: H2442–2451.

Inoguchi T, Battan R, Handler E, *et al.* (1992) Preferential elevation of protein kinase C isoform beta II and diacylglycerol levels in the aorta and heart of diabetic rats: Differential reversibility to glycemic control by islet cell transplantation. *Proc Natl Acad Sci USA* **89**: 11059–11063.

Ishii H, Jirousek MR, Koya D, *et al.* (1996) Amelioration of vascular dysfunctions in diabetic rats by an oral PKC beta inhibitor. *Science* **272**: 728–731.

Ivan M, Kondo K, Yang H, *et al.* (2001) HIF alpha targeted for VHL-mediated destruction by proline hydroxylation: Implications for O2 sensing. *Science* **292**: 464–468.

Jaakkola P, Mole DR, Tian YM, *et al.* (2001) Targeting of HIF-alpha to the von Hippel-Lindau ubiquitylation complex by O2-regulated prolyl hydroxylation. *Science* **292**: 468–472.

Jakeman LB, Winer J, Bennett GL, *et al.* (1992) Binding sites for vascular endothelial growth factor are localized on endothelial cells in adult rat tissues. *J Clin Invest* **89**: 244–253.

Jirousek MR, Gillig JR, Gonzalez CM, *et al.* (1996) (S)-13-[(dimethylamino)methyl]-10,11,14,15-tetrahydro-4,9:16, 21-dimetheno-1H, 13H-dibenzo[e,k]pyrrolo[3,4-h][1,4,-13]oxadiazacyclohexadecene-1,3(2H)-dione (LY333531)

and related analogues: Isozyme selective inhibitors of protein kinase C beta. *J Med Chem* **39**: 2664–2671.

Kador PF, Akagi Y, Takahashi Y, *et al.* (1990) Prevention of retinal vessel changes associated with diabetic retinopathy in galactose-fed dogs by aldose reductase inhibitors. *Arch Ophthalmol* **108**: 1301–1309.

Karpen, CW, Cataland S, O'Dorisio TM, Panganamala RV. (1985) Production of 12-hydroxyeicosatetraenoic acid and vitamin E status in platelets from type I human diabetic subjects. *Diabetes* **34**: 526–531.

Kennedy L, Baynes JW. (1984) Non-enzymatic glycosylation and the chronic complications of diabetes: An overview. *Diabetologia* **26**: 93–98.

Kern TS, Engerman RL. (1996) A mouse model of diabetic retinopathy. *Arch Ophthalmol* **114**: 986–990.

Klein R. (1995) Hyperglycemia and microvascular and macrovascular disease in diabetes. *Diabetes Care* **18**: 258–268.

Klein R, Klein BE, Moss SE. (1989) The Wisconsin epidemiological study of diabetic retinopathy: A review. *Diabetes Metab Rev* **5**: 559–570.

Knight RJ, Kofoed KF, Schelbert HR, Buxton DB. (1996) Inhibition of glyceraldehyde-3-phosphate dehydrogenase in post-ischaemic myocardium. *Cardiovasc Res* **32**: 1016–1023.

Kowluru RA, Jirousek MR, Stramm L, *et al.* (1998) Abnormalities of retinal metabolism in diabetes or experimental galactosemia: V. Relationship between protein kinase C and ATPases. *Diabetes* **47**: 464–469.

Koya D, King GL. (1998) Protein kinase C activation and the development of diabetic complications. *Diabetes* **47**: 859–866.

Krogsaa B, Lund-Andersen H, Mehlsen J, Sestoft L. (1987) Blood-retinal barrier permeability versus diabetes duration and retinal morphology in insulin dependent diabetic patients. *Acta Ophthalmol. (Copenh)* **65**: 686–692.

Kumagai AK. (1999) Glucose transport in brain and retina: implications in the management and complications of diabetes. *Diabetes Metab Res Rev* **15**: 261–273.

Kumagai AK, Glasgow BJ, Pardridge WM. (1994) GLUT1 glucose transporter expression in the diabetic and nondiabetic human eye. *Invest Ophthalmol Vis Sci* **35**: 2887–2894.

Kumagai AK, Vinores SA, Pardridge WM. (1996) Pathological upregulation of inner blood-retinal barrier

Glut1 glucose transporter expression in diabetes mellitus. *Brain Res* **706**: 313–317.

Kwong LK, Sohal RS. (1998) Substrate and site specificity of hydrogen peroxide generation in mouse mitochondria. *Arch Biochem Biophys* **350**: 118–126.

Lee AY, Chung SS. (1999) Contributions of polyol pathway to oxidative stress in diabetic cataract. *Faseb J* **13**: 23–30.

Leto G, Pricci F, Amadio L, *et al.* (2001) Increased retinal endothelial cell monolayer permeability induced by the diabetic milieu: Role of advanced non-enzymatic glycation and polyol pathway activation. *Diabetes Metab Res Rev* **17**: 448–458.

Liao DF, Monia B, Dean N, Berk BC. (1997) Protein kinase C-zeta mediates angiotensin II activation of ERK1/2 in vascular smooth muscle cells. *J Biol Chem* **272**: 6146–6150.

Lieth E, Barber AJ, Xu B, *et al.* (1998) Glial reactivity and impaired glutamate metabolism in short-term experimental diabetic retinopathy. Penn State Retina Research Group. *Diabetes* **47**: 815–820.

Lipton SA, Rosenberg PA. (1994) Excitatory amino acids as a final common pathway for neurologic disorders. *N Engl J Med* **330**: 613–622.

Lu M, Kuroki M, Amano S, *et al.* (1998) Advanced glycation end products increase retinal vascular endothelial growth factor expression. *J Clin Invest* **101**: 1219–1224.

Lutty GA, McLeod DS, Merges C, *et al.* (1996) Localization of vascular endothelial growth factor in human retina and choroid. *Arch Ophthalmol* **114**: 971–977.

Lynch JJ, Ferro TJ, Blumenstock FA, *et al.* (1990) Increased endothelial albumin permeability mediated by protein kinase C activation. *J Clin Invest* **85**: 1991–1998.

Mamputu JC, Renier G. (2002) Advanced glycation end products increase, through a protein kinase C-dependent pathway, vascular endothelial growth factor expression in retinal endothelial cells. Inhibitory effect of gliclazide. *J Diabetes Complications* **16**: 284–293.

Mandarino LJ, Finlayson J, Hassell JR. (1994) High glucose downregulates glucose transport activity in retinal capillary pericytes but not endothelial cells. *Invest Ophthalmol Vis Sci* **35**: 964–972.

Mantych GJ, Hageman GS, Devaskar SU. (1993) Characterization of glucose transporter isoforms in the adult and developing human eye. *Endocrinology* **133**: 600–607.

Marano CW, Garulacan LA, Ginanni N, Mullin JM. (2001) Phorbol ester treatment increases paracellular permeability across IEC-18 gastrointestinal epithelium in vitro. *Dig Dis Sci* **46**: 1490–1499.

Marfella R, Verrazzo G, Acampora R, *et al.* (1995) Glutathione reverses systemic hemodynamic changes induced by acute hyperglycemia in healthy subjects. *Am J Physiol* **268**: E1167–E1173.

Masson N, Willam C, Maxwell PH, *et al.* (2001) Independent function of two destruction domains in hypoxia-inducible factor-alpha chains activated by prolyl hydroxylation. *Embo J* **20**: 5197–5206.

Maxwell PH, Wiesener MS, Chang GW, *et al.* (1999) The tumour suppressor protein VHL targets hypoxia-inducible factors for oxygen-dependent proteolysis. *Nature* **399**: 271–275.

McCaleb ML, McKean ML, Hohman TC, *et al.* (1991) Intervention with the aldose reductase inhibitor, tolrestat, in renal and retinal lesions of streptozotocin-diabetic rats. *Diabetologia* **34**: 695–701.

McLellan AC, Thornalley PJ, Benn J, Sonksen PH. (1994) Glyoxalase system in clinical diabetes mellitus and correlation with diabetic complications. *Clin Sci (Lond)* **87**: 21–29.

Mitch WE, Bailey JL, Wang X, *et al.* (1999) Evaluation of signals activating ubiquitin-proteasome proteolysis in a model of muscle wasting. *Am J Physiol* **276**: C1132–C1138.

Mizutani M, Gerhardinger C, Lorenzi M. (1998) Muller cell changes in human diabetic retinopathy. *Diabetes* **47**: 445–449.

Mizutani M, Kern TS, Lorenzi M. (1996) Accelerated death of retinal microvascular cells in human and experimental diabetic retinopathy. *J Clin Invest* **97**: 2883–2890.

Monnier VM. (1989) Towards a Maillard theory of ageing. In: Baynes JW, Monnier VM. (eds.), *The Maillard Reaction in Aging, Diabetes and Nutrition*, Alan R. Liss, New York, pp. 1–22.

Mueckler M. (1994) Facilitative glucose transporters. *Eur J Biochem* **219**: 713–725.

Mueckler M, Caruso C, Baldwin SA, *et al.* (1985) Sequence and structure of a human glucose transporter. *Science* **229**: 941–945.

Murata Y, Kim HG, Rogers KT, *et al.* (1994) Negative regulation of Sp1 trans-activation is correlated with the binding of cellular proteins to the amino terminus of the Sp1 trans-activation domain. *J Biol Chem* **269**: 20674–20681.

Nakamura S, Makita Z, Ishikawa S, *et al.* (1997) Progression of nephropathy in spontaneous diabetic rats is prevented by OPB-9195, a novel inhibitor of advanced glycation. *Diabetes* **46**: 895–899.

Newton AC, Johnson JE. (1998) Protein kinase C: A paradigm for regulation of protein function by two membrane-targeting modules. *Biochim Biophys Acta* **1376**: 155–172.

Nishikawa T, Edelstein D, Brownlee M. (2000a) The missing link: A single unifying mechanism for diabetic complications. *Kidney Int. Suppl* **77**: S26–S30.

Nishikawa T, Edelstein D, Du XL, *et al.* (2000b) Normalizing mitochondrial superoxide production blocks three pathways of hyperglycaemic damage. *Nature* **404**: 787–790.

Nor JE, Christensen J, Mooney DJ, Polverini PJ. (1999) Vascular endothelial growth factor (VEGF)-mediated angiogenesis is associated with enhanced endothelial cell survival and induction of Bcl-2 expression. *Am J Pathol* **154**: 375–384.

Nourooz-Zadeh J, Pereira P. (1999) Age-related accumulation of free polyunsaturated fatty acids in human retina. *Ophthalmic Res* **31**: 273–279.

O'Rahilly S. (2002) Insights into obesity and insulin resistance from the study of extreme human phenotypes. *Eur J Endocrinol* **147**: 435–441.

O'Rahilly S, Barroso I, Wareham NJ. (2005) Genetic factors in type 2 diabetes: The end of the beginning? *Science* **307**: 370–373.

Oya T, Hattori N, Mizuno Y, *et al.* (1999) Methylglyoxal modification of protein. Chemical and immunochemical characterization of methylglyoxal-arginine adducts. *J Biol Chem* **274**: 18492–18502.

Papapetropoulos A, Fulton D, Mahboubi K, *et al.* (2000) Angiopoietin-1 inhibits endothelial cell apoptosis via the Akt/survivin pathway. *J Biol Chem* **275**: 9102–9105.

Parekh DB, Ziegler W, Parker PJ. (2000) Multiple pathways control protein kinase C phosphorylation. *Embo J* **19**: 496–503.

Park CW, Kim JH, Lee JH, *et al.* (2000a) High glucose-induced intercellular adhesion molecule-1 (ICAM-1) expression through an osmotic effect in rat mesangial cells is PKC-NF-kappa B-dependent. *Diabetologia* **43**: 1544–1553.

Park JY, Takahara N, Gabriele A, *et al.* (2000b) Induction of endothelin-1 expression by glucose: An effect of protein kinase C activation. *Diabetes* **49**: 1239–1248.

Phillips SA, Mirrlees D, Thornalley PJ. (1993) Modification of the glyoxalase system in streptozotocin-induced diabetic rats. Effect of the aldose reductase inhibitor Statil. *Biochem Pharmacol* **46**: 805–811.

Poulsom R, Prockop DJ, Boot-Handford RP. (1990) Effects of long-term diabetes and galactosaemia upon lens and retinal mRNA levels in the rat. *Exp Eye Res* **51**: 27–32.

Price SR, Bailey JL, Wang X, *et al.* (1996) Muscle wasting in insulinopenic rats results from activation of the ATP-dependent, ubiquitin-proteasome proteolytic pathway by a mechanism including gene transcription. *J Clin Invest* **98**: 1703–1708.

Quinn M, Angelico MC, Warram JH, Krolewski AS. (1996) Familial factors determine the development of diabetic nephropathy in patients with IDDM. *Diabetologia* **39**: 940–945.

Rao GN, Cotlier E. (1986) Free epsilon amino groups and 5-hydroxymethylfurfural contents in clear and cataractous human lenses. *Invest Ophthalmol Vis Sci* **27**: 98–102.

Rasmussen H, Chu KW, Campochiaro P, *et al.* (2001) Clinical protocol. An open-label, phase I, single administration, dose-escalation study of ADGVPEDF.11D (ADPEDF) in neovascular age-related macular degeneration (AMD). *Hum Gene Ther* **12**: 2029–2032.

Robinson GS, Pierce EA, Rook SL, *et al.* (1996) Oligodeoxynucleotides inhibit retinal neovascularization in a murine model of proliferative retinopathy. *Proc Natl Acad Sci USA* **93**: 4851–4856.

Robison WG Jr., Tillis TN, Laver N, Kinoshita JH. (1990) Diabetes-related histopathologies of the rat retina prevented with an aldose reductase inhibitor. *Exp Eye Res* **50**: 355–366.

Roos MD, Su K, Baker JR, Kudlow JE. (1997) O glycosylation of an Sp1-derived peptide blocks known Sp1 protein interactions. *Mol Cell Biol* **17**: 6472–6480.

Roy S. (1996) Distribution and expression of GLUT1 in the retina of galactose-fed rat. [ARVO abstract]. *Invest Ophthalmol Vis Sci* **37**: S970.

Sander B, Larsen M, Engler C, *et al.* (1994) Early changes in diabetic retinopathy: Capillary loss and blood-retina barrier permeability in relation to metabolic control. *Acta Ophthalmol (Copenh)* **72**: 553–559.

Shapiro R, McManus MJ, Zalut C, Bunn HF. (1980) Sites of nonenzymatic glycosylation of human hemoglobin A. *J Biol Chem* **255**: 3120–3127.

Shiba T, Inoguchi T, Sportsman JR, *et al.* (1993) Correlation of diacylglycerol level and protein kinase C activity in rat retina to retinal circulation. *Am J Physiol* **265**: E783–E793.

Shinohara M, Thornalley PJ, Giardino I, *et al.* (1998) Overexpression of glyoxalase-I in bovine endothelial cells inhibits intracellular advanced glycation endproduct formation and prevents hyperglycemia-induced increases in macromolecular endocytosis. *J Clin Invest* **101**: 1142–1147.

Sokol S, Moskowitz A, Skarf B, *et al.* (1985) Contrast sensitivity in diabetics with and without background retinopathy. *Arch Ophthalmol* **103**: 51–54.

Soulis-Liparota T, Cooper M, Papazoglou D, *et al.* (1991) Retardation by aminoguanidine of development of albuminuria, mesangial expansion, and tissue fluorescence in streptozocin-induced diabetic rat. *Diabetes* **40**: 1328–1334.

Spitaler MM, Graier WF. (2002) Vascular targets of redox signalling in diabetes mellitus. *Diabetologia* **45**:476–494.

Stellmach V, Crawford SE, Zhou W, Bouck N. (2001) Prevention of ischemia-induced retinopathy by the - natural ocular antiangiogenic agent pigment epithelium-derived factor. *Proc Natl Acad Sci USA* **98**: 2593–2597.

Stevens VJ, Rouzer CA, Monnier VM, Cerami A. (1978) Diabetic cataract formation: Potential role of glycosylation of lens crystallins. *Proc Natl Acad Sci USA* **75**: 2918–2922.

Stitt AW, Bhaduri T, McMullen CB, *et al.* (2000) Advanced glycation end products induce blood-retinal barrier dysfunction in normoglycemic rats. *Mol Cell Biol Res Commun* **3**: 380–388.

Stitt AW, Li YM, Gardiner TA, *et al.* (1997) Advanced glycation end products (AGEs) co-localize with AGE receptors in the retinal vasculature of diabetic and of AGE-infused rats. *Am J Pathol* **150**: 523–531.

Stratton IM, Adler AI, Neil HA, *et al.* (2000) Association of glycaemia with macrovascular and microvascular complications of type 2 diabetes (UKPDS 35): Prospective observational study. *BMJ* **321**: 405–412.

Sutter CH, Laughner E, Semenza GL. (2000) Hypoxia-inducible factor 1alpha protein expression is controlled by oxygen-regulated ubiquitination that is disrupted by deletions and missense mutations. *Proc Natl Acad Sci USA* **97**: 4748–4753.

Suzuki K, Koh YH, Mizuno H, *et al.* (1998) Overexpression of aldehyde reductase protects PC12 cells from the cytotoxicity of methylglyoxal or 3-deoxyglucosone. *J Biochem (Tokyo)* **123**: 353–357.

Suzuma K, Takahara N, Suzuma I, *et al.* (2002) Characterization of protein kinase C beta isoform's action on retinoblastoma protein phosphorylation, vascular endothelial growth factor-induced endothelial cell proliferation, and retinal neovascularization. *Proc Natl Acad Sci USA* **99**: 721–726.

Swamy MS, Abraham EC. (1987) Lens protein composition, glycation and high molecular weight aggregation in aging rats. *Invest Ophthalmol Vis Sci* **28**: 1693–1701.

Takagi H, King GL, Aiello LP. (1998) Hypoxia upregulates glucose transport activity through an adenosine-mediated increase of GLUT1 expression in retinal capillary endothelial cells. *Diabetes* **47**: 1480–1488.

Takata K, Hirano H, Kasahara M. (1997) Transport of glucose across the blood-tissue barriers. *Int Rev Cytol* **172**: 1–53.

Takata K, Kasahara T, Kasahara M, *et al.* (1990) Erythrocyte/HepG2-type glucose transporter is concentrated in cells of blood-tissue barriers. *Biochem Biophys Res Commun* **173**: 67–73.

Takata K, Kasahara T, Kasahara M, *et al.* (1992) Ultracytochemical localization of the erythrocyte/HepG2-type glucose transporter (GLUT1) in cells of the blood-retinal barrier in the rat. *Invest Ophthalmol Vis Sci* **33**: 377–383.

Tesfamariam B, Cohen RA. (1992) Free radicals mediate endothelial cell dysfunction caused by elevated glucose. *Am J Physiol* **263**: H321–326.

Thornalley PJ. (1990) The glyoxalase system: New developments towards functional characterization of a metabolic pathway fundamental to biological life. *Biochem J* **269**: 1–11.

Tolentino MJ, McLeod DS, Taomoto M, *et al.* (2002) Pathologic features of vascular endothelial growth factor-induced retinopathy in the nonhuman primate. *Am J Ophthalmol* **133**: 373–385.

Tran J, Rak J, Sheehan C, *et al.* (1999) Marked induction of the IAP family antiapoptotic proteins survivin and XIAP by VEGF in vascular endothelial cells. *Biochem Biophys Res Commun* **264**: 781–788.

Vorwerk CK, Lipton SA, Zurakowski D, *et al.* (1996) Chronic low-dose glutamate is toxic to retinal ganglion cells. Toxicity blocked by memantine. *Invest Ophthalmol Vis Sci* **37**: 1618–1624.

Wallace DC. (1992) Diseases of the mitochondrial DNA. *Annu Rev Biochem* **61**: 1175–1212.

Watanabe T, Mio Y, Hoshino FB, *et al.* (1994) GLUT2 expression in the rat retina: Localization at the apical ends of Muller cells. *Brain Res* **655**: 128–134.

White MF. (2002) IRS proteins and the common path to diabetes. *Am J Physiol Endocrinol. Metab* **283**: E413–E422.

Williams B, Gallacher B, Patel H, Orme C. (1997) Glucose-induced protein kinase C activation regulates vascular permeability factor mRNA expression and peptide production by human vascular smooth muscle cells in vitro. *Diabetes* **46**: 1497–1503.

Williamson JR, Chang K, Frangos M, *et al.* (1993) Hyperglycemic pseudohypoxia and diabetic complications. *Diabetes* **42**: 801–813.

Wise GN. (1956) Retinal neovascularization. *Trans Am Acad Ophthalmol Otolaryngol* **54**: 729–826.

Wolff SP, Dean RT. (1987) Glucose autoxidation and protein modification. The potential role of 'autoxidative glycosylation' in diabetes. *Biochem J* **245**: 243–250.

Xia P, Aiello LP, Ishii H, *et al.* (1996) Characterization of vascular endothelial growth factor's effect on the activation of protein kinase C, its isoforms, endothelial cell growth. *J Clin Invest* **98**: 2018–2026.

Xia P, Kramer RM, King GL. (1995) Identification of the mechanism for the inhibition of Na+,K(+)-adenosine triphosphatase by hyperglycemia involving activation of protein kinase C and cytosolic phospholipase A2. *J Clin Invest* **96**: 733–740.

## 4.2. Cell Factors

### António Francisco Ambrósio

The complications of diabetes are mainly related to vascular alterations in the heart, kidney, legs and retina. The clinical signs have supported the view that vascular endothelial cells are particularly susceptible to hyperglycemia, and that changes occurring in endothelial cells underlie functional abnormalities in various organs and tissues.

Diabetic retinopathy (DR) has been considered a disease that affects principally retinal microvessels (Cunha-Vaz, 1993; 2001). Several clinical evidences, such as the formation of microaneurysms and cotton-wool spots, hemorrhages, macular edema and neovascularization, are indicative that retinal microvascular cells are susceptible to hyperglycemia. However, other retinal cell types, such as neurons, Muller cells, astrocytes and microglial cells may also be affected by diabetes. In recent years, a large body of evidence has clearly demonstrated that other cell types are affected by diabetes in the retina (Gardner *et al.*, 2000; Lorenzi and Gerhardinger, 2001), and alterations occurring in each cell type can potentially affect other cells. However, it is not clear yet which cell types might be affected first. This chapter will focus on past and present evidences demonstrating the involvement of several cell types of the retina in the pathogenesis of DR. Since platelets and leukocytes have also been linked to retinal dysfunction caused by diabetes, the pathogenic mechanisms involving both platelets and leukocytes will also be addressed. It is important to mention that this chapter will deal with cell changes relevant to early non-proliferative retinopathy, the initial stages of the retinopathy, when individual cell changes can still be identified and their relative value considered. Later changes occurring at the proliferative phase are essentially due to retinal ischemia and appear to be mainly independent of the systemic diabetic disease.

### 4.2.1. Cell Changes Relevant to Blood-Retinal Barrier Breakdown

Breakdown of the blood-retinal barrier is a hallmark of DR. It has been shown that both inner and outer BRB are affected by diabetes, but the inner retinal vasculature appears to be the primary site of leakage in diabetic humans and rats (Vinores *et al.*, 1989, 1993; Carmo *et al.*, 1998). Most of research in this field has been addressed to inner BRB, and, therefore, most data are related with retinal microvasculature and endothelial cells.

### 4.2.2. Tight Junctions

The retina is separated from blood circulation by two barriers, the inner blood-retinal barrier (BRB), confined to endothelial cells from retinal blood vessels, and the outer BRB, located at retinal pigment epithelial cells (Shakib and Cunha-Vaz, 1966). The barrier properties are due to the presence of junctional structures between cells. These structures, named tight junctions (TJ), prevent solutes from moving between cells, thus, regulating paracellular permeability, and provides retina with a selective mechanism to regulate its environment (osmotic balance and nutrients).

Regarding the molecular architecture of TJ, several structural proteins have been identified in both endothelial and epithelial cells in various tissues. Occludin, a 65 kDa protein, was the first transmembrane protein identified as a component of TJ (Furuse *et al.*, 1993). It was also shown that a family of multiple integral membrane proteins called

claudins, smaller than occludin (about 22 kDa), is also localized in TJ (Furuse *et al.*, 1998; Morita *et al.*, 1999). Confocal and immunoelectron microscopy have shown that another integral membrane protein, called junctional adhesion molecule (JAM), co-distributes with tight junction components (Martin-Padura *et al.*, 1998). Intracellular non-transmembrane proteins on the cytosolic leaflet have also been identified as components of TJ: zonula occludens-1 (ZO-1) (Stevenson *et al.*, 1986), ZO-2 (Jesaitis *et al.*, 1994); ZO-3 (Haskins *et al.*, 1998); cingulin (Citi *et al.*, 1988) 7H6 (Zhong *et al.*, 1993) and symplekin (Keon *et al.*, 1996). ZO-1, ZO-2 and ZO-3 have a high capacity for multiple protein-protein interactions and may function to couple extracellular signaling pathways to the cytoskeleton, thus, suggesting a role for cytoskeleton regulation of TJ (Wittchen *et al.*, 1999).

### 4.2.3. Alterations in Tight Junctions Expression and Phosphorylation

The increase in BRB permeability is the first clinically evident sign of DR (Cunha-Vaz *et al.*, 1975). Considering that tight junction proteins have a predominant role in regulating BRB permeability, changes in tight junction proteins expression and localization in endothelial or epithelial cells, due to diabetes, may account for increased permeability properties. The first evidence demonstrating that the content of occludin decreases in the retinas of streptozotocin (STZ)-induced diabetic rats in comparison to control animals was reported by Antonetti *et al.* (1998). The immunoreactivity of occludin decreased in the retinas of diabetic animals, as demonstrated by immunoblot analysis and immunohistochemistry. In addition, occludin was differentially distributed in the blood vessels. In diabetic retinas, occludin immunoreactivity decreased in the capillaries and it was redistributed in the arterioles from continuous cell border to punctate immunoreactivity. Treatment with insulin, only for 48 hours, reversed the pattern of occludin immunoreactivity in diabetic retinas, clearly demonstrating that this is not an irreversible process (Barber *et al.*, 2000). The reduction of occludin immunoreactivity was not accompanied by a reduction in claudin-5 immunoreactivity, suggesting that occludin might play a prominent role in this process (Barber and Antonetti, 2003). However, recently, two studies have demonstrated that the mRNA expression and protein content of claudin-5 are decreased in the retinas of STZ-induced diabetic rats (Bucolo *et al.*, 2009; Klaassen *et al.*, 2009). Moreover, Leal and colleagues (2007) found that the levels of ZO-1, in addition to occludin levels, are also decreased in diabetic mice retinas.

Vascular endothelial growth factor (VEGF) has been largely implicated in the pathogenesis of DR and has been shown to have an important role in regulating vessel permeability (Wilkinson-Berka, 2004), but it is not completely clear yet how VEGF regulates paracellular permeability. Treatment of cultured bovine retinal endothelial cells (BRECs) with VEGF for six hours significantly reduces the content of occludin (Antonetti *et al.*, 1998). VEGF also increases BRB permeability soon after injection into the vitreous, and this effect is mediated by the activation and translocation of protein kinase C (PKC) (Aiello *et al.*, 1997). VEGF induces a rapid phosphorylation of occludin, 15 min after intravitreal injection, probably mediated by PKC, but other kinases may be involved (Antonetti *et al.*, 1999). This observation was accompanied by a rapid increase in occludin content, which decreased after 90 min. Similar results were found when BRECs were exposed to VEGF.

In addition to occludin phosphorylation, VEGF also rapidly increases the phosphorylation of ZO-1 in tyrosine residues, contrary to occludin, which seems to be predominantly phosphorylated in serine or threonine residues. These results indicate that the phosphorylation of tight junction proteins might promote an increase in tight junction permeability or signal a long-term decrease in tight junction proteins content. It has been hypothesized that in addition to VEGF other growth factors can promote an increase in

barrier permeability by redistribution of tight junction proteins. Confirming this hypothesis, it was found that platelet-derived growth factor (PDGF) increases the permeability to dextran and alters the distribution of both occludin and ZO-1 from the cell border to the cytoplasm in MDCK cells (Harhaj *et al.*, 2002). On the opposite, corticosteroids can increase barrier properties. Treatment of BRECs with hydrocortisone decreased the transport of water and solutes across cell monolayers. Hydrocortisone increased the protein and mRNA content of occludin and increased both occludin and ZO-1 staining at cell borders. In addition, occludin phosphorylation was significantly reduced, pointing out again that occludin phosphorylation is an important process in the regulation of barrier permeability (Antonetti *et al.*, 2002). In human umbilical vein endothelial cells (HUVECs) monolayers treated with hydrogen peroxide, it was observed an increase in occludin phosphorylation on serine residues, redistribution of occludin on the cell surface and dissociation of occludin from ZO-1. In addition to serine phosphorylation, tyrosine phosphorylation of occludin was found to reduce its ability to bind both ZO-1 and ZO-2 (Kale *et al.*, 2003). Also, the inhibition of tyrosine phosphatase, which prevents protein dephosphorylation at tyrosine residues, induced disruption of endothelial barrier integrity in porcine brain capillary endothelial cells and proteolysis of occludin, but not ZO-1 and claudin-5 (Lohmann *et al.*, 2004).

This group of results, obtained in experimental models, clearly demonstrates that BRB permeability is associated with changes in the expression, phosphorylation and localization of tight junction proteins in endothelial cells, principally occludin and ZO-1, but more recent evidences also point a role for claudin-5. VEGF, a potential key player in the pathogenesis of DR, was also found to regulate the expression and phosphorylation of tight junction proteins, probably through protein kinase C.

The evidence presented here shows that the increase in BRB permeability is essentially due to an increase in paracellular flux, i.e. flux between cells. The possibility that transcellular flux, i.e. flux occurring through the cells, might also contribute to increased barrier permeability cannot be ruled out, but there is no clear evidence demonstrating the contribution of transcellular permeability to BRB breakdown.

### 4.2.4. Microvascular Cell Death

Retinal diabetic microangiopathy is characterized by BRB breakdown, basement membrane thickening of retinal vessels, formation of microaneurysms, hemorrhages, cotton-wool spots, capillary obliteration and acellular capillaries, which ultimately lead to retinal ischemia and neovascularization (Cunha-Vaz, 1978). Some of these events occur because retinal vascular cells, namely pericytes and endothelial cells, die prematurely during diabetes. Microvascular cells may become dysfunctional and undergo apoptosis due to hyperglycemia.

Pericytes are embedded in basement membrane and are considered to regulate capillary and arteriolar lumen size due to their contractile properties. Pericytes also have a lower capacity for replication and are, apparently, more susceptible to stress conditions than endothelial cells (Sharma *et al.*, 1985; Archer, 1999). It is known since several decades ago that pericyte loss is an early event in diabetic retinas (Addison *et al.*, 1970; Papachristodoulou *et al.*, 1976). More recently, Mizutani *et al.* (1996) have shown, using the TUNEL technique, which detects cells undergoing apoptosis *in situ*, that diabetes causes accelerated death of both retinal pericytes and endothelial cells in diabetic patients and rats. The early apoptosis in retinal microvascular cells, detected after 6 to 8 months of diabetes, predicts the development of the histologic lesions, characteristic of DR, which appear several months later (Kern *et al.*, 2000). Li *et al.* (1997) also found a significant decrease in the ratio pericytes/endothelial cells in human diabetic retinas, indicating that pericytes are more susceptible to diabetes than endothelial cells. In galactose-fed dogs, which develop retinal capillary changes similar to those observed in DR, there is also a selective degeneration of retinal pericytes (Kador *et al.*, 1988).

Consistent with the fact that apoptosis of pericytes and retinal endothelial cells appears to be the mechanism of retinal capillary cells loss, it was shown that caspase-3, an executioner apoptotic enzyme, is activated in diabetic rat retinas and in retinal capillary cells exposed to high glucose (Kowluru and Koppolu, 2002; Mohr *et al.*, 2002; Busik *et al.*, 2008). Caspase-10 (initiator caspase), caspase-3 and caspase-9 (effector caspases) were also shown to be involved in the apoptosis of pericytes, since selective inhibition of these caspases inhibited annexin V staining, an indicator of early apoptosis (Lecomte *et al.*, 2004). In mice retinas, several caspases, including caspase-1, -2, -6, -8, and -9, were activated as early as two months of diabetes. With increasing duration of diabetes, the pattern of caspase activity changed. Similar results were obtained with retinas from patients with type 2 diabetes, with significant increases in the activities of caspase-1, -3, -4 and -6 (Mohr *et al.*, 2002). The expression of another regulator of apoptosis, the pro-apoptotic protein Bax, is also significantly increased in postmortem retinas of diabetic donors. Several pericytes, as well as neural cells, presented intense Bax staining, often in conjunction with DNA fragmentation. Cultured retinal pericytes exposed to high levels of glucose also showed elevated levels of Bax and annexin V staining (Podestà *et al.*, 2000), and high glucose increased the translocation of Bax into the mitochondria and the release of cytochrome C into the cytosol in both pericytes and endothelial cells (Kowluru and Abbas, 2003). Moreover, some evidences support the involvement of caspase-independent apoptotic processes in retinal cells, particularly through apoptosis inducing factor (AIF). An upregulation of AIF levels was found in the retinas of diabetic patients (Abu El-Asrar *et al.*, 2007), and elevated glucose-induced apoptosis in retinal endothelial cells was associated with AIF translocation from the mitochondria to the nucleus (Leal *et al.*, 2009).

Microvascular cells apoptosis might be triggered or mediated by different processes and molecules. Advanced glycation end products (Denis *et al.*, 2002; Yamagishi *et al.*, 2002) and increased activity of aldose reductase (Murata *et al.*, 2002) have been linked to retinal pericytes apoptosis. The activation of the nuclear factor (NF)-*kappaB* also triggers an apoptotic program in cultured retinal pericytes exposed to high glucose, but not in endothelial cells. The number of pericytes with positive nuclei for NF-*kappaB* also increased in retinal capillaries of diabetic patients, and this observation correlated well with microvascular cell apoptosis and acellular capillaries. In both control and diabetic retinas from human donors, endothelial cells were not positive for NF-*kappaB* (Romeo *et al.*, 2002). Oxidative stress also seems to have a role in microvascular cells apoptosis. Incubating isolated retinal capillary cells exposed to high glucose with antioxidants and feeding diabetic rats with a diet supplemented with various antioxidants inhibited the activation of retinal caspase-3 and apoptosis of endothelial cells and pericytes (Kowluru and Koppolu, 2002). Scavenging superoxides also inhibit the release of cytochrome C from mitochondria and the translocation of Bax to mitochondria (Kowluru and Abbas, 2003).

The enzyme poly(ADP-ribose)polymerase (PARP) also seems to have an important role in the development of diabetic retinopathy and in microvascular cells apoptosis. The activity of PARP is increased in whole retinas, in endothelial cells and pericytes of diabetic rats. Treatment with a PARP inhibitor inhibited NF-*kappaB* activation, microvascular cell death and the development of the characteristic histopathologic lesions of diabetic retinas (Zheng *et al.*, 2004).

This group of findings clearly shows that hyperglycemia causes apoptosis in microvascular cells and that retinal pericytes seem to be more susceptible than endothelial cells to stress conditions triggered by diabetes. However, it must be noted that it is easier to identify an apoptotic pericyte *in situ* than an apoptotic endothelial cell. Pericytes are surrounded by the basement membrane, and, therefore, it is much more difficult to eliminate its debris, whereas, dying endothelial cells are easily removed by blood flow and substituted by another endothelial cell. It is obvious that microvascular cell death will have consequences on capillary architecture and function and will compromise BRB properties.

## 4.2.5. Neuronal Dysfunction and Death

As mentioned before, DR has been considered a microvascular disease since several decades ago. The clinical evidences indicate that there is an increased capillary permeability and capillary occlusion, which are responsible for edema and neovascularization. However, various important findings have also implicated neuronal and glial components in the pathophysiology of DR. Thus, DR can now be considered a neurodegenerative disease of the eye, in addition to a microvascular disease (Barber, 2003).

Although neural retina is responsible for light-sensing, integration and transmission of information, little attention was given to the possible involvement of neurons and glial cells in the pathogenesis of DR, probably because the retina is transparent and the neural components are not as easily revealed as microvasculature with the techniques and methods used in clinical practice and research. However, vision loss is always due to impaired neuronal function. Indeed, several decades ago, it was reported that there is loss of all types of retinal neurons in diabetic retinas, being retinal neurons located in the inner retina the most affected (Wolter, 1961; Bloodworth, 1962). These studies presented evidence for pyknosis of neuronal cell bodies in postmortem retinas of diabetic patients. Changes in the electroretinogram obtained from patients with DR (Simonsen, 1974; Uccioli *et al.*, 1995) and alterations in color vision and contrast sensitivity (Daley *et al.*, 1987) also reveal an abnormal function of the visual system. The amplitude and latency of oscillatory potentials is reduced in the retina of diabetic patients or STZ-induced diabetic rats (Simonsen, 1974; Frost-Larsen *et al.*, 1981;

Sakai *et al.*, 1995). Interestingly, these alterations in electroretinograms can be reversed by treatment with aldose reductase inhibitors (Funada *et al.*, 1987; Lowitt *et al.*, 1993; Segawa *et al.*, 1988), indicating not only that the increased activity of the polyol pathway is involved in the development of these abnormalities, but also suggesting that the neural function is not irreversibly compromised.

Since these functional changes may be often identified before detection of microvascular lesions (Lopes de Faria *et al.*, 2001), it seems that diabetes directly compromises the function of neural retina, even before it might be further affected by the alteration in the permeability of BRB.

More recently, several reports confirmed the studies of Wolter (1961) and Bloodworth (1962) showing that neuronal apoptosis is also a hallmark of DR. Evidence of programmed cell death in retinal ganglion cells (RGC) and Muller cells was found in the retinas of early diabetic rats. Treatment with nerve growth factor (NGF) prevented apoptosis in RGC and Muller cells, suggesting that neurotrophic factors may be useful therapeutic agents in DR (Hammes *et al.*, 1995). A very important study, which may have changed the concept of DR, was published by Barber and colleagues (1998) a decade ago. This study was the first quantitative report showing an increase in neural cell apoptosis in the diabetic retina. It was demonstrated that the thickness of the inner plexiform and inner nuclear layers are reduced upon 7.5 months of STZ-induced diabetes, and that the number of ganglion cells is also decreased. Using the TUNEL assay, it was shown that the number of apoptotic nuclei was increased just one month after induction of diabetes, and the amount of apoptotic nuclei remained constant during the entire duration of diabetes. The TUNEL-positive cells were not associated with blood vessels and did not colocalize with the specific antigen for endothelial cells, von Willebrand factor, clearly indicating that most of the cells undergoing apoptosis were not vascular cells. In a small number of postmortem human retinas, an increase in TUNEL-positive cells was also observed. This group of evidences supports the idea that diabetes induces a chronic neurodegeneration in the retina.

Since then, several studies have corroborated these findings. In diabetic rats, the number of cells labeled with a neuronal specific marker, NeuN, was reduced in both ganglion cell layer and inner nuclear layer, with this layer being more affected (Zeng *et al.*, 2000). A slight reduction in the thickness of the inner retina was also found by Park and colleagues (2003), but more important, a remarkable reduction was seen in the outer nuclear layer 24 weeks after the onset of diabetes. Just four weeks after the induction of diabetes, a few photoreceptors exhibited characteristics of apoptosis, which increased with time. Moreover, necrotic ganglion, horizontal and amacrine cells were also observed. More recently, *in vitro* studies have also demonstrated that high glucose increases the number of apoptotic cells in neural retinal cell cultures (Santiago *et al.*, 2007; Fig. 4.4).

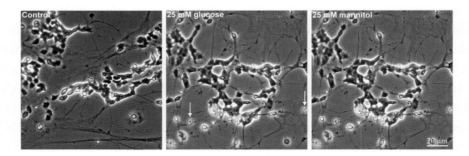

**Fig. 4.4.** High glucose-induced apoptosis in retinal neural cells. The number of TUNEL-positive cells (apoptotic cells — arrows) increases in primary cultures of retinal cells exposed to high glucose (30 mM) for seven days, but not to mannitol, the osmotic control.

Sorbinil, an inhibitor of aldose reductase, decreased the number of apoptotic neurons in the inner retina of STZ-induced diabetic rats. Insulin treatment prevented most abnormalities induced by diabetes. Diabetic mice, which are known to have much lower activity of aldose reductase and do not accumulate sorbitol, did not exhibit neuronal apoptosis. These findings point to a role of polyol pathway in retinal neurodegeneration (Asnaghi *et al.*, 2003). Although Asnaghi and colleagues did not found significant apoptosis in the retinas of diabetic mice, a reduction in the number of ganglion cells in C57Bl/6 diabetic mice was found. A decrease in the thickness of inner and outer nuclear layers was also observed. Particularly in the ganglion cell layer, it was demonstrated that ganglion cells were dying by apoptosis dependent on caspase-3 activation (Martin *et al.*, 2004). In the retinas obtained from human subjects with diabetes it was recently shown that ganglion cells express several proapoptotic markers (Abu-El-Asrar *et al.*, 2004), suggesting that these cells are particularly vulnerable, which is in agreement with some previous studies using diabetic animals. Moreover, it was found that elevated glucose induces apoptosis in retinal neural cells by a caspase-independent pathway involving AIF translocation from the mitochondria to the nucleus (Santiago *et al.*, 2007).

The discrepancy of the results obtained by several groups, mostly regarding the type of retinal cells that are most affected, may reflect the use of different strains of rats and different methods to analyze the preparations. However, all these evidences clearly demonstrate that neuronal apoptosis is present in DR, occurring before or at the same time the BRB is affected. The exposure of neural retinal cells, which are known to have an intense metabolic activity and a low regenerative capacity, to hyperglycemic conditions, associated with the lack of trophic factors, such as insulin, may render these cells more susceptible than microvascular cells to stress conditions, and, thus, become the primary target of diabetes. However, it must be emphasized that the functional capacity of

retinal neurons might be affected, although its integrity may be preserved, in some cases.

## 4.2.6. Glial Cells Reactivity and Changes

The retina has two types of macroglial cells: Muller cells that are only encountered in the retina and span all retinal layers, and astrocytes that migrate into the retina from the optic nerve and are located at the nerve fiber layer being less abundant than Muller cells. Both cell types envelope retinal vessels, the initial segments of ganglion cells axons and neurons as well. These cells have rather important functions in the retina. They provide structural and metabolic support for retinal neurons and blood vessels and are essential to retinal homeostasis (Bringmann and Reichenbach, 2001). Among other important functions they regulate the expression of tight junction proteins and control the permeability of BRB (Tout *et al.*, 1993; Gardner *et al.*, 1997).

Alterations in Muller cells, with possible implications in BRB, have been reported more than two decades ago in STZ-induced diabetic rats (Hori and Mukai, 1980). The accumulation of highly electron-dense bodies, which resembled lysosomes, in the cytoplasm of Muller cells, was correlated with metabolic alterations in the retina. Changes in the nucleus, consistent with apoptotic features, were also observed in Muller cells in the retinas of diabetic rats (Schellini *et al.*, 1995). The pioneer work of Hammes and colleagues (1995) clearly showed that, in addition to neurons and microvascular cells, Muller cells exhibit apoptotic features and increase the expression of the intermediate glial fibrillary acidic protein (GFAP). This observation was accompanied by an increase in the expression of the low-affinity NGF receptor p75NGFR, and treatment with NGF prevented apoptosis in Muller cells, indicating that neurotrophins may be useful in the treatment of DR. NGF also prevented pericyte loss and the appearance of acellular occluded capillaries.

More recently, it was shown that high glucose induces apoptosis in transformed rat Muller cells and in isolated human Muller cells. This effect was correlated with the translocation of glyceraldehyde-3-phosphate dehydrogenase (GAPDH) from the cytosol to the nucleus. The presence of R-(-)-deprenyl in cells treated with high glucose prevented nuclear translocation of GAPDH and Muller cells apoptosis (Kusner *et al.*, 2004). Exposure of Muller cells to high glucose for 72 hours also significantly inactivated Akt and induced apoptosis. A significant dephosphorylation of Akt was also observed in Muller cells in the retina of diabetic rats, suggesting that high glucose may cause cell death, at least in part due to the downregulation of Akt pathway, which is known to be a survival pathway (Xi *et al.*, 2005).

Abnormalities of the b-wave, which also originates from Muller cells, registered in the electroretinograms (ERG) of insulin-controlled juvenile diabetics (Lovasik *et al.*, 1988) and in diabetic or galactosemic animals (Segawa *et al.*, 1988; Hotta *et al.*, 1995; Li *et al.*, 2002) have been associated with retinal Muller cell dysfunction. Treatment of diabetic animals with TAT, an aldose reductase inhibitor, significantly improved the prolongation of the peak latency of oscillatory potentials in the b-wave of the ERG, demonstrating that the polyol pathway is involved in Muller cell dysfunction caused by diabetes.

There are also evidences demonstrating that astrocytes and Muller cells react differently to diabetes (Barber *et al.*, 2000). The immunoreactivity against GFAP is limited to astrocytes in control retinas, and two months after induction of diabetes with STZ, the GFAP immunoreactivity is reduced in astrocytes and increased in Muller cells. After four months, the astrocytes do not express GFAP, but Muller cells have intense staining. Similar changes were observed in BB/Wor diabetic rats. It is also an interesting fact that the expression of occludin in retinal vessels decreases in the same areas where GFAP is reduced. This observation suggests that the alterations in glial cells may contribute to increased permeability of the BRB. It is also important to note that treatment with insulin for only 48 hours reverses the pattern of GFAP expression, indicating that these changes may be reversible and also suggesting that the lack of trophic factors, such as insulin, may have an important role in

glial reactivity. The protective effect of insulin was confirmed by Asnaghi and colleagues (2003), which have also reported that the inhibition of aldose reductase prevents glial cell changes.

In addition to alterations in b-wave and GFAP expression in diabetic retinas, there are other evidences consistent with glial cell malfunction. An increase in GABA immunoreactivity in Muller cells in diabetic rat retinas was observed, while no apparent changes were found in glycine immunoreactivity. The activity of glutamic acid decarboxylase (GAD) was increased, while the activity of GABA transaminase (GABA-T) decreased (Ishikawa *et al.*, 1996). Pathologic accumulation of GABA in Muller cells was also evidenced by immunogold (Ishikawa *et al.*, 1996). These results indicate that there are changes in GABA metabolism in diabetic retinas and Muller cells are clearly involved in this process.

These alterations in Muller cells and astrocytes are indicative of an increase in metabolic stress, but it is not clear yet what these changes mean. Because Muller cells produce factors capable of modulating blood flow, vascular permeability and cell survival and their processes surround blood vessels in the retina, a possible role of these cells in the pathogenesis of retinal microangiopathy deserves to be investigated.

### 4.2.7. Glutamate Excitotoxicity in Diabetic Retinopathy: Involvement of Neurons and Glial Cells

Glutamine synthetase, the enzyme responsible for converting glutamate into glutamine, is only expressed in Muller cells in the retina (Newman and Reichenbach, 1996). The ability of diabetic rat retinas to convert glutamate into glutamine is decreased when compared to control retinas (Lieth *et al.*, 1998), due to a reduction in the activity and content of glutamine synthetase (Mizutani *et al.*, 1998; Lieth *et al.*, 2000). The oxidation of glutamate is also significantly reduced in diabetic retinas (Lieth *et al.*, 2000). These results indicate that diabetes induces at least two enzymatic abnormalities in the glutamate metabolism pathway: transamination to $\alpha$-ketoglutarate and amination to glutamine. Insulin restored the activity of glutamine synthetase, suggesting that some glial changes may be due to hypoinsulinemia.

The glutamate content increased by 1.6-fold (Lieth *et al.*, 1998) or 40% (Kowluru *et al.*, 2001) in diabetic retinas. Excessive glutamate may cause excitotoxicity, and, therefore, may be responsible for neural degeneration in the retina during diabetes. The administration of antioxidants inhibited the increase in retinal glutamate content caused by diabetes (Kowluru *et al.*, 2001). Increased levels of GABA and glutamate were also found in the vitreous of patients with proliferative DR (Ambati *et al.*, 1997).

In addition to a decrease in the activity of glutamine synthetase in diabetic retinas, it was reported that Muller cells freshly isolated from diabetic rats have a lower ability to remove glutamate from the extracellular space, when compared to Muller cells isolated from normal rats (Li and Puro, 2002). The activity of the glutamate transporter, which was monitored using the patch-clamp technique, significantly decreases in Muller cells isolated from diabetic retinas. This effect is due to oxidation since the exposure to a disulfide-reducing agent restores the activity of the glutamate transporter. This decrease in the activity of glutamate transporter may also contribute to disrupt glutamate homeostasis, increasing the levels of glutamate in the retina, which may be excitotoxic to retinal neurons. Although this group of results indicates that glutamate levels are increased in diabetic retinas and may cause a chronic glutamate excitotoxicity, it was also reported that experimental diabetes produces a generalized fall in the content of free amino acids, including glutamate, in the retina (Vilchis and Salceda, 1996). This discrepancy of the results may reflect the use of different models and techniques to measure the levels of amino acids. Although in some cases glutamate levels are not increased, we cannot exclude the possibility of increased glutamate levels in defined regions,

particularly at the synaptic cleft, that might cause neural apoptosis.

Some additional evidences also point to the involvement of glutamate in retinal neural degeneration in DR. The evoked release of [$^3$H]-D-aspartate, which mimics glutamate behavior and is not metabolized, is significantly increased in retinal neural cell cultures exposed to high glucose for seven days and in the retinas of diabetic animals at four weeks of diabetes (Santiago *et al.*, 2006a). [$Ca^{2+}$]$_i$ also changes stimulated by kainate, which is an ionotropic glutamate receptor agonist, are increased in retinal cultures treated with high glucose when compared to non-treated cultures or with cultures exposed to mannitol, the osmotic control. In addition, [$Ca^{2+}$]$_i$ does not recover to basal levels during the period of the experiment, clearly indicating that high glucose impairs $Ca^{2+}$ homeostasis (Santiago *et al.*, 2006b). Therefore, both the increase in glutamate release and the $Ca^{2+}$ deregulation observed in retinal neural cultures might be strictly correlated to retinal neural apoptosis caused by diabetes.

Recent findings also indicate that the expression of glutamate receptors and calcium-binding proteins (calbindin and parvalbumin) in the retina and retinal cell cultures are altered by diabetes or elevated glucose (Ng *et al.*, 2004; Santiago *et al.*, 2006b; Santiago *et al.*, 2008). Alterations in the content of several ionotropic glutamate receptor subunits, and particularly the content of GluR2 subunit, which controls AMPA receptor permeability to $Ca^{2+}$, is substantially increased in retinal cultures treated with high glucose, and consequently AMPA receptors are less permeable to $Ca^{2+}$ (Santiago *et al.*, 2006b). These alterations in the expression of glutamate receptors may have consequences in synaptic transmission and affect cell-to-cell communication, causing physiological changes in the retina.

At present, it is not yet clear whether glutamate excitotoxicity is responsible for neural cell apoptosis in diabetic retinas. However, there is no doubt that glutamate metabolism, glutamate levels and the expression of glutamate receptors are altered by diabetes, and at least, this will have consequences at the level of neurotransmission and the retinal function. Whether BRB might be affected by these changes is not known.

### 4.2.8. Microglia

Retinal microglial cells can be found in every layer of the human retina and may be of two types. One form originates from hematopoietic cells and the other is derived from the optic nerve mesenchyme. Microglial cells play an important role against invading microorganisms, in immunoregulation and tissue repair. Normally, microglial cells are quiescent, but in certain conditions, such as diabetes, they may be activated.

Several evidences have shown that microglial cells might be involved in the pathophysiology of DR. The increase in microglial density and the alterations in the shape of microglial cells, as an indication of functional activation, were found in the retinas of diabetic animals (Rungger-Brandle *et al.*, 2000; Gaucher *et al.*, 2007; Yang *et al.*, 2009). Zeng and colleagues (2000) have shown that microglial cells are activated and appear hypertrophic, just one month after inducing diabetes in rats. The number of microglial cells was increased, and some cells appeared in the outer plexiform layer at four months. At 14 and 16 months, reactive microglial cells were detected in the outer nuclear and photoreceptor layer. Also, in retinas of patients with diabetic retinopathy microglia is markedly increased in number and are hypertrophic at different stages of the disease (Zeng *et al.*, 2008).

These changes may be elicited by neural cell death occurring in ganglion cell layer and inner nuclear layer, as well as by some alterations in photoreceptors. Although the evidences in the literature related to the involvement of microglial cells in the pathogenesis of DR are not abundant, these reports clearly demonstrate that retinal microglial cells are activated by diabetes, and suggests that inflammation has a role in the pathogenesis of DR.

### 4.2.9. The Outsiders: Leukocytes and Platelets

Leukocytes and platelets do not belong to the retina, but they can be encountered in the retinal blood circulation. Past and present evidences have been considering microthrombosis and inflammation important players in DR, where platelets and leukocytes are key elements.

### 4.2.10. Low-Grade Chronic Inflammation

Several evidences point to a role of inflammation in the development of DR, and the adhesion of leukocytes to retinal vessels has been linked to the breakdown of BRB. Leukocytes are large cells, which have high cytoplasmic rigidity and capacity to generate free radicals and proteolytic enzymes. In diabetes, leukocytes are more activated and less deformable, and, therefore, may be involved in capillary non-perfusion, endothelial cell damage and vascular leakage in the retinas.

Miyamoto and colleagues (1998) demonstrated for the first time an increase in leukostasis, *in vivo*, in the retinas of diabetic rats. Retinal leukostasis was correlated with increased expression of intercellular adhesion molecule-1 (ICAM-1) and vascular leakage, since the blockade of ICAM-1 with a monoclonal antibody prevented both leukostasis and vascular leakage (Miyamoto *et al.*, 1999). The adhesion of leukocytes was also shown to be temporally and spatially associated with endothelial cell death in experimental diabetes. Again, the neutralization with specific antibodies of ICAM-1 and the leukocyte integrin CD18 prevented leukocyte adhesion and endothelial cell death (Joussen *et al.*, 2001).

The apoptosis of endothelial cells, which ultimately leads to BRB breakdown, is dependent on a *Fas-FasL* interaction, which is mediated by leukocytes. The inhibition of *FasL* reduces endothelial cell injury and BRB breakdown, but does not decrease the adhesion of leukocytes to the retinal vasculature (Joussen *et al.*, 2002).

Also, the neutrophils from diabetic animals express higher levels of the surface integrins CD11a, CD11b and CD18 and exhibit higher integrin-mediated adhesion to endothelial cells. *In vivo* experiments also showed that the blockade of CD18 decreases leukostasis in retinal microvessels, pointing to a role of integrin adhesion molecules in DR (Barouch *et al.*, 2000). Experiments with mice deficient in the genes encoding for the adhesion molecules ICAM-1 and CD18 have shown that ICAM-/- and CD18-/- diabetic mice exhibit fewer adherent leukocytes to the retinal vasculature than non-diabetic animals. This observation was correlated with less vascular leakage and a reduced number of damaged endothelial cells (Joussen *et al.*, 2004).

The inhibition of beta isoform of protein kinase C (PKC), which has been shown to play a key role in the pathogenesis of DR (Curtis and Scholfield, 2004), prevented the adhesion of leukocytes to retinal vessels (Nonaka *et al.*, 2000). Advanced-glycation end-products, VEGF and nitric oxide produced by endothelial nitric oxide synthase (eNOS) also seem to play important roles in the adhesion of leukocytes to retinal vessels, thus suggesting that these players are potentially good targets in the treatment of early DR (Joussen *et al.*, 2002; Moore *et al.*, 2003; Mamputu and Renier, 2004). More recently, evidences have demonstrated that nitric oxide produced by inducible NOS (iNOS) appears to have a predominant role in leukostasis and BRB breakdown (Leal *et al.*, 2007; Zheng *et al.*, 2007) (Fig. 4.5).

This group of results clearly demonstrates that leukocytes have a predominant role in the early stages of diabetic complications in the retina, and DR can be characterized as a chronic, low-grade, inflammatory process, that may be responsible for vascular lesions occurring in retinal vessels.

Analyzing the profile of gene expression in the retinas of diabetic and normal rats, using cDNA microarrays, it was found that most of the genes that are upregulated are correlated with an inflammatory response (Joussen *et al.*, 2001). The levels of the pro-inflammatory cytokine IL-1beta and the activity of NOS are also increased in the retinas of STZ-induced diabetic rats (Carmo *et al.*, 1999). The administration of an anti-inflammatory drug, cyclosporin A, inhibited the production of IL-1beta and the expression of inducible NOS and cyclooxygenase-2 (COX-2). These observations were correlated with a decrease in the permeability of BRB (Carmo *et al.*, 2000). The use of an antioxidant therapy prevented the increase in the levels of IL-1beta in the retinas of diabetic rats (Kowluru and Odenbach, 2004). Injection of IL-1beta into the vitreous also increased the number of apoptotic cells in retinal microvessels and the number of acellular capillaries. This observation was correlated with increased levels of nitric oxide and 8-hydroxy-2′-deoxyguanosine (an indicator of oxidative stress).

*In vitro* experiments have shown that high glucose increases the expression of IL-1beta in bovine retinal endothelial cells. Incubation of retinal cells with

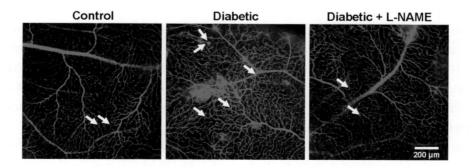

**Fig. 4.5.**   Leukocyte adhesion to retinal vessels. The increase in the number of adherent leukocytes (green spots) to retinal vessels of diabetic mice is inhibited by treatment with L-NAME, a NOS inhibitor.

IL-1beta increased NO levels, activated NF-kappa B and increased the activity of caspase-3 and apoptosis. The addition of the interleukin-1 receptor antagonist (IL-1ra) significantly decreased endothelial cell apoptosis (Kowluru and Odenbach, 2004).

TNF-$\alpha$ has also been implicated in the pathogenesis of DR. The levels of TNF-$\alpha$ were found to be increased in the serum and vitreous patients with proliferative DR (Schram *et al.*, 2005; Demircan *et al.*, 2006; Gustavsson *et al.*, 2008) and in retinas of diabetic rats (Joussen *et al.*, 2002; Krady *et al.*, 2005; Behl *et al.*, 2008). Moreover, TNF-$\alpha$ increases leukocyte adhesion to retinal vessels (Ben-Mahmud *et al.*, 2004) and BRB permeability (Saishin *et al.*, 2003), and inhibition of TNF-$\alpha$ with etanercept inhibits leukostasis and BRB breakdown in the retina of diabetic animals (Joussen *et al.*, 2002).

All these evidences demonstrate that IL-1beta and TNF-$\alpha$ may play important roles in the early stages of DR and further implicates inflammation in the pathogenesis of DR.

### 4.2.11. Microthrombosis

Capillary nonperfusion and eventual obliteration can be the consequence of retinal microthrombosis. Increased platelet adhesiveness and aggregation have been documented in diabetic patients since at least three decades ago (Heath *et al.*, 1971; Bensoussan *et al.*, 1975). In experimental diabetes, the formation of microthrombi by electron microscopy in retinal vessels obtained from diabetic rats was observed (9 to 12 months). These microthrombi were mainly composed of aggregated platelets and fibrin strands (Ishibashi *et al.*, 1981). Boeri and colleagues (2001) demonstrated, after isolating the intact vascular network from postmortem retinas obtained from diabetic and nondiabetic donors, and using antibodies to fibrin cross-linking factor XIII and platelet glycoprotein (GP)-IIIa to identify fibrin-platelet thrombi, that

diabetic retinas present a greater than normal number and size of platelet-fibrin thrombi in the retinal capillaries. There was also a topographical association of microthrombosis with apoptotic cells in both diabetic and nondiabetic vessels.

In some clinical studies the use of an inhibitor of platelet aggregation proved to be useful in the treatment of DR. Trifusal, a platelet antiaggregant drug, decreased the leakage of fluorescein and the number of microaneurysms, while in the untreated group both parameters were increased (Esmatjes *et al.*, 1989). Treatment of diabetic rats with aspirin plus dipyridamole also inhibited the production of thromboxane B2 by platelets and decreased the synthesis of prostacyclin (De la Cruz *et al.*, 1997). These observations clearly indicate that platelets are involved in microthrombosis, although leukocytes may also be involved, which seems to play an important role in the pathogenesis of DR. The molecular mechanisms involved in the formation of microthrombi are not yet completely understood, but this deserves a particular attention, since it might be a promising therapeutic target.

### 4.2.12. Concluding Remarks

In recent years, important steps have been taken in the process of improved understanding of the pathogenic mechanisms underlying DR. Its pathology should no longer be only considered a microvascular disease, although microvascular alterations predominate. Indeed, in addition to alterations in retinal microvessels, essentially due to functional changes or apoptosis of endothelial cells and pericytes, other retinal cells are affected: neurons, Muller cells, astrocytes and microglial cells (Fig. 4.6). In addition, the involvement of leukocytes and platelets should not be forgotten.

Some evidences suggest that neurons and glial cells might be affected first by hyperglycemia and not

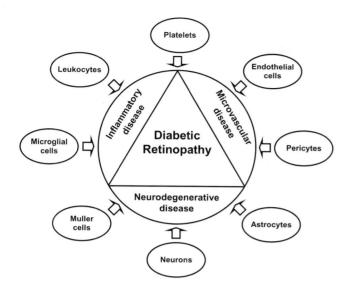

**Fig. 4.6.** Schematic representation of the processes and cell types involved in the pathogenesis of Diabetic Retinopathy.

microvascular cells, but this question remains unsolved. In fact, in some experimental models the breakdown of BRB occurs very early, and this event may influence retinal neural function. Although several questions remain unanswered, it is reasonable to accept that alterations in any cell type will affect other types of cells, since any retinal cell is directly or indirectly linked to the others. Therefore, we must look to the retina as a whole and future therapeutic strategies must take this into account.

In conclusion, with the present level of knowledge DR should be considered both a microvascular, inflammatory and neurodegenerative disease.

# References

Abu-El-Asrar AM, Dralands L, Missotten L, *et al.* (2004) Expression of apoptosis markers in the retinas of human subjects with diabetes. *Invest Ophthalmol Vis Sci* **45**: 2760–2766.

Abu El-Asrar AM, Dralands L, Missotten L, *et al.* (2007) Expression of antiapoptotic and proapoptotic molecules in diabetic retinas. *Eye* **21**: 238–245.

Addison DJ, Garner A, Ashton N. (1970) Degeneration of intramural pericytes in diabetic retinopathy. *Br Med J* **1**: 264–266.

Aiello LP, Bursell SE, Clermont A, *et al.* (1997) Vascular endothelial growth factor-induced retinal permeability is mediated by protein kinase C *in vivo* and suppressed by an orally effective beta-isoform-selective inhibitor. *Diabetes* **46**: 1473–1480.

Ambati J, Chalam KV, Chawla DK, *et al.* (1997) Elevated gamma-aminobutyric acid, glutamate, and vascular endothelial growth factor levels in the vitreous of patients with proliferative diabetic retinopathy. *Arch Ophthalmol* **115**: 1161–1166.

Antonetti DA, Barber AJ, Hollinger LA, *et al.* (1999) Vascular endothelial growth factor induces rapid phosphorylation of tight junction proteins occludin and zonula occluden 1. A potential mechanism for vascular permeability in diabetic retinopathy and tumors. *J Biol Chem* **274**: 23463–23467.

Antonetti DA, Barber AJ, Khin S, *et al.* (1998) Vascular permeability in experimental diabetes is associated with reduced endothelial occludin content: Vascular endothelial growth factor decreases occludin in retinal endothelial cells. Penn State Retina Research Group. *Diabetes* **47**: 1953–1959.

Antonetti DA, Wolpert EB, DeMaio L, *et al.* (2002) Hydrocortisone decreases retinal endothelial cell water and solute flux coincident with increased content and decreased phosphorylation of occludin. *J Neurochem* **80**: 667–677.

Archer DB. Bowman Lecture 1998. (1999) Diabetic retinopathy: Some cellular, molecular and therapeutic considerations. *Eye* **13**: 497–523.

Asnaghi V, Gerhardinger C, Hoehn T, *et al.* (2003) A role for the polyol pathway in the early neuroretinal apoptosis and glial changes induced by diabetes in the rat. *Diabetes* **52**: 506–511.

Barber AJ. (2003) A new view of diabetic retinopathy: A neurodegenerative disease of the eye. *Prog Neuropsychopharmacol Biol Psychiatry* **27**: 283–290.

Barber AJ, Antonetti DA, Gardner TW. (2000) Altered expression of retinal occludin and glial fibrillary acidic protein in experimental diabetes. *Invest Ophthalmol Vis Sci* **41**: 3561–3568.

Barber AJ, Antonetti DA. (2003) Mapping the blood vessels with paracellular permeability in the retinas of diabetic rats. *Invest Ophthalmol Vis Sci* **44**: 5410–5416.

Barber AJ, Lieth E, Khin SA, *et al.* (1998) Neural apoptosis in the retina during experimental and human diabetes. Early onset and effect of insulin. *J Clin Invest* **102**: 783–791.

Barouch FC, Miyamoto K, Allport JR, *et al.* (2000) Integrin-mediated neutrophil adhesion and retinal leukostasis in diabetes. *Invest Ophthalmol Vis Sci* **41**: 1153–1158.

Behl Y, Krothapalli P, Desta T, *et al.* (2008) Diabetes-enhanced tumor necrosis factor-alpha production promotes apoptosis and the loss of retinal microvascular cells in type 1 and type 2 models of diabetic retinopathy. *Am J Pathol* **172**: 1411–1418.

Ben-Mahmud BM, Mann GE, Datti A, *et al.* (2004) Tumor necrosis factor-alpha in diabetic plasma increases the activity of core 2 GlcNAc-T and adherence of human leukocytes to retinal endothelial cells: Significance of core 2 GlcNAc-T in diabetic retinopathy. *Diabetes* **53**: 2968–2976.

Bensoussan D, Levy Toledano S, Passa P, *et al.* (1975) Platelet hyperaggregation and increased plasma level of Von Willebrand factor in diabetics with retinopathy. *Diabetologia* **11**: 307–312.

Bloodworth JM Jr (1962). Diabetic retinopathy. *Diabetes* **11**: 1–22.

Boeri D, Maiello M, Lorenzi M. (2001) Increased prevalence of microthromboses in retinal capillaries of diabetic individuals. *Diabetes* **50**: 1432–1439.

Bresnick GH, Palta M. (1987). Predicting progression to severe proliferative diabetic retinopathy. *Arch Ophthalmol* **105**: 810–814.

Bringmann A, Reichenbach A. (2001). Role of Muller cells in retinal degenerations. *Front Biosci* **6**: E72–E92.

Bucolo C, Ward KW, Mazzon E, *et al.* (2009) Protective Effects of a Coumarin Derivative in Diabetic Rats. *Invest Ophthalmol Vis Sci* Mar 11 [Epub ahead of print].

Busik JV, Mohr S, Grant MB, *et al.* (2008). Hyperglycemia-induced reactive oxygen species toxicity to endothelial cells is dependent on paracrine mediators. *Diabetes* **57**: 1952–1965.

Carmo A, Cunha-Vaz JG, Carvalho AP, *et al.* (2000) Effect of cyclosporin-A on the blood — retinal barrier permeability in streptozotocin-induced diabetes. *Mediators Inflamm* **9**: 243–248.

Carmo A, Cunha-Vaz JG, Carvalho AP, *et al.* (1999) L-arginine transport in retinas from streptozotocin diabetic rats: Correlation with the level of IL-1 beta and NO synthase activity. *Vision Res* **39**: 3817–3823.

Carmo A, Ramos P, Reis A, *et al.* (1998) Breakdown of the inner and outer blood retinal barrier in streptozotocin-induced diabetes. *Exp Eye Res* **67**: 569–575.

Citi S, Sabanay H, Jakes R, *et al.* (1988) Cingulin, a new peripheral component of tight junctions. *Nature* **333**: 272–276.

Cunha-Vaz JG. (2001). Initial alterations in nonproliferative diabetic retinopathy. *Ophthalmologica* **215**: 7–13.

Curtis TM, Scholfield CN. (2004). The role of lipids and protein kinase Cs in the pathogenesis of diabetic retinopathy. *Diabetes Metab Res Rev* **20**: 28–43.

Daley ML, Watzke RC, Riddle MC, *et al.* (1987). Early loss of blue-sensitive color vision in patients with type I diabetes. *Diabetes Care* **10**: 777–781.

De la Cruz JP, Moreno A, Munoz M, *et al.* (1997) Effect of aspirin plus dipyridamole on the retinal vascular pattern in experimental diabetes mellitus. *J Pharmacol Exp Ther* **280**: 454–459.

Denis U, Lecomte M, Paget C, *et al.* (2002) Advanced glycation end-products induce apoptosis of bovine retinal pericytes in culture: Involvement of diacylglycerol/ceramide production and oxidative stress induction. *Free Radic Biol Med* **33**: 236–247.

Demircan N, Safran BG, Soylu M, *et al.* (2006) Determination of vitreous interleukin-1 (IL-1) and tumour necrosis factor (TNF) levels in proliferative diabetic retinopathy. *Eye* **20**: 1366–1369.

Esmatjes E, Maseras M, Gallego M, *et al.* (1989) Effect of treatment with an inhibitor of platelet aggregation on the evolution of background retinopathy: 2 years of follow-up. *Diabetes Res Clin Pract* **7**: 285–291.

Frost-Larsen K, Larsen HW, Simonsen SE. (1981). Value of electroretinography and dark adaptation as prognostic tools in diabetic retinopathy. *Dev Ophthalmol* **2**: 222–234.

Funada M, Okamoto I, Fujinaga Y, *et al.* (1987) Effects of aldose reductase inhibitor (M79175) on ERG oscillatory potential abnormalities in streptozotocin fructose-induced diabetes in rats. *Jpn J Ophthalmol* **31**: 305–314.

Furuse M, Fujita K, Hiiragi T, *et al.* (1998) Novel integral membrane proteins localizing at tight junctions with no sequence similarity to occludin. *J Cell Biol* **141**: 1539–1550.

Furuse M, Hirase T, Itoh M, *et al.* (1993) Occludin: A novel integral membrane protein localizing at tight junctions. *J Cell Biol* **123**: 1777–1788.

Gardner TW, Antonetti DA, Barber AJ, *et al.* (2000) New insights into the pathophysiology of diabetic retinopathy: Potential cell-specific therapeutic targets. *Diabetes Technol Ther* **2**: 601–608.

Gardner TW, Lieth E, Khin SA, *et al.* (1997) Astrocytes increase barrier properties and ZO-1 expression in retinal vascular endothelial cells. *Invest Ophthalmol Vis Sci* **38**: 2423–2427.

Gaucher D, Chiappore JA, Paques M, *et al.* (2007) Microglial changes occur without neural cell death in diabetic retinopathy. *Vision Res* **47**: 612–623.

Gustavsson C, Agardh E, Bengtsson B, *et al.* (2008) TNF-alpha is an independent serum marker for proliferative retinopathy in type 1 diabetic patients. *J Diabetes Complications* **22**: 309–316.

Hammes HP, Federoff HJ, Brownlee M. (1995). Nerve growth factor prevents both neuroretinal programmed cell death and capillary pathology in experimental diabetes. *Mol Med* **1**: 527–534.

Harhaj NS, Barber AJ, Antonetti DA. (2002) Platelet-derived growth factor mediates tight junction redistribution and increases permeability in MDCK cells. *J Cell Physiol* **193**: 349–364.

Haskins J, Gu L, Wittchen ES, *et al.* (1998) ZO-3, novel member of the MAGUK protein family found at the tight junction, interacts with ZO-1 and occludin. *J Cell Biol* **141**: 199–208.

Heath H, Brigden WD, Canever JV, *et al.* (1971) Platelet adhesiveness and aggregation in relation to diabetic retinopathy. *Diabetologia* **7**: 308–315.

Hori S, Mukai N. (1980) Ultrastructural lesions of retinal pericapillary Muller cells in streptozotocin-induced diabetic rats. *Albrecht Von Graefes Arch Klin Exp Ophthalmol* **213**: 1–9.

Hotta N, Koh N, Sakakibara F, *et al.* (1995) An aldose reductase inhibitor, TAT, prevents electroretinographic abnormalities and ADP-induced hyperaggregability in streptozotocin-induced diabetic rats. *Eur J Clin Invest* **25**: 948–954.

Ishibashi T, Tanaka K, Taniguchi Y. (1981). Platelet aggregation and coagulation in the pathogenesis of diabetic retinopathy in rats. *Diabetes* **30**: 601–606.

Ishikawa A, Ishiguro S, Tamai M. (1996) Accumulation of gamma-aminobutyric acid in diabetic rat retinal Muller cells evidenced by electron microscopic immunocytochemistry. *Curr Eye Res* **15**: 958–964.

Ishikawa A, Ishiguro S, Tamai M. (1996) Changes in GABA metabolism in streptozotocin-induced diabetic rat retinas. *Curr Eye Res* **15**: 63–71.

Jesaitis LA, Goodenough DA. (1994). Molecular characterization and tissue distribution of ZO-2, a tight junction protein homologous to ZO-1 and the Drosophila discs-large tumor suppressor protein. *J Cell Biol* **124**: 949–961.

Joussen AM, Huang S, Poulaki V, *et al.* (2001) In vivo retinal gene expression in early diabetes. *Invest Ophthalmol Vis Sci* **42**: 3047–3057.

Joussen AM, Murata T, Tsujikawa A, *et al.* (2001) Leukocyte-mediated endothelial cell injury and death in the diabetic retina. *Am J Pathol* **158**: 147–152.

Joussen AM, Poulaki V, Le ML, *et al.* (2004) A central role for inflammation in the pathogenesis of diabetic retinopathy. *FASEB J* **18**: 1450–1452.

Joussen AM, Poulaki V, Mitsiades N, *et al.* (2003) Suppression of Fas-FasL-induced endothelial cell apoptosis prevents diabetic blood-retinal barrier breakdown in a model of streptozotocin-induced diabetes. *FASEB J* **17**: 76–78.

Joussen AM, Poulaki V, Mitsiades N, *et al.* (2002) Nonsteroidal anti-inflammatory drugs prevent early diabetic retinopathy via TNF-alpha suppression. *FASEB J* **16**: 438–440.

Joussen AM, Poulaki V, Qin W, *et al.* (2002) Retinal vascular endothelial growth factor induces intercellular adhesion molecule-1 and endothelial nitric oxide synthase expression and initiates early diabetic retinal leukocyte adhesion *in vivo*. *Am J Pathol* **160**: 501–509.

Kador PF, Akagi Y, Terubayashi H, *et al.* (1988) Prevention of pericyte ghost formation in retinal capillaries of galactose-fed dogs by aldose reductase inhibitors. *Arch Ophthalmol* **106**: 1099–1102.

Kale G, Naren AP, Sheth P, *et al.* (2003) Tyrosine phosphorylation of occludin attenuates its interactions with ZO-1, ZO-2, and ZO-3. *Biochem Biophys Res Commun* **302**: 324–329.

Keon BH, Schafer S, Kuhn C, *et al.* (1996) Symplekin, a novel type of tight junction plaque protein. *J Cell Biol* **134**: 1003–1018.

Kern TS, Tang J, Mizutani M, *et al.* (2000) Response of capillary cell death to aminoguanidine predicts the development of retinopathy: Comparison of diabetes and galactosemia. *Invest Ophthalmol Vis Sci* **41**: 3972–3978.

Kevil CG, Oshima T, Alexander B, *et al.* (2000) H(2)O(2)-mediated permeability: Role of MAPK and occludin. *Am J Physiol Cell Physiol* **279**: C21–C30.

Klaassen I, Hughes JM, Vogels IM, *et al.* (2009) Altered expression of genes related to blood-retina barrier disruption in streptozotocin-induced diabetes. *Exp Eye Res* **89**: 4–15.

Kowluru RA, Abbas SN. (2003) Diabetes-induced mitochondrial dysfunction in the retina. *Invest Ophthalmol Vis Sci* **44**: 5327–5334.

Kowluru RA, Engerman RL, Case GL, *et al.* (2001) Retinal glutamate in diabetes and effect of antioxidants. *Neurochem Int* **38**: 385–390.

Kowluru RA, Koppolu P. (2002). Diabetes-induced activation of caspase-3 in retina: Effect of antioxidant therapy. *Free Radic Res* **36**: 993–999.

Kowluru RA, Odenbach S. (2004). Role of interleukin-1beta in the development of retinopathy in rats: Effect of antioxidants. *Invest Ophthalmol Vis Sci* **45**: 4161–4166.

Kowluru RA, Odenbach S. (2004). Role of interleukin-1beta in the pathogenesis of diabetic retinopathy. *Br J Ophthalmol* **88**: 1343–1347.

Krady JK, Basu A, Allen CM, *et al.* (2005) Minocycline reduces proinflammatory cytokine expression, microglial activation, and caspase-3 activation in a rodent model of diabetic retinopathy. *Diabetes* **54**: 1559–1565.

Kusner LL, Sarthy VP, Mohr S. (2004) Nuclear translocation of glyceraldehyde-3-phosphate dehydrogenase: A role in high glucose-induced apoptosis in retinal Muller cells. *Invest Ophthalmol Vis Sci* **45**: 1553–1561.

Leal EC, Aveleira CA, Castilho AF, *et al.* (2009) High glucose and oxidative/nitrosative stress conditions induce apoptosis in retinal endothelial cells by a caspase-independent pathway. *Exp Eye Res* **88**: 983–991.

Leal EC, Manivannan A, Hosoya K, *et al.* (2007) Inducible nitric oxide synthase isoform is a key mediator of leukostasis and blood-retinal barrier breakdown in diabetic retinopathy. *Invest Ophthalmol Vis Sci* **48**: 5257–5265.

Lecomte M, Denis U, Ruggiero D, *et al.* (2004) Involvement of caspase-10 in advanced glycation end-product-induced apoptosis of bovine retinal pericytes in culture. *Biochim Biophys Acta* **1689**: 202–211.

Li Q, Puro DG. (2002). Diabetes-induced dysfunction of the glutamate transporter in retinal Muller cells. *Invest Ophthalmol Vis Sci* **43**: 3109–3116.

Li Q, Zemel E, Miller B, *et al.* (2002) Early retinal damage in experimental diabetes: Electroretinographical and morphological observations. *Exp Eye Res* **74**: 615–625.

Li W, Yanoff M, Liu X, Ye X. (1997). Retinal capillary pericyte apoptosis in early human diabetic retinopathy. *Chin Med J (Engl)* **110**: 659–663.

Lieth E, Barber AJ, Xu B, *et al.* (1998) Glial reactivity and impaired glutamate metabolism in short-term experimental diabetic retinopathy. *Diabetes* **47**: 815–820.

Lieth E, LaNoue KF, Antonetti DA, *et al.* (2000) Diabetes reduces glutamate oxidation and glutamine synthesis in the retina. *Exp Eye Res* **70**: 723–730.

Lobo CL, Bernardes RC, de Abreu JR, *et al.* (2001) One-year follow-up of blood-retinal barrier and retinal thickness alterations in patients with type 2 diabetes mellitus and mild nonproliferative retinopathy. *Arch Ophthalmol* **119**: 1469–1474.

Lohmann C, Krischke M, Wegener J, *et al.* (2004) Tyrosine phosphatase inhibition induces loss of blood-brain barrier integrity by matrix metalloproteinase-dependent and -independent pathways. *Brain Res* **995**: 184–196.

Lopes de Faria JM, Katsumi O, Cagliero E, *et al.* (2001) Neurovisual abnormalities preceding the retinopathy in patients with long-term type 1 diabetes mellitus. *Graefes Arch Clin Exp Ophthalmol* **239**: 643–648.

Lorenzi M, Gerhardinger C. (2001). Early cellular and molecular changes induced by diabetes in the retina. *Diabetologia* **44**: 791–804.

Lovasik JV, Spafford MM. (1998). An electrophysiological investigation of visual function in juvenile insulin-dependent diabetes mellitus. *Am J Optom Physiol Opt* **65**: 236–253.

Lowitt S, Malone JI, Salem A, *et al.* (1993) Acetyl-L-carnitine corrects electroretinographic deficits in experimental diabetes. *Diabetes* **42**: 1115–1118.

Mamputu JC, Renier G. (2004) Advanced glycation end-products increase monocyte adhesion to retinal endothelial cells through vascular endothelial growth factor-induced ICAM-1 expression: Inhibitory effect of antioxidants. *J Leukoc Biol* **75**: 1062–1069.

Martin-Padura I, Lostaglio S, Schneemann M, *et al.* (1998) Junctional adhesion molecule, a novel member of the immunoglobulin superfamily that distributes at intercellular junctions and modulates monocyte transmigration. *J Cell Biol* **142**: 117–127.

Martin PM, Roon P, Van Ells TK, *et al.* (2004) Death of retinal neurons in streptozotocin-induced diabetic mice. *Invest Ophthalmol Vis Sci* **45**: 3330–3336.

Miyamoto K, Hiroshiba N, Tsujikawa A, *et al.* (1998) *In vivo* demonstration of increased leukocyte entrapment in retinal microcirculation of diabetic rats. *Invest Ophthalmol Vis Sci* **39**: 2190–2194.

Miyamoto K, Khosrof S, Bursell SE, *et al.* (1999) Prevention of leukostasis and vascular leakage in streptozotocin-induced diabetic retinopathy via intercellular adhesion molecule-1 inhibition. *Proc Natl Acad Sci USA* **96**: 10836–10841.

Mizutani M, Gerhardinger C, Lorenzi M. (1998) Muller cell changes in human diabetic retinopathy. *Diabetes* **47**: 445–449.

Mizutani M, Kern TS, Lorenzi M. (1996) Accelerated death of retinal microvascular cells in human and experimental diabetic retinopathy. *J Clin Invest* **97**: 2883–2890.

Mohr S, Xi X, Tang J, *et al.* (2002) Caspase activation in retinas of diabetic and galactosemic mice and diabetic patients. *Diabetes* **51**: 1172–1179.

Moore TC, Moore JE, Kaji Y, *et al.* (2003) The role of advanced glycation end products in retinal microvascular leukostasis. *Invest Ophthalmol Vis Sci* **44**: 4457–4464.

Morita K, Furuse M, Fujimoto K, *et al.* (1999) Claudin multigene family encoding four-transmembrane domain protein components of tight junction strands. *Proc Natl Acad Sci USA* **96**: 511–516.

Murata M, Ohta N, Fujisawa S, *et al.* (2002) Selective pericyte degeneration in the retinal capillaries of galactose-fed dogs results from apoptosis linked to aldose reductase-catalyzed galactitol accumulation. *J Diabetes Complications* **16**: 363–370.

Newman E, Reichenbach A. (1996) The Muller cell: A functional element of the retina. *Trends Neurosci* **19**: 307–312.

Ng YK, Zeng XX, Ling EA. (2004) Expression of glutamate receptors and calcium-binding proteins in the retina of streptozotocin-induced diabetic rats. *Brain Res* **1018**: 66–72.

Nonaka A, Kiryu J, Tsujikawa A, *et al.* (2000) PKC-beta inhibitor (LY333531) attenuates leukocyte entrapment in retinal microcirculation of diabetic rats. *Invest Ophthalmol Vis Sci* **41**: 2702–2706.

Papachristodoulou D, Heath H, Kang SS. (1976) The development of retinopathy in sucrose fed and streptozotocin-diabetic rats. *Diabetologia* **12**: 367–374.

Park SH, Park JW, Park SJ, *et al.* (2003) Apoptotic death of photoreceptors in the streptozotocin-induced diabetic rat retina. *Diabetologia* **46**: 1260–1268.

Podesta F, Romeo G, Liu WH, *et al.* (2000) Bax is increased in the retina of diabetic subjects and is associated with pericyte apoptosis *in vivo* and *in vitro*. *Am J Pathol* **156**: 1025–1032.

Romeo G, Liu WH, Asnaghi V, *et al.* (2002) Activation of nuclear factor-kappaB induced by diabetes and high glucose regulates a proapoptotic program in retinal pericytes. *Diabetes* **51**: 2241–2248.

Rungger-Brandle E, Dosso AA, Leuenberger PM. (2000) Glial reactivity, an early feature of diabetic retinopathy. *Invest Ophthalmol Vis Sci* **41**: 1971–1980.

Sakai H, Tani Y, Shirasawa E, *et al.* (1995) Development of electroretinographic alterations in streptozotocin-induced diabetes in rats. *Ophthalmic Res* **27**: 57–63.

Saishin Y, Saishin Y, Takahashi K, *et al.* (2003) Inhibition of protein kinase C decreases prostaglandin-induced breakdown of the blood-retinal barrier. *J Cell Physiol* **195**: 210–219.

Santiago AR, Cristovao AJ, Santos PF, *et al.* (2007) High glucose induces caspase-independent cell death in retinal neural cells. *Neurobiol Dis* **25**: 464–472.

Santiago AR, Hughes JM, Kamphuis W, *et al.* (2008) Diabetes changes ionotropic glutamate receptor subunit expression level in the human retina. *Brain Res* **1198**: 153–159.

Santiago AR, Pereira TS, Garrido MJ, *et al.* (2006a) High glucose and diabetes increase the release of [3H]-D-aspartate in retinal cell cultures and in rat retinas. *Neurochem Int* **48**: 453–458.

Santiago AR, Rosa SC, Santos PF, *et al.* (2006b) Elevated glucose changes the expression of ionotropic glutamate receptor subunits and impairs calcium homeostasis in retinal neural cells. *Invest Ophthalmol Vis Sci* **47**: 4130–4137.

Schellini SA, Gregorio EA, Spadella CT, *et al.* (1995) Muller cells and diabetic retinopathy. *Braz J Med Biol Res* **28**: 977–980.

Schram MT, Chaturvedi N, Schalkwijk CG, *et al.* (2005) Markers of inflammation are cross-sectionally associated with microvascular complications and cardiovascular disease in type 1 diabetes — the EURODIAB Prospective Complications Study. *Diabetologia* **48**: 370–378.

Segawa M, Hirata Y, Fujimori S, *et al.* (1998) The development of electroretinogram abnormalities and the possible role of polyol pathway activity in diabetic hyperglycemia and galactosemia. *Metabolism* **37**: 454–460.

Sharma NK, Gardiner TA, Archer DB. (1985) A morphologic and autoradiographic study of cell death and regeneration in the retinal microvasculature of normal and diabetic rats. *Am J Ophthalmol* **100**: 51–60.

Simonsen SE. (1974) Prognostic value of ERG (oscillatory potential) in juvenile diabetics. *Acta Ophthalmol Suppl* **123**: 223–224.

Stevenson BR, Siliciano JD, Mooseker MS, *et al.* (1986) Identification of ZO-1: A high molecular weight polypeptide associated with the tight junction (zonula occludens) in a variety of epithelia. *J Cell Biol* **103**: 755–766.

Tout S, Chan-Ling T, Hollander H, *et al.* (1993) The role of Muller cells in the formation of the blood-retinal barrier. *Neuroscience* **55**: 291–301.

Uccioli L, Parisi V, Monticone G, *et al.* (1995) Electrophysiological assessment of visual function in newly-diagnosed IDDM patients. *Diabetologia* **38**: 804–808.

Vilchis C, Salceda R. (1996) Effect of diabetes on levels and uptake of putative amino acid neurotransmitters in rat retina and retinal pigment epithelium. *Neurochem Res* **21**: 1167–1171.

Vinores SA, Gadegbeku C, Campochiaro PA, *et al.* (1989) Immunohistochemical localization of blood-retinal barrier breakdown in human diabetics. *Am J Pathol* **134**: 231–235.

Vinores SA, Van Niel E, Swerdloff JL, *et al.* (1993) Electron microscopic immunocytochemical demonstration of blood-retinal barrier breakdown in human diabetics and its association with aldose reductase in retinal vascular endothelium and retinal pigment epithelium. *Histochem J* **25**: 648–663.

Wilkinson-Berka JL. (2004) Vasoactive factors and diabetic retinopathy: Vascular endothelial growth factor, cycoloxygenase-2 and nitric oxide. *Curr Pharm Des* **10**: 3331–3348.

Wittchen ES, Haskins J, Stevenson BR. (1999) Protein interactions at the tight junction. Actin has multiple binding partners, and ZO-1 forms independent complexes with ZO-2 and ZO-3. *J Biol Chem* **274**: 35179–35185.

Wolter JR. (1961) Diabetic retinopathy. *Am J Ophthalmol* **51**: 1123–1141.

Xi X, Gao L, Hatala DA, *et al.* (2005) Chronically elevated glucose-induced apoptosis is mediated by inactivation of Akt in cultured Muller cells. *Biochem Biophys Res Commun* **326**: 548–553.

Yamagishi S, Amano S, Inagaki Y, *et al.* (2002) Advanced glycation end products-induced apoptosis and overexpression of vascular endothelial growth factor in bovine retinal pericytes. *Biochem Biophys Res Commun* **290**: 973–978.

Yang LP, Sun HL, Wu LM, *et al.* (2009) Baicalein reduces inflammatory process in a rodent model of diabetic retinopathy. *Invest Ophthalmol Vis Sci* **50**: 2319–2327.

Zeng XX, Ng YK, Ling EA. (2000) Neuronal and microglial response in the retina of streptozotocin-induced diabetic rats. *Vis Neurosci* **17**: 463–471.

Zeng HY, Green WR, Tso MO. (2008) Microglial activation in human diabetic retinopathy. *Arch Ophthalmol* **126**: 227–232.

Zheng L, Szabo C, Kern TS. (2004) Poly(ADP-ribose) polymerase is involved in the development of diabetic retinopathy via regulation of nuclear factor-kappaB. *Diabetes* **53**: 2960–2967.

Zheng L, Du Y, Miller C, *et al.* (2007) Critical role of inducible nitric oxide synthase in degeneration of retinal capillaries in mice with streptozotocin-induced diabetes. *Diabetologia* **50**: 1987–1996.

Zhong Y, Saitoh T, Minase T, *et al.* (1993) Monoclonal antibody 7H6 reacts with a novel tight junction-associated protein distinct from ZO-1, cingulin and ZO-2. *J Cell Biol* **120**: 477–483.

## 4.3. Neovascularization in Diabetic Retinopathy

### Ermelindo Leal and António Francisco Ambrósio

Diabetic retinopathy is characterized by progressive alterations in the retinal microvasculature, leading to vascular hyperpermeability, vascular occlusion and, eventually, neovascularization. Neovascularization refers to the process of generating new capillary blood vessels from a pre-existing vascular bed. Physiological exceptions, in which neovascularization occurs, are found during embryonic development, menstrual cycle and wound healing (Hyder *et al.*, 1999).

Unregulated neovascularization occurs in several pathologies, such as tumor growth (Hanahan, 1998), rheumatoid arthritis (Koch, 1998), psoriasis (Kuroda *et al.*, 2001), arteriosclerosis (Bishop *et al.*, 2001) and various retinal diseases, including diabetic retinopathy (Ferrara *et al.*, 1999). Retinal neovascularization is a major complication of diabetic retinopathy (proliferative diabetic retinopathy) and often leads to loss of vision. In the eye, neovascularization is different from elsewhere, at least at the beginning of the process, because the development of new retinal vessels occurs almost devoid of accompanying cells and it degrades visual function and retinal anatomy due to intravitreal hemorrhage, retinal detachment and neovascular glaucoma.

### 4.3.1. Ischemia and Neovascularization in Diabetic Retinopathy

In retinal development, growing vessels were noted to invade areas of newly formed retina. These observations suggested that a diffusible growth factor stimulated by oxygen deprivation might induce this blood vessel growth. Neovascularization of the retina, in the development of retinal vasculature and retinal disease, is preceded temporally and associated spatially by retinal capillary non-perfusion (Michaelson, 1948; Henkind, 1978). In experimental diabetic retinopathy, the first histologically detectable lesions are capillary wall thickening, pericyte and endothelial cell loss and leukocyte adhesion to the vessel wall. These processes result in vascular hyperpermeability and occlusion, which induce respectively retinal oedema and ischemia.

Diverse processes may lead to retinal ischemia, including central retinal vein occlusion, progressive deterioration of vascular function due to prolonged hyperglycemia and obliteration of newly formed retinal vessels in premature neonates subjected to hyperoxia. All these processes, which have retinal ischemia in common, may culminate in the development of neovascularization. Once insufficient perfusion of the retina and a critical level of ischemia have been achieved, the different forms of retinopathy seem to converge to the hypoxia-induced formation of morphologically abnormal vessels. This is the dominant link in the formation of new vessels in the retina.

Ischemia when reaching a certain threshold induces neovascularization. We will review here the various growth factors that may play a role in the development of neovascularization in the retina and result from the occurrence of retinal ischemia.

### 4.3.2. Growth Factors

Growth factors are small proteins originally named for their common property of inducing mitosis. They can also have other biological activities, such as cell differentiation, extracellular matrix synthesis and chemotaxis. Michaelson (1948) postulated from histologic and clinical observations that neovascularization was due to the release of a diffusible factor from the ischemic retina. Such factor should be secreted and freely diffusible, so that it could stimulate vessel growth in adjacent retinal tissue. Hypoxia, another component of ischemia, should induce the expression of this molecule at either the protein synthesis or secretion level, and retinal endothelial cells should possess receptors for this factor. In addition, intraocular levels of this factor should be increased during active intraocular neovascularization. Finally, inhibition of this factor should prevent neovascularization. This concept still remains accepted today.

Several growth factors, such as basic fibroblast growth factor (bFGF), insulin-like growth factor (IGF), platelet-derived growth factor (PDGF) and vascular endothelial growth factor (VEGF) have been implicated in retinal neovascularization.

### 4.3.3. Basic Fibroblast Growth Factor (bFGF)

Basic and acidic fibroblast growth factors belong to the fibroblast growth factor (FGF) family. Basic fibroblast growth factor (bFGF) was named because of its mitogenic effect on fibroblasts and its high (basic) isoelectric point (9.6), which distinguishes it from acidic FGF (aFGF; pI = 5.6). bFGF is angiogenic both *in vitro* and *in vivo* (Javerzat *et al.*, 2002; Ribatti *et al.*, 2002), and it stimulates endothelial cell proliferation and migration. bFGF also induces capillary endothelial cells to migrate into three dimensional collagen matrices to form capillary-like tubes (Montesano, 1986; Eliceiri *et al.*, 1999). bFGF was the first growth factor found in the retina and was long suspected to play an important role in proliferative DR. However, the role of bFGF in ocular angiogenesis was difficult to define. For example, bFGF does not possess a signal sequence for secretion. However, bFGF mRNA and protein levels were reported to be elevated in several models, including the retinas of newborn mice exposed to hyperoxia (Nyberg *et al.*, 1990), and the retinal pigment epithelium (RPE) of retinas following laser injury (Zhang *et al.*, 1993). Studies of bFGF presence in the eyes of patients with proliferative DR were inconsistent. A histopathologic study of retinal neovascular membranes from patients with proliferative DR revealed no bFGF in active neovascular zones (Hanneken *et al.*, 1991). Conversely, bFGF mRNA, bFGF peptide and FGF receptor-1 were found in epiretinal membranes of proliferative DR patients, but

not in all patients (Hueber *et al.*, 1996). In another study, it was demonstrated that bFGF levels were significantly increased in the vitreous of patients with proliferative DR (Boulton *et al.*, 1997). bFGF expression was also found in the retinal vasculature of diabetic rats (Song *et al.*, 2004), and it was predominantly expressed during the phase of maximum angiogenesis in the mouse model of proliferative retinopathy (Chavakis *et al.*, 2002). More recently, an association of new polymorphisms in bFGF with proliferative DR was found. Significantly higher frequencies of 754C allele of the new 754C/G polymorphism were found in patients with proliferative DR comparing to a nondiabetic group. The bFGF plasma level in proliferative DR group was also significantly higher than in groups with nonproliferative DR and without diabetes. Moreover, those levels were significantly higher for CC and GC genotypes of 754C/G polymorphism in proliferative DR group (Beranek *et al.*, 2008). These findings support a possible role of bFGF in proliferative diabetic retinopathy.

### 4.3.4. Insulin-Like Growth Factors (IGF)

Insulin-like growth factors (IGF-I and IGF-II) are peptides with multiple biological effects (LeRoith and Roberts, 1993). IGF-I and IGF-II mRNAs are expressed in several tissues. However, IGF-II predominates during fetal development, and IGF-I is primarily expressed postnatally. The IGF peptides interact mostly with the IGF-I receptor, a transmembrane receptor with tyrosine kinase activity and with structural similarity to the insulin receptor. IGF action is also influenced by IGF-binding proteins, which have been found in the circulation and in extracellular fluids and affect IGF half-life and receptor interactions (LeRoith and Roberts, 1993).

The concept that growth hormone may influence the course of DR arose from a clinical observation of proliferative DR regression following tissue death of the pituitary gland during pregnancy (Sheehan's syndrome) and from the fact that proliferative DR does not occur before puberty (Poulsen, 1953). It was also shown that hypophysectomy in humans and animals led to a regression of DR (Luft *et al.*, 1955; Sharp *et al.*, 1987). However, the complications of hypophysectomy were frequent, severe and often lethal. Indeed, an association between growth hormone abnormalities and DR was demonstrated (Poulsen, 1966; Merimee, 1978) and it was shown that growth hormone mediated many of its effects via the production of insulin-like growth factors IGF-I and IGF-II.

Several *in vitro* studies support a role for IGF-I in retinal neovascularization. IGF-I stimulates migration and proliferation of endothelial cell lines, retinal capillary endothelial cells (Grant *et al.*, 1986; 1987) and RPE cells (Grant *et al.*, 1990). IGF-I receptors are widely distributed in the eye (Lambooij *et al.*, 2003), and treatment of mice, undergoing ocular ischemia with an IGF-I receptor antagonist, prevents retinal neovascularization (Smith *et al.*, 1999), which suggests a key role of IGF-I in this process. Furthermore, following hypoxia, vascular endothelial cell-specific IGF-I receptor knockout mice showed reduced retinal neovascularization (Kondo *et al.*, 2003). Also, in humans, mutations in growth-hormone receptor, IGF-I or IGF-I receptor genes reduce retinal vascularization (Hellstrom *et al.*, 2002).

IGF-I has been shown to be angiogenic *in vivo* at high doses (Grant *et al.*, 1993). IGF-I levels in vitreous and serum of patients with proliferative DR were increased compared with controls (Dills *et al.*, 1991; Inokuchi *et al.*, 2001). Vitreous IGF-II levels were not significantly different between diabetic patients and controls (Grant *et al.*, 1986). Recently, it was shown that normoglycemic/normoinsulinemic transgenic mice overexpressing IGF-I in the retina developed most alterations seen in human diabetic eye disease suggesting a role of IGF-I in the development of ocular complications in long-term diabetes (Ruberte *et al.*, 2004).

In DR, IGF-I has not been found to have a causative role but may act as an aggravating factor rather than the main angiogenic factor. The amount of IGF-I receptor present and/or its sensitivity might be

important, as some patients may be more sensitive to the angiogenic action of IGF-I than others.

### 4.3.5.  Platelet-Derived Growth Factor (PDGF)

PDGF is composed of two distinct but homologous chains (PDGF A-chain and PDGF B-chain) that can form homodimers or heterodimers and bind to specific $\alpha$ and $\beta$ tyrosine kinase receptors (Heldin *et al.*, 1998). PDGF can elicit proliferation and migration of several cell types, such as fibroblasts, vascular smooth muscle cells and chondrocytes, and is a potent chemoattractant and activator of neutrophils, monocytes and fibroblasts *in vitro* (Heldin *et al.*, 1998). PDGF and hypoxia were found to upregulate VEGF expression in rabbit (Stavri *et al.*, 1995) and human (Brogi *et al.*, 1994) smooth muscle cells. These experiments suggested that PDGF could enhance angiogenesis indirectly via an action on other cells that subsequently could affect endothelial cells. *In vivo*, PDGF plays a critical pathogenic role in tumorigenesis, atherosclerosis, fibrosis and inflammatory disorders (Rosenkranz, 1999).

PDGF and its receptors are present in the developing rodent retina (Mudhar *et al.*, 1993) and in vitreous and retinas of diabetic patients with proliferative DR (Robbins *et al.*, 1994; Freyberger *et al.*, 2000). However, in a murine model of ischemic retinopathy it was demonstrated that only VEGF antagonists, but not PDGF antagonists, are sufficient to inhibit neovascularization (Ozaki *et al.*, 2000).

Although bFGF, IGF and PDGF might play a role in DR neovascularization, they seem not to be the primary ocular angiogenic growth factor. bFGF, lacking a signal sequence for secretion, may not be secreted rapidly from the cell in response to ischemic changes, but released secondary to cell injury. IGF appears to have a role in angiogenesis, but may not be sufficient to produce neovascularization in the absence of other growth factors, since high concentrations are required to stimulate neovascularization. PDGF also seems not to be sufficient to promote neovascularization.

### 4.3.6. Vascular Endothelial Growth Factor (VEGF)

VEGF, also known as vascular permeability factor, is a 35–45 kDa homodimeric protein (Keck *et al.*, 1989; Leung *et al.*, 1989). VEGF is a highly conserved protein existing in four isoforms in humans, resulting from RNA splicing (Ferrara *et al.*, 1991; Houck *et al.*, 1991; Shima *et al.*, 1996).

VEGF is an endothelial cell-specific mitogen and it is strongly upregulated by hypoxia (Plate *et al.*, 1992; McColm *et al.*, 2004). The expression of VEGF is induced in tumors (Kim *et al.*, 1993; Winkler *et al.*, 2004), and its inhibition can dramatically reduce tumor growth *in vivo* (Kim *et al.*, 1993). VEGF mRNA expression and binding was found during normal vascular development (Breier *et al.*, 1992; Millauer *et al.*, 1993) and high levels of VEGF mRNA are involved in ovulation (Ferrara *et al.*, 1991), suggesting a physiological role of VEGF in processes involving angiogenesis.

VEGF acts by interacting with a family of tyrosine kinase receptors, more specific for endothelial cells, that include VEGFR-1 (Flt-1), VEGFR-2 (Flk-1) and VEGFR-3 (Flt-4). All VEGF receptors have specific high affinity binding sites for VEGF (De Vries *et al.*, 1992; Millauer *et al.*, 1993; Joukov *et al.*, 1996).

Several reports have provided strong evidences that VEGF plays a role in retinal angiogenic processes (Saishin *et al.*, 2003; Sarlos *et al.*, 2003). VEGF is expressed in the retina (McGookin *et al.*, 1992) and the observation that hypoxia induces VEGF production (Shweiki *et al.*, 1992) suggested that VEGF might be an ideal candidate to mediate the hypoxia-induced intraocular neovascular response. VEGF is involved in retinal neovascularization and increased vasopermeability noted within the eyes of patients with ischemic retinopathy (Vinores *et al.*, 1997). In addition, unlike bFGF, VEGF possesses a signal sequence (Houck *et al.*, 1991; Tischer *et al.*, 1991) and is secreted.

Within the retina, VEGF can be produced by several cells, such as pigment epithelial cells (Yang *et al.*, 1994), pericytes (Simorre *et al.*, 1994), endothelial cells (Aiello *et al.*, 1995), glial cells, Müller cells (Pierce *et al.*, 1995) and ganglion cells (Shima *et al.*, 1996). In addition, *in vitro*, hypoxia causes a dramatic upregulation of both mRNA and protein levels of VEGF in many of these cell types (Shima *et al.*, 1995; Eichler *et al.*, 2000), and VEGF induces retinal endothelial cell growth in a dose-dependent manner (Thieme *et al.*, 1995).

Since VEGF seemed to be a mediator of ischemia-induced ocular neovascularization, investigators tried to demonstrate that VEGF functions as a primary ocular angiogenesis factor *in vivo*. In a mouse model of retinopathy of prematurity, VEGF expression was elevated prior to the development of retinal neovascularization. The levels of VEGF remained high during the period of retinal neovascularization and gradually regressed when the new vessels became atrophic (Pierce *et al.*, 1995). In a primate model of retinal venous occlusion, intravitreal VEGF levels were increased in the ischemic eye just before iris neovascularization and reached the peak of expression during the neovascular stage (Miller *et al.*, 1994). In the retinas of diabetic animals, the increase in the expression of VEGF has been extensively demonstrated (Murata *et al.*, 1996; Hammes *et al.*, 1998; Cukiemik *et al.*, 2004).

In humans, the levels of VEGF are elevated in the vitreous and aqueous humor of patients with proliferative DR (Adamis *et al.*, 1994; Aiello *et al.*, 1994; Saishin *et al.*, 2003), and the levels of VEGF decrease in aqueous humor after laser treatment (Aiello *et al.*, 1994). In addition, in another study, where the presence of angiogenic growth factors was evaluated, it was found that only VEGF was consistently detected in neovascular membranes obtained from patients with proliferative DR (Malecaze *et al.*, 1994). Increased VEGF levels were also found in the retinas of patients with non-proliferative diabetic retinopathy (Lutty *et al.*, 1996; Amin *et al.*, 1997).

VEGF injection in the vitreous can induce intraretinal and iris neovascularization (Tolentino *et al.*, 1996).

The blockade of VEGF has been tested in different neovascularization models. The injection of soluble VEGF receptors suppressed iris neovascularization in monkeys undergoing retinal vein occlusion (Adamis *et al.*, 1996). This finding suggested that compounds inhibiting VEGF action might be useful clinically in suppressing intraocular neovascularization and diminishing visual loss from ischemic retinopathies. Several approaches to inhibit VEGF action were considered. One approach consists in the injection of relatively large inhibitors, such as aptamers or Fab fragments of anti-VEGF antibodies, directly into the eye (Kwak *et al.*, 2000; The EyeTech Study Group, 2002). Other approach is the administration of small molecules acting as VEGF antagonists (Ozaki *et al.*, 2000; Bainbridge *et al.*, 2002; Krzystolik *et al.*, 2002). Soluble VEGF receptors can reduce, in a specific way, VEGF bioavailability, but they are rapidly cleared. However, it was found that when ligand-binding domains of VEGF receptors linked to the Fc portion of IgG are used, the clearance of soluble VEGF receptors slows and neovascularization is suppressed (Saishin *et al.*, 2003). In addition, the inhibition of tyrosine kinase activity of VEGF receptors can be promising, not only in cancer therapy, but also in the treatment of proliferative DR. Studies using mouse models of oxygen-induced retinopathy and ischemia-induced retinopathy demonstrated that treatment with specific receptor kinase inhibitors decrease retinal neovascularization (Nauck *et al.*, 1998; Maier *et al.*, 2005).

In recent years, anti-VEGF agents have emerged as new approaches for the treatment of diabetic ocular complications. Although more clinical trials are needed in the diabetic population, because of the very good results reported in neovascular age-related macular degeneration (Nagpal *et al.*, 2007), this treatment is currently being used by many ophthalmologists in proliferative diabetic retinopathy and diabetic macular edema (Simo and Hernandez, 2008). Pegaptanib (Macugen), ranibizumab (Lucentis) and bevacizumab (Avastin) are the currently available anti-VEGF

agents. Pegaptanib is a neutralizing RNA aptamer, which binds with high specificity and affinity to human VEGF165 (Yasukawa *et al.*, 2004). Ranibizumab is the antigen-binding domain (Fab) derived from a full-length monoclonal antibody (mAb) directed against human VEGF (Kim *et al.*, 1992). However, whereas ranibizumab is a 48 kDa Fab fragment, bevacizumab is a complete 149 kDa antibody and, therefore, possesses two antigen-binding domains (Kaiser, 2006). In contrast to pegaptanib, ranibizumab and bevacizumab bind and inhibit the biological activity of all isoforms of human VEGF.

Several studies using these anti-VEGF drugs reported very promising results in patients with diabetes. In a prospective, double-blind, multicentre, dose-ranging, controlled trial that included 172 patients with DME, participants treated with pegaptanib had better visual acuity, were more likely to show a reduction in central retinal thickness and were less likely to need additional therapy with photocoagulation (Cunningham *et al.*, 2005). In addition, most of the participants with retinal neovascularization showed a regression of neovascularization (Adamis *et al.*, 2006). Studies using ranibizumab and bevacizumab have also found a rapid regression of retinal neovascularization, an improvement in visual acuity and a decrease in retinal thickness, even in non-responders to conventional treatment (Avery *et al.*, 2006; Nguyen *et al.*, 2006; Spaide and Fisher, 2006). Nevertheless, larger studies are needed to investigate the effectiveness of these anti-VEGF drugs in the diabetic population.

It is important to mention that VEGF does not act alone. Other factors that regulate or are regulated by VEGF might also be considered good molecular targets, since it will also be possible indirectly to block, totally or partially, VEGF action.

### 4.3.7. Conclusions

Proliferative diabetic retinopathy is the most severe stage of DR pathology. It is characterized by the growth of new vessels, often leading to blindness. Neovascularization is an indirect effect of hyperglycemia, which leads to pericyte and endothelial cell loss, progressive vascular damage, widespread capillary occlusion and subsequent retinal ischemia. It is the ischemia that induces neovascularization of the retina. Several growth factors, such as bFGF, IGF, PDGF and VEGF, are upregulated by ischemia, and these molecules are responsible for the growth of new vessels. However, several evidences suggest that VEGF may be the most important mediator of ischemic ocular angiogenesis, and, therefore, VEGF seems to be one of the best targets in the treatment of proliferative DR. The inhibition of VEGF may be approached at several levels, including regulation of transcription, protein activity, receptor action or intracellular signal transduction.

# References

Adamis A, Bernal MT, D'Amico D, *et al.* (1994) Increased Vascular Endothelial Growth Factor levels in the vitreous of eyes with proliferative diabetic retinopathy. *Am J Ophthalmol* **11**: 445–450.

Adamis AP, Shima DT, Tolentino MJ, *et al.* (1996) Inhibition of vascular endothelial growth factor prevents retinal ischemia-associated iris neovascularization in a nonhuman primate. *Arch Ophthalmol* **114**: 66–71.

Adamis AP, Altaweel M, Bressler NM, *et al.* (2006) Changes in retinal neovascularization after pegaptanib (Macugen) therapy in diabetic individuals. *Ophthalmol* **113**: 23–28.

Aiello LP, Avery RL, Arrigg PG, *et al.* (1994) Vascular Endothelial Growth Factor in ocular fluid of patients with diabetic retinopathy and other retinal disorders. *New Engl J Med* **331**: 1480–1487.

Aiello L, Northup J, Keyt B, *et al.* (1995) Hypoxic regulation of vascular endothelial growth factor in retinal cells. *Arch Ophthalmol* **113**: 1538–1544.

Amin RH, Frank RN, Kennedy A, *et al.* (1997) Vascular endothelial growth factor is present in glial cells of the retina and optic nerve of human subjects with nonproliferative diabetic retinopathy. *Invest Ophthalmol Vis Sci* **38**: 36–47.

Avery RL, Pearlman J, Pieramici DJ, *et al.* (2006) Intravitreal bevacizumab (Avastin) in the treatment of proliferative diabetic retinopathy. *Ophthalmol* **113**: 1695 e1–e15.

Bainbridge JW, Mistry A, De Alwis M, *et al.* (2002) Inhibition of retinal neovascularisation by gene transfer of soluble VEGF receptor sFlt-1. *Gene Ther* **9**: 320–326.

Beranek M, Kolar P, Tschoplova S, *et al.* (2008) Genetic variation and plasma level of the basic fibroblast growth factor in proliferative diabetic retinopathy. *Diabetes Res Clin Pract* **79**: 362–367.

Bishop GG, McPherson JA, Sanders JM, *et al.* (2001) Selective alpha(v)beta(3)-receptor blockade reduces macrophage infiltration and restenosis after balloon angioplasty in the atherosclerotic rabbit. *Circulation* **103**: 1906–1911.

Boulton M, Gregor Z, McLeod D, *et al.* (1997) Intravitreal growth factors in proliferative diabetic retinopathy: Correlation with neovascular activity and glycaemic management. *Br J Ophthalmol* **81**: 228–233.

Breier G, Albrecht U, Sterrer S, *et al.* (1992) Expression of vascular endothelial growth factor during embryonic angiogenesis and endothelial cell differentiation. *Development* **114**: 521–532.

Brogi E, Wu T, Namiki A, *et al.* (1994) Indirect angiogenic cytokines upregulate VEGF and bFGF gene expression in vascular smooth muscle cells, whereas hypoxia upregulates VEGF expression only. *Circulation* **90**: 649–652.

Chavakis E, Riecke B, Lin J, *et al.* (2002) Kinetics of integrin expression in the mouse model of proliferative retinopathy and success of secondary intervention with cyclic RGD peptides. *Diabetologia* **45**: 262–267.

Cukiernik M, Hileeto D, Evans T, *et al.* (2004) Vascular endothelial growth factor in diabetes induced early retinal abnormalities. *Diabetes Res Clin Pract* **65**: 197–208.

Cunningham ET Jr., Adamis AP, Altaweel M, *et al.* (2005) A phase II randomized double-masked trial of pegaptanib, an anti-vascular endothelial growth factor aptamer, for diabetic macular edema. *Ophthalmology* **112**: 1747–1757.

De Vries C, Escobedo JA, Ueno H, *et al.* (1992) The fms-like tyrosine kinase, a receptor for vascular endothelial growth factor. *Science* **255**: 989–991.

Dills DG, Moss SE, Klein R, *et al.* (1991) Association of elevated IGF-1 levels with increased retinopathy in late-onset diabetes. *Diabetes* **40**: 1725–1730.

Eichler W, Kuhrt H, Hoffmann S, *et al.* (2000) VEGF release by retinal glia depends on both oxygen and glucose supply. *Neuroreport* **11**: 3533–3537.

Eliceiri BP, Paul R, Schwartzberg PL, *et al.* (1999) Selective requirement for Src kinases during VEGF-induced angiogenesis and vascular permeability. *Mol Cell* **4**: 915–924.

Ferrara N, Houck KA, Jakeman LB, *et al.* (1991) The vascular endothelial growth factor family of polypeptides. *J Cell Biochem* **47**: 211–218.

Ferrara N, Alitalo K. (1999) Clinical applications of angiogenic growth factors and their inhibitors. *Nat Med* **5**: 1359–1364.

Freyberger H, Brocker M, Yakut H, *et al.* (2000) Increased levels of platelet-derived growth factor in vitreous fluid of patients with proliferative diabetic retinopathy. *Exp Clin Endocrinol Diabetes* **108**: 106–109.

Grant M, Russell B, Fitgerald C, *et al.* (1986) Insulin-like growth factors in vitreous: Studies in control and diabetic subjects with neovascularization. *Diabetes* **35**: 416–420.

Grant M, Jerdan J, Merimee TJ. (1987) Insulin-like growth factor-I modulates endothelial cell chemotaxis. *J Clin Endocrinol Metab* **65**: 370–371.

Grant MB, Guay C, Marsh R. (1990) Insulin-like growth factor I stimulates proliferation, migration and plasminofen activator release by human retinal pigment epithelial cells. *Curr Eye Res* **9**: 323–335.

Grant MB, Mames RN, Fitgerald C, *et al.* (1993) Insulin-like growth factor I as an angiogenic agent: *In vivo* and *in vitro* studies. *Ann N Y Acad Sci* **692**: 230–242.

Hammes HP, Lin J, Bretzel RG, *et al.* (1998) Upregulation of the vascular endothelial growth factor/vascular endothelial growth factor receptor system in experimental background diabetic retinopathy of the rat. *Diabetes* **47**: 401–406.

Hanahan D. (1998) A flanking attack on cancer. *Nat Med* **4**: 13–14.

Hanneken A, de Lutty G, Fox G, *et al.* (1991) Altered distribution of basic fibroblast growth factor in diabetic retinopathy. *Arch Ophthalmol* **109**: 1005–1011.

Heldin CH, Ostman A, Ronnstrand L. (1998) Signal transduction via platelet-derived growth factor receptors. *Biochim Biophys Acta* **1378**: F79–F113.

Hellstrom A, Carlsson B, Niklasson A, *et al.* (2002) IGF-I is critical for normal vascularization of the human retina. *J Clin Endocrinol Metab* **87**: 3413–3416.

Henkind P. (1978) Ocular neovascularization. *Am J Ophthalmol* **85**: 287–301.

Houck K, Ferrara N, Winer J, *et al.* (1991) The vascular endothelial growth factor family: Identification of a fourth molecular species and characterization of alternative splicing. *Mol Endocrinol* **5**: 1806–1814.

Hueber A, Wiedemann P, Esser P, *et al.* (1996–97). Basic fibroblast growth factor mRNA, bFGF peptide and FGF receptor in epiretinal membranes of intraocular proliferative disorders (PVR and PDR). *Int Ophthalmol* **20**: 345–350.

Hyder SM, Stancel GM. (1999) Regulation of angiogenic growth factors in the female reproductive tract by estrogens and progestins. *Mol Endocrinol* **13**: 806–811.

Inokuchi N, Ikeda T, Imamura Y, *et al.* (2001) Vitreous levels of insulinlike growth factor-I in patients with proliferative diabetic retinopathy. *Curr Eye Res* **23**: 368–371.

Javerzat S, Auguste P, Bikfalvi A. (2002) The role of fibroblast growth factors in vascular development. *Trends Mol Med* **8**: 483–489.

Joukov V, Pajusola K, Kaipainen A, *et al.* (1996) A novel vascular endothelial growth factor, VEGF-C, is a ligand for the Flt4 (VEGFR-3) and KDR (VEGFR-2) receptor tyrosine kinases. *EMBO J* **15**: 290–298.

Kaiser PK. (2006) Antivascular endothelial growth factor agents and their development: Therapeutic implications in ocular diseases. *Am J Ophthalmol* **142**: 660–668.

Keck PJ, Hauser SD, Krivi G, *et al.* (1989) Vascular permeability factor, an endothelial cell mitogen related to PDGF. *Science* **246**: 1309–1312.

Kim KJ, Li B, Houck K, *et al.* (1992) The vascular endothelial growth factor proteins: Identification of biologically relevant regions by neutralizing monoclonal antibodies. *Growth Factors* **7**: 53–64.

Kim KJ, Li B, Winer J, *et al.* (1993) Inhibition of vascular endothelial growth factor-induced angiogenesis suppresses tumour growth *in vivo*. *Nature* **362**: 841–844.

Koch AE. (1998) Review: Angiogenesis: Implications for rheumatoid arthritis. *Arthritis Rheum* **41**: 951–962.

**150** *Diabetic Retinopathy*

Kondo T, Vicent D, Suzuma K, *et al.* (2003) Knockout of insulin and IGF-1 receptors on vascular endothelial cells protects against retinal neovascularization. *J Clin Invest* **111**: 1835–1842.

Krzystolik MG, Afshari MA, Adamis AP, *et al.* (2002) Prevention of experimental choroidal neovascularization with intravitreal anti-vascular endothelial growth factor antibody fragment. *Arch Ophthalmol* **120**: 338–346.

Kuroda K, Sapadin A, Shoji T, *et al.* (2001) Altered expression of angiopoietins and Tie2 endothelium receptor in psoriasis. *J Invest Dermatol* **116**: 713–720.

Kwak N, Okamoto N, Wood JM, *et al.* (2000) VEGF is major stimulator in model of choroidal neovascularization. *Invest Ophthalmol Vis Sci* **41**: 3158–3164.

Lambooij AC, van Wely KH, Lindenbergh-Kortleve DJ, *et al.* (2003) Insulin-like growth factor-I and its receptor in neovascular age-related macular degeneration. *Invest Ophthalmol Vis Sci* **44**: 2192–2198.

LeRoith D, Roberts CT Jr. (1993) Insulin-like growth factors. *Ann N Y Acad Sci* **692**: 1–9.

Leung DW, Cachianes G, Kunang WJ, *et al.* (1989) Vascular endothelial growth factor is a secreted angiogenic mitogen. *Science* **246**: 1306–1309.

Luft R, Olivecrona H, Ikkos D, *et al.* (1955) Hypophysectomy in man: Further experiences in severe diabetes mellitus. *Br Med J* **2**: 752–756.

Lutty GA, McLeod DS, Merges C, *et al.* (1996) Localization of vascular endothelial growth factor in human retina and choroid. *Arch Ophthalmol* **114**: 971–977.

Maier P, Unsoeld AS, Junker B, *et al.* (2005) Intravitreal injection of specific receptor tyrosine kinase inhibitor PTK787/ZK222 584 improves ischemia-induced retinopathy in mice. *Graefes Arch Clin Exp Ophthalmol* **243**: 593–600.

Malecaze F, Clamens S, Simorre-Pinatel V, *et al.* (1994) Detection of VEGF mRNA and VEGF-like activity in proliferative diabetic retinopathy. *Arch Ophthalmol* **112**: 1476–1480.

McColm JR, Geisen P, Hartnett ME. (2004) VEGF isoforms and their expression after a single episode of hypoxia or repeated fluctuations between hyperoxia and hypoxia: Relevance to clinical ROP. *Mol Vis* **10**: 512–520.

McGookin E, Stopa E, Kuo-LeBlanc, *et al.* (1992) Vascular endothelial growth factor (VEGF) has a different distribution than basic fibroblast growth factor (bFGF) in the adult human retina. *Invest Ophthalmol Vis Sci* **33**: 651.

Merimee T. (1978) A follow-up study of vascular disease in growth-hormone-deficient dwarfs with diabetes. *N Engl J Med* **298**: 1217–1222.

Michaelson IC. (1948) The mode of development of the vascular system of the retina, with some observations on its significance for certain retinal disease. *Trans Ophthalmol Soc UK* **68**: 137–180.

Millauer B, Wizigmann-Voos S, Schnurch H, *et al.* (1993) High affinity VEGF binding and developmental expression suggest Flk-1 as a major regulator of vasculogenesis and angiogenesis. *Cell* **72**: 835–846.

Miller JW, Adamis AP, Shima DT, *et al.* (1994) Vascular endothelial growth factor/vascular permeability factor is temporally and spatially correlated with ocular angiogenesis in a primate model. *Am J Pathol* **145**: 574–584.

Montesano R, Vassali JD, Baird A, *et al.* (1986) Basic fibroblast growth factor induces angiogenesis *in vitro*. *Proc Natl Acad Sc* **83**: 7297–7301.

Mudhar HS, Pollock RA, Wang C, *et al.* (1993) PDGF and its receptors in the developing rodent retina and optic nerve. *Development* **118**: 539–552.

Murata T, Nakagawa K, Khalil A, *et al.* (1996) The relation between expression of vascular endothelial growth factor and breakdown of the blood-retinal barrier in diabetic rat retinas. *Lab Invest* **74**: 819–825.

Nagpal M, Nagpal K, Nagpal PN. (2007) A comparative debate on the various anti-vascular endothelial growth factor drugs: Pegaptanib sodium (Macugen), ranibizumab (Lucentis) and bevacizumab (Avastin). *Indian J Ophthalmol* **55**: 437–439.

Nauck M, Karakiulakis G, Perruchoud AP, *et al.* (1998) Corticosteroids inhibit the expression of the vascular endothelial growth factor gene in human vascular smooth muscle cells. *Eur J Pharmacol* **341**: 309–315.

Nguyen QD, Tatlipinar S, Shah SM, *et al.* (2006) Vascular endothelial growth factor is a critical stimulus for diabetic macular edema. *Am J Ophthalmol* **142**: 961–969.

Nyberg F, Hahnenberger R, Jakobson AM, *et al.* (1990) Enhancement of FGF-like polypeptides in the retinae of newborn mice exposed to hyperoxia. *FEBS Lett* **267**: 75–77.

Ozaki H, Seo MS, Ozaki K, *et al.* (2000) Blockade of vascular endothelial cell growth factor receptor signaling is sufficient to completely prevent retinal neovascularization. *Am J Pathol* **156**: 697–707.

Pierce EA, AR Foley ED, Aiello LP, *et al.* (1995) Vascular Endothelial Growth Factor/Vascular Permeability Factor expression in a mouse model of retinal neovascularization. *Proc Natl Acad Sci USA* **91**: 905–909.

Plate KH, Breier G, Weich HA, *et al.* (1992) Vascular endothelial growth factor is a potential tumour angiogenesis factor in human gliomas *in vivo*. *Nature* **359**: 845–848.

Poulsen JE. (1953) The Houssay phenomenon in man: Recovery from retinopathy in a case of diabetes with Simmonds' disease. *Diabetes* **2**: 7–12.

Poulsen J. (1966) Diabetes and anterior pituitary insufficiency: Final course and postmortem study of a diabetic patient with Sheehan's syndrome. *Diabetes* **15**: 73–77.

Robbins SG, Mixon RN, Wilson DJ, *et al.* (1994) Platelet-derived growth factor ligands and receptors immunolocalized in proliferative retinal diseases. *Invest Ophthalmol Vis Sci* **3**: 3649–3663.

Ribatti D, Presta M. (2002) The role of fibroblast growth factor-2 in the vascularization of the chick embryo chorioallantoic membrane. *J Cell Mol Med* **6**: 439–446.

Rosenkranz S, Kazlauskas A. (1999) Evidence for distinct signaling properties and biological responses induced by the PDGF receptor alpha and beta subtypes. *Growth Factors* **16**: 201–216.

Ruberte J, Ayuso E, Navarro M, *et al.* (2004) Increased ocular levels of IGF-1 in transgenic mice lead to diabetes-like eye disease. *J Clin Invest* **13**: 1149–1157.

Saishin Y, Saishin Y, Takahashi K, *et al.* (2003) VEGF-TRAP(R1R2) suppresses choroidal neovascularization and VEGF-induced breakdown of the blood-retinal barrier. *J Cell Physiol* **195**: 241–248.

Sarlos S, Rizkalla B, Moravski CJ, *et al.* (2003) Retinal angiogenesis is mediated by an interaction between the angiotensin type 2 receptor, VEGF, and angiopoietin. *Am J Pathol* **163**: 879–887.

Sharp P, Fallon T, Brazier O, *et al.* (1987) Long-term follow-up of patients who underwent yttrium-90 pituitary implantation for treatment of proliferative diabetic retinopathy. *Diabetologia* **30**: 199–207.

Shima D, Adamis A, Ferrara N, *et al.* (1995) Hypoxic induction of endothelial cell growth factors in retinal cells: Identification and characterization of vascular endothelial growth factor (VEGF) as the mitogen. *Mol Med* **2**: 182–193.

Shima D, Gougos A, Miller J, *et al.* (1996) Cloning and mRNA expression of VEGF in ischemic retinas of *Macaca fascicularis*. *Invest Ophthalmol Vis Sci* **37**: 1334–1340.

Shima D, Kuroki M, Deutsch U, *et al.* (1996) The mouse gene for vascular endothelial growth factor: Genomic structure, definition of the transcriptional unit, characterization of transcriptional and post-transcriptional regulatory sequences. *J Biol Chem* **271**: 1–7.

Shweiki D, Itin A, Soffer D, *et al.* (1992) Vascular endothelial growth factor induced by hypoxia may mediate hypoxia-initiated angiogenesis. *Nature* **359**: 843–845.

Simo R, Hernandez C. (2008) Intravitreous anti-VEGF for diabetic retinopathy: Hopes and fears for a new therapeutic strategy. *Diabetologia* **51**: 1574–1580.

Simorre P, Guerrin M, Chollet P, *et al.* (1994) Vasculotropin–VEGF stimulates retinal capillary endothelial cells through an autocrine pathway. *Invest Ophthalmol Vis Sci* **35**: 3393–3400.

Smith LE, Shen W, Perruzzi C, *et al.* (1999) Regulation of vascular endothelial growth factor-dependent retinal neovascularization by insulin-like growth factor-1 receptor. *Nat Med* **5**: 1390–1395.

Song E, Dong Y, Han LN, *et al.* (2004) Diabetic retinopathy: VEGF, bFGF and retinal vascular pathology. *Chin Med J (Engl)* **117**: 247–251.

Spaide RF, Fisher YL. (2006) Intravitreal bevacizumab (Avastin) treatment of proliferative diabetic retinopathy complicated by vitreous hemorrhage. *Retina* **26**: 275–278.

Stavri GT, Hong Y, Zachary IC, *et al.* (1995) Hypoxia and platelet-derived growth factor-BB synergistically upregulate the expression of vascular endothelial growth factor in vascular smooth muscle cells. *FEBS Lett* **358**: 311–315.

The EyeTech Study Group. (2002) Preclinical and phase 1A. Clinical evaluation of an Anti-VEGF Pegylated Aptamer (EYE001) for the treatment of exudative age-related macular degeneration. *Retina* **22**: 143–152.

Thieme H, Aiello L, Takagi H, *et al.* (1995) Comparative analysis of vascular endothelial growth factor receptors on retinal and aortic vascular endothelial cells. *Diabetes* **44**: 98–103.

Tischer E, Mitchell R, Hartman T, *et al.* (1991) The human gene for vascular endothelial growth factor: Multiple protein forms are encoded through alternative exon splicing. *J Biol Chem* **266**: 11947–11954.

Tolentino MJ, Miller JW, Gragoudas ES, *et al.* (1996) Intravitreous injections of vascular endothelial growth factor produce retinal ischemia and microangiopathy in an adult primate. *Ophthalmology* **103**: 1820–1828.

Vinores SA, Youssri AI, Luna JD, *et al.* (1997) Upregulation of vascular endothelial growth factor in ischemic and non-ischemic human and experimental retinal disease. *Histol Histopathol* **12**: 99–109.

Winkler F, Kozin SV, Tong RT, *et al.* (2004) Kinetics of vascular normalization by VEGFR2 blockade governs brain tumor response to radiation: Role of oxygenation, angiopoietin-1, and matrix metalloproteinases. *Cancer Cell* **6**: 553–563.

Yang Q, Zwijsen A, Slegers H, *et al.* (1994) Purification and characterization of VEGF/VPF secreted by human retinal pigment epithelial cells. *Endothelium* **2**: 73–85.

Yasukawa T, Ogura Y, Tabata Y, *et al.* (2004) Drug delivery systems for vitreoretinal diseases. *Prog Retin Eye Res* **23**: 253–281.

Zhang NL, Samadani EE, Frank RN. (1993) Mitogenesis and retinal pigment epithelial cell antigen expression in the rat after krypton laser photocoagulation. *Invest Ophthalmol Vis Sci* **34**: 2412–2424.

# 4.4. Candidate Genes of Diabetic Retinopathy

## Alda Ambrósio

### 4.4.1. Molecular Genetics Approaches to Gene Mapping in Complex Human Disease

Disease gene mapping in humans has a long history, predating even the identification of DNA as the genetic molecule. The positional candidate gene analysis has been proposed as a powerful tool to identify genetic variants of complex diseases (Horikawa *et al.*, 2000). Concerning statistical genetics, several methods have been proposed for linkage analysis of complex traits, including parametric and nonparametric linkage approaches (Ott and Hoh, 2000; Hoh and

Ott, 2004). Parametric linkage analysis (LOD score) in Mendelian disorders test the co-segregation of a genetic marker with the disease, which is dependent on the physical distance between the marker and the disease gene, measured by the recombination fraction. This method (LOD score) uses all the data available and is extremely powerful when the true model is used, as, for example, in the case of monogenic diseases. However, much of its power is lost in complex disorders, indicating a need for alternative approaches.

To avoid some problems of model specification in complex disorders, nonparametric methods of linkage analysis that do not require specification of mode of inheritance were developed and were called affected sib pair (ASP) and affected pedigree member (APM) methods (Weeks and Lange, 1988). However, in these methods, only sibpairs or other pairs of affected relatives are investigated and the power of seeing alleles segregating in large pedigrees is lost. Moreover, Kruglyak *et al.* (1996) developed a computer package named GENEHUNTER that analyzes moderate size pedigrees in their entirety. This program does not require specification of a genetic model (although this program can also perform parametric linkage analysis) and, therefore, is considered the most appropriate method to use for the linkage analysis of diabetic retinopathy (DR). However, susceptibility genes may be difficult to map by linkage analysis because of the limited power to detect genes of small effect (Risch and Merikangas, 1996).

Genetic association studies examine the relationship of variants in candidate genes or genomic regions with vulnerability to disease. Although they provide a potentially powerful way of identifying genes of small effect, case-control association studies can generate false positives as a result of population stratification. This problem can be addressed by the Haplotype Relative Risk (HRR) (Terwilliger and Ott, 1992) and Transmission Disequilibrium Test (TDT) (Spielman *et al.*, 1993) strategies, in which association or linkage disequilibrium is tested in nuclear families. For these strategies, DNA is collected both from patient and from their parents, and parental chromosomes not transmitted to affected individuals serve as ethnically matched controls (Risch and Merikangas, 1996; Collins *et al.*, 1997). In the genome era, there is great hope that genetic approaches, such as linkage disequilibrium mapping, can be used to study common human disorders using a case-control population association study design (Varilo and Peltonen, 2004). Thus, linkage disequilibrium mapping is a powerful alternative to linkage analysis for the mapping and detection of genes involved in DR. The parental chromosomes are marked so that chromosomal regions in the form of haplotypes are compared in these studies to increase the power of association, and the haplotypes in a diploid individual is a major technical challenge in genetic studies of complex trait (Salisbury *et al.*, 2003). For example, linkage disequilibrium detectable with microsatellites in disease alleles over wide genetic intervals in population isolates (Varilo and Peltonen, 2004) has facilitated mapping and positional cloning of numerous disease genes.

Genetic variation in the human genome occurs predominantly as single nucleotide polymorphisms (SNPs), based on the single nucleotide variations at the genomic level, which distributes widely across the human genome and have become the primary markers for genetic studies to identify susceptible genes for complex diseases (Kendal, 2003). Until now, tens of thousands SNPs have been discovered among the human genome and our DNA may contain as many as ten million SNPs, of which three million or more are likely to differ between any two unrelated individuals. SNPs are viewed as ideal markers for large-scale genome-wide association studies to discover genes in common complex diseases, such as DR, because of their dense distribution across the genome. These variants used in fine-scale genetic mapping and genome-wide association studies may predispose individuals to illnesses, such as diabetes, hypertension or cancer or affect disease progression (Kwok and Chen, 2003). Moreover, these three million genetic differences make a significant contribution to the observed variation in complex human phenotypes, such as disease susceptibility and our responses to drugs or environmental chemicals.

With the development of identification and analysis techniques for SNPs, especially in combination with DNA chips (Hoh and Ott, 2004), SNPs are gradually fitable for fine-scale mapping of diseases, especially susceptibility genes of complex diseases and they will eventually substitute the most commonly used microsatellite markers presently.

The number of SNP genotyping methods has exploded in recent years and many robust methods are currently available. SNP detection technologies have evolved from labor intensive, time consuming and expensive processes to some of the most highly automated, efficient and relatively inexpensive methods (Kwok and Xiao, 2004). Despite the considerable gains over the last decade, new approaches must be developed to lower the cost and increase the speed of SNP detection. Recently, to identify genetic variants that might confer susceptibility to diabetic nephropathy, a genome-wide analysis of gene-based SNPs in a large cohort of Japanese diabetic patients was performed. The results obtained suggested the existence of several distinct regions as good candidates for the susceptibility to diabetic nephropathy (Maeda, 2004). Studies like these are needed to identify the susceptibility genes involved in DR.

## 4.4.2. Genetic Susceptibility in Diabetic Retinopathy

Hyperglycemia occurs in every patient with diabetes mellitus and it is the most important factor in the development of diabetic complications (Chakrabarti *et al.*, 2000). Several studies have provided evidence that good diabetes control is important to prevent diabetic retinopathy, but some groups of patients develop diabetic retinopathy despite good control, while others escape retinopathy despite poor control. In addition, the onset, intensity and the progression of diabetic complications show large interindividual variations (Rogus *et al.*, 2002). Furthermore, aggregation in families and specific ethnic groups and the lack of complications in some diabetics with poor metabolic control indicate a genetic predisposition to develop some diabetic complications, such as retinopathy (Warpeha and Chakravarthy, 2003).

Family and twin studies have been used to determine the degree to which a disease is heritable. Family studies establish risk ratio for different types of relatives of affected individuals. The risk for illness are much higher in close relatives of patients than in general population, and increase with the degree of relationship. Twin studies have also indicated a higher heritability for DR, since identical twins are nearly always concordant (Leslie and Pyke, 1982). Taking this into account, it is evident that genetic factors play an important role in the pathogenesis of DR, but to date association studies have, thus, failed to implicate causative genetic variants consistently (Warpeha and Chakravarthy, 2003). The identification of genes involved, however, has proven to be a difficult task, because DR is characterized by a etiologic heterogeneity, uncertainty about the number of loci involved and about their interactions and also the interaction between genes and environmental factors.

Considering that DR is a complex multifactorial illness and given the heterogeneity of this disorder, it is important to investigate susceptibility genes in genetically homogenous populations (Varilo and Peltonen, 2004). The identification of DR susceptibility loci should reveal new therapeutic targets, but it requires accurate phenotyping. Careful phenotyping is necessary to reduce population heterogeneity and this can be achieved by using endophenotypes, a strategy that increases the likelihood of identifying DR related genes.

Two approaches can be used to find genetic factors in multifactorial complex disorders, including genome scans for markers linked to disease and candidate genes (Hoh and Ott, 2004). Relatively to DR,

there is just one genome scan study with families using sib-pair linkage analysis (Imperatore *et al.*, 1998). An alternative and complementary strategy to a random genome search is to analyze genes with potential involvement in the disease. Thus, a candidate gene can be identified by its position in a chromosomal area that has been implicated in a prior genome scan or alternatively can be selected based upon evidence that the gene product plays a role in the pathophysiology of the disease (Hoh and Ott, 2004). Whereas linkage analysis tests for cosegregation of a gene marker and disease phenotype in families, association studies can use either families or unrelated controls and examine the co-occurrence of a marker and the disease at the population level (Risch and Merikangas, 1996).

## 4.4.3. Candidate Genes in Diabetic Retinopathy

Diabetic retinopathy is the leading cause of blindness in adults aged 30 to 65 years. However, 20% of the diabetic population does not develop significant retinopathy. Late complications of diabetes mellitus include a variety of clinical pictures, mainly related to the involvement of the arterial wall of both large vessels (macroangiopathy) and small vessels (microangiopathy) (Chakrabarti *et al.*, 2000). Their presence in almost all types of diabetes indicates that there is a common pathogenic mechanism. Poor metabolic control, hemodynamic factors and long duration of diabetes may predispose to the development of DR. Hyperglycemia leads to some metabolic abnormalities, i.e. non-enzymatic glycosylation of proteins and increased polyol pathway activity.

Some evidence indicates that a genetic background may predispose to the development of DR or protect from its onset. The aldose reductase pathway, glucose transporters, cell communication and extracellular matrix related genes, among others, are often considered the leading candidate genes to be examined and association studies have been commonly used. Because association studies are largely concerned with genes of minor effect, studies of large statistically powerful samples may produce more compelling results than the more typical small-scale studies that have been done.

## 4.4.4. Aldose Reductase Gene

Alterations in the aldose reductase (AR) pathway have long been linked to the pathophysiology of DR. Inhibitors of AR (ARIs) have been shown to be effective in preventing some of the diabetic complications in animal models (Yamaoka *et al.*, 1995; Chung and Chung, 2003). However, clinical trials using these drugs were disappointing (Chung and Chung, 2003), casting doubt on the role of AR in this disease.

Genes involved in AR pathway are being studied in a number of population samples as candidates for DR. The AR is encoded by the AR2 gene and is involved in the conversion of glucose to sorbitol, acting as the rate-limiting enzyme of the polyol pathway (Chakrabarti *et al.*, 2000). For example, diabetic patients with microvascular disease have increased gene expression and enzyme activity of AR, which may be due to variants in the AR gene. The gene coding for AR2 has been localized to chromosome 7q35 and to date several polymorphisms in AR gene were identified and investigated in a number of population samples with inconsistent results (Ko *et al.*, 1995; Chistyakov *et al.*, 1997; Fujisawa *et al.*, 1999; Kao *et al.*, 1999; Ichikawa *et al.*, 1999; Ikegishi *et al.*, 1999; Demaine *et al.*, 2000; Olmos *et al.*., 2000; Lee *et al.*, 2001; Kumaramanickavel *et al.*, 2003; Santos *et al.*, 2003; Wang *et al.*, 2003). This inconsistency could be attributed to genetic heterogeneity, diagnostic uncertainties, differences in allele frequencies across ethnic populations and small sample size. Concerning this gene, the only genetic marker associated with risk of DR is an (AC)n dinucleotide repeat sequence, upstream of the transcription start site of this gene (Taverna, 2004). One of the alleles (Z-2)

was found to be associated with early onset of retinopathy in patients with non-insulin-dependent diabetes (Kumaramanickavel *et al.*, 2003), suggesting that AR or a gene in the close vicinity may be involved in the pathogenesis of this diabetic complication.

## 4.4.5. VEGF Gene

Angiogenesis is a major feature in diabetic retinopathy (Ferrara, 1999) and several protein factors crucial for regulation of angiogenesis have been identified. Among these factors, vascular endothelial growth factor (VEGF) is considered to be the most important regulator for vascular endothelial cell growth and differentiation, both in physiological and pathological conditions (Chakrabarti *et al.*, 2000; Koyama *et al.*, 2002; Iida *et al.*, 2002).

VEGF is a member of a large family of proteins and is produced by retinal pigment epithelial cells, ganglion cells, Muller cells and pericytes. VEGF exists in three main splice variants, characterized by 121 amino acids (VEGF 121), 165 amino acids (VEGF 165) and 189 amino acids (VEGF 189) and acts via two specific receptors: VEGF-R1 or Flt-1 and VEGF-R2 or KDR (Ferrara and Davissmyth, 1997). Hypoxia has been shown to be a major inducer of VEGF gene transcription and VEGF has been established as an important mediator of increased retinal vascular permeability, acting via a PKC dependent mechanism (Aiello *et al.*, 1997). Indeed, several studies indicate that VEGF may play a significant role in the pathogenesis of diabetic complications (Knott *et al.*, 1999; Ishida *et al.*, 2000; Awata *et al.*, 2002; Lu and Adamis, 2002; Caldwell *et al.*, 2003; Bortoloso *et al.*, 2004; Cooper *et al.*, 2004; Ray *et al.*, 2004; Roybal *et al.*, 2004; Sall *et al.*, 2004). Therefore, VEGF represents an exciting target for therapeutic intervention in DR.

Several polymorphisms of the VEGF gene have been identified. Awata *et al.* (2002), using a screening study, identified seven polymorphisms in both the promoter region, 5′-untranslated region (UTR) and 3′-UTR of the VEGF gene and examined the genetic variations of the VEGF gene to assess its possible relation to DR in type 2 diabetic patients. Among those seven common polymorphisms, the C(-634)G polymorphism in the 5′-UTR of the VEGF gene was associated with DR in Japanese type 2 diabetic patients. Ray *et al.* (2004) also investigated whether two polymorphisms in the promoter region of the VEGF gene were associated with the susceptibility to DR in UK Caucasians with diabetes. These authors found association between the T(-460)C polymorphism in the promoter region of the VEGF gene and proliferative DR. These results are promising, but additional studies with a larger sample size in different populations in the world are needed to clarify the role of the VEGF gene in DR.

### 4.4.6. RAGE Gene

The advanced glycation end products (AGEs) are generated during long term diabetes and have been considered to have an important role in the pathogenesis of DR (Chakrabarti *et al.*, 2000). AGEs result from the nonenzymatic glycation of proteins and lipids (Brownlee, 1995) and accumulate in the tissues as a function of time as a result of hyperglycemia. The mechanisms by which AGEs may cause pathologic changes include intracellular alteration of protein function, interference with extracellular matrix function and free radical formation through interactions with several AGE specific receptors (AGE-Rs), AGE-R1-3, RAGE, as well as the scavenger receptors ScR-II and CD-36 that are present on vascular, renal, hemopoietic and neuronal/glial cells that serve in the regulation of AGE removal (Stitt, 1999).

In susceptible individuals, the AGE-R expression/function may be subject to environmental or gene-related modulation, which in turn may influence tissue-specific gene functions. Furthermore, altered expression and activity of AGE-R components has recently been found in both mouse diabetic models and humans with diabetic complications (Lu *et al.*, 1998; Chakrabarti *et al.*, 2000; Treins *et al.*, 2001; Okamoto *et al.*, 2002; Yamagishi *et al.*, 2002).

Several converging lines of evidence suggest a role of the RAGE gene in DR. Various groups have investigated the role of the RAGE gene, located on chromosome 6p21.3A, in DR, but the results are controversial. Globocnik-Petrovic *et al.* (2003) found no association of the −429 T/C and the −374 T/A gene polymorphisms of the RAGE gene and DR, using a case-control association design in Caucasians with type 2 diabetes. Conversely, positive findings were reported for the Gly82Ser polymorphism in the RAGE gene in Asian Indian patients with type 2 diabetes (Kumaramanickavel *et al.*, 2002). Additionally, Hudson *et al.* (2001) have identified eight novel polymorphisms of the RAGE gene and found that the prevalence of the − 429C allele is increased in the retinopathy group.

### 4.4.7. Angiotensin-Converting Enzyme Gene

The genes of the renin-angiotensin system are an important group of candidate genes in the pathogenesis of DR. *In vitro*, angiotensin II stimulates the expression of VEGF, a permeability-inducing and endothelial cell specific angiogenic factor, which has been implicated in the pathogenesis of DR in humans and in experimental animals, as mentioned previously (Gilbert *et al.*, 2000; Kida *et al.*, 2003). Treatment of diabetic rats with angiotensin-converting enzyme (ACE) inhibitors reduces diabetes-associated changes in VEGF gene expression and vascular permeability. These findings implicate the renin-angiotensin system in the VEGF overexpression and hyperpermeability, which accompany DR and provide a potential mechanism for the beneficial effects of ACE inhibition in diabetic retinal disease (Chakrabarti *et al.*, 2000). Indeed, ACE inhibition has been recently suggested to have retinoprotective actions in diabetic patients (Taverna, 2004), although the mechanism of this effect is not known.

Since substantial experimental evidence implicates ACE gene in DR, this gene has been considered another candidate gene predisposing to the development of DR. Several groups investigated the relationship between the ACE gene and DR and have not shown conclusive results (Fujisawa *et al.*, 1995; Gutierrez *et al.*, 1997; Fujisawa *et al.*, 1998; Globocnik-Petrovic *et al.*, 2003), although one of its polymorphisms insertion/deletion seems to be associated with long-term diabetic complications (Naji *et al.*, 1995; Matsumoto *et al.*, 2000).

### 4.4.8. PAI-1 Gene

A number of other candidate genes less explored, involved in cellular communication and extracellular matrix, have also been implicated in DR. Among these, in particular the plasminogen activator-inhibitor 1 (PAI-1) gene has long been hypothesized in the pathophysiology of DR, because PAI-1 is a key regulator of fibrinolytic pathway and extracellular matrix turnover (Taverna, 2004). Since changes in gene expression could play a central role in the phenotypic abnormalities of the retinal vascular cells observed in DR Cagliero *et al.* (1991) measured the gene expression of PAI-1 in human retinal microvessels by using hybridization studies. They found that the PAI-1 mRNA levels in retinal microvessels isolated from type 2 diabetic patients were significantly higher than those in vessels isolated from age-matched controls. Also, a study was done to identify the relationship between PAI-1 gene and DR in 327 Caucasian diabetic type 2 subjects and 123 Caucasian control subjects (Mansfield *et al.*, 1994). The results obtained indicate that there is no evidence of association between PAI-1 gene

and DR in patients with diabetes mellitus. Globocnik-Petrovic *et al.* (2003) investigated the relationship between the insertion/deletion PAI-1 gene polymorphism and the development of DR in a group of Caucasian subjects with type 2 diabetes, using an association study, and found no association between this polymorphism and DR either in non proliferative, proliferative or severe proliferative DR. Additionally, other studies yielded variable results (Nagi *et al.*, 1997; Tarnow *et al.*, 2000; Santos *et al.*, 2003, Murata *et al.*, 2004).

### 4.4.9. Endothelin Genes

More recently, it has been suggested that endothelin (ET), which belongs to a family of vasoactive peptides, has an important role in several disorders of the microvasculature, as, for example, DR (Lam *et al.*, 2003; Chakrabarti *et al.*, 2004). The ET family comprises three unique isoforms known as ET-1, ET-2 and ET-3. In the human genome there are three endothelin genes, EDN1, EDN-2 and EDN-3, which are located in different chromosomes. ET-1 and ET-2 are both strong vasoconstrictors, whereas ET-3 is a weaker vasoconstrictor compared to the other two isoforms. ET-1 also acts as a mitogen on the vascular smooth muscle (Chakrabarti *et al.*, 2000).

Evidence for the involvement of the endothelin genes in DR can be found in animal studies. Chakrabarti *et al.* (1998) demonstrated that diabetic rat retinas show an increase in ET-1, ET-3 and in ET(A) and ET(B) receptor mRNA expression, when compared to control rats. An increased ocular and retina tissue levels of ET-1 in diabetic rats has also been reported.

To date only two studies have been performed with endothelin genes, namely EDN-1 gene and DR, and negative results were obtained. Warpeha *et al.* (1999) reported no significant differences in allele frequencies for the 4127G/A polymorphism between the patients who had retinopathy and the patients without retinopathy. The relationship between EDN-1 gene and proliferative DR in diabetes type 2 was also investigated in a set of 246 Caucasian subjects (Kankova *et al.*, 2001). This group have not demonstrated association at this locus. Although negative results were obtained, more independent studies are needed with this polymorphism and others in the same gene to clarify its role in DR.

### 4.4.10. Nitric Oxide Synthase Genes

A large body of evidence have also implicated the nitric oxide synthase/nitric oxide (NOS/NO) system in the pathogenesis of DR (Warpeha *et al.*, 1999; Morris *et al.*, 2002; Santilli *et al.*, 2004). It was shown that the expression of NOS is altered in the retinal vasculature in the early stages of diabetic retinopathy (Chakravarthy *et al.*, 1998; Moris *et al.*, 2002). Therefore, intervention targeting any of the pathways involved in the NOS/NO system cascade may also prove potential therapeutic targets in the prevention of DR.

NO is produced by endothelial cells, as well as by other cells in the body. In humans, there are three isoforms of NOS, the enzyme that oxidizes arginine to citrulline and produces NO (Nathan and Xie, 1994), each of which is encoded by a distinct gene. The NOS isoforms include endothelial NOS, which is encoded by NOS3 gene, inducible NOS encoded by NOS2A gene and neuronal NOS encoded by NOS1 gene. Since NO regulates endothelial function, genes encoding nitric oxide synthases could confer susceptibility and are good candidates genes to DR. Warpeha *et al.* (1999) investigated the allele distribution of (CCTTT)n repeat within the 5′ upstream promoter region of the NOS2A gene in diabetic patients from Northern Ireland and found that the 14-repeat allele of the NOS2A marker was significantly associated with the absence of DR. This finding suggests that the 14-repeat allele may confer selective advantages in

diabetic individuals, which may delay or prevent microvascular complications of diabetes. The relationship between NOS3 gene and DR was also investigated in a sample of individuals with 15 years of type 2 diabetes and severe retinopathy and no association was obtained (Warpeha *et al.*, 1999). This data suggest that the genetic variant of NOS3 gene does not appear to have a major role in the pathogenesis of DR.

### 4.4.11. Other Candidate Genes

Other studies have also investigated the role of various genes, including TNF-beta (Kankova *et al.*, 2001), TNF-alpha (Hawrami *et al.*, 1996; Beránek *et al.*, 2002), B-3 adrenergic receptor (Sakane *et al.*, 1997), Paraoxonase 1 (Kao *et al.*, 1998; Mackness *et al.*, 2000; Murata *et al.*, 2004), $\alpha 2\beta 1$integrin (Matsubara *et al.*, 2000), collagen IV$\alpha$1 (Alcolado *et al.*, 1993), GLUT1 (Gutierrez *et al.*, 1998), Neuropeptide Y (Niskanen *et al.*, 2000), calpain-10 (Cassell *et al.*, 2002; Fingerlin *et al.*, 2002) and sorbitol dehydrogenase (Amano *et al.*, 2003) in the pathogenesis of DR, but most of the data appear to be inconclusive and require further confirmation.

### 4.4.12. Concluding Remarks

Several lines of evidence suggest that the pathogenesis of DR is a complex phenomenon. Multiple clinical and pathophysiological studies, as well as genetic analysis, suggest that DR is a consequence of interactions between environmental factors, especially hyperglycemia, and several genetic factors.

It is now widely accepted that genetic factors contribute to the onset and progression of chronic diabetic complications, but the gene or genes conferring susceptibility to DR remain to be identified. A large body of evidence have implicated different genes, such as AR, VEGF, RAGE, PAI-1, END, NOS2A, NOS3, PAI-1, ACE, TNF-beta, TNF-alpha, B-3AR, PON1, $\alpha 2\beta 1$, IV$\alpha$, GLUT1, Neuropeptide Y, calpain-10 and SDH in the pathogenesis of DR. Association approaches have unequivocally identified susceptibility genes for DR, but conflicting results have arisen due to complex inheritance, which leads to reduced power of the samples studied to detect small effect genes. Using homogenous populations (Varilo and Peltonen, 2004) and mixed approaches, namely linkage, association and linkage disequilibrium (Hoh and Ott, 2004) is the best way to detect susceptibility genes in DR.

As mentioned previously, SNP is considered the best genetic marker to investigate susceptibility genes in DR, because a SNP is a change of a single base pair within a gene sequence that can sometimes influence the function of the gene product (Kwok and Xiao, 2004). The new era of human genetic analyses has began with the end of the human genome project, and the discovery of the complete sequence of human DNA showed surprisingly small differences between the genetic materials of randomly chosen people. Furthermore, to increase the power of sample is important to investigate more SNPs in the same gene. Extended linkage disequilibrium can be detected readily, even across several haplotypes, thus potentially reducing the number of SNPs for future whole-genome scans (Kwok and Xiao, 2004). In fact, a molecular approach to haplotyping is, therefore, highly desirable. Accumulated evidence also indicates that responses to drugs are, at least to some extent, under genetic control. Thus, pharmacogenetics, the study of variability in drug responses attributed to hereditary factors in different populations, may significantly assist in providing answers towards meeting this challenge (Schmith *et al.*, 2003). Furthermore, pharmacogenetics mostly relies on associations between a specific genetic marker like SNPs and a particular response to drugs. However, previously, this type of studies has been mostly limited to *a priori* selected candidate gene due to restricted genotyping and analytical capacities. Nowadays, considering the large number of SNPs available and the newly developed technologies, such as automated genotyping and bioinformatics (Clifford *et al.*, 2004), it is possible to investigate more than 200,000 SNPs distributed over the entire human genome. Indeed, bioinformatics can play an important role in SNP discovery and analysis. It is possible to use computational methods to identify SNPs and to predict whether they are likely to be neutral or deleterious.

The use of novel techniques, such as DNA microarrays (DNA chip) (Sklar *et al.*, 1999) and the high density SNP (Wang *et al.*, 1998; Kwok and Xiao, 2004) in combination with sophisticated statistical analyses (Hoh and Ott, 2000; 2004), will allow to identify susceptibility genes in DR. Considering the complexity of DR the optimal study design must include linkage and association methods, meta-analyses and analytical models. Finally, since DR is a complex disorder and environmental and genetic factors are deeply involved, it is important to investigate the interaction between genes among them and between these and environmental factors.

# References

Aiello LP, Bursell SE, Clermont A, *et al.* (1997) Vascular endothelial growth factor-induced retinal permeability is mediated by kinase C *in vivo* and suppressed by an orally effective beta-isoform-selective inhibitor. *Diabetes* **46**: 1473–1480.

Alcolado JC, Baroni MG, Li SR, *et al.* (1993) Genetic variation around the collagen-IV 1A gene locus and proliferative retinopathy in type 2 diabetes-mellitus. *Hum Hered* **43**: 126–130.

Amano S, Yamagishi S, Koda Y, *et al.* (2003) Polymorphisms of sorbitol dehydrogenase (SDH) gene and susceptibility to diabetic retinopathy. *Med Hypotheses* **60**(4): 550–551.

Awata T, Inoue K, Kurihara S, *et al.* (2002) A common polymorphism in the 5′-untranslated region of the VEGF gene is associated with diabetic retinopathy in type 2 diabetes. *Diabetes* **51**(5): 1635–1639.

Beránek M, Kanková K, Benes P, *et al.* (2002) Polymorphism R25P in the encoding transforming growth factor-beta (TGF-$\beta$1) in a newl identified risk factor for proliferative diabetic retinopathy. *Am J Med Genet* **106**: 278–283.

Bortoloso E, Del Prete D, Dalla Vestra M, *et al.* (2004) Quantitative and qualitative changes in vascular endothelial growth factor gene expression in glomeruli of patients with type 2 diabetes. *Eur J Endocrinol* **150**(6): 799–807.

Brownlee M. (1995) Advanced protein glycosylation in diabetes and aging. *Annu Rev Med* **46**: 223–234.

Cagliero E, Grant MB, Lorenzi M. (1991) Measurement of gene expression in human retinal microvessels by solution hybridisation. *Invest Ophthalmol Vis Sci* **32**(5):1439–1445.

Caldwell RB, Bartoli M, Behzadian MA, *et al.* (2003) Vascular endothelial growth factor and diabetic retinopathy: Pathophysiological mechanisms and treatment perspectives. *Diabetes Metab Res Rev* **19**(6): 442–455.

Cassell PG, Jackson AE, North BV, *et al.* (2002) Haplotype combinations of calpain-10 gene polymorphisms associated with increased risk of impaired glucose tolerance and type 2 diabetes in South Indians. *Diabetes* **51**: 1622–1628.

Chakrabarti S, Cukiernik M, Hileeto D, *et al.* (2000) Role of vasoactive factors in the pathogenesis of early changes in diabetic retinopathy. *Diabetes Metab Res Ver* **16**: 393–407.

Chakrabarti S, Gan XT, Merry A, *et al.* (1998) Augmented retinal endothelin-1, endothelin-3, endothelinA and endothelinB gene expression in chronic diabetes. *Curr Eye Res* **17**(3): 301–307.

Chakrabarti S, Khan ZA, Cukiernik M, *et al.* (2004) C-peptide and retinal microangiopathy in diabetes. *Exp Diabesity Res* **5**(1): 91–96.

Chakravarthy U, Hayes RG, Stitt AW, *et al.* (1998) Constitutive nitric oxide synthase expression in retinal vascular endothelial cells is suppressed by high glucose and advanced glycation end products. *Diabetes* **47**: 945–952.

Chistjakov DA, Turakulov RI, Gorashko NM, *et al.* (1997) Polymorphism of a dinucleotide repeat within the aldose reductase gene in normalcy and insulin-dependent diabetes with vascular complications. *Mol Biol* **31**: 660–664.

Chung SS, Chung SK. (2003) Genetic analysis of aldose reductase in diabetic complications. *Curr Med Chem* **10**(15): 1375–1387.

Clifford RJ, Edmonson MN, Nguyen C, *et al.* (2004) Bioinformatics tools for single nucleotide polymorphism discovery and analysis. *Ann N Y Acad Sci* **1020**: 101–109.

Collins FS, Guyer MS, Chakravarti A. (1997) Variations on the theme: Cataloging human DNA aequence variation. *Science* **278**: 1580–1581.

Cooper ME, Vranes D, Youssef S, *et al.* (1999) Increased renal expression of vascular endothelial growth factor (VEGF) and its receptor VEGFR-2 in experimental diabetes. *Diabetes* **48**: 2229–2239.

Demaine A, Cross D, Millward A. (2000) Polymorphisms of the aldose reductase gene and susceptibility to retinopathy in type I diabetes mellitus. *Invest Ophthalmol Vis Sci* **41**: 4064–4068.

Ferrara N, Davissmyth T. (1997) The biology of vascular endothelial growth factor. *Endocrine Rev* **18**: 4–25.

Ferrara N. (1999) Role of vascular endothelial growth factor in the regulation of angiogenesis. *Kidney Int* **56**(3): 794–814.

Fingerlin TE, Erdos MR, Watanabe RM, *et al.* (2002) Variation in three single nucleotide polymorphisms in the calpain-10 gene not associated with type 2 diabetes in a large Finnish cohort. *Diabetes* **51**: 1644–1648.

Fujisawa T, Ikegami H, Kawaguchi Y, *et al.* (1998) Meta-analysis of association of insertion/deletion polymorphism of angiotensin I converting enzyme gene with diabetic nephropathy and retinopathy. *Diabetologia* **41**: 47–53.

Fujisawa T, Ikegami H, Kawaguchi Y, *et al.* (1999) Length rather than a specific allele of dinucleotide repeat in the 5′ upstream region of the aldose reductase gene is associated with diabetic retinopathy. *Diabet Med* **16**(12): 1044–1047.

Fujisawa T, Ikegami H, Shen GQ, *et al.* (1995) Angiotensin I converting enzyme gene polymorphism is associated with myocardial infraction, but not with retinopathy or nephropathy, in NIDDM. *Diabetes Care* **18**: 983–985.

Gilbert RE, Kelly DJ, Cox AJ, *et al.* (2000) Angiotensin converting enzyme inhibition reduces retinal over-expression of vascular endothelial growth factor and hyperpermeability in experimental diabetes. *Diabetologia* **43**(11): 1360–1367.

Globocnik-Petrovic M, Steblovnik K, Peterlin B, *et al.* (2003) The −429 T/C and −374 T/A gene polymorphisms of the receptor of advanced glycation end products gene are not risk factors for diabetic retinopathy in Caucasians with type 2 diabetes. *Klin Monatsbl Augenheilkd* **220**(12): 873–876.

Globocnik-Petrovic M, Hawlina M, Peterlin B, *et al.* (2003) Insertion/deletion plasminogen activator inhibitor 1 and insertion/deletion angiotensin-converting enzyme gene polymorphisms in diabetic retinopathy in type 2 diabetes. *Ophthalmologica* **217**(3): 219–224.

Gutierrez C, Vendrell J, Pastor R, *et al.* (1998) GLUT1 gene polymorphism in non-insulin-dependent diabetes mellitus: Genetic susceptibility relationship with cardiovascular risk factors and microangiopathic complications in a Mediterranean population. *Diabetes Res Clin Pract* **41**: 113–120.

Gutierrez C, Vendrell J, Pastor R, *et al.* (1997) Angiotensin I converting enzyme an angiotensinogen gene polymorphisms in non-insulin-dependent diabetes mellitus. Lack of relationship with diabetic nephropathy and retinopathy in a Caucasian Mediterranean population. *Metab Clin Exp* **46**: 976–980.

Hanyu O, Hanawa H, Nakagawa O, *et al.* (1998) Polymorphism of the angiotensin converting enzyme gene in diabetic nephropathy in Type II diabetic patients with proliferative retinopathy. *Renal Failure* **20**: 125–133.

Hawrami K, Hitman GA, Rema N, *et al.* (1996) An association study in non-insulin dependent diabetes mellitus subjects between susceptibility to retinopathy and tumor necrosis factor polymorphism. *Hum Immunol* **46**: 49–54.

Heesom AE, Hibberd ML, Millward A, *et al.* (1997) Polymorphism in the 5′-end of the aldose reductase gene is strongly associated with the development of diabetic nephropathy in type I diabetes. *Diabetes* **46**: 287–291.

Hoh J, Ott J. (2004) Genetic dissection of diseases: Design and methods. *Cur Opin Genet Develp* **14**: 229–232.

Hoh J, Ott J. (2000) Scan statistics to scan markers for susceptibility genes *PNAS* **97**: 9615–9617.

Horikawa Y, Oda N, Cox NJ, *et al.* (2000) Genetic variation in the gene encoding calpain-10 is associated with type 2 diabetes mellitus. *Nat Genet* **26**: 163–175.

Hudson BI, Stickland MH, Futers TS, *et al.* (2001) Effects of novel polymorphisms in the RAGE gene on transcriptional regulation and their association with diabetic retinopathy. *Diabetes* **50**(6): 1505–1511.

Ichikawa F, Yamada K, Ishiyama-Shigemoto S, *et al.* (1999) Association of an (A-C)n dinucleotide repeat polymorphic marker at the 5′-region of the aldose reductase gene with retinopathy but not with nephropathy or neuropathy in Japanese patients with Type 2 diabetes mellitus. *Diabet Med* **16**(9): 744–748.

Iida K, Kawakami Y, Sone H, *et al.* (2002) Vascular endothelial growth factor gene expression in a retinal pigmented cell is up-regulated by glucose deprivation through 3′ UTR. *Life Sci* **71**(14): 1607–1614.

Ikegishi Y, Tawata M, Aida K, *et al.* (1999) Z-4 allele upstream of the aldose reductase gene is associated with proliferative retinopathy in Japanese patients with NIDDM, and elevated luciferase gene transcription in vitro. *Life Sci* **65**: 2061–2070.

Imperatore G, Hanson RL, Pettitt DJ, *et al.* (1998) Sib pair linkage analysis for susceptibility genes for microvascular complications among Pima Indians with type 2 diabetes. *Diabetes* **47**: 821–830.

Ishida S, Shinoda K, Kawashima S. (2000) Coexpression of VEGF receptors VEGF-R2 and neuropilin-1 in proliferative diabetic retinopathy. *Invest Ophthalmol Vis Sci* **41**(7): 1649–1656.

Kankova K, Muzik J, Karaskova J, *et al.* (2001) Duration of non-insulin-dependent diabetes mellitus and the TNF-beta NcoI genotype as predictive factors in proliferative diabetic retinopathy. *Ophthalmologica* **215**(4): 294–298.

Kao YL, Donaghue K, Chan A, *et al.* (2000) Low paraoxonase activity in type II diabetes mellitus complicated by retinopathy. *Clin. Sci* **98**: 335–363.

Kao YL, Donaghue K, Chan A, *et al.* (1999) An aldose reductase intragenic polymorphism associated with diabetic retinopathy. *Diabetes Res Clin Pract* **46**(2): 155–160.

Kendal WS. (2003) An exponential dispersion model for the distribution of human single nucleotide polymorphisms. *Mol Biol Evol* **20**(4): 579–590.

Kida T, Ikeda T, Nishimura M, *et al.* (2003) Renin-angiotensin system in proliferative diabetic retinopathy and its gene expression in cultured human muller cells. *Jpn J Ophthalmol* **47**(1): 36–41.

Knott RM, Pascal MM, Ferguson C, *et al.* (1999) Regulation of transforming growth factor-beta, basic fibroblast growth factor, and vascular endothelial cell growth factor mRNA in peripheral blood leukocytes in patients with diabetic retinopathy. *Metabolism* **48**(9): 1172–1178.

Ko BC, Lam KS, Wat NM, *et al.* (1995) An (A-C)n dinucleotide repeat polymorphic marker at the 5′ end of the aldose reductase gene is associated with early-onset diabetic retinopathy in NIDDM patients. *Diabetes* **44**(7): 727–732.

Koyama S, Takagi H, Otani A, *et al.* (2002) Inhibitory mechanism of vascular endothelial growth factor (VEGF) by bucillamine. *Br J Pharmacol* **137**(6): 901–909.

Kruglyak L, Daly MJ, Reeve-daly MR, *et al.* (1996) Parametric and non-parametric analysis: A unified multipoint approach. *Am J Hum Genet* **59**: 1347–1363.

Kumaramanickavel G, Ramprasad VL, Sripriya S, *et al.* (2002) Association of Gly82Ser polymorphism in the RAGE gene with diabetic retinopathy in type II diabetic Asian Indian patients. *J. Diabetes Complications* **16**(6): 391–394.

Kumaramanickavel G, Sripriya S, Ramprasad VL, *et al.* (2003) Z-2 aldose reductase allele and diabetic retinopathy in India. *Ophthalmic Genet* **24**(1): 41–48.

Kwok PY, Chen X. (2003) Detection of single nucleotide polymorphisms. *Curr Issues Mol Biol* **5**(2): 43–60.

Kwok PY, Xiao M. (2004) Single-molecule analysis for molecular haplotyping. *Hum Mutat* **23**(5): 442–446.

Lam HC, Lee JK, Lu CC, *et al.* (2003) Role of endothelin in diabetic retinopathy. *Curr Vasc Pharmacol* **1**(3): 243–250.

Lander ES, Schork NJ. (1994) Genetic dissection of complex traits. *Science* **265**: 2037–2048.

Lee SC, Wang Y, Ko GT, *et al.* (2001) Association of retinopathy with a microsatellite at 5′ end of the aldose reductase gene in Chinese patients with late-onset Type 2 diabetes. *Ophthalmic Genet* **22**(2): 63–67.

Leslie RDG, Pyke DA. (1982) Diabetic retinopathy in identical twins. *Diabetes* **31**: 19–21.

Lu M, Adamis AP. (2002) Vascular endothelial growth factor gene regulation and action in diabetic retinopathy. *Ophthalmol Clin North Am* **15**(1): 69–79.

Lu M, Kuroki M, Amano S, *et al.* (1998) Advanced glycation end products increase retinal vascular endothelial growth factor expression. *J Clin Invest* **101**(6): 1219–1224.

Mackness B, Durrington PN, Abuashia B, *et al.* (2000) Low paraoxonase activity in type 2 diabetes mellitus complicated by retinopathy. *Clin. Sci. (Lond.)* **98**(3): 355–363.

Maeda S. (2004) Genome-wide search for susceptibility gene to diabetic nephropathy by gene-based SNP. *Diabetes Res Clin Pract* **1**: S45–S47.

Mansfield MW, Stickland MH, Carter AM, *et al.* (1994) Polymorphisms of the plasminogen activator inhibitor-1 gene in type 1 and type 2 diabetes, and in patients with diabetic retinopathy. *Thromb. Haemost* **71**(6): 731–736.

Matsubara Y, Murata M, Maruyama T, *et al.* (2000) Association between diabetic retinopathy and genetic variations in $\alpha 2\beta 1$ integrin, a platelet receptor for collagen. *Blood* **95**: 1560–1564.

Matsumoto A, Iwashima Y, Abiko A, *et al.* (2000) Detection of the association between a deletion polymorphism in the gene encoding angiotensin I-converting enzyme and advanced diabetic retinopathy. *Diabetes Res Clin Pract* **50**(3): 195–202.

Morris BJ, Markus A, Glenn CL, *et al.* (2002) Association of a functional inducible nitric oxide synthase promoter variant with complications in type 2 diabetes. *J Mol Med* **80**(2): 96–104.

Murata M, Maruyama T, Suzuki Y, *et al.* (2004) Paraoxonase 1 Gln/Arg polymorphism is associated with the risk of microangiopathy in type 2 diabetes mellitus. *Diabet Med* **21**(8): 837–844.

Nagi DK, Mansfield MW, Stickland MH, *et al.* (1995) Angiotensin converting enzyme (ACE) insertion/deletion (I/D) and dibetic retinopathy in subjects with IDDM and NIDDM. *Diabetes Med* **12**: 997–1001.

Nagi DK, McCormack LJ, Mohamed-Ali V, *et al.* (1997) Diabetic retinopathy, promoter (4G/5G) polymorphism of PAI-1 gene, and PAI-1 activity in Pima Indians with type 2 diabetes. *Diabetes Care* **20**(8):1304–1309.

Nathan C, Xie Z. (1994) Nitric oxide synthases: Roles, toll, and controls. *Cell* **78**: 915.

Nielsen R. (2004) Population genetic analysis of ascertained SNP data. *Hum Genomics* **1**(3): 218–224.

Niskanen L, Voutilainen-Kaunisto R, Terasvirta M, *et al.* (2000) Leucine 7 to proline 7 polymorphism in the neuropeptide y gene is associated with retinopathy in type 2 diabetes. Exp Clin Endocrinol. *Diabetes* **108**: 235–236.

Okamoto T, Yamagishi S, Inagaki Y, *et al.* (2002) Angiogenesis induced by advanced glycation end products and its prevention by cerivastatin. *FASEB J* **16**(14): 1928–1930.

Olmos P, Futers S, Acosta AM, *et al.* (2000) (AC)23 [Z-2] polymorphism of the aldose reductase gene and fast progression of retinopathy in Chilean type 2 diabetics. *Diabetes Res Clin Pract* **47**(3): 169–176.

Ott J. (1990) Genetic linkage and complex disease: A comment. *Genet Epidemiol* **7**: 35–36.

Ray D, Mishra M, Ralph S, *et al.* (2004) Association of the VEGF gene with proliferative diabetic retinopathy but not proteinuria in diabetes. *Diabetes* **53**(3): 861–864.

Risch N, Merikangas K. (1996) The future of the genetic studies of complex human disease. *Science* **273**: 1516–1517.

Rogus JJ, Warram JH, Krolewski AS. (2002) Perspectives in diabetes. Genetic studies of late diabetic complications. The overlooked importance of diabetes duration before complications onset. *Diabetes* **51**: 1655–1662.

Roybal CN, Yang S, Sun C-W, *et al.* (2004) Homocysteine increases the expression of vascular Endothelial Growth Factor by a mechanism involving endoplasmic reticulum stress and transcription factor ATF4. *J Biological Chemistry* **279**: 14844–14852.

Sakane N, Yoshida K, Kondo M, *et al.* (1997) Beta(3)-adrenoreceptor gene polymorphism: A newly defined risk factor for proliferative retinopathy in NIDDM patients. *Diabetes* **46**: 1633–1636.

Salisbury BA, Pungliya M, Choi JY, *et al.* (2003) SNP and haplotype variation in the human genome. *Mutat Res* **526**(1–2): 53–61.

Sall JW, Klisovic DD, O'Dorisio MS, *et al.* (2004) Somatostatin inhibits IGF-1 mediated induction of VEGF in human retinal pigment epithelial cells. *Exp Eye Res* (2004) **79**(4): 465–476.

Santilli F, Cipollone F, Mezzetti A, *et al.* (2004) The role of nitric oxide in the development of diabetic angiopathy. *Horm Metab Res* **36**(5): 319–335.

Santos KG, Tschiedel B, Schneider J, *et al.* (2003) Diabetic retinopathy in Euro-Brazilian type 2 diabetic patients: Relationship with polymorphisms in the aldose reductase, the plasminogen activator inhibitor-1 and the methylenetetrahydrofolate reductase genes. *Diabetes Res Clin Pract* **61**(2): 133–136.

Schmith VD, Campbell DA, Sehgal S, *et al.* (2003) Pharmacogenetics and disease genetics of complex diseases. *Cell Mol Life Sci* **60**(8): 1636–1646.

Sklar P, Altshuler D, Cargill M, *et al.* (1999) DNA microarrays for polymorphism detection and genotyping: Utility in the understanding of complex neuropsychiatric diseases. *CNS Spectrums* **4**: 59–74.

Spielman RS, McGinnis RE, Ewens WJ. (1993) Transmission test for linkage desequilibrium: The insulin gene region and insulin-dependent diabetes mellitus (IDDM). *Am J Hum Genet* **52**: 506–516.

Stitt AW, HE C, Vlassara H. (1999) Characterisation of the advanced glycation end-product receptor complex in human vascular endothelial cells. *Biochem Biophys Res Commun* **256**: 549–556.

Tarnow L, Stehouwer CD, Emeis JJ, *et al.* (2000) Plasminogen activator inhibitor-1 and apolipoprotein E gene polymorphisms and diabetic angiopathy. *Nephrol Dial Transplant* **15**: 625–630.

Taverna MJ. (2004) Genetics of diabetic complications: Retinopathy. *Ann Endocrinol* (*Paris*). Feb; **65**(Suppl. 1): S17–S25.

Terwilliger JD, Ott J. (1992) A haplotype-based "Haplotype Relative Risk" approach to detecting allelic associations. *Hum Hered* **42**: 337–346.

Treins C, Giorgetti-Peraldi S, Murdaca J, *et al.* (2001) Regulation of vascular endothelial growth factor expression by advanced glycation end products. *J Biol Chem* **276**(47): 43836–43841.

Varilo T, Peltonen L. (2004) Isolates and their potential use in complex gene mapping efforts. *Curr Opin Genet Dev* **14**(3): 316–323.

Vlassara H. (2001) The AGE-receptor in the pathogenesis of diabetic complications. *Diabetes Metab Res Rev* **17**(6): 436–443.

Wang DG, Fan JB, Siao CJ, *et al.* (1998) Large scale identification, mapping and genotyping of single nucleotide polymorphisms in the human genome. *Science* **280**: 1077–1082.

Wang Y, Ng MC, Lee SC, *et al.* (2003) Phenotypic heterogeneity and associations of two aldose reductase gene polymorphisms with nephropathy and retinopathy in type 2 diabetes. *Diabetes Care* **26**(8): 2410–2415.

Warpeha KM, Ah-Fat F, Harding S, *et al.* (1999) Dinucleotide repeat polymorphisms in EDN1 and NOS3 are not associated with severe diabetic retinopathy in type 1 or type 2 diabetes. *Eye* **13**: 174–178.

Warpeha KM, Crakravarthy U. (2003) Molecular genetics of microvascular disease in diabetic retinopathy. *Eye* **17**: 305–311.

Warpeha KM, Xu W, Liu L, *et al.* (1999) Genotyping and functional analysis of a polymorphic (CCTTT)(n) repeat of NOS2A in diabetic retinopathy. *FASEB J* **13**(13): 1825–1832.

Weeks DE, Lange K. (1988) The affected-pedigree-member method of linkage analysis. *Am J Hum Genet* **42**: 315–326.

Yamagishi S, Amano S, Inagaki Y, *et al.* (2002) Advanced glycation end products-induced apoptosis and overexpression of vascular endothelial growth factor in bovine retinal pericytes. *Biochem Biophys Res Commun* **290**(3): 973–978.

Yamaoka T, Nishimura C, Yamashita K, *et al.* (1995) Acute onset of diabetic pathological changes in transgenic mice with human aldose reductase cDNA. *Diabetologia* **38**(3): 255–261.

Yang B, Cross DF, Ollerenshaw M, *et al.* (2003) Polymorphisms of the vascular endothelial growth factor and susceptibility to diabetic microvascular complications in patients with type 1 diabetes mellitus. *J Diabetes Complications* **17**(1): 1–6.

# Chapter 5

# Epidemiology

## José Rui Faria Abreu

Diabetes, particularly diabetic retinopathy, is the leading cause of new cases of blindness in persons aged 20 to 74 years in the U.S. (Kahn and Hiller, 1974). It is estimated that in the U.S. more than 12% of new cases of blindness are attributable to diabetes.

## 5.1. Prevalence of Visual Impairment

Prevalence is the proportion of cases or events (visual impairment) in the total population at risk (diabetic patients) in a fixed time. The definition of blindness, however, varies between countries. For example, in the U.S. legal blindness is a visual acuity less or equal than 6/60, whereas in Iceland and Sweden is less than 6/60 and in Germany 1/50 or less. A patient with 6/60 is blind in U.S. but not blind in Sweden or Germany and a patient with 2/50 is blind in Iceland but not in Germany. The World Health Organization (WHO) has found 65 different definitions of blindness used by clinicians, scientists and governments and recommended a standardized definition of blindness and visual impairment that was incorporated into the International Classification of Disease (ICD). In this classification:

1. Low vision — is defined as a visual acuity less than 6/18 (3/10 or 20/60) but equal to or better than 3/60 (0.5/10 or 20/400).
2. Blindness — is defined as a visual acuity of less than 3/60 (0.5/10 or 20/400) in the better eye with best possible correction and a field loss in each eye of less than 10° from fixation.

Blindness and visual impairment restrict daily activities. The Impact Visual Impairment (IVI) evaluation describes and quantifies these restrictions (0 = not at all; 1 = rarely; 2 = little; 3 = fair amount; 4 = a lot and 5 = can't do because of eye). For blind diabetics the highest restriction was found to be for leisure and work (3.0), mobility/obstructed locomotion (2.8) and social interaction domains (2.8) compared with emotional reaction to vision loss (2.3), household and personal care domains (2.1), for $p < 0.005$ (Lamoureux et al., 2004).

The WHO database shows a large variety of prevalence of blindness among adults in Europe: 2/1000 (France–1985), 25/1000 (Malta–1989), 7/1000 (UK–1991). The reported values are, 5/1000 (Cedrone et al., 2003) and 2/1000 in Denmark (Buch et al., 2004). In U.S. the general prevalence is 3/1000, being 6.5 times more prevalent in those of 65 or more years (Rodriguez et al., 2002).

Vision loss due to diabetic retinopathy results from macular edema, macular nonperfusion, vitreous hemorrhage, fibrous tissue distorting the retina leading to retinal detachment and neovascular glaucoma. Diabetic retinopathy is overall the third cause of visual impairment.

In 1988 the U.S. Nation Society to Prevent Blindness estimated that 7.9% of persons, who were legally blind, reported diabetes as the cause of their blindness. In population over 65 years, 15.8% of blindness and 19.6% of visual impairment was ascribable to diabetic retinopathy (Prasad et al., 2001).

Age-related diseases are the major causes of blindness and low vision. Cataract is the leading cause of blindness in the world (Thylefors *et al.*, 1995). In industrialized countries, cataract blindness is usually prevented by surgery. In U.S. cataract care consumes approximately 60% of the Medicare Budget for vision (Ellwein *et al.*, 2002). Diabetes is associated with increased risk of cataract (Congdon, 2001). Age-related macular degeneration (ARMD) causes irreversible loss of central vision and is the leading cause of blindness among European-derived individuals older than 65 years — more than 15% in people in the ninth decade of life (The Eye Disease Prevalence Study Group, 2004). In Sweden only few elderly diabetic patients were blind from other causes (cataract and glaucoma) in contrast to France (Delcourt *et al.*, 1995) and U.S. (Klein *et al.*, 1984).

## Age

The global estimated prevalence of blindness is 44 times more in patients of 60 or more years of age than in those of 44 or less years (Thylefors *et al.*, 1994). Visual impairment is lower between 20–64 years, but between 65–84 years is nine times more prevalent ($p < 0.001$) and 64 times for those between 80–84 years age (Buch *et al.*, 2004). The prevalence of blindness in type 1 diabetes is 0% in patients of 24 years or less, but is superior to 10% in patients of 55 or more years.

Some studies determine blindness due to diabetes only in people of 15 or more years (Jerneld, 1988), but others consider all ages (Klein *et al.*, 1984). These can explain some different prevalence in literature.

## Socioeconomic Situation and Ethnics

In sub-Saharian Africa, prevalence of blindness (14/1000) is five times the European prevalence (3/1000). In Baltimore, in an urban population, *blacks* had on average a twofold excess prevalence of blindness and visual impairment than *whites* (Tielsch *et al.*, 1990). In Gambia, 92% of blindness was due to cataract and trachoma, and diabetes is not referred as a cause of visual impairment (Faahl *et al.*, 1989).

## Sex

In the U.S. *non-white* diabetic women (Hispanics included) were three times more likely to become blind than non-white men.

## Data from Epidemiological Studies

In Leicester, the rate of blindness in the general population of 65 or more years of age due to diabetic retinopathy was 0.2/1000 in 1975 and 0.04/1000 in 1985 (a 80% drop). This may be due to the increasing use of laser treatment and the introduction of specialized retinal services. On the other hand, this is responsible for the increasing rate of partial sight registration, more 30% (Thompson *et al.*, 1989).

In type 1 diabetics, the 20-years cumulative prevalence of blindness, has fallen from 3.5% in patients with onset in 1965–1969 to 0% in those with onset in 1979–1984 ($p < 0.001$) due to improved glycemic control, early aggressive antihypertensive treatment and laser treatment (Hovind *et al.*, 2003).

It is impossible to compare data from different *centers* for many reasons:

(a) Each center has its own definition. For example, *categorizing* diabetes according to the age of onset. Subjects diagnosed before 30 years (Klein *et al.*, 1984; Kristinsson *et al.*, 1994); at 30 or less years (Nielsen, 1984); less than 36 years (Porta *et al.*, EURODIAB); 40 or less years (Jerneld *et al.*, 1983); less than 40 years (Aroca *et al.*, 1994; Fernandez–Vigo *et al.*, 1992).

(b) Roy *et al.* (2000) considers a type "1–1/2" for those patients with an acute onset of diabetes before 30 years but not currently taking insulin.

(c) There are studies to characterize prevalence of retinopathy that include the entire follow-up periods (Klein *et al.*, 1984); other studies, in patients with type 1, included only those with 10 or more years of follow-up (Cahill *et al.*, 2000).

(d) There are *centers* that consider all ages, but other exclude patients with less than 15 years of age (Ling *et al.*, 2002) or 18 years (Fong *et al.*, 2002). Others only consider patients with 40 or more years (Dimitrov *et al.*, 2003).

(e) The blindness in diabetics may result from other causes (cataract; glaucoma and ARMD) and these are not reported or accounted for. For example, in Spain, the prevalence of blindness in diabetic patients was reported to be 11.3% but only 54% of them were due to retinopathy (Aroca *et al.*, 1996). In the U.S. 23.5% of type 1 diabetic patients have visual impairment and 16.7% were blind due to other causes (Klein *et al.*, 1984). This is even more so in type 2 diabetics that show other causes in 83.7% of those with partial sight and 48.5% of those with registered legal blindness. In Denmark, Nielsen *et al.* (1982) referred rates of legal blindness from other causes in 11.1% of the insulin treated patients and in 20% of the patients treated with oral hypoglycemic agents.

(f) The incidence of proliferative retinopathy and maculopathy has declined due to improved glycemic control and more aggressive antihypertensive treatment and the generalization of laser treatment in the last decades.

The Steno Group has shown that in diabetic patients type 1 (onset before 40 years age) followed for 20 or more years the cumulative incidence of proliferative diabetic retinopathy after 20 years of diabetes presented a dramatic decrease from 31.1% in those with onset in the period 1965–1969 to 12.5% in those diagnosed between 1979 and 1984, 40%

reduction ($p < 0.001$). The cumulative incidence of maculopathy also declined from 18.6% to 7.4%, also a 40% reduction ($p = 0.03$, Hovind *et al.*, 2003).

In type 1 diabetic patients the incidence increased significantly with higher values of glycosylated hemoglobin, presence of gross proteinuria, hypertension, pack/years smoked, so the prevalence of blindness and low vision was different according to the decade of the epidemiological study (Moss *et al.*, 1998).

The number of newly registered blind patients referred to low vision rehabilitation centers in Stokolm County — Sweden, decreased by one third during a 15-year period after a mass mailing to diabetics (Backlund *et al.*, 1997).

On the contrary, Porta *et al.* (1995) were unable to demonstrate a decrease in registration of blindness in the northwest Italy, between 1967 and 1991, despite the introduction of screening programmes for diabetic retinopathy. However, in 2001, Porta *et al.*, reported a decreased incidence of blindness in type 1 although in type 2, particularly among elderly patients, it remained constant.

Grey *et al.* (1989), in Avon, Great Britain found an increase in prevalence of blindness in diabetics between 1959–1960 and 1985–1986. During the past 20 years the prevalence of blindness in type 1 diabetes in Denmark has gone from 4% to 2.2% (Sjolie *et al.*, 1995).

It is, however, generally accepted that diabetic retinopathy is the major cause of blindness in people of working age (Grey *et al.*, 1989; Foster *et al.*, 1990), accounting for 90% of blindness (Prasad *et al.*, 2001).

Prevalence of blindness has been reported to be 5.5 times (Cerrulli *et al.*, 1988, Italy), 20 times (Nielsen *et al.*, 1982, Denmark) or 25 times (Palmberg 1977, USA) higher in diabetics than in a nondiabetic population.

In Europe, the percentage of blindness due to diabetes among adults was found to be less than 8% in Netherlands, Scotland, Bulgaria, and Slovakia

(Kokur *et al.*, 2002). In 1988 the U.S. Nation Society to Prevent Blindness survey estimated that 7.9% of persons, who were legally blind, reported diabetes as the cause of their blindness.

### 5.1.1. Prevalence of Visual Impairment in Diabetic Patients

In Europe, the prevalence of visual impairment varies widely, showing differences of 12 times even between two Scandinavian countries, 1.1% in Sweden (Buch *et al.*, 2004) and 13.3% in Norway (Hapnes *et al.*, 1996) (Table 5.1).

#### *Type 1*

According to The EURODIAB Complications Study, in 31 diabetes centers in Europe the prevalence of visual impairment (VA — 0.3 to > 0.1) is 1.4% (ranging between 0% and 10%) (Sjolie *et al.*, 1997) (Table 5.2).

**Table 5.1    Prevalence of Visual Impairment in Diabetes**

| Spain | Aroca *et al.*, 1996 | 7.7% |
|---|---|---|
| UK | Prasad *et al.*, 2001 | 2.84% |
| | Ling *et al.*, 2002 | 3.7% |
| Denmark | Nielsen *et al.*, 1982 | 9.4% |
| | Buch *et al.*, 2004 | 2.7% |
| Norway | Hapnes *et al.*, 1996 | 13.3% |
| Sweden | Henricsson *et al.*, 1996 | 1.1% |
| USA | Fong *et al.*, 2002 | 6.7% |

**Table 5.2    Prevalence of Visual Impairment in Diabetes Type 1**

| Sweden | Jerneld, 1988 | 4.9% |
|---|---|---|
| | Henricsson *et al.*, 1996 | 0.2% |
| Norway | Hapnes *et al.*, 1996 | 6.3% |
| Iceland | Kristinsson *et al.*, 1994 | 3% |
| USA | Klein *et al.*, 1984 | 4.7% |

#### *Type 2*

In type 2 diabetic patients the prevalence of visual impairment varies between 1.2% and 14.6% (Table 5.3).

### 5.1.2. Prevalence of Blindness in Diabetic Patients

The prevalence of blindness in diabetic patients may vary from 0.03% in Sweden (Hapnes *et al.*, 1996) to 8.1% in Norway (Hapnes *et al.*, 1996) even in countries with the same degree of development (Table 5.4).

**Table 5.3    Prevalence of Visual Impairment in Diabetes Type 2**

| Sweden | Jerneld, 1988 | 7.2% |
|---|---|---|
| | Henricsson *et al.*, 1996 | 1.2% |
| Norway | Hapnes *et al.*, 1996 | 14.6% |
| Iceland | Kristinsson *et al.*, 1994 | 7% |
| UK | Chadran *et al.*, 2002 | 1.7% |
| Australia | Dimitov *et al.*, 1994 | 4% |
| USA | Klein *et al.*, 1984 | 6.5% |

**Table 5.4    Prevalence of Blindness in Diabetic Patients**

| Spain | Aroca, 1996 | 6.1% |
|---|---|---|
| | Martin *et al.*, 1992 | 3.75% |
| Portugal | DGCSP, 1991 | 4.9% |
| Italy | Cerruli *et al.*, 1988 | 2.12% |
| Sweden | Henricsson *et al.*, 1986 | 0.03% |
| Norway | Hapnes *et al.*, 1996 | 8.1% |
| Denmark | Nielsen, 1982 | 7.2% |
| | Buch *et al.*, 2004 | 0.2% |
| UK | Committee Blindness, 1955–1952 | 2% |
| | Broadbent *et al.*, 1990 | 0.8% |
| | Sparrow, 1993 | 4% |
| | Prasad *et al.*, 2001 | 0.75% |
| USA | Fong *et al.*, 2002 | 1.5% |

## Type 1

In Europe, the prevalence of blindness in type 1 diabetes, according to EURODIAB is 2.3%, ranging from 0.0% to 6.5% Sjolie *et al.* (1997) (Table 5.5).

The prevalence of blindness varies with the levels of care. In Sweden the prevalence of blindness dropped 95% (4.4% to 0.24%) between 1988 and 1996 (Jerneld *et al.*, 1988; Ericsson *et al.*, 1996) and in Denmark at the 20-years cumulative prevalence of blindness has fallen from 3.5% in patients with onset in the period 1965–1969 to 0% in those with onset 1979–1984 ($p < 0.001$), due to improved glycemic control, early aggressive antihypertensive treatment and laser treatment (Hovind *et al.*, 2003).

The duration of diabetic disease is an important variable in the prevalence of legal blindness: 4.2% in patients with 15–19 years duration and 17.1% in patients with 22–24 years duration of diabetes, four times more (Roy *et al.*, 2000).

## Type 2

Prevalence of blindness in type 2 diabetic patients varies between 0.35% and 9%, about 26 times (Table 5.6).

## 5.2. Incidence of Visual Impairment

Incidence is the proportion between the number of new cases (visual impairment) occurring in a given period (1, 2, 4 years) and the total population at risk

**Table 5.5 Prevalence of Blindness in Diabetes Type 1**

| Spain | Vigo *et al.*, 1991 | 8.7% |
|---|---|---|
| Sweden | Nielsen *et al.*, 1982 | 5.7% |
| | Sjolie *et al.*, 1987 | 3.4% Males |
| | | 2.6% Females |
| Norway | Hapnes *et al.*, 1996 | 9.4% |
| Denmark | Nielsen, 1982 | 5.7% |
| UK | McLeod *et al.*, 1988 | 1.5% |
| | Chadran *et al.*, 2002 | 0.6% |
| USA | Klein *et al.*, 1984 | 3.2% |

**Table 5.6 Prevalence of Blindness in Diabetes Type 2**

| Spain | Vigo *et al.*, 1991 | 4.1% |
|---|---|---|
| Portugal | GGSP, 1991 | 1% |
| France | Cathalinau *et al.*, 1993 | 0.37% |
| UK | McLeod *et al.*, 1988 | 1.5% |
| | Comack *et al.*, 2001 | 0.21% |
| | Chadran *et al.*, 2002 | 0.47% |
| Norway | Hapnes *et al.*, 1996 | 9% |
| Sweden | Henricsson *et al.*, 1996 | 0.35% |
| Denmark | Nielsen *et al.*, 1982 | 5.7% |
| Iceland | Kristinsson *et al.*, 1994 | 1.6% |
| USA | Klein *et al.*, 1984 | 1.2% |
| Australia | Dimitrov *et al.*, 2003 | 4% |

(all diabetics or only those with diabetic retinopathy, Nielsen, 1984) at the beginning of the period or sometimes at the end of the follow-up period. So, diabetic patients with no impaired visual acuity are followed upon annually to determine occurrences of partial sight loss or blindness.

Incidence is a better measure of occurrence than prevalence, because it depends not only on the prevalence but also on the levels of care, such as introduction of $HbA_{1C}$ testing, self-monitoring of blood glucose, improvement in blood pressure therapy, surgery rate (cataract and vitrectomy) and death rate (Minassian, 2003).

Incidence rates of visual impairment must be reported at intervals longer than one year, because yearly incidence is difficult to determine accurately. The annual incidence of blindness in diabetic patients is relatively low, about 4/1000/year. The cumulative 20-year incidence of blindness after diabetes diagnosis (6.6% were IDDM) was determined to be 8.2% (in most cases, 91.8%, due to others causes than retinopathy, e.g. cataract and macular degenerative accounting for 63.2% (Dwyer *et al.*, 1985).

During the last decades the incidence of blindness in diabetic patients has decreased significantly, probably due to early detection of sight-threatening retinopathy, proliferative retinopathy and macular edema, improved management of hypertension and hyperglycemia and generalized use of laser and vitrectomy treatments.

(a) Backlund *et al.* (1995) reported in Stockholm County a 30% fall in the incidence of blindness between 1984–1988 and 1989–1993 periods.
(b) In the WEDRS study (Moss *et al.*, 1988; 1994; 1998) the annual incidence of blindness also decreased during three different 4-year periods of follow-up. Periods between 1980/1982 and 1984/1986; 1984/1986 and 1988/1992 and 1990/1992 and 1994/1996 (Table 5.7).

## 5.2.1. Visual Impairment

Only few population-based studies on the incidence of visual impairment in diabetic patients are available. Earlier studies have been hospital-based, retrospective or only based on a few patients.

An association between occurrence of blindness and visual impairment and high levels of $HbA_{1C}$ was found regularly by different authors (Moss *et al.*, 1988; 1994; 1998 and Henricsson *et al.*, 1996).

### 5.2.1.1. *Type 1 diabetes*

It is noteworthy that the reported incidence of visual impairement varies more than 40 times depending on the epoch that the study was performed.

**Denmark**

The annual incidence of visual impairment in insulin-treated patients (46% diagnosed before the age of

30 years) in the Island of Falster was 3.7% (Nielsen, 1984).

**Sweden**

The known diabetic population with less than 75 years of age in the country and city of Helsingborg — Sweden, had an annual incidence of 4.6/1000 persons/year (3.0–6.6 –95% CI) due to diabetic retinopathy (Henricsson *et al.*, 1996).

**U.S.**

The 14 years incidence of visual impairment was found to be 14.2% with an annual incidence of about 1.01%. These values have decreased in more recent periods (1980–1986, 1.19%; 1984–1992, 0.85%; 1990–1996, 0.90%).

The decline registered in rates of vision loss followed by a partial return to higher levels of vision loss may be explained in different ways:

(a) The initial decline is due to improved detection and treatment of threatening retinopathy followed by an increase due to the increased age of cohort.
(b) It represents a random variation over time in the incidence of vision loss.
(c) Losses due to death or non-participation. A proportion of the patients that participated in the initial four years (1980/1982–1984/1986) died or did not participate in the follow-up examinations, so an underestimation of the true rates might be possible. In effect the rate of blindness in patients who died during the follow-up period was three times the rate of survivors (Sjolie *et al.*, 1987).

In conclusion, when considering population-based studies the annual incidence of visual impairment in type 1 diabetic patients varies between 5 and 9/1000. Nielsen found a higher value 20 years ago, before generalization of better glycemic and hypertension control and laser treatment and it corresponded to a sample including more than 50% true type 2 diabetes.

**Table 5.7 Annual Incidence of Blindness in the WESDRS Study**

|  | 1980/2–1984/86 | 1984/6–1990/2 | 1990/2–1995/6 |
|---|---|---|---|
| Type 1 | 0.38% | 0.05% | 0.18% |
| Type 2 |  |  |  |
| (a) Insulin | 0.82% | 0.14% |  |
| (b) Non insulin | 0.67% | 0.37% |  |

### 5.2.1.2. *Type 2 diabetes*

**Denmark**

Annual incidence of visual impairment among all diabetic patients treated by oral hypoglycemia agents was 44/1000, 50% due to diabetic retinopathy (Nielsen, 1984).

**Sweden**

In the nineties, after the introduction of a screening program in population based studies, the annual incidence decreased. In the known diabetic population with less than 75 years of age in the county and city of Helsingborg the annual incidence was 5.0/1000 (Henricsson *et al.*, 1996) and the 8-year incidence of visual impairment (VA ≤ 0.5) was 70/1000 (9/1000/year) higher in insulin-treated patients (Hansson-Lundblad *et al.*, 2002).

**U.S.-WESDR**

The annual incidence in insulin-treated patients with diabetes type 2 has fallen from 46/1000 in 1988 to 37/1000 in 1994. In those not taking insulin, the incidence did not vary, 21/1000 to 24/1000 (Moss *et al.*, 1988, 1994).

In conclusion, in type 2 diabetes the incidence of visual impairment is about six times higher than in type 1 diabetic patients. Type 2 diabetic patients are older. At baseline only 18.4% of type 2 patients had less than 45 years compared with 88.2% in type 1, and it must be kept in mind that all age-related ocular diseases also occur in diabetic patients.

### 5.2.2. Blindness

### 5.2.2.1. *Type 1 diabetes*

**Denmark**

Even in the same country it is possible to find extremely different values. From a reported value of 37/1000 in "insulin-treated" patients (only 46% were truly type 1, i.e. diagnosed before 30 years age) in the Island of Falster (Nielsen, 1984) to an annual

incidence of 0.95/1000 in males and 1.25/1000 in females for the other regions (Sjolie *et al.*, 1987).

**Sweden**

In the known diabetic population with less than 75 years age in the county and city of Helsingborg, Sweden, Henricsson *et al.* (1996) reported a low annual incidence.

**England**

The annual incidence of blindness in type 1 patients (onset at age 20 years or less) was found to be approximately 0.1/1000. The 10-year incidence of blindness in diabetic patients with onset at age 20 years or less was 1/1000, the 20-years incidence, 16/1000 and 30-years incidence 35/1000 (Caird *et al.*, 1969).

**Wisconsin, U.S.**

The 14-year incidence of blindness was low, 2.4/1000. The annual incidence dropped from 3.8/1000 in 1986 to 0.5/1000 in 1992 and 1.8/1000 in 1996 (Moss *et al.*, 1998).

In conclusion, considering only population based studies, the incidence of blindness in type 1 diabetic patients varies between 0 and 2.4/1000.

Nielsen found a much higher value in a sample with more than 50% with true type 2 diabetics, 37/1000, 20 years ago before generalization of better care in diagnosis, prevention with intensive glycemic and hypertension control, laser treatment and vitrectomy.

### 5.2.2.2. *Type 2 diabetes*

**Island of Falster, Denmark**

Patients treated with oral hypoglycemic agents and/or diet alone had an annual incidence of 19/1000 (Nielsen, 1984).

**Sweden**

After the introduction of a screening program in a population based study in Sweden, diabetic patients of less than 75 years of age had an annual incidence of 1.3/1000 (Henricsson *et al.*, 1996) and the 8-year incidence of blindness in another study was similar 8/1000 (Hansson-Lundblad *et al.*, 2002).

**UK**

Diabetic patients at the age of 60 or more years had an annual incidence of 8/1000 (Cohen *et al.*, 1991).

**U.S.**

The WEDRS annual incidence varies between 3/1000 (a 4-year follow-up) and −4/1000 (a 10-year follow-up) in patients taking insulin. In those not taking insulin it is lower — 1.75/1000 (4-year follow-up) and 4.8/1000 (10-year follow-up).

In conclusion, the incidence of blindness is similar in both types of diabetic patients, suggesting a better prognosis for type 2 patients who are older (Moss *et al.*, 1988; 1994).

## 5.3. Risk Factors for Visual Loss

The risk of visual impairment and blindness is substantially reduced by programmes that combine methods for early detection with timely treatment.

### 5.3.1. Sex

The WEDRS (Moss *et al.*, 1994) showed that in type 1 diabetic patients, sex was not associated with the 10-year incidence of legal blindness, but on the contrary, type 2 diabetic women had worse prognosis for blindness in those not taking insulin, 5.8% vs 3.6% in men and also in those taking insulin, 5.4% vs 2.3% in men.

### 5.3.2. Race

The Baltimore Eye Survey, showed that patients aged 40 or more years, had no significant difference in

prevalence of blindness between whites, 6%, and blacks, 5% (Sommer *et al.*, 1991).

### 5.3.3. Age

The 4-year incidence of blindness increased significantly with increasing age in all diabetic patients.

**Type 1 diabetes**

The incidence of blindness increased from 1.8% in the third decade to 2.1% in the fourth and to 3.1% in the fifth.

**Type 2 diabetes**

The incidence of blindness increased with age (Moss *et al.*, 1988) (Table 5.8).

### 5.3.4. Duration of Diabetes

The 4-year incidence of blindness increases significantly with duration of diabetes in those taking insulin, type 1 and 2, but does not increase in those with type 2 not taking insulin (Moss *et al.*, 1988) (Table 5.9).

### 5.3.5. Severity of Retinopathy

The preliminary report of DRS (1976) showed that the 2-years cumulative event rate of visual acuity

**Table 5.8 Incidence of Blindness Due to Diabetes vs. Age**

| Age | Taking insulin | Not taking insulin |
|---|---|---|
| 30–44 | 0.0% | 0.0% |
| 45–54 | 1.2% | 1.9% |
| 55–64 | 1.5% | 2.7% |
| 65–74 | 3.1% | 0.0% |
| 75+ | 12.5% | 8.5% |

(Moss *et al.*, 1988).

**Table 5.9   Four-Year Incidence of Blindness vs. Duration of Diabetes**

| Duration (Years) | Type 1 | Type 2 Taking Insulin | Type 2 not Taking Insulin |
|---|---|---|---|
| 0–9 | 0.0% | 1.9% | 2.5% |
| 10–19 | 2.9% | 3.3% | 3.7% |
| 20–29 | 3.7% | 4.9% | 0.0% |
| 30+ | 0.0% | 5.9% | — |

**Table 5.10   Four-Year Incidence of Blindness and Retinopathy at Baseline (WEDRS Study)**

| | Younger-onset | Older-onset | |
|---|---|---|---|
| | | Insulin | Not Insulin |
| (a) No apparent retinopathy (Level 1) | 0.3% | 4.5% | 3.2% |
| (b) Non proliferative Mild / Moderate (Level 1, 5–3) | 4.2% | 6.8% | 5.1% |
| Severe (Level 4–5) | 4.4% | 12.3% | 24.2% |
| (c) Proliferative | 9.4% | 5.7% | — |

**Table 5.11   Four-Year Incidence of Visual Loss vs. Macular Edema**

| | Younger-onset | Older-onset | |
|---|---|---|---|
| | | Insulin | Not Insulin |
| No macular edema | 5.4% | 13.9% | 9.6% |
| Macular edema | 19.1% | 39.2% | 53.3% |

### 5.3.7.  Metabolic Control

Intensive glycemic control decreases risk of vision loss according to different studies.

#### Type 1 diabetes

The DCCT investigated the effect of intensive diabetes management to obtain near-euglycemic control (three or more daily injections or a continuous subcutaneous infusion) vs conventional treatment, (i.e. only one or two daily injections), and found that intensive control reduces the risk of incidence and progression of retinopathy.

#### Type 2 diabetes

The UK Prospective Diabetes Study (UKPDS, 1998) demonstrated that improved blood glucose control (FPG < 6 mmol/L) reduced the 5.5-years overall rate of microvascular complications by 25%. In patients receiving intensive vs conventional therapy it reduced significantly the incidence of sight threatening retinopathy ($p = 0.003$).

In Sweden, in type 2 diabetic patients, regular fundus photographic screening showed that those with sight-threatening retinopathy had higher $HbA_{1C}$ levels (Hansson-Lunblad *et al.*, 2002). The association between occurrence of blindness and higher $HbA_{1C}$ levels is found in various epidemiological studies

less than 5/200 is worse when more severe retinopathy is present: no new vessels (2.4%); new vessels elsewhere (9.6%); new vessels in the disk (24.5%).

In the WEDRS, the 4-year incidence of blindness showed a significant correlation with retinopathy level at baseline (Moss *et al.*, 1988) (Table 5.10).

### 5.3.6.  Macular Edema

The WEDRS showed that the presence of macular edema is a significant factor of risk in the 4-year incidence of visual loss (doubling the visual angle) (Table 5.11).

(Moss, 1988, 1994; Henricsson *et al.*, 1996; Krolewski *et al.*, 1995; Warram *et al.*, 1995).

### 5.3.8. Hypertension

#### Type 1 diabetes

Higher ocular perfusion pressure was associated with greater incidence of progression to proliferative diabetic retinopathy, probably because systolic blood pressure plays a major role in the intravascular pressure rise (Moss *et al.*, 1994).

#### Type 2 diabetes

The UKPDS (1998) found that patients with tight control of their blood pressure (< 150/85 mm Hg), using either an ACE inhibitor or a Beta-blocker, had a 34% reduction in progression of retinopathy ($p = 0.004$), a 47% reduced risk of three or more lines in the ETDRS chart of visual acuity ($p = 0.004$) and a 38.6% reduced risk per year in the need of photocoagulation as compared with those with less tight control (< 180/105), after a period of 7.5 years follow-up.

However, in one randomized trial performed in hypertensive diabetic patients (diastolic blood pressure $\geq 90$ mm Hg) it was found, that after 5.3 years of appropriate blood pressure control either with nisolpidine or enalapril that there was no difference with regard to progression of diabetic retinopathy between those receiving intensive control (diastolic BP < 75 mm Hg) vs those treated with moderate BP control (diastolic BP 80–89 mm Hg) (Estacio, 2000).

### 5.3.9. Nephropathy

In Sweden, regular photographic screening in type 2 diabetic patients evidenced that those with sight-threatening retinopathy had higher s-creatinine levels ($p = 0.032$) (Hansson-Lunblad *et al.*, 2002).

## 5.4. Economic Costs of Visual Impairment and Blindness

Vision impairment is linked with restriction of participation in daily life activities, social isolation and reduced physical activities in general (Lamoureux *et al.*, 2004).

The WHO (1998) refers to a study in the United Kingdom that indicates that visually disabled people were poorer on average, had lower educational levels, lower employment and less social life compared to sighted persons. It is referred that in Africa, blind persons die earlier compared to sighted people.

Blindness and visual impairment have enormous emotional, social and political costs. Direct costs include long term residential and nurse care, homecare workers, costs to the governments in the form of disability payments and social welfare programs.

Indirect costs are due to loss of working days due to disability, loss of employment opportunities and reduced quality of life. In the WESDR prospective study, younger-onset men aged 25 or more years, who had PDR and who were employed at baseline, were more likely to become unemployed four years later. There is also Intangible costs like pain, anxiety, discrimination and loss of self-esteem. Younger-onset women who were married and had impaired vision at baseline had an increased 4-year incidence of divorce (Klein *et al.*, 1994).

Several questionnaires have been developed to measure patients' quality of life. For example, the Center for Eye Research in Australia (Lamoureux *et al.*, 2004) had developed a questionnaire, the Impact Vision Impairment (IVI), that measures patients' quality of life, people restriction of participation in daily activities in 32 items under five domains: leisure and work, consumer and social interaction, household and personal care — the least restrictive in diabetic patients, mobility and emotional reaction to visual loss.

Participants in Lamoureux study reported that the functional life domains causing the greatest restriction were leisure and work, mobility, consumer and social interaction. Nineteen of the 20 most restrictive items originating from these three domains were compared with the emotional reaction to visual loss, household and personal care domains.

The economic and social costs of visual impairment must be considered from the perspective of the disabled individual and the country as a whole.

Physical and psychosocial implications of visual impairment cannot be accurately quantified in monetary terms. The estimate costs vary widely from country to country.

The cost estimated by the U.S. federal government, not including reduced productivity, output loss, societal burdens of rehabilitation and other local expenses, was $12,769 per person per year in working age and US$833 for those aged 65 or more years (Chiang *et al.*, 1992). In the U.S. the average blind person receives $6,900 annually from Social Security Disability Insurance (Javitt *et al.*, 1989).

The annual cost for partial sight loss associated with macular edema was $3150 (Dasbach *et al.*, 1991).

## 5.5. Prevalence of Retinopathy

On the basis of both, ETDRS and WEDRS studies, the American Academy of Ophthalmology launched a project to develop consensus regarding a classification scheme. A group of 31 individuals from 16 countries achieved a consensus and classification was simplified to only 3 grades with grade 2 subdivided in 3 sub-groups and macular edema also in 3 grades (Wilkinson *et al.*, 2003). However, the data available is based in previous classifications, which do not match well between the different studies.

### 5.5.1. Type 1 Diabetes

As stated previously, the prevalence of retinopathy in different studies is difficult to compare because samples are different. For Klein *et al.* (1984), type 1 diabetes should have the age of onset of diabetes before 30 years age and before the 40 years to Jerneld *et al.* (1983). The Klein study is a populational study, the numbers of Jerneld are from a screening study and consider only patients at risk of 15 years age or older. All studies are based in fundus photographs although Jerneld study included angiography. The study of Henricsson *et al.* (1996) only considers diabetics with 10 years diabetes mellitus duration. Some studies are made using seven field stereo photographes (Klein *et al.*, 1984; Jerneld *et al.* 1985), whereas, others used single photographs and ophthalmoscopy (Ling *et al.*, 2002).

Absence of retinopathy was found in 29.6% (Klein *et al.*, 1984) and in 65.5% (Hapnes *et al.*, 1996) and proliferative retinopathy in 1.8% (Henricsson *et al.*, 2003) and in 21.5% (Klein *et al.* 1984) (Table 5.12).

Prevalence of macular edema also varies. Klein *et al.* (1984) found no macular edema before five years duration but in patients with 20 or more years duration it was detected in 29%. In the overall diabetic population, prevalence of macular edema was about 11.1%. Kristinsson *et al.* (1994) found 9.8%; Ling *et al.* (2002) 11.5% and in Spain, Aroca *et al.* (1996) found a value of 10.5% in patients with 15 or more years duration of diabetes.

### 5.5.2. Type 2 Diabetes

The reported values of prevalence in diabetes type 2 also varies because samples are different. The percentage of patients free of retinopathy varies between 45.6% in U.S. (Klein *et al.*, 1984) and 89.8% in Norway (Hapnes *et al.*, 1996) (Table 5.13).

The percentage of those with proliferative diabetic retinopathy varies between 0.6% in Norway

**Table 5.12    Prevalence of Retinopathy in Diabetes Type 1**

|  | No Retinopathy | Nonproliferative | Proliferative |
|---|---|---|---|
| (1) USA |  |  |  |
| a. Klein *et al.*, 1984 | 29.6% | 48.3% | 21.5% |
| b. Roy, 2000 | 36.1% | 45% | 18.9% |
| (2) EURODIAB | 54% | 33% | 13% |
| Sjolie *et al.*, 1997 |  |  |  |
| (3) DENMARK | 52% | 35% | 13% |
| Sjolie, 1985 |  |  |  |
| (4) SEWEDEN |  |  |  |
| Jerneld *et al.*, 1985 | 53% | 34% | 13% |
| *et al.*, 1988 | 32% | 50% | 18% |
| Henricsson *et al.*, 2003 | 61.4% | 37.8% | 1.8% |
| (5) ICELAND |  |  |  |
| Kristinsson *et al.*, 1994 | 48% | 39% | 13% |
| (6) NORWAY |  |  |  |
| Hapnes *et al.*, 1996 | 65.6% | 21.9% | 12.5% |
| (7) UNITED KINGDOM |  |  |  |
| Ling *et al.*, 2002 | 51% | 40.3% | 8.7% |

**Table 5.13    Prevalence of Retinopathy in Diabetes Type 2**

|  | No Retinopathy | Nonproliferative | Proliferative |
|---|---|---|---|
| (1) USA |  |  |  |
| a. Klein *et al.*, 1984 | 45.6% | 45.6% | 8.5% |
| (2) UK |  |  |  |
| Lee *et al.*, 2003 |  |  | 3.8% |
| Ling *et al.*, 2002 | 69.7% | 21.4% | 2.8% |
| (3) SWEDEN |  |  |  |
| Jerneld *et al.*, 1985 | 83% | 19.8% | 1.9% |
| Jerneld, 1988 | 83% | 19.9% | 1.4% |
| (4) ICELAND |  |  |  |
| Kristinsson *et al.*, 1994 | 59% | 48% | 7% |
| (5) NORWAY |  |  |  |
| Hapnes *et al.*, 1996 | 89.8% | 9.6% | 0.6% |
| (6) DENMARK |  |  |  |
| Hove *et al.*, 2002 | 68.1% |  |  |
| (7) FINLAND |  |  |  |
| Hirvela *et al.*, 1997 | 79% |  |  |
| (8) SPAIN |  |  |  |
| Martin *et al.*, 1992 |  |  | 5.7% |

(Hapnes *et al.*, 1996) and 8.5% in U.S. (Klein *et al.*, 1984) (Table 5.13).

The severity of retinopathy varies with the existence of risk factors like the duration of diabetes. Prevalence of proliferative retinopathy is reported to be 2% in persons with diabetes for less than five years and 15.5% in persons who had diabetes for 15 or more years (Klein *et al.*, 1984).

Prevalence also depends on the type of treatment. Proliferative retinopathy is reported to be present in 14.1% of insulin treated diabetic patients (Aroca *et al.*, 1996) and in 3.9% (Ling *et al.*, 2002) comparing with prevalences of 2.9% (Aroca *et al.*, 1996) and 1.3% (Ling *et al.*, 2002) in patients not receiving insulin.

**Macular edema**

In populational studies prevalence of clinically significant macular edema (CSME) appears to vary widely (Table 5.14).

Prevalence of CSME is absent a negligible shortly by after diagnosis but increases to more than 10% after 25 years of the disease (Klein *et al.*, 1994).

In Spain, prevalence of CSME is 4.5% before five years duration and 25.8% after 15 years duration (Aroca *et al.*, 1996). The prevalence of macular edema also differs with the type of treatment: 9.1% in

patients receiving insulin vs 4.1% in diabetic patients not needing insulin (Ling *et al.*, 2002).

# 5.6. Risk Factors of Retinopathy

Primary prevention serves to avoid risk factors of retinopathy. It is necessary to identify risk factors and modify them when possible to prevent the onset and the progression of retinopathy early in its course, so that patients can remain well.

## 5.6.1. Type 1 Diabetes

### 5.6.1.1. *Duration of diabetes*

Duration is probably the major predictor for development and progression of retinopathy.

The prevalence of any type of retinopathy increases from 8% at three years to 25% at five years, to 60% at 10 years and to 80% at 15 years among younger onset diabetic patients. Proliferative diabetic retinopathy is not observed in the first three years but after 15 years a quarter of diabetic patients have retinopathy (Klein *et al.*, 1984).

The 4-year incidence of proliferative diabetic retinopathy (PDR) is 0% during the first five years of evolution but PDR occurs in 27.9% of diabetic

**Table 5.14  Prevalence of Clinically Significant Macular Edema**

| Klein *et al.*, 1995 | Insulin | 15.2% |
|---|---|---|
| | Non insulin | 3.7% |
| | Total | 8.4% |
| Fristinsson *et al.*, 1997 | | 10% |
| Aroca *et al.*, 1996 | <5 years 4.5% | |
| | >15 years 25.8% | |
| Ling *et al.*, 2002 | | 6.1% |
| Hirvela *et al.*, 2002 | | 8% |
| Lee *et al.*, 2003 | | 2.1% (65 years or over) |

patients in a 4-year interval after 13–14 years evolution of diabetes; although after 15 years the incidence appears to remain stable (Klein *et al.*, 1989).

In the EURODIAB Study, duration (years) was shown to be a significant risk factor for incidence of retinopathy (Porta *et al.*, 2003). However, in Ireland, Cahill *et al.* (2000) found no association between presence of DR with duration of diabetes ($p = 0.438$) in patients with 10 or more years duration of the disease.

Total duration, as a continuous variable, showed that the prepubertal years of diabetes are significant for the development of retinopathy, however, there is an increasing delay on the onset of complications in those with longer prepubertal duration (Knowles *et al.*, 1965; Murphy *et al.*, 1990; Faria de Abreu *et al.*, 1994; Donaghue *et al.*, 2002). Growth hormone rises after gonadarche onset and may be the major accelerator of diabetic retinopathy.

### 5.6.1.2. *Age at diagnosis*

In 1965, Knowles *et al.* reported that the years before puberty do not appear to influence the development of retinopathy. Similar findings were published by Murphy *et al.*, 1990; Faria de Abreu *et al.*, 1994, Dane *et al.*, 1997 and Donaghue *et al.*, 2003.

In a 10-years incidence study of proliferative diabetic retinopathy (WESDRS, Klein *et al.*, 1994) it was found that proliferative diabetic retinopathy was less likely to have developed in patients who were under 10 years of age at diagnosis, suggesting that prepubertal years might have a neutral effect on progression. Similar observations were reported by Olsen *et al.*, 1999.

There is, however, some evidence suggesting that the prepubertal duration of diabetes may be of significance in the development of retinopathy. In patients with the same postpubertal diabetes duration it was found a significantly higher prevalence of retinopathy than in patients with onset of diabetes before 10 years of age (Goldstein *et al.*, 1993).

The EURODIAB patients diagnosed before puberty showed a higher risk of progression to proliferative diabetic retinopathy and prepubertal evolution could even be considered a predictor for progression of the retinopathy (Porta *et al.*, 2001).

### 5.6.1.3. *Glycemic control*

Patients with worse metabolic control show, in general, high risk of developing retinopathy, progression and sight threatening complications.

Kullberg *et al.* (1994) found that patients with mean values of $HbA_{1C} > 8\%$ showed higher relative risk compared to those with $HbA_{1C} < 7\%$. $HbA_{1C}$ was monitored closely during five or more years.

In Ireland, Cahill *et al.* (2000) found that the presence of DR is associated with poorer diabetic control.

The EURODIAB study patients who progressed to proliferative retinopathy had higher levels of $HbA_{1C}$, $8.3 \pm 0.2$, compared with the patients who did not progress to proliferative retinopathy, $6.3 \pm 0.1$ (Porta *et al.*, 2001).

In a nationwide population incidence study in Sweden patients who developed retinopathy had worse metabolic control, $HbA_{1C}$ 8.1% vs 6.8% (Henricsson *et al.*, 2003). Similarly, in a longitudinal study ($11.2 \pm 2.5$ years) the proportion of individuals with preproliferative or laser treated retinopathy had a significantly higher mean $HbA_{1C}$ over the follow-up period (Bryden *et al.*, 2003).

In a prospective 12-year study of 420 individuals with insulin dependent diabetes mellitus Goldstein *et al.* (1993) found that retinopathy developed approximately two years later in subjects with $HbA_{1C}$ less than to 7.5%, compared to those with higher values and also that the mean $HbA_{1C}$ was higher in patients who developed proliferative diabetic retinopathy.

In the WESDRS, Klein *et al.* (1995) found that the 10-year incidence of macular edema (20.1%) and clinically significant macular edema (13.6%) was associated with higher levels of $HbA_{1C}$ (Odds ratio 1.56–95% CI 1.38–1.76). The 10-year incidence of macular edema was 8.7% in patients with $HbA_{1C}$ ranging between 5.6–9.4%, but increased to 28.1% in those with $HbA_{1C}$ ranging between 12.1–19.5%. In the 14-year incidence and progression of diabetic retinopathy study WESDRS (Klein *et al.*, 1998) the presence of macular edema and proliferative retinopathy were associated with increases in glycosilated hemoglobin levels. Lower glycosilated hemoglobin levels, however, were associated with improvement in retinopathy. A 1% decrease in the glycosilated hemoglobin level from baseline to 4-year follow-up would be expected to lead to a 25% decrease in the 14-year incidence of proliferative diabetic retinopathy and a 24% decrease in the incidence of macular edema.

Lower levels of $HbA_{1C}$ even later in the course of diabetes may modify the risk of macular edema (Klein *et al.*, 1998).

The DCCT, a multicenter intervention study, also showed that intervening to obtain a good metabolic control is effective in reducing the incidence and gravity of retinal lesions. Intensive management with three or more daily injections or continuous subcutaneous infusion of insulin compared with "conventional treatment" (one or two daily injections) reduced in 76% the mean risk of retinopathy incidence, in 63% the risk of progression, in 47% the risk of developing severe nonproliferative diabetic retinopathy or proliferative diabetic retinopathy, in 23% the risk of clinically significant macular edema and in 56% the risk in the need for laser treatment (DCCT, 1993).

The benefit persisted four years after the period of intensive control: 75% risk reduction in the progression of retinopathy ($p < 0.001$), 69% risk reduction in development of severe nonproliferative diabetic retinopathy and proliferative diabetic retinopathy, 58% risk reduction in development of clinically significant macular edema and 52% reduction in the need for laser treatment (DCCT, 2000).

The beneficial effects of "tight" blood glucose control did not appear until approximately two and half years after initiation of this type of management (DCCT, 2000). About 10% of the patients with preexisting retinopathy had a transient worsening of their retinopathy after the institution of tight blood glucose control (DCCT, 1998). The number of hypoglycemic control, values below 65 mg/dl, seems to be an important risk factor in those patients who have retinopathy progression during normo-glycemic reentry (Sebag, 1993).

### 5.6.1.4. *Blood pressure control*

The WESDRS found that patients with type 1 diabetes had a 17% prevalence of hypertension at baseline and a 25% incidence after 10 years of diabetes duration (Klein *et al.*, 1996). Increased blood pressure, through an effect on blood flow, has been hypothesized to damage the retinal capillary endothelial cells contributing to development and progression of retinopathy. In prospective studies, blood pressure was found generally to be a risk factor increasing the incidence of retinal disease. Chase *et al.* (1990) found, over a 2 to 3 years period, that the presence of high blood pressure resulted in higher incidence of retinopathy and progression of preexisting retinopathy ($p < 0.05$) in patients 14 years of age or more and insulin-dependent diabetes mellitus for five years or longer. In the WESDRS diastolic blood pressure was a significant predictor of the 14-year progression of diabetic retinopathy and incidence of proliferative diabetic retinopathy, even after controling for other risk factors (Klein *et al.*, 1998). In patients with 10 or more years of diabetes duration there is also a significant association of severity of retinopathy and diastolic blood pressure (Klein *et al.*, 1985).

In an interventional 2-year randomized doubleblind placebo-controlled trial (EUCLID), one inhibitor of angiotensin-converting enzyme, lisinopril, reduced in 50% progression of retinopathy in nonhypertensive or mildly hypertensive patients when compared to the placebo group even when adjusted for glycemic control. However, patients assigned to lisinopril had a significantly lower $HbA_{1C}$ at baseline (Chaturvedi *et al.*, 1998).

### 5.6.1.5. *Pregnancy*

The levels of progesterone are higher in pregnancy and that may induce intraocular production of VEGF

(Sone *et al.*, 1996). VEGF has been implicated in the pathogenesis of macular edema and neovascularization. Pregnancy is considered a risk factor of development and/or progression of retinopathy. The severity of retinopathy has been associated with $HbA_{1C}$ before ($p < 0.01$) and after ($p < 0.01$) pregnancy but not during it. The women who had progression of retinopathy during pregnancy had a significantly earlier onset of diabetes than those with improvement or no progression ($p < 0.01$). During pregnancy no association was found between the progression of retinopathy and blood pressure or adverse perinatal outcomes (Bek *et al.*, 2002).

Retinopathy can progress rapidly during pregnancy (Moloney *et al.*, 1982), usually only a transient progression and the long-term risk does not appear to be increased by pregnancy (DCCT, 2000). When planning pregnancy, women with preexisting diabetes should have a comprehensive eye examination and should be counseled on the risk of development and progression of diabetic retinopathy. When pregnant they should have an eye examination in the first trimester and close follow-up throughout pregnancy (Aiello *et al.*, 2001).

### 5.6.1.6. Height, weight and body mass index (BMI)

Chen *et al.* (1992) in a population-based study found no significant association between BMI and retinopathy. The EURODIAB study found that progression to proliferative diabetic retinopathy was associated with low height ($p = 0.0004$) and low weight ($p = 0.03$), but not with BMI ($p = 0.8$) (Porta, 2001). On the contrary, Dorchy *et al.* (2002) in a longitudinal study found that patients who developed proliferative diabetic retinopathy had significantly higher BMI (27 vs 22 $Kg/m^2$; $p = 0.04$).

In a nationwide population-based cohort of young adult patients with 10 or more years diabetes duration in Sweden, the prevalence and severity of diabetic retinopathy had a correlation with high BMI $p = 0.001$ (Henricsson *et al.*, 2003).

### 5.6.1.7. Serum lipid levels

Chen *et al.* (1992), in a population-based study, found, by multivariate analysis, that cholesterol levels were not correlated with retinopathy. On the contrary, however, Dorchy *et al.* (2002) found that patients with high levels of cholesterol (> 200 mg/dl) were more prone to develop proliferative diabetic retinopathy. The EURO-DIAB study found that higher levels of triglyceride ($p = 0.0001$) and LDL (0.003) were risk factors for proliferative diabetic retinopathy (Porta *et al.*, 2001).

### 5.6.1.8. Proteinuria

Patients with 10 or more years of diabetes duration have a significant association between severity of retinopathy and the presence of proteinuria, $p < 0.0001$ (Klein *et al.*, 1985). Proteinuria was associated with 14-year progression to proliferative retinopathy ($p < 0.001$) and to the incidence of macular edema (Klein *et al.*, 1998).

In Ireland, Cahill *et al.* (2000) found that presence of diabetic retinopathy was not associated with microalbuminuria levels. In Spain, Aroca *et al.* (2003) found in a 10 years prospective study that the incidence of retinopathy was associated with the presence of microalbuminuria but microalbuminuria was also correlated with diabetes duration, age and hypertension. However, discriminant analysis of the data showed that microalbuminuria was not a risk factor of retinopathy.

### 5.6.1.9. Cigarette smoking

The ischemic effects of smoking on the circulation, such as increased carbon monoxide, increased platelet aggregation and vasoconstriction have been proposed to have a deleterious effect on diabetic retinopathy. Nielsen *et al.* (1978), in a longitudinal study of five or more years, found no relation between smoking, even in heavy smokers and retinopathy in females, but found a positive correlation in males. Dornan *et al.* (1982), found no association in the incidence of retinopathy and progression to proliferative between smokers and nonsmokers. Klein *et al.* (1983) in a population-base study, found no excess risk of retinopathy in smokers or ex-smokers when contrasted with those who never smoke. Similarly, Chen *et al.* (1992) in a population-based study found that smoking had no significant association with retinopathy. Marshall *et al.* (1993) in an institutional study did not find a significant association between smoking and diabetic retinopathy.

Kullberg *et al.* (1994) in a longitudinal study of on average of 9.2 years in type 1 diabetes found no negative effect of smoking in the severity of retinopathy. Finally, Moss *et al.* (1996) found in a longitudinal 4-year and 10-year examination population-based study that neither smoking status nor pack-years smoking showed significant association with increased risk in incidence or progression of the diabetic retinopathy. The absence of a clear deleterious effect of smoking on the incidence or progression of diabetic retinopathy does not imply that diabetic patients, who smoke, should not stop, since smoking is a definite risk factor for cardiovascular disease.

### 5.6.1.10. *Alcohol*

Chen *et al.* (1992) in a population-based study found that alcohol had no significant association with retinopathy and Moss *et al.* (1992) found that the average alcohol consumption was inversely associated with prevalence of proliferative diabetic retinopathy (odds ratio — 0.49).

### 5.6.1.11. *Physical activity*

In a retrospective study no association was found between physical activity and the severity of diabetic retinopathy (Orchard *et al.*, 1990). Cruickshanks *et al.* (1995) in a 6-year longitudinal study from the WESDRS found that measurements of physical activity levels did not appear to be associated with either a two-step increase or decrease in the risk of progression of retinopathy or development of proliferative retinopathy.

### 5.6.1.12. *Myopia*

Myopia (> –2.00 d) was protective for progression to proliferative diabetic retinopathy in younger-onset persons with an odd ratio of 0.40 (95% LI 0.18–0.86) (Moss *et al.*, 1995).

## 5.6.2. Type 2 Diabetes

### 5.6.2.1. *Duration of diabetes*

An increasing frequency of retinopathy has been found in association with increasing duration of diabetes in both noninsulin-taking persons (prevalence rose from 23% in those who had diabetes for less than two years to 57.5% in persons with disease for 15 or more years) and in insulin-taking persons (rates rose from 30% to 84.5%). Three percent of non-insulin-taking patients and 4% of insulin-taking patients had proliferative retinopathy at 0–4 years after diagnosis, compared with 4.3% and 20.1% after 15 or more years (Klein *et al.*, 1984). In noninsulin-taking patients the prevalence of macular edema rose from 3% in persons with diabetes of less than three years duration to 28% in those with 21–22 years duration (Klein *et al.*, 1984).

### 5.6.2.2. *Age at examination*

A consistent positive relation was found between macular edema and age at examination. About 7.3% of patients with 30–44 years of age had severe non-proliferative or proliferative diabetic retinopathy vs 11.5% of those with 75 or more years, and the prevalence of macular edema, which was 4.3% between 30–44 years, rose to 8.9% at 45 or more years of age (Klein *et al.*, 1984).

Henricsson *et al.* (1996) in a population-based study in Sweden using multiple regression analysis also found a relationship between age at diagnosis, severity of retinopathy and macular edema ($p < 0.05$).

### 5.6.2.3. *Treatment*

The prevalence and severity of retinopathy are worse in insulin-taking than in non-insulin-taking diabetic patients. Retinopathy was absent in only 29.8% of diabetic patients taking insulin in comparison with 45.6% in diabetic patients not taking insulin. The prevalence of proliferative retinopathy was 14.1% in insulin-taking diabetic patients vs 2.9% in non-insulin-taking (Klein *et al.*, 1984). Insulin-taking patients had an higher overall rate of macular edema than non-insulin-taking patients, 15% vs 3.7% (Klein *et al.*, 1984).

Henricsson *et al.* (1996) in a population-based study in Sweden also found using multiple regression analysis, a relationship between insulin treatment and the incidence and severity of retinopathy and macular edema ($p < 0.05$).

In a 6-month prospective study of noninsulin-dependent patients with presexisting retinopathy, the change to conventional insulin therapy increased the risk of progression of diabetic retinopathy by 10 times (Roysarkar *et al.*, 1993).

### 5.6.2.4. *Glycemic control*

Klein *et al.* (1984) in a population-based study found that severity of retinopathy was related with higher glycosilated hemoglobin levels using the Cox regression model.

Similarly, Jerneld *et al.* (1985) found a significant relation to levels of $HbA_{1C}$, using multiple logistic regression analysis.

Henricsson *et al.* (1996) in a population-based study in Sweden also found a relationship between $HbA_{1C}$ levels and the incidence and severity of retinopathy and macular edema ($p < 0.05$). Patients with maculopathy had significantly higher $HbA_{1C}$ ($p < 0.005$) than those with no retinopathy (Knudsen *et al.*, 2002).

Prospective longitudinal studies are expected to provide more accurate information on the interaction between glycemic control and diabetic retinopathy. Klein *et al.* (1995) in the WESDRS found that over a 10-year period the incidence of macular edema was 25.4% in those taking insulin and 13.9% in the group not taking insulin. The incidence was associated with higher levels of $HbA_{1C}$ at baseline. The 10-year incidence was 3.7% in those with $HbA_{1C}$ ranging from 5.6–9.4% and increased to 39.7% in those with $HbA_{1c}$ ranging from 12.1–19.5%.

Ohkubo *et al.* (1995) in a randomized 6-year prospective study in Japanese patients found that those treated with multiple insulin injection treatment vs conventional insulin injection treatment had a significant decrease in the incidence of retinopathy ($p = 0.039$) and in the progression of retinopathy ($p = 0.049$).

The United Kingdom Prospective Study (UKPDS 33, 1998) demonstrated that improved blood glucose control reduced the overall rate of microvascular complications by 25% in patients receiving intensive (maintaining fast plasma glucose — FPG < 6 mmol/L) vs conventional treatment (maintaining FPG < 15 mmol/L without symptoms of hyperglycemia). For every percentage point decrease in $HbA_{1C}$ (vg from 8 to 7%) there was a 37% reduction in the risk of microvascular complications. There was a 29% reduction in the need of retinal photocoagulation ($p = 0.003$) and 17% risk reduction for progression of retinopathy ($p = 0.012$).

Gaede *et al.* (1999) from the Steno Group found in type 2 microalbuminuric diabetic patients submitted to intensive treatment a significantly lower rate of progression of retinopathy compared with standard treatment.

In a 2-year longitudinal study of Japanese patients with "mild preproliferative diabetic retinopathy" scattered soft exsudates without other nonperfused areas or venous beading –27% developed proliferative diabetic retinopathy and they presented a mean value of $HbA_{1C}$ of 9.4%. Among those who had not developed proliferative retinopathy the mean $HbA_{1C}$ was 7.6% ($p < 0.0004$). The proportion of eyes developing proliferative diabetic retinopathy was 48% among those with $HbA_{1C}$ values of 8.6% or more by comparison with only 8% progressing to proliferative retinopathy among those with mean $HbA_{1C}$ values below 8.6% ($p < 0.04$). The proportion of developing proliferative diabetic retinopathy was estimated to approximately double with each 1% increase in the mean $HbA_{1C}$ value (Sato *et al.*, 2001).

### 5.6.2.5. *Blood pressure*

Hypertension is common in patients with type 2 diabetes, with a prevalence of 40–60% over the age range of 45 to 75 (UKPDS, 1998). In the U.S. diabetic patients had a two-fold excess incidence of in hypertension regardless of gender (Krolewski *et al.*, 1985).

Klein *et al.*, (1984) in a population-based study, using a Cox regression model, found that severity of retinopathy was related to higher systolic blood pressure in patients with less than 15 years duration of their diabetes.

However, in studies of 4-year incidence, progression to proliferative diabetic retinopathy was not associated with blood pressure (Moss *et al.*, 1994). Klein *et al.* (1995) did not find any consistent association of blood pressure and retinopathy in 4 and a 10-year incidence studies.

Klein *et al.* (1995) found that over a 10-year period the incidence of macular edema was 14.4% in males and 22.1% in females. The incidence of macular edema was associated with increased diastolic pressure. The 10-year incidence was 15.4% in those with diastolic blood pressure ranging from 42–71 mm Hg, which increased to 27.1% in those ranging from 86–117 mm Hg.

The UKPDS was a large (1148 patients) randomized prospective (median 8.4 years) clinical trial of hypertensive diabetic patients, evaluating the effects of tight blood pressure control with an angiotensin converting enzyme inhibitor or a beta-blocker (< 150/85 mm Hg) with less tight control (< 180/105 mm Hg). A 34% reduction was observed in progression of retinopathy by two steps, using the modified ETDRS scale ($p = 0.004$), a 47% reduction in the risk of doubling visual angle using the ETDRS chart and a 35% reduction in the need of retinal photocoagulation ($p = 0.02$). These effects were independent of glycemic control (UKPDS, 38, 1998).

However, in another randomized trial of 470 hypertensive patients — baseline diastolic pressure => 90 mm Hg, The Appropriate Blood Pressure Control in Diabetes (ABCD) (Estacio *et al.*, 2000) did not find any difference for a mean 5.3 years follow-up between intensive control (diastolic < 75 mm Hg) and moderate control (80–89 mm Hg) with regard to progression of diabetic retinopathy.

### 5.6.2.6. *Cholesterol and triglycerides*

Klein *et al.* (1991) found no relation between severity of diabetic retinopathy and per quartile levels of total and HDL-cholesterol. They only found, in insulin-taking diabetic patients, a relationship between total-cholesterol and the presence of hard exudates in univariate analysis, but this effect was not apparent in multivariate analysis, maybe due to the fact that total-cholesterol is highly correlated with duration of diabetes and diastolic blood pressure.

Olivarius *et al.* (2001) in newly diagnosed middle-aged and elderly diabetic patients from a Danish population-based study found an intriguing inverse relationship between diabetic retinopathy and fasting triglycerides in microalbuminuric patients, but no such relationship in normoalbuminuric and albuminuric patients. Finally, Knudsen *et al.* (2002) found that patients with maculopathy had higher cholesterol levels than those without retinopathy ($p < 0.005$).

### 5.6.2.7. *Renal involvement*

Olivarius *et al.* (2001) in newly diagnosed middle-aged and elderly diabetic patients from a Danish population-based study found that diabetic retinopathy and the urinary albumin/creatinine ratio were strongly positively associated. Similarly, Knudsen *et al.* (2002) found that patients with maculopathy had higher urinary albumin excretion rate than those without retinopathy ($p < 0.001$).

### 5.6.2.8. *Body mass index (BMI)*

Jerneld *et al.* (1985) found, by single logistic regression analysis, a significant correlation ($p < 0.05$) between a high BMI and low prevalence of diabetic retinopathy in patients treated with oral antihypertensive agents, especially in women, probably indicating that obese patients, particularly women with mild diabetes, are less prone to complications. Olivarius *et al.* (2001) in newly diagnosed middle-aged and elderly diabetic patients from a Danish population-based study found that diabetic retinopathy was associated with a high BMI.

### 5.6.2.9. *Cigarette smoking and alcohol*

Klein *et al.* (1983) in a population-base study found no excess risk of retinopathy in smokers or ex-smokers when contrasted with those who never smoke. Sparrow *et al.* (1993) in a population-based study from a city of Leicestershire in the United Kingdom found that non-insulin treated diabetic patients current cigarette smokers had a "marginal" high risk ($p = 0.073$) for retinopathy and maculopathy.

Moss *et al.* (1996) found in longitudinal 4 and 10-year examination population based study that neither smoking status nor pack-years smoked showed a significant association with increased risk in incidence or progression of diabetic retinopathy. They even found, in those not taking insulin, by univariate analysis, a weak protective effect of smoking on the progression to proliferative diabetic retinopathy ($p < 0.05$) that disappeared, however, in the multivariate analysis. Similarly, Moss *et al.* (1992) found that average alcohol consumption was not associated with the prevalence of any retinopathy or proliferative diabetic retinopathy.

### 5.6.2.10. *Physical activity*

A prospective study of 198 subjects suggested that "inadequate exercise" might be related to the development of retinopathy (Rasmiddatta *et al.*, 1998). However, it has been recommended that diabetics with proliferative diabetic retinopathy should avoid anaerobic exercise or any type of exercise that involves straining, jarring, near maximal isometric contractions ore valsalva-type manoeuvres (Aiello *et al.*, 2001).

### 5.6.2.11. *Cataract extraction*

Progression of diabetic retinopathy has been described after intracapsular and extracapsular cataract extraction (Jaffe *et al.*, 1988, 1992; Pollack *et al.*, 1991; Benson *et al.*, 1993) and also after phacoemulsification (Henricsson *et al.*, 1996; Dowler *et al.*, 2000; Mittra *et al.*, 2000). Others have found no significant progression (Wagner *et al.*, 1996; Squirrell *et al.*, 2002; Krepler *et al.*, 2002; Schrey *et al.*, 2002).

## 5.7. Retinopathy, Comorbidity and Mortality

### 5.7.1. Comorbidity

Comorbidity indicates an association between retinopathy and other disorders that is more than coincidental. Patients with diabetic retinopathy have higher risk of: cardiovascular disease, nephropathy and neovascular glaucoma. Patients with type 1 diabetes (Margonato *et al.*, 1986) and with type 2 diabetes (Estacio *et al.*, 1998) with severe diabetic retinopathy have impaired cardiovascular response to exercise and heart attack. Stroke and amputation occurs more frequently in patients with proliferative diabetic retinopathy (Klein *et al.*, 1986).

American type 1 diabetic patients with diabetic nephropathy have a sixfold increase risk of developing proliferative diabetic retinopathy than normoalbuminuric patients (Rossing *et al.*, 1998). Similar findings were noted among Europeans (Esmatjes *et al.*, 1996). Half of all type 1 diabetic patients with proliferative diabetic retinopathy with 10 or more years of duration had concomitant proteinuria (Klein *et al.*, 1986).

Cahill *et al.* (2000), in United Kingdom, in juvenile patients with diabetes of 10 or more years, found no significant association between the prevalence of diabetic retinopathy and microalbuminuria levels.

In Portugal, Genro *et al.* (1987) in an institutional study found a "correlation" between retinopathy and nephropathy in type 1 diabetic patients ($p < 0.001$). Pinto-Figueiredo *et al.* (1992) also found a "close association" between retinopathy and nephropathy ($p < 0.001$).

Jerneld (1988) in a Swedish diabetic population-based study found that serum creatinine concentration was correlated to the degree of retinopathy. Retinopathy was present in 59% of the patients with proteinuria and the percentage of patients with retinopathy increased with higher degrees of proteinuria.

The presence of proteinuria is significantly associated with macular edema in type 1 diabetes ($p < 0.0001$) and in type 2 diabetic insulin-taking patients ($p = 0.041$) (Klein *et al.*, 1984). This association between proteinuria at baseline and the incidence of macular edema was confirmed in a 14-year incidence and progression study of type 1 diabetic patients (Klein *et al.*, 1998).

Nearly all type 1 patients and two third of type 2 patients on dialysis have some form of retinopathy, the majority of which is proliferative diabetic retinopathy (Watanabe *et al.*, 1993).

In a population-based study, Olivarius *et al.* (2001), found that diabetic retinopathy and renal involvement, as expressed by urinary albumin/creatinine ratio, were strongly positively associated.

Overall, it may be stated that association between nephropathy and retinopathy is more clear when in presence of proliferative diabetic retinopathy.

Neovascular glaucoma occurs usually in eyes with more severe forms of retinopathy, in those with proliferative diabetic retinopathy and in those that have had vitrectomy (Klein *et al.*, 2003).

### 5.7.2. Mortality

Cardiovascular disease is the most common cause of death in diabetic patients. About 75% die from coronary heart disease (Chait *et al.*, 1994).

The increased risk of severe retinopathy with cardiovascular disease is consistant with decreased survival over a 5-year period in both younger and older-onset groups. The 5-year survival rate for type 1 diabetes without retinopathy was 99% compared with only 76% for those with proliferative retinopathy and in type 2 the 5-year survival rate was 77%

for those without retinopathy and 53% for those with proliferative diabetic retinopathy (Klein *et al.*, 1989).

Blindness from diabetes is associated with higher mortality than most other causes of blindness (Khan *et al.*, 1974). The 10-year survival for diabetic blind persons, by age at registration, is 21% for men and 23% for women under 65 years age and 17% for men and 14% for women for those with 65 years or more (Rogot *et al.*, 1966). It was found by Helbig *et al.* (1996) that five years after vitreous surgery the survival rate was only 68%.

## 5.8. Health Care Delivery

Most of an estimated of 45 million blind people around the world have lost their sight due to diseases that are treatable or preventable. Vision loss is one of the ten most common causes of disability in the developed world and there is scientific evidence showing that early detection and treatment can prevent much of vision loss. Even in the developed world many diabetics become unnecessarily blind.

Vision loss by retinopathy is a public health problem. Vision loss affects a lot of people, imposes a large burden on individuals and society in terms of morbidity, quality of life and costs. It is a problem that is expected to increase in the future.

In the WESDRS, 25% of younger onset diabetic patients and 36% of older-onset diabetic patients had never had an ophthalmological examination (Witkin *et al.*, 1984).

In the U.S. according to NHIS (1989) of all adults with diabetes, 55% reported that they had not been seen by an ophthalmologist in the past 12 months (Klein *et al.*, 2000).

In the Wisconsin epidemiological study, roughly 1/3 of diabetics had not had an ophthalmic examination in the previous two years (Moss *et al.*, 1994) and in Melbourne nearly half diabetic patients had never had an ophthalmic examination (Lee *et al.*, 1995).

In 1989, the World Health Organization and the European Regional Committee of the International Diabetes Federation held a joint meeting in St. Vincent, Italy. Conclusions were published as the St. Vincent Declaration claiming that it is possible to reduce the progression to blindness by detecting, in due time, sight threatening retinopathy and performing laser treatment. Indeed, an analysis of the combined results of scatter and focal laser treatment shows that with rigorous treatment and follow-up up to 98% of severe vision loss or blindness related to diabetic retinopathy can be prevented or delayed (Ferris, 1993).

There is general agreement that widespread screening to detect those patients who require treatment could substantially reduce the impact of diabetic retinopathy. Such screening has been shown to be feasible.

Diabetic retinopathy fulfils the WHO criteria for a screening programme to detect up to 10% with sight threatening diabetic retinopathy (severe or very severe nonproliferative retinopathy, proliferative retinopathy and clinically significant macular edema). Diabetic retinopathy has a long period of evolution before vision loss, is treatable and screening may be performed by noninvasive, sensitive and specific techniques.

At present, there are two principal screening options: fundoscopy and fundus photography. Ophthalmoscopy is the most commonly used technique to screen for diabetic retinopathy, but the gold standard procedure for the detection and classification of diabetic retinopathy is stereoscopic color fundus photographs in seven standard fields. However, this last technique is labor intensive, time consuming and uncomfortable to the patient. A review of 22 cohort screening studies concluded that nonmydriatic retinal 45° photography provides the most effective screening procedure for sight-threatening retinopathy (Hutchinson *et al.*, 2000). Two digital photographies compared well with sensitivity > 80% and specificity of > 92%, against seven fields stereophotography (Scanlon *et al.*, 2003). The use of mydriatics improved the sensitivity of nonmydriatic cameras (Jones *et al.*, 1988; Ryder *et al.*, 1991; Lairson *et al.*, 1992; Pugh *et al.*, 1993). Murgatroyd *et al.* (2004) found that mydriasis reduces the proportion of ungradable photographs from 26% to 5% /$p < 0.001$). There are available digital cameras capable of producing instantaneous 45°–50° photos of the retina allowing immediate assessment of their quality. Digital image is considered superior for detecting retinopathy, considering advantages regarding storage, accessibility, image enhancement and analysis (George *et al.*, 1998). Digitized systems offer the possibility of central assessment by electronically transferring to remote Reading Centers, facilitating the screening of large numbers of patients. Sensitivity for detection of sight threatening retinopathy — clinically significant macular edema and proliferative retinopathy — is respectively 87% and 100% and specificity 96%, although there is the possibility of missing severe nonproliferative diabetic retinopathy beyond the standard of field 45° photography (Ryder *et al.*, 1991).

It is possible to use 2–3 field nonstereo-photos as used in Liverpool and Coimbra (James *et al.*, 2000; Faria de Abreu *et al.*, 2003).

According to Saari *et al.* (2004) digital red-free black and white imaging is more sensible and has higher specificity than digital color to detect mild nonproliferative diabetic retinopathy. Microaneurysms and IRMAS were more clearly visualized.

The European Retinopathy Working Party recommended examinations at least every two years after diagnosis and at least yearly or more if retinopathy developed. The American Diabetes Association advised yearly or more frequent intervals in type 2 patients and the American Academy of Ophthalmology recommended yearly screening for no or minimum retinopathy and 6–12 months for more severe retinopathy. The United Kingdom National screening guidelines indicate a screening every 2–3 years for those with no retinopathy (Younis *et al.*, 2003).

## 5.8.1. Economy

In 1970, the total health care expenditure in the U.S. was approximately US$73,1 billion or 7% of the gross domestic product (GDP). With health care costs rising due to the advent of new technologies, in the year 2001 the total costs in health care had risen to US$1,425 billion or 14.1% of the GDP (Brown *et al.*, 2004).

Medical care may be an effective societal investment rather than merely a public expense and become increasingly financed by corporate and government entities with costs and gains having expanding significance in legislative policy decisions. It is clearly necessary to inform health authorities of the potential savings that can be achieved by early treatment of diabetic retinopathy. All resources from publicly and privately funded healthcare schemes worldwide are finite, so all healthcare financing systems operate under some form of budgetary constraint. The limited availability of resources and the impossibility to satisfy all our desires and wants implies that choices must be constantly made. The value of a resource must be the best for the society in order to gain broad acceptance by legislative and regulatory agencies. There is a clear need of an information system to compare the value (improvement in length of life and/or quality of life) on different medical interventions to the patient for the resources available.

Economy is the science of making choices between different resources allocation pathways. Consequently, the drive to allocate resources in the most efficient and effective manner is imperative.

Health economists developed models that simulate patients with diabetes from diagnosis to dead, including the occurrence of progressive complications, such as nephropathy, retinopathy and neuropathy.

The economic and social costs of visual impairment must be considered from the perspective of the disabled individual and the country as a whole. A person who is blind and his or her family faces important constraints.

### 5.8.1.1. *Identification of costs of screening and treatment*

*Costs of a Health Programme*

Health system costs or direct costs are those associated with organization and operating costs within the health sector including graders, clinical assistance, photographers, auxillary nurses, clerical workers, film, medical and surgical (drops, sundries, etc.), capital charges and depreciation, van, camera, computer, camera maintenance, petrol, overheads and external quality control.

Costs of systematic screening in Liverpool using three nonstereo photos was £21.00 per patient/per year. The cost effectiveness, total costs of screening divided by the number of cases detected is £209.00 per year (Broadbent *et al.*, 1999). Javitt *et al.* (1989) calculated the charges of screening (US$62) and photocoagulation treatment of both eyes (US$1980) for a total of US$2042.

*Patient-based costs*

Costs born by patients and their families are expenses, patient and family input into treatment, time lost from work and "physical costs" attributed to pain and suffering and non-medical costs, such as transportation, ancillary workers, homecare workers and other out of pocket expenses.

*Costs of illness and visual impairment*

Cost of illness is the measure of the economic burden due to a given disease, such as lost productivity and medical expenses for its treatment.

In the U.S. the annual federal budgetary costs for diabetic type 1 blind patients, younger than 65 years, in 1990 prices, was calculated as US$15,205, including US$6615 in combined Social Security Disability Insurance (SSDI) and Social Security Insurance (SSI) payments, US$150 in tax expenditures, US$3204 in tax losses and US$5236 in Medicare and Medicaid payments.

These costs do not take into account costs associated with rehabilitation, welfare or other expenditures incurred at the state or local level.

Federal expenditure with blindness in patients with 65 years or older has been estimated at $484 per year. The annual costs for visual impairment have been estimated at 50% of the value associated with blindness (Javit *et al.*, 1989, 1991).

### 5.8.1.2. *Quality of life*

Clinical activities should have a positive impact on how a person functions and lives. This concept has been referred to as health-related quality of life, health state or functional state. Questionnaires have been developed to measure patients' quality of life.

The Center for Eye Research in Australia (Lamoureux *et al.*, 2004), for example, has developed a questionnaire — The Impact Vision Impairment — IVI — that measures patients' quality of life in function of the person restriction of participation in daily activities, in 32 items under five domains: leisure and work, consumer and social interaction, household and personal care (the least restrictive in diabetic patients), mobility and emotional reaction to vision loss.

The cost estimates to improve the quality of life vary widely from country to country. Physical and psychosocial implications of visual impairment cannot be accurately quantified in monetary terms. It is necessary to translate the cost of a benefit into a monetary unit, to measure costs per unit of health effect.

The Euro-QOL (quality of life) uses five parameters: mobility, self-care, usual activity, pain and anxiety/depression. Within each of these parameters there are three levels: 1 — some, 2 — moderate, 3 — severe. Using a combination of these parameters there are a total of 243 possible health states.

Utility value evaluates "objectively" the quality of life. In essence, the measurement of a utility value allows the degree of a patient's impairment, in regard to functioning in everyday activities of life, caused by health state. By convention, a utility value of 1.0 implies a perfect health state and the closer the utility value is to 1.0, the better a person can function in the activities of daily life, whereas a utility state of 0.0 signifies death and the closer to 0.0 the more difficulty a person has in dealing with the activities of life.

Utilities can be assessed by different methods:

(a) Time trade-off (TTO). The number of years a patient willing to trade in return to improved quality of life divided by estimated number of years of remaining life.

    Utility value = 1 – Time trade/time of remaining of life.

(b) Standard gamble (SG). A patient is asked to suppose that there is a technology that can return his eyesight to normal in both eyes for the rest of his life, but that this technology has a risk of death. So results are death or perfect vision.

What is the highest risk of death (%) that any patient is willing to accept before refusing the treatment in return to a perfect health state.

Utility value = 1 – risk of death (%) the patient is willing to assume in return to normal.

Vision loss by diabetic retinopathy is associated with a substantial decrease in a patient's quality of life. Utility values were calculated by Brown *et al.* (1999) in 100 consecutive diabetic patients with retinopathy and according to visual acuity in the better eye. Utility value was evaluated in five groups by both methods (Table 5.15).

Using TTO, patients in group 1 were willing to trade 15% of their remaining years of life in return to perfect vision, but patients in the group 5 traded 41% of their remaining years of life in return to perfect vision. There was no difference in the degree of education (+ or – than 12th grade education) and no difference between genders. With SG, however, men considered to have significantly less quality of life with the same acuity ($p = 0.005$).

**Table 5.15  Utility Values for Visual Loss Due to Diabetic Retinopathy**

| Best Corrected VA in the Better Eye | TTO | SG |
|---|---|---|
| Group 1 — 20/20–20/25 (10/10–8/10) | 0.85 | 0.90* |
| Group 2 — 20/30–20/50 (7/10–4/10) | 0.78 | 0.92** |
| Group 3 — 20/60–20/100 (3/10–2/10) | 0.78 | 0.84* |
| Group 4 — 20/200–20/400 (1/10–0.5/10) | 0.64 | 0.71* |
| Group 5 — < 20/400 (<0.5/10) | 0.59 | 0.70* |

*p - NS
**p < 0.000008

### 5.8.1.3.  *Health care economic analyses*

Prevention programmes may improve eye care with substantial public budgetary savings. There are several types of economic analysis in health care.

Cost-benefit analysis measure both costs and outcomes of alternative intervention in terms of resources. Experience in a Denmark community, for example, suggested that the savings associated with preventing just one case of blindness during the first year of a systemic screening would almost pay for the cost of the entire screening programme (Williams, 1999).

Cost-effectiveness analysis relies on the calculation of both costs and effectiveness of heath care intervention in the same monetary unit. It is necessary to translate the cost of a benefit into a monetary unit to measure costs per unit of health effect. Cost-effectiveness ratio is a measure of the cost per unit of sight years saved from vision loss and blindness or the cost for each diabetic screened and treated and the benefit calculated by utilities values.

Cost-utility analysis is the most sophisticated. It measures resources (cost of screening and therapy in dollars) spent for the total value gained from an intervention, quantified "objectively" as the degree of a patient benefit (utility) and the length of the rest of life (years), The Quality Adjust Life Years — QALY; the Handicap Adjust Life Year — HALI; the Disability Adjust Life Year — DALY.

Quality-adjusted life years is an utility value conferred by a medical intervention in screening and therapy multiplied by the number of years over which that therapy has a beneficial effect. The results are expressed using cost per quality-adjusted life-years — $/QALY.

Example, if utility value increased with laser treatment from 0.6 (no treatment) to 0.8 (laser treatment) there is a 0.2 gradation improvement. If a patient has a life expectancy of 30 years, the number of QALY gained would be 30 × 0.2-6.

Treatment costs and effectiveness (QALY) can be applied to arrive at a measure of cost-effectiveness (dollars expended per quality adjusted life years). Individuals with diabetes have a QALY estimated at 0.85 but if they had severe visual loss is 0.59 (Smith, 2000).

Rehabilitation also has costs and benefits. Drummond (1987) estimated that a year of blindness for well adjusted rehabilitated corresponds to 0.48 QALY and for the poorly adjusted after rehabilitation efforts corresponds to 0.36 QALY.

Screening and treatment of eye disease in patients with diabetes mellitus US costs $3190 per QALY saved.

### 5.8.1.4.  *Cost-effectiveness in diabetic retinopathy*

Several simulation models calculate the total years of sight loss, moderate or severe, with and without treatment when both eyes are affected. Despite appropriate screening and laser treatment at the earliest indication the model predicts that ultimately 28% will suffer severe visual loss (SVL) vs 54% if no treatment is administrated.

The model predicts that 22% of patients will suffer a doubling of their visual angle from macular edema compared with 34% of those without treatment.

The total QALY from person-year in diabetic retinopathy was calculated in type 1 to be US$1996/QALY (Javitt, 1996), in type 2 noninsulin taker, US$2933/QALY (Javitt, 1996) and in type 2 insulin treated, $3530/QALY (Javitt, 1996).

**Table 5.16   Cost-Effectiveness of Screening and Treatment of Diabetic Retinopathy**

| | (1) Cost of Screening and Treatment per Person/Year of Saved Sight | (2) Cost of Screening and Treatment per QALY for the Average Person |
|---|---|---|
| All diabetics | US$1557 | US$3190 |
| IDDM | US$1099 | US$1996 |
| No IDDM | US$1839 | US$3339 |
| Insulin | US$1616 | US$2933 |
| Non-insulin | US$1944 | US$3530 |

Health interventions, which are under US$20000/QALY, are worthy of implementation by society (Laupacics *et al.*, 1992).

If screening and treatments are delivered as recommended, the model predicts an average of four years of sight saved per each patient, who receives panretinal photocoagulation (cost of US$966) and an average of five years benefit to each patient with focal photocoagulation (cost of US$1118).

The annual cost of welfare benefits per patient with severe visual loss due to diabetic retinopathy is nearly seven times the cost per patient per year, far less expensive than to pay the consequences of disability (Javitt *et al.*, 1989).

Using a modeling system based on Monte Carlo techniques of analyse is events and costs incurred during the lifetime course of Americans who developed type 1 diabetes, US$101 millions are annually saved by screening programmes (Javitt *et al.*, 1991).

Maberley *et al.* (2003) from data of a screening program in Western James Bay area of Northern Ontario, using Monte Carlo modeling to generate probability distribution, calculated the cost per year vision saved as US$3900 and over 10 years as US$15,000.

Average Medicare charges in 1990 are increasingly becoming the basis for medical care reimbursement for indemnity and managed care insurance plans. Even from a health insurer's perspective, screening and treating diabetic retinopathy are cost-effective according to two methods (Table 5.16).

Prevention programmes for blindness due to diabetic retinopathy are cost-effective, because early detection and treatment prevent visual impairment and the costs managing the effects of severe visual loss can be effectively reduced.

According to the American Diabetes Association (1998) screening for diabetic retinopathy saves vision at a relatively low cost, and even this cost is often less than the disability payments provided to people who would go blind in the absence of screening programmes (Younis *et al.*, 2003).

# References

Aiello LP, Cahill MT. (2001) Systemic considerations in the management of diabetic retinopathy. *Am J Ophthalmol* **132**: 770–776.

American Diabetes Association. (1998) Diabetic retinopathy. *Diabetes Care* **21**: 157–160.

Anderson S, Broadbent DM, Swain JYS, *et al.* (2003) Ambulatory photographic screening for diabetic retinopathy in nursing homes. *Eye* **17**: 711–717.

Angioi-Duprez K, Gresset J, Olivier S, *et al.* (2002) Are non-mydriatic cameras a valuable tool for diabetic retinopathy screening. The Montreal HMR Centre results. *Eur J Ophthalmol* **12**: 161.

Angioi-Duprez K, Maalouf T, Boucher MC. (2002) Opinion of French ophthalmologists on screening for diabetic retinopathy and the use of non-mydriatic cameras: A nation-wide survey. *Eur J Ophthalmol* **12**: 162.

Aroca R, Dejardin DC. (1996) Estudio de prevalencia de retinopatía diabética en la población del Baix Camp (Tarragona). *Arch Soc Esp Oftalmol* **71**: 261–268.

Arun CS, Ngugi N, Lovelock L, Taylor E. (2003) Effectiveness of screening in preventing blindness due to diabetic retinopathy. *Diabet Med* **20**: 186–190.

Backlund LB, Algreve PV, Rosenqvist U. (1995) Five-year incidence of new blindness in diabetes reduced by one third in an urban region. In: Proceedings of EASD 31th annual meeting. European Association for the Study of Diabetes.

Backlund LB, Algreve PV, Rosenqvist U. (1997) New blindness in diabetes reduced by more than one third in Stockholm County. *Diabetes Care* **14**: 732–740.

Bailey C. (2001) Screening for diabetic retinopathy. Focus Issue 15, Summer 2001.

Batcelder T, Barricks M. (1995) The Wisconsin Epidemiological Study of Diabetic Retinopathy. *Am J Ophthalmol* **113**: 702–703.

Bek T, Lauszus F, Klebe JG. (2002) Diabetic retinopathy in pregnancy during tight metabolic control. *Eur J Ophthalmol* **12**: 142.

Benson WE, Brown GC, Tasman W, *et al.* (1993) Extracapsular cataract extraction with placement of posterior chamber lens in patients with diabetic retinopathy. *Ophthalmology* **100**: 730–738.

Blankenship GW, Machmer R. (1985) Long-term diabetic vitrectoy results. Report of 10 years follow-up. *Ophthalmology* **92**: 503–506.

Boivin JF, McGregor M, Archer C. (1996) Cost effectiveness of screening for primary open angle glaucoma. *J Med Screening* **3**: 154–163.

Brahams D. (1992) Medicine and the law: Eye monitoring in diabetes. *Lancet* **339**: 863–864.

Broadbent DM, Scott JA, Vora JP, Harding SP. (1999) Prevalence of diabetes eye disease in an inner-city population; The Liverpool diabetic eye study. *Eye* **13**: 160–165.

Brown MM, Brown GC, Sharma S, Shah G. (1999) Utility values and diabetic retinopathy. *Am J Ophthalmol* **128**: 324–330.

Brown GC, Brown MM, Shama S. (2004) Heath care economic analyses. *Retina* **24**: 139–146.

Bryden KS, Dunger DB, Mayou RA, *et al.* (2003) Poor prognosis of young adults with type 1 diabetes. *Diabetes Care* **26**: 1052–1057.

Buch H, Vinding T, Cour M, *et al.* (2004) Prevalence and causes of visual impairment and blindness among 9980 scandinavian adults. The Copenhagen City Eye Study. *Ophthalmology* **111**: 53–61.

Burnett S, Hurwitz B, Davey C, *et al.* (1998) The implementation of prompted retinal screening for diabetic eye disease by accredited optometrists in an inner-city district of North London: A quality of care study. *Diabetic Med* **15**: S38–S43.

Buxton EM, Sculpher MJ, Ferguson B, *et al.* (1991) Screening for treatable diabetic retinopathy: A comparison of different methods. *Diabetic Med* **8**: 371–377.

Cahill M, Wallace D, Travers S, *et al.* (2000) Detection and prevalence of early diabetic retinopathy in juvenile diabetics with diabetes for 10 years or more. *Eye* **14**: 847–850.

Caird FI, Pirie A, Ramsell TG. (1969) Diabetes and the Eye. Blackwell Scientific Publications, Oxford, pp. 72–100.

Caird FI, Burditt AF, Drapper GJ. (1974) Blindness caused by diabetic retinopathy. *Am J Ophthalmol* **78**: 58–67.

Caro JJ, Ward AJ, O'Brien JA. (2002) Lifetime costs of complications resulting from type 2 diabetes in US. *Diabetes Care* **25**: 476–481.

Carvican L, Clowes J, Gillow T. (2000) Preservation of sight in diabetes: Developing a national risk reduction programme. *Diabetic Med* **17**: 627–634.

Cathelineau B, Delcourt C, Jellal M, *et al.* (1993) Epidemiology of ocular complications in diabetes multicentre prospective study (CODIAB). EASDEC, April, 1993.

Cedrone C, Culasso F, Cesareo M, *et al.* (2003) Incidence of blindness in a sample population. The Priverno eye study, Italy. *Ophthalmology* **110**: 584–588.

Cerulli LCC. (1988) Cecitá da diabete e retinopatia diabetica. In: Brancato R, Pozza G (eds.), *La Retinopatia Diabetica*. Milano, pp. 239–249.

Chait A, Bierman EL. (1994) Pathogenesis of macrovascular diseases in diabetes. In: Khan CR, Weier GC (eds.), *Joslin's Diabetes Mellitus*. Lea & Febiger, Philadelphia, pp. 648–664.

Chandran S, Broadbent DM, Younis N, *et al.* (2002) Visual acuity in patients with type 1 diabetes at entry into a systematic eye screening programme: The Liverpool diabetic eye study. *Eur J Ophthalmol* **12**: 160.

Chandran S, Broadbent DM, Younis N, *et al.* (2002) Visual acuity in patients with type 1 diabetes at entry into a systematic eye screening programme: The Liverpool diabetic eye study. *Eur J Ophthalmol* **12**: 161.

Chase HP, Garg SK, Jackson WE, *et al.* (1990) Blood pressure and retinopathy in type 1 diabetes. *Ophthalmology* **97**: 155–159.

Chaturvedi N, Sjolie AK, Stephenson JM, *et al.* (1998) Effect of lisinopril on progression of retinopathy in normotensive people with type 1 diabetes. *Lancet* **351**: 28–31.

Chen M-S, Kao C-S, Chang C-J, *et al.* (1992) Prevalence and risk factors of diabetic retinopathy among noninsulin-dependent diabetic subjects. *Am J Ophthalmol* **114**: 723–730.

Chew EY, Mills JL, Metzger BE, *et al.* (1995) Metabolic control and progression of retinopathy. The diabetes in early pregnancy study. National Institute of Child Health and Human Development Diabetes in Early Pregnancy Study. *Diabetes Care* **18**: 631–637.

Chiang YP, Bassi LJ, Javitt JC. (1992) Federal budgetary costs of blindness. *Milbank Q* **70**: 319–340.

Cohen DL, Neil HAW, Thorogood M, Mann JI. (1991) A population-based study of the incidence of complications associated with type 2 diabetes in elderly. *Diab Med* **8**: 928–933.

Congdon NG. (2001) Prevention strategies for age-related cataract: Present limitations and future possibilities. *Br J Ophthalmol* **85**: 516–520.

Cormack TGM, Grant B, Macdonald MJ, *et al.* (2001) Incidence of blindness due to eye disease in Fife 1990–1999. *Br J Ophthalmol* **85**: 354–356.

Cruickshanks KJ, Moss SE, Klein R, Klein BE. (1992) Physical activity and proliferative retinopathy in people diagnosed with diabetes before age 30 years. *Diabetes Care* **15**: 1267–1272.

Cruickshanks KJ, Moss SE, Klein R, Klein BE. (1995) Physical activity and the risk of progression of retinopathy or the development of proliferative retinopathy. *Ophthalmo-logy* **102**: 1177–1182.

Danielsen D, Jonasson F, Helgason T. (1982) Prevalence of retinopathy and proteinuria in type 1 diabetics in Iceland. *Acta Med Scand* **212**: 277–280.

Dane T, Kordonouri O, Hovener G, Weber B. (1977) Diabetic angiopathy in children. *Diabet Med* **14**: 1012–1025.

Dasbach EJ, Frybach DG, Newcomb PA, *et al.* (1991) Cost effectiveness of strategies for detecting diabetic retinopathy. *Med Care* **29**: 20–39.

Deckert T, Simonsen SE, Poulsen JE. (1967) Prognosis of proliferative retinopathy in juvenile diabetics. *Diabetes* **16**: 728–733.

Delcourt C, Villatte-Cathelineau B, Vauzelle-Kervroedan F, *et al.* (1995) Visual impairment in type 2 diabetic patients. *Acta Ophthalmol Scand* **73**: 293–298.

Dimitrov PN, Mukesh BN, McCarty MA, Taylor HR. (2003) Five-year incidence of bilateral cause-specific visual impairment in the Melbourne visual impairment project. *Invest Ophthalmol Vis Sci* **44**: 5075–5081.

Direcção Geral dos Cuidados de Saúde Primários. (1991) Divisão de saúde dos adultos. Rastreio da retinopatia diabética no concelho do Cartaxo. Abril/Maio.

Dorchy H, Claes C, Verougstraete C. (2002) Risk factors of developing proliferative diabetic retinopathy in type 1 diabetic patients. *Diabetes Care* **24**: 789–799.

Dornan T, Mann JI, Turner R. (1982) Factors protective against retinopathy in insulin-dependent diabetics free of retinopathy for 30 years. *Br Med J* **285**: 1073–1077.

Donaghue KC, Fairchild JM, Craig ME, *et al.* (2003) Do all prepubertal years of diabetic duration contribute equally to diabetes complications. *Diabetes Care* **26**: 1224–1229.

Dowler JG, Hykin PG, Hamilton AM. (2000) Phacoemulsification versus ECCE in patients with diabetes. *Ophthalmology* **107**: 457–462.

Drummond M: Consultant Report to the National Eye Institute. (1987) Available from National Eye Institute, Building 31, Room 6A-06, Bethesda, MD 20892.

Dwyer MS, Melton III LJ, Ballard DJ, *et al.* (1985) Incidence of diabetic retinopathy and blindness: A population-based study in Rochester, Minnesota. *Diabetes Care* **8**: 316–322.

Ellewein LB, Urato CJ. (2002) Use of eye care and associated charges among the Medicare populations. *Arch Ophthalmol* **120**: 804–811.

Esmatjes E, Castell C, Gonzalez T, *et al.* (1996) Epidemiology of renal involvement in type II (NIDDM) in Catalonia. The Catalan Diabetic Nephropathy Study Group. *Diabetes Res Clin Pract* **32**: 157–163.

Estacio RO, Regensteiner JG, Wolfel EE, *et al.* (1998) The association between diabetic complications and exercise capacity in NIDDM patients. *Diabetes Care* **21**: 291–295.

Estacio RO, Jeffers BW, Gifford N, Schriet RW. (2000) Effect of blood pressure control on diabetic microvascular complications in patients with hypertension and type 2 diabetes. *Diabetes Care* **23**(Suppl. 2): B54–B64.

Fahal H, Minassian D, Sowa S, Foster A. (1989) National survey of blindness and low vision in the Gambia: Results. *Br J Ophthalmol* **73**: 82–87.

Faria de Abreu JR, Silva R, Cunha-Vaz JG. (1994) The blood retinal barrier in diabetes during puberty. *Arch Ophthalmol* **112**: 1334–1338.

Fernandez-Vigo J, Macho JS, Rey AD, *et al.* (1993) The prevalence of retinopathy in Northwest Spain. *Acta Ophthalmol* **71**: 22–26.

Ferris LL. (1993) How effective are treatments for diabetic retinopathy. *JAMA* **269**: 1290–1291.

Flack AAK, Kaar M-L, Laatikainen LT. (1993) Prevalence and risk factors of retinopathy in children with diabetes. A population-based study on Finnish children. *Acta Ophthalmol* **71**: 801–809.

Fong DS, Sharza M, Chen W, *et al.* (2002) Vision loss among diabetics in a group model health maintenance organization (HMO). *Am J Ophthalmol* **133**: 236–241.

Foster A, Johnson G. (1990) Magnitude and causes of blindness in the developing world. *Int Ophthalmol* **14**: 135–140.

Gaede P, Vedel P, Parving H-H, Pedersen O. (1999) Intensified multifactorial intervention in patients with type 2 diabetes mellitus and microalbuminuria: The Steno type 2 randomised study. *Lancet* **353**: 617–622.

Genro V, Laires R, Vinagre MM, *et al.* (1987) Análise de 1082 diabéticos observados consecutivamente no departamento de prevenção e controlo da retinopatia diabética da Associação Protectora dos Diabéticos de Portugal. *Rev Soc Port Oftalmol* XIII: 37–44.

George LD, Halliwell M, Hill R, *et al.* (1998) A comparison of digital image and 35 mm colour transparencies in detecting and grading diabetic retinopathy. *Diab Med* **15**: 250–253.

Gillow JT, Gray JA. (2001) The national screening committee review of diabetic retinopathy screening. *Eye* **15**: 1–2.

Goldstein DE, Blinder KJ, Ide CH, *et al.* (1993) Glycemic control and development of retinopathy in young-onset insulin dependent diabetes mellitus. Results of a 12-year longitudinal study. *Ophthalmology* **100**: 1125–1132.

Grey RHB, Burns-Cox CJ, Hughes A. (1989) Blindness and partial sight registration in Avon. *Br J Ophthalmol* **73**: 88–94.

Hansson-Lumdblad C, Holm K, Agardh C-D, Agardh E. (2002) A small number of older type 2 diabetic patients end up visual acuity impaired despite regulat photographic screening and laser treatment for diabetic retinopathy. *Acta Ophthalmol Scand* **80**: 310–315.

Hapnes R, Bergrem H. (1996) Diabetic eye complications in a medium sized municipality in southwest Norway. *Acta Ophthalmol* **74**: 497–500.

Harding SP, Broadbent DM, Neoh C, *et al.* (1995) Sensitivity and specificity of photography and direct ophthalmoscopy in screening for sight threatening eye disease: The Liverpool diabetic eye study. *Br Med J* **311**: 1131–1135.

Helbig H, Kellner U, Bornfeld N, Foerster MH. (1996) Life expectancy of diabetics patient undergoing vitreous surgery. *Br J Ophthalmol* **80**: 640–643.

Henricsson M, Heijl A, Janzon L. (1996) Diabetic retinopathy before and after cataract surgery. *Br J Ophthalmol* **80**: 789–793.

Henricsson M, Nilsson A, Groop L, *et al.* (1996) Prevalence of diabetic retinopathy in relation to age of onset of diabetes, treatment, duration and glycemic control. *Acta Ophthalmol Scand* **74**: 523–527.

Henricsson M, Tyrberg M, Heijl A, Janzon L. (1996) Incidence of blindness and visual impairment in diabetic patients participating in an ophthalmological control and screening programme. *Acta Ophthalmol Scand* **74**: 533–538.

Henricsson M, Nystrom L, Blohmé G, *et al.* (2003) The incidence of retinopathy after diagnosis in young adult people with diabetes. Result from the nationwide population-based diabetes incidence study in Sweden (DISS). *Diabetes Care* **26**: 349–354.

Herbert HM, Jordan K, Flanagan DW. (2003) Is screening with digital imaging using one retinal view adequate? *Eye* **17**: 497–500.

Hirvela H, Laatikainen L. (1997) Diabetic retinopathy in people aged 70 years or older. The Oulu eye study. *Br J Ophthalmol* **81**: 214–217.

Houston A. (1982) Retinopathy in the Poole area: An epidemiological study inquiry. In: Eschwege E (ed.), *Advances in Diabetes Epidemiology*. Elsevier, Amsterdam, pp. 199–206.

Hove MN, Kristensen JK, Lauritzen T, Bek T. (2004) The prevalence of retinopathy in an unselected population of type 2 diabetic patients from Arhus County, Denmark. *Acta Ophthalmol Scan* **82**: 443–448.

Hovind P, Tarnow L, Rossing P, *et al.* (2002) Decreasing incidence of diabetic retinopathy and proliferative retinopathy in type 1 diabetes. *Eur J Ophthalmol* **12**: 142.

Hovind P, Tarnow L, Rossing K, *et al.* (2003) Decreasing incidence of severe diabetic microangiopathy in type 1 diabetes. *Diabetes Care* **26**: 1258–1264.

Hutchinson A, McIntosh A, Peters J, *et al.* (2000) Effectiveness of screening and monitoring tests for diabetic retinopathy — a systematic review. *Diab Med* **17**: 495–506.

Icks A, Trautner C, Haastert B, *et al.* (1997) Blindness due to diabetes: Population based age and sex specific incidence rates. *Diab Med* **14**: 571–575.

Jackson W. (2002) Improving diabetic retinopathy screening. *Diabetes Care* **8**: 1477–1478.

Jaffe GJ, Burton TC, Kuhn E, *et al.* (1992) Progression of non-proliferative diabetic retinopathy and visual outcome after extracapsular cataract extraction and intraocular lens implantation. *Am J Ophthalmol* **114**: 448–456.

James M, Turner DA, Broadbent DM, *et al.* (1989) Cost effectiveness analysis screening for sight threatening diabetic eye disease. *Br Med J* **320**: 1627–1631.

Javitt JC, Canner JK, Sommer A. (1989) Cost effectiveness of current approaches to control of retinopathy in type 1 diabetics. *Ophthalmology* **96**: 255–264.

Javitt JC, Aiello LP, Bassi LJ, *et al.* (1991) Detecting and treating retinopathy in patients with type 1 diabetes mellitus. Savings associated with improved implementation of current guidelines. *Ophthalmology* **98**: 1565–1574.

Javitt JC, Aiello LP. (1996) Cost-effectiveness of detecting and treating diabetic retinopathy. *Ann Inter Med* **124**: 164–169.

Jerneld B, Algevere P. (1984) Prevalence of retinopathy in insulin-dependent juvenile–onset diabetes mellitus — A fluorescein-angiographic study. *Acta Ophthalmol* **62**: 617–630.

Jerneld B, Algevere P. (1985) Prevalence of retinopathy in diabetes mellitus treated with oral antihyperglycaemic agents. *Acta Ophthalmol* **63**: 535–540.

Jerneld B, Algevere P. (1985) Relationship of duration and onset of diabetes to prevalence of diabetic retinopathy. *Am J Ophthalmol* **102**: 431–437.

Jerneld B, Algevere P. (1987) Visual acuity in a diabetic population. *Acta Ophthalmol* **65**: 170–177.

Jerneld B. (1988) Prevalence of diabetic retinopathy. A population study from the swedish island of Gotland. *Acta Ophthalmol* **118**: 66.

Jones D, Dolben J, Owens DR, *et al.* (1988) Non-mydriatic Polaroid photography in screening diabetic retinopathy: evaluation in clinical setting. *BMJ* **296**: 1029–1030.

Khan HA, Hiller R. (1974) Blindness caused by diabetic retinopathy. *Am J Ophthalmol* **78**: 58–67.

Klein R, Moss SE, Klein BEK, Demots DL. (1989) Relation of ocular and systemic factors to survival in diabetes. *Arch Intern Med* **149**: 266–272.

Klein R, Klein BEK, Davies MD. (1983) Is cigarette smoking associated with diabetic retinopathy? *Am J Epidemiol* **118**: 228–238.

Klein R, Klein BEK, Moss SE, *et al.* (1984) The Wisconsin epidemiologic study of diabetes retinopathy. II Prevalence and risk of diabetic retinopathy when age at diagnosis is less than 30 years. *Arch Ophthalmol* **102**: 520–526.

Klein R, Klein BEK, Moss SE, *et al.* (1984) The Wisconsin epidemiologic study of diabetes retinopathy. III Prevalence and risk of diabetic retinopathy when age at diagnosis is 30 or more years. *Arch Ophthalmol* **102**: 527–532.

Klein R, Klein BEK, Moss SE. (1985) A population-based study of diabetes retinopathy in insulin-using patients diagnosed before 30 years of age. *Diabetes Care* **8**: 71–76.

Klein R, Klein BEK, Moss SE *et al.* (1986) The Wisconsin epidemiological study of diabetic retinopathy: V. Proteinuria and retinopathy in a population of diabetic persons diagnosed prior to 30 years of age. In: Friedman EA, L'Esperance Jr FA (eds.), *Diabetic Renal-Retinal Syndrome 3*, Grune & Stratton, Orlando.

Klein R, Moss SE, Klein BEK, *et al.* (1989) Relation of ocular and systemic factors to survival in diabetes. *Arch Int Med* **149**: 266–272.

Klein BEK, Moss SE, Jlein R, Surawicz TS. (1991) The Wisconsin Epidemiologic Study of diabetic retinopathy XII. Relationship of serum cholesterol to retinopathy and hard exudates. *Ophthalmology* **98**: 1261–1265.

Klein R, Klein BEK, Moss SE, Linton KLP. (1992) The Beaver Dam eye study. Retisnopathy in adults with newly discovered and previously diagnose diabetes retinopathy. *Ophthalmology* **99**: 58–62.

Klein R, Klein BEK, Moss SE. (1992) The epidemiology of proliferative diabetic retinopathy. *Diabetes Care* **15**: 1875–1891.

Klein R, Klein BEK, Jensen SC, Moss SE. (1994) The relation of socio-economic factors to the incidence of proliferative diabetic retinopathy and loss of vision. *Ophthalmology* **101**: 68–76.

Klein R, Klein BEK, Moss SE, Cruickshanks KJ. (1994) The Wisconsin epidemiologic study of diabetic retinopathy: XIV. Ten-year incidence and progression of diabetic retinopathy. *Arch Ophthalmol* **112**: 1217–1228.

Klein R, Klein BEK, Moss SE, Cruickshanks KJ. (1995) The Wisconsin epidemiologic study of diabetic retinopathy: XV. The long term incidence of macular edema. *Ophthalmology* **102**: 7–16.

Klein R, Klein BEK, Lee KE, Cruickshanks KJ. (1996) The incidence of hypertension in insulin dependent diabetes. *Arch Inter Med* **156**: 622–627.

Klein R, Klein BEK, Moss SE, Cruickshanks KJ. (1998) The Wisconsin epidemiologic study of diabetic retinopathy: XVII. The 14-year incidence and progression of diabetic retinopathy and associated risk factors in type 1 diabetes. *Ophthalmology* **105**: 1801–1815.

Klein R, Klein BEK. (2000) Epidemiology of eye disease in diabetes. In: Flyn HW, Smiddy WE (eds.), *Diabetes and Ocular Disease. Past, Present and Future Therapies.* The Foundation of the American Academy of Ophthalmology, San Francisco, pp. 19–67.

Klein BEK, Klein R. (2003) Diabetic Retinopathy. In: Johnson GJ, Minassian DC, Weale RA, West SK (eds.), *The Epidemiology of Eye Disease*, 2nd ed. Oxford, University Press, Oxford, Chap. 20, pp. 341–355.

Kokur I, Resnikoff S. (2002) Visual impairment and blindness in Europe and their prevention. *Br J Ophthalmol* **86**: 716–722.

Knowles HC, Guest GM, Lampe J, *et al.* (1965) The course of juvenile diabetes treated with unmeasured diet. *Diabetes* **14**: 239–273.

Knudsen ST, Bek T, Poulsen PL, *et al.* (2002) Macular edema reflects generalized vascular hypermeability in type 2 diabetic patients with retinopathy. *Eur J Ophthalmol* **12**: 145.

Kristinsson JK, Stéfansson E, Jónasson F, *et al.* (1994) Systematic screening for diabetic eye disease in insulin dependent diabetes. *Acta Ophthalmol* **72**: 72–78.

Kristinsson JK, Stéfansson E, Jónasson F, *et al.* (1994) Screening for eye disease in type 2 diabetes mellitus. *Acta Ophthalmol* **72**: 341–346.

Krolewski AS, Warram JH, Cupples A, *et al.* (1985) Hypertension, orthostatic hypotension and microvascular complications of diabetes. *J Chron Dis* **38**: 319–326.

Krolewski AS, Laffel LMB, Krolewski M, *et al.* (1995) Glycosylated hemoglobin and the risk of microalbuminuria in patients with insulin-dependent diabetes mellitus. *N Engl J Med* **332**: 1251–1255.

Kullberg CE, Finnstrom K, Arnqvist HJ. (1994) Severity of background retinopathy in type 1 diabetes increases with the level of long-term glycated haemoglobin. *Acta Ophthalmol* **72**: 181–188.

Laing SP, Swerdlow AJ, Slater SD, *et al.* (1999) The British diabetic Association cohort study, I: All cause mortality in patients with insulin-treated diabetes. *Diabet Med* **16**: 459–465.

Lairson DR, Pugh JA, Kapadia AS, *et al.* (1992) Cost-effectiveness of alternative methods for diabetic retinopathy screening. *Diabetes Care* **15**: 1369–1377.

Lamoureux EL, Hassel JB, Keeffe JE. (2004) The impact of diabetic retinopathy on participation in daily living. *Arch Ophthalmol* **122**: 84–88.

Larsen N, Godt J, Grunkin M, *et al.* (2003) Automated detection of diabetic retinopathy in a fundus photographic screening population. *Invest Ophthalmol Vis Sci* **44**: 767–771.

Larsen M, Godt J, Larsen N, *et al.* (2003) Automated detection of fundus photographic red lesions in diabetic retinopathy. *Invest Ophthalmol Vis Sci* **44**: 761–766.

Laupacics A, Feeny D, Detsky AS, *et al.* (1992) How attractive does a technology have be to warrant adoption and utilization? Tentative guideline for using clinical and economic evaluation. *Can Med Assoc* **146**: 473–481.

Laursen ML, Moller F, Green A, Sjolie AK. (2002) Incidence of blindness, visual impairment and progression of retinopathy after introducing a screening programme for diabetic retinopathy. *Eur J Ophthalmol* **12**: 159.

Lee PL, Feldman ZW, Ostermann J, *et al.* (2003) Longitudinal prevalence of major eye disease. *Arch Ophthalmol* **121**: 1303–1310.

Leese GP, Ahmed S, Newton RW, *et al.* (1993) Use of mobile screening unit for diabetic retinopathy in rural and urban areas. *Br Med J* **306**: 187–189.

Ling R, Ramsewak V, Taylor D, Jacob J. (2002) Longitudinal study of cohort of people with diabetes screened by the Exter diabetic retinopathy screening program. *Eye* **14**: 140–145.

Maberley D, Walker H, Koushik A, Cruess A. (2003) Screening for diabetic retinopathy in James Bay, Ontario: A cost-effectiveness analysis. *CMAJ* **168**(2): 160–164.

Margonato A, Gerundini P, Vicedomini G, *et al.* (1986) Abnormal cardiovascular response to exercise in young asymptomatic diabetic patients with retinopathy. *Am Heart J* **112**: 554–560.

Marshall G, Gargs SK, Jackson WE, *et al.* (1993) Factors influencing the onset and progression of diabetic retinopathy in subjects with insulin-dependent diabetes mellitus. *Ophthalmology* **100**: 1133–1139.

Marques MM. (1993) Rastreio de Retinopatia diabética no Concelho do Cartaxo. *Rev Port Clin Geral* **10**: 42–49.

Martin C, Fernandez-Vigo J, Fernandez J, *et al.* (1992) Prevalencia de retinopatia diabetica: Estudio comparativo de dos poblaciones no seleccionadas en Galicia y Extremadura. *Arch Soc Españ Oftalmol* **62**: 389–394.

McLeod BK, Thompson JR, Rosenthal AR. (1988) The prevalence of retinopathy in the insulin requiring diabetic patients of an English country town. *Eye* **2**: 424–430.

Minassian DC. (2003) Epidemiological research methods: an outline. In: Johnson GJ, Minassian DC, Weale RA, West SK (eds.), *The Epidemiology of Eye Disease*, 2nd ed. Oxford University Press, Oxford, pp. 31–41.

Mittra RA, Borrillo JL, Dev S, *et al.* (2000) Retinopathy progression and visual outcomes after phacoemulsification in patients with diabetes mellitus. *Arch Ophthalmol* **118**: 912–917.

Moloney JB, Drury MI. (1982) The effect of pregnancy on the natural course of diabetic retinopathy. *Am J Ophthalmol* **93**: 745–756.

Moss SE, Klein R, Klein BEK. (1988) The incidence of visual loss in a diabetic population. *Ophthalmology* **95**: 1340–1348.

Moss SE, Klein R, Klein BEK. (1994) Ten-year incidence of visual loss in a diabetic population. *Ophthalmology* **101**: 1061–1070.

Moss SE, Klein R, Klein BEK. (1994) Ocular factors in the incidence and progression of diabetic retinopathy. *Ophthalmology* **101**: 77–83.

Moss SE, Klein R, Klein BEK. (1996) Cigarette smoking and ten-year progression of diabetic retinopathy. *Ophthalmology* **103**: 1438–1442.

Moss SE, Klein R, Klein BEK. (1998) The 14-year incidence of visual loss in a diabetic population. *Ophthalmology* **105**: 998–1003.

Murgatroyd H, Ellingford A, Cox A, *et al.* (2004) Effect of mydriasis and different field strategies on digital image screening of diabetic eye disease. *Br J Ophthalmol* **88**: 920–924.

Murphy RP, Nanda M, Plotnick L, *et al.* (1990) The relationship of puberty to diabetic retinopathy. *Arch Ophthalmol* **108**: 215–218.

National Eye Health Education Program. (1988) Congressional record, National Department of Labor, Health and Human services, education, and related agencies. *Appropriation Bill* 100–189.

National Society to Prevent Blindness. (1980) Vision problems in US. Data analysis, definitions, data sources, detailed data tables, analysis, interpretations. New York: National Society to Prevent Blindness.

Nielsen MM, Hjollund E. (1978) Smoking and diabetic retinopathy. *Lancet* 533–534.

Nielsen NV. (1982) The prevalence and causes of impaired vision in diabetics. An epidemiological study of diabetes mellitus on the Island of Falster, Denmark. *Acta Ophthalmol* **60**: 677–691.

Nielsen NV. (1984) Diabetic retinopathy I. The course of retinopathy in insulin-treated diabetics. A one year epidemiological cohort study of diabetes mellitus. The Island of Falster, Denmark. *Acta Ophthalmol* **62**: 256–265.

Nielson NV. (1984) Diabetic retinopathy: The course of retinopathy in diabetics treated with oral hypoglycaemic agents and diet regime alone: A one year epidemiological cohort study of diabetes mellitus: The Island of Falster, Denmark. *Acta Ophthalmol* **62**: 266–273.

Nishimura R, LaPorte RE, Dorman JS, *et al.* (2001) Mortality trends in type 1 diabetes: The Allegheny County (Pennsylvania) Registry 1965–1999. *Diabetes Care* **24**: 823–827.

Ohkubo Y, Kishikawa H, Araki E, *et al.* (1995) Intensive insulin therapy prevents the progression of diabetic microvascular complications in Japanese patients with non-insulin dependent diabetes mellitus: A randomised prospective 6-year study. *Diabetes Res Cin Pract* **28**: 103–117.

Olivarius NF, Nielsen NV, Andreasen AH. (2001) Diabetic retinopathy in newly diagnosed middle-aged and elderly diabetic patients. Prevalence and interrelationship with microalbuminuria and triglycerides. *Graefe's Arch Clin Exp Ophthalmol* **239**: 664–672.

Olsen BS, Johannesen J, Sjolie AK, *et al.* and the Danish study group of diabetes in childhood. (1999) Metabolic control and prevalence of microvascular complications in young Danish patients with type 1 diabetes mellitus. *Diabet Med* **16**: 79–85.

Orchard TJ, Dorman JS, Maser RE, *et al.* (1990) Factors associated with avoidance of severe complications after 25 years of IDDM; Pittsburgh epidemiology of diabetes complications study I. *Diabetes Care* **13**: 741–747.

Palmberg P. (1977) Diabetic Retinopathy. *Diabetes* **26**: 703–709.

Pinto-Figueiredo L, Moita J, Genro V, *et al.* (1992) Diabetic retinopathy in a population of 1302 insulin dependent diabetics (IDDM) diagnosed before 30 years of age. *Int Ophthalmol* **16**: 429–437.

Pollack A, Dotan S, Oliver M. (1991) Progression of diabetic retinopathy after cataract extraction. *Br J Ophthalmol* **75**: 547–551.

Porta M, Tomalino MG, Santoro F, *et al.* (1995) Diabetic retinopathy as a cause of blindness in the province of Turin, Northwest Italy in 1967–1991. *Diab Med* **12**: 355–361.

Porta M, Bruno G, Pietragalla G, *et al.* (2001) Decreasing incidence of diabetes-related blindness in working age in the province of Turin. Age-period-cohort analysis of temporal trends in 1968–97. *Diabetologia* **44**(1): 187.

Prasad S, Kamath GG, Jones K, *et al.* (2001) Prevalence of blindness and visual impairment in a population of people with diabetes. *Eye* **13**: 640–643.

Pugh JA, Jacobson JM, Van Heuven WA, *et al.* (1993) Screening for diabetic retinopathy. The wide angle camera. *Diabetes Care* **16**: 889–895.

Rasmidatta S, Khunsuk-Mengrai K, Warunyuwong C. (1998) Risk factors of diabetic retinopathy in non-insulin dependent diabetes mellitus. *J Med Assoc Thai* 169–174.

Retinopathy Working Party. (1991) A protocol for screening for diabetic retinopathy in Europe. *Diab Med* **8**: 263–267.

Reuterving CO, Johansson LT, Wachtmeister L, Stenlund H. (2002) Incidence of blindness in diabetes mellitus. A five-year follow-up. *Eur J Ophthalmol* **12**: 163.

Rodriguez J, Sanchez R, Munoz B, *et al.* (2002) Causes of Blindness and visual impairment in a population-based sample of US Hispanics. *Ophthalmology* **109**: 737–743.

Rogot E. (1965) Survivorship among the age blinds — The New Outlook **29**: 333.

Rogot E, Goldberg ID, Goldstein H. (1966) Survivorship and causes of death among the blinds. *J Chronic Dis* **19**: 179.

Rossing K, Jacobsen P, Rossing P, *et al.* (1998) Improved visual function in IDDM patients with unchanged cumulative incidence of sight-threatening diabetes retinopathy. *Diabetes Care* **21**: 2007–2015.

Roy MS. (2000) Diabetic retinopathy in African Americans with type 1 diabetes: The New Jersey 725.I Methodology, population, frequency of retinopathy and visual impairment. *Arch Ophthalmol* **118**: 97–107.

Roysarkar TK, Gupta A, Dash RJ, Dogra MR. (1993) Effect of insulin therapy on progression of retinopathy in noninsulin-dependent diabetes mellitus. *Am J Ophthalmol* **115**: 569–574.

Ryder REJ, Vira JP, Atica JA, *et al.* (1985) A possible new method to improve the detection of diabetic retinopathy: Polaroid non-mydriatic retinal photography. *BMJ* **291**: 1256–1257.

Ryder REJ, Griffiths H, Moriarty KT, *et al.* (1991) Superimposing retinal photography with a 4 mm pupil camera on existing retinopathy screening services in the diabetic clinic. *Practical Diabetes* **8**: 151–153.

Ryder REJ, Close CF, Gray MD, *et al.* (1994) Fail safe retinopathy detection and categorisation by experienced ophthalmic opticians combining dilated retinal photography with ophthalmoscopy. *Diabetic Med* *11* **2**: S44.

Ryder REJ, Kong N, Bates AS, *et al.* (1998) Instant electronic imaging systems superior to Polaroid as detecting sight-threatening diabetic retinopathy. *Diab Med* **15**: 254–258.

Saari JM, Summanen P, Kievela T, Saari KM. (2004) Sensitivity and specificity of digital retinal images in grading diabetic retinopathy. *Acta Ophthalmol Scand* **82**: 126–130.

Sato Y, Lee Z, Hayashi Y. (2001) Subclassification of preproliferative diabetic retinopathy and glycemic control: Relationship between mean hemoglobin $A_{1C}$ value and development of proliferative diabetic retinopathy. *Jpn J Ophthalmol* **45**: 523–527.

Scanlon PH, Malhotra R, Greenwood RH, *et al.* (2003) Comparison of two reference standards in validating two field mydriatic digital photographs as a method of screening for diabetic retinopathy. *Br J Ophthalmol* **87**: 1258–1263.

Schrey S, Krepler K, Biowski R, Wedrich A. (2002) Midterm visual outcome and progression of diabetic retinopathy following cataract surgery. *Ophthalmologica* **216**: 337–340.

Sebag J, Charles MA, Selam JL. (1993) Effect of insulin therapy on progression of retinopathy in noninsulin-dependent diabetes mellitus. *Am J Ophthalmol* **116**: 516–517.

Singer DE, Nathan DM, Fogel HA, Schachat AP. (1992) Screening for diabetic retinopathy. *Ann Intern Med* **116**: 660–671.

Sjolie AK. (1985) Ocular complications in insulin treated diabetes mellitus. An epidemiological study. *Acta Ophthalmol* **172**: 1–76.

Sjolie AK, Greene A. (1987) Blindness in insulin-treated diabetic patients with age at onset < 30 years. *J Cron Dis* **40**: 215–220.

Sjolie AK, Green A. (1995) Epidemiological surveillance of diabetes related blindness In Proceedings of the XXXII Nordic Congress of Ophthalmology in, Odense.

Sjolie AK, Stephenson J, Aldington S, *et al.* and the EURODIAB IDDM complications study group. (1997) Retinopathy and vision loss in insulin-dependent diabetes in Europe. *Ophthalmology* **104**: 252–260.

Sjolie AK. (2000) Retinopathy screening: The key to prevention. Proceedings of a Round Table Meeting. *Pract Diab Int* **17**(1): S2–S3.

Smith AF, Brown GC. (2000) Understanding cost effectiveness: A detailed review. *Br J Ophthalmol* **94**: 794–798.

Smith SE, Smith SA, Brown PM, *et al.* (1978) Papillary signs in autonomic neuropathy. *BMJ* **2**: 924–927.

Smith SA, Shilling JS, Hull DA, *et al.* (1994) Two year audit of primary care eye screening service in diabetes. *Diabetic Med* **11**(1): S23.

Sommer A, Tielsch JM, Katz J, *et al.* (1991) Racial differences in the cause-specific prevalence of blindness in east Baltimore. *N Eng J Med* **325**: 1412–1417.

Sone H, Okuda Y, Kawakami Y, *et al.* (2005) Progestrone induces vascular endothelial growth factor on retinal pigment epithelium cells in culture. *Life Sci* **59**: 21–25.

Sparrow JM, McLeod BK, Smith TD, *et al.* (1993) The prevalence of diabetic retinopathy and maculopathy and their risk factors in the non-insulin-treated diabetic patients of an English Town. *Eye* **7**: 158–163.

Squirrell D, Bhola R, Bush J, *et al.* (2002) A prospective, case control study of the natural history of diabetic retinopathy and maculopathy after uncomplicated phacoemlsification cataract surgery in patients with type 2 diabetes. *Br J Ophthalmol* **86**: 565–571.

Thompson JR, Du L, Rosenthal AR. (1989) Recent trends in the registration of blindness and partial sight in Leicester. *Br J Ophthalmol* **73**: 95–99.

The Diabetes Control and Complications Trial Research Group. The effect of intensive treatment of diabetes on the development and progression of long-term complications in insulin-dependent diabetes mellitus. *N Eng J Med* **329**: 977–986.

The DCCT. (1998) Early worsening of diabetic retinopathy in the diabetes control and complications trial. *Arch Ophthalmol* **116**: 874–876.

The Diabetes Control and Complications Trial Research Group Epidemiology of diabetes intervention and complications research group. (2000) Retinopathy and nephropathy in patients with type-1 diabetes four years after a trial of intensive therapy. *N Eng J Med* **342**: 381–389.

The Diabetic Retinopathy Study Research Group. (1976) Preliminary report on effects of photocoagulation therapy. *Am J Ophthalmol* **81**: 383–396.

The DCCT Research Group. (1990) Effect of pregnancy on the progression of diabetic retinopathy. *Diabetes Care* **13**: 34–40.

The Eye Disease Prevalence Research Group. (2004) Causes and prevalence of visual impairment among adults in the United States. *Arch Ophthalmol* **122**: 477–485.

Thompson JR, Du L, Rosenthal AR. (1989) Recent trends in the registration of blindness and partial sight in Leicester. *Br J Ophthalmol* **73**: 95–99.

Thylefors B, Negrel AD, Pararajasegaram R, Dadzie KY. (1995) Global data on blindness. *Bull World Health Organization* **73**: 115–121.

Tielsch JM, Sommer A, Witt K, *et al.* and the Baltimore Eye Survey Research Group. (1990) Blindness and visual impairment in an American Urban population. *Arch Ophthalmol* **108**: 286–290.

UK Prospective Diabetes Study (UKPDS) Group. (1998) Intensive blood-glucose control with sulphonylureas or insulin compared with conventional treatment and risk of complications in patients with type 2 diabetes (UKPDS 33). *Lancet* **352**: 837–853.

UK Prospective Diabetes Study Group. (1998) Effect of intensive blood glucose control with metformine on complications of overweight patients with type 2 diabetes (UKPDS 34). *Lancet* **12**: **358**: 854–865.

UK Prospective Diabetes Study Group. (1998) Tight blood pressure control and risks of macrovascular and microvascular complications in type 2 diabetes (UKPDS 38). *BJM* **317**: 708–713.

Vigo JF, Sandez J, Castro J, *et al.* (1991) Etude épidémiologic sur la cécité chez des patients diabétiques. Prévalence dans un étude sur la population de Galicie, Espagne. *Ophtalmologie* **5**: 484–488.

Vijan S, Hofer TP, Hayward RA. (2000) Cost-utility analysis of screening intervals for diabetic retinopathy in patients with type 2 diabetes mellitus. *JAMA* **283**: 889–896.

Vinicor F. (1994) Is diabetes a public health disorder? *Diabetes Care* **17**(1): 22–27.

Wagner T, Knaflic D, Rauber M, *et al.* (1996) Influence of cataract surgery on diabetic eye: A prospective study. *Ger J Ophthalmol* **5**: 79–83.

Watanabe Y, Yuzawa Y, Mizumoto D, *et al.* (1993) Long term follow-up study of 268 diabetic patients undergoing haemodialysis, with special attention to visual acuity and heterogeneity. *Nephrol Dial Transplant* **8**: 725–734.

Warram JH, Manson JE, Krolewski AS. (1995) Glycosylated hemoglobin and the risk of microalbuminuria in patients with insulin-dependent diabetes mellitus (letter). *N Engl J Med* **332**: 1305–1306.

Wilkinson CP, Ferris FL, Klein RE, *et al.* (2003) Proposed international clinical diabetic retinopathy and diabetic macular edema disease severity scales. *Ophthalomology* **40**(9): 1675–1676.

Williams AS. (1999) Visual impairment with diabetes: Estimate of lower and upper limits of prevalence in United States. *Diabetes Educ* **25**: 23–24, 27–28.

Witkin SR, Klein B. (1984) Ophthalmologic care for persons with diabetes. *J Am Assoc* **251**: 2534–2537.

World Health Organization Europe, European Region of International Diabetes Federation. The St Vincent Declaration 1989.

Younis N, Broadbent DM, Vora JP, *et al.* (2003) Incidence of sight-threatening retinopathy in patients with type 2 diabetes in Liverpool Diabetic Eye Study; a co-hort study. *Lancet* **361**: 195–200.

Zhang L, Krzentowski G, Albert A, Levebrte PJ. (2001) Risk of developing retinopathy in diabetes control and complications trial type 1 diabetic patients with good and poor control. *Diabetes Care* **24**: 1273–1279.

# Chapter 6

# Major Clinical Trials on Treatment for Diabetic Retinopathy

**Luisa Ribeiro**

Diabetic retinopathy has been and probably remains one of the four major causes of blindness in the U.S. (Kalin and Hiller, 1974; Kalin and Bradley, 1975).

In its earliest stages, diabetic retinopathy usually has no symptoms. However, there are some retinal lesions that indicate risk of progression to retinopathy and vision loss. The first clinical signs of diabetic retinopathy are microaneurysms. Hemorrhages (intraretinal hemorrhages) result from rupture of microaneurysms, decompensated capillaries and intraretinal microvascular abnormalities. Intraretinal microvascular abnormalities (IRMAs) are preexisting dilated vessels with endothelial cell proliferation that became "shunts" through areas of nonperfusion. IRMAs reveal a severe stage of nonproliferative retinopathy and within a short time frank neovascularization may appear on the surface of the retina or optic disk. Venous caliber abnormalities (venous dilatation, venous beading or loop formation) indicate severe retinal hypoxia.

Proliferative retinopathy is defined by proliferating endothelial cells tubules that grow at or near the optic disk, neovascularization of the disk (NVD), or elsewhere in the retina, neovascularization elsewhere (NVE). Adjacent to these new vessels fibrous tissue often appears.

Patients with high-risk of proliferative diabetic retinopathy (PDR) require immediate laser photocoagulation. One or more of the following lesions characterize high-risk PDR: NVD that is approximately one-quarter to one-third disk area or more in size, NVD less than one-quarter disk area in size if fresh vitreous or preretinal hemorrhage are present, NVE greater than or equal to one-half disk area in size if fresh vitreous or preretinal hemorrhage are present.

## Clinical Trials

Insulin changed the treatment of diabetes and extended the lives of people with this disease. The increased longevity assures more time to develop late complications, such as retinopathy. Vision loss and blindness are real problems, without completely successful means of treatment.

The growing number of people with diabetes who survive long enough to develop retinopathy and the lack of a truly effective treatment justifies the quest for convincing evidence regarding the available therapeutical approaches. The level of evidence that needs to be achieved involves large randomized clinical trials.

In fact, in the last 40 years, verify the effectiveness of the available treatments of diabetic retinopathy, a series of large randomized, multicenter and prospective clinical trials, mainly funded by the National Eye Institute (NEI) of the National Institutes of Health (NIH), were performed in the U.S.

Three randomized clinical trials in particular have given a major contribution to determine the strategies for clinical management of patients with diabetic retinopathy.

The DRS (Diabetic Retinopathy Study) demonstrated the value of panretinal photocoagulation. The ETDRS (Early Treatment Diabetic Retinopathy Study) gave important information about the timing of panretinal laser surgery and demonstrated the importance of focal photocoagulation for clinically significant macular edema (CSME) to reduce the risk of moderate visual loss. The DRVS (Diabetic Retinopathy Vitrectomy Study) provided guidelines for the correct time to consider vitrectomy surgery in diabetic patients and vitreous hemorrhage.

The great importance of metabolic control and the relationship between blood sugar levels and diabetic retinopathy were well demonstrated in large multicenter clinical trials. The Diabetes Control and Complications Trials (DCCT) and the United Kingdom Prospective Diabetes Control and Complications Trials (UKPDS), this last randomized clinical trial showing that blood pressure lowering helps slowing the progression of retinopathy.

The large, multicenter, randomized clinical trials, although restricted by their well-defined design, gave us an important contribution to our understanding regarding many aspects of the treatment of diabetic retinopathy. Appropriate management of diabetic patients can only be achieved after knowing the main recommendations and findings of these clinical trials.

# 6.1. Photocoagulation

Treatments of diabetic retinopathy must be aimed at preventing development and progression of the retinopathy and finally at reducing the risk of blindness. During the 1960s there was no clear tested treatment for diabetic retinopathy, which led with the advent of photocoagulation to the design of two large clinical trials to test the efficacy of photocoagulation on diabetic retinopathy.

## 6.1.1. Diabetic Retinopathy Study (DRS)

The Diabetic Retinopathy Study (DRS) was designed to test whether photocoagulation reduced the occurrence of severe visual loss in patients with either proliferative or severe nonproliferative diabetic retinopathy (Diabetic Retinopathy Study Research Group, 1976; 1978; 1979; 1981a; 1981b).

The 1742 patients enrolled in this clinical trial had one eye randomized to either argon laser or xenon photocoagulation. The major eligibility criteria in the DRS were the following: visual acuity $\geq$ 20/100 in each eye; proliferative diabetic retinopathy in at least one eye or severe nonproliferative diabetic retinopathy in both, and both eyes suitable for photocoagulation.

The major design features were the following: one eye of each patient was randomly assigned to photocoagulation (scatter, panretinal), local (direct confluent treatment of surface new vessels) and focal (for macular edema) as appropriate. The other eye was assigned to follow-up without photocoagulation.

The eye assigned to treatment was then randomly assigned to argon laser or xenon photocoagulation. The DRS conclusively demonstrated that scatter (panretinal) photocoagulation significantly reduces the risk of severe visual loss (SVL), visual acuity < 5/200 at two consecutive completed 4-month follow-up visits from proliferative diabetic retinopathy (PDR), particularly when high-risk PDR is present.

Photocoagulation reduced risk of severe visual loss by 50% or more (SVL).

There were modest risks of a slight loss in visual acuity and visual field loss (these risks were greater with xenon than argon photocoagulation).

Treatment benefits were shown to outweigh risks for eyes with high risk proliferative diabetic retinopathy (50% 5-year rate of SVL in the eyes without treatment was reduced to 20% by treatment).

The DRS showed that scatter laser treatment or xenon light photocoagulation treatment reduced severe visual loss by 50% or more in patients with proliferative diabetic retinopathy (PDR) who had high-risk characteristics.

Indications for Scatter Laser Treatment of PDR were established as the presence of NVD was equal to or greater than that shown in the standard photograph 10A, which is about ¼ to ⅓ disk area in extent with or without vitreous or preretinal hemorrhage and vitreous or preretinal hemorrhage with any NVD (even less than that shown in DRS standard photograph 10A) or hemorrhage with NVE greater than ½ disk area in extent.

After 24 months of follow-up in the DRS, the rates of severe visual loss for eyes with high-risk characteristics in the control group and treated group were 26% and 11%, respectively. Eyes with PDR, but without high-risk characteristics, had a much lower risk of developing severe visual loss by two years in both the control group and the treated group (7% and 3% respectively). These rates were even lower for the eyes with nonproliferative diabetic retinopathy. The side effects of treatment were greater in the xenon group when compared with the argon group.

The DRS demonstrated that some patients may not develop high-risk PDR even after five years of follow-up. However, clinical evaluation must still be used for the decision whether to treat, always according to the recommendations of the results of DRS. There are many factors that have influence on the decision for photocoagulation treatment, such as the degree of retinopathy, poor compliance, course of fellow eye, systemic diseases (renal, hypertension, etc.), pregnancy and pending cataract surgery.

DRS concluded that scatter (panretinal) photocoagulation was an effective treatment for proliferative diabetic retinopathy and demonstrated that 60% of reduction in the development of severe visual loss was obtained for eyes with severe nonproliferative or proliferative retinopathy randomly assigned to scatter photocoagulation compared with eyes assigned to no photocoagulation. Eyes with proliferative retinopathy and vitreous hemorrhage or new vessels on the disk, greater than approximately one fourth to one third disk area, had a high risk of severe visual loss without treatment.

## 6.1.2. Early Treatment Diabetic Retinopathy Study (ETDRS)

The Early Treatment Diabetic Retinopathy Study (ETDRS) is a multicenter collaborative clinical trial sponsored by the National Eye Institute. Its main objective was to evaluate photocoagulation and aspirin treatment in diabetic patients who had mild-to-severe nonproliferative or early proliferative diabetic retinopathy (Diabetic Retinopathy Study Research Group, 1979). The motivation of the study design was based on three questions:

1. When in the course of diabetic retinopathy is it most effective to initiate photocoagulation therapy?
2. Is photocoagulation an effective treatment of macular edema?
3. Is aspirin effective to improve the course of diabetic retinopathy?

The study enrolled 3711 patients with mild-to-severe nonproliferative or early proliferative diabetic retinopathy in both eyes. The major eligibility criteria included: visual acuity ≥ 20/40 (≥ 20/400 if reduction caused by macular edema); mild NPDR to non-high-risk PDR, with or whithout macular edema and both eyes suitable for photocoagulation. The patients were randomly assigned to either aspirin (650 mg per day) or placebo. One eye of each patient was assigned to early argon laser photocoagulation and the other to deferral of photocoagulation. The visits were performed every four months.

Eyes selected to early photocoagulation received one of four different combinations of scatter (panretinal) and focal treatment, depending on retinopathy status at baseline, differing in retinopathy severity and the presence or absence of macular edema (The Early Treatment Diabetic Retinopathy Study Research Group, 1991). The strategies for photocoagulation were established according to the following categories: eyes without macular edema, eyes with macular edema and less severe retinopathy or eyes with macular edema and more severe retinopathy.

The major contributions of ETDRS were the following: focal photocoagulation (direct laser for focal leaks and grid laser for diffuse leaks) reduced the risk of moderate visual loss (doubling of visual angle) by 50% or more and increased the chance of a small improvement in visual acuity; both early scatter with or without focal photocoagulation and deferral were followed by low rates of severe visual loss (5-year rates in deferral subgroups were 2–10%; in early photocoagulation groups these rates were 2–6%); focal photocoagulation should be considered for eyes with clinically significant macular edema.

Scatter (pan retinal) photocoagulation is not indicated for mild to moderate NPDR but should be considered as retinopathy approaches the high-risk stage and usually should not be delayed when the high-risk stage is present.

The ETDRS gave us available information concerning the timing of scatter (pan retinal) laser surgery for advancing diabetic retinopathy and demonstrated that focal photocoagulation for clinically significant macular edema (CSME) reduces the risk of moderate visual loss by 50% or more.

Early treatment, compared with deferral of photocoagulation, was associated with a small reduction in the incidence of severe visual loss (visual acuity less than 5/200 at two consecutive visits) but 5-year rates were low in both the early treatment and deferral group 2.6% and 3.7%, respectively, (Early Treatment Diabetic Retinopathy Study Research Group, 1991).

Adverse effects of scatter photocoagulation were most evident in the months following treatment and were less in eyes assigned to less extensive scatter photocoagulation. This was well demonstrated by visual acuity testing and visual field examinations.

ETDRS results provided important information and demonstrated that for eyes with macular edema focal photocoagulation is effective in decreasing the risk of moderate visual loss but that panretinal photocoagulation is not. The major advantages of focal photocoagulation seem to be the decrease in frequency of persistent macular edema, the possibility to increase the visual acuity only with minor visual field losses. Panretinal photocoagulation should be considered and usually should not be delayed if the eyes are at high-risk of proliferative diabetic retinopathy.

The ETDRS provided all the patients with aspirin or placebo to verify whether the anti-platelet effects of aspirin would affect the microcirculation of the retina and slow the development of proliferative diabetic retinopathy (Early Treatment Retinopathy Study Research Group, 1991). This component of the study showed that aspirin did not affect the progression of retinopathy and/or visual acuity and the drug did not increase the risk of vitreous hemorrhage. On the other hand, the use of aspirin reduced the risk of cardiovascular morbidity and mortality.

Early scatter photocoagulation results from ETDRS demonstrated that early scatter photocoagulation resulted in small reduction in risk of severe visual loss (< 5/200 for at least four months), however, it is not indicated for eyes with mild-to-moderate diabetic retinopathy and seems to be more effective in patients with type 2 diabetes.

The analysis of ETDRS data suggests that early scatter treatment for eyes with severe nonproliferative diabetic retinopathy or early proliferative diabetic retinopathy is effective in reducing severe visual loss in patients with type 2 diabetes.

In conclusion, the ETDRS showed also that laser treatment (focal photocoagulation) of the posterior fundus was of value in preventing vision loss from macular edema and also increased the chance of moderate visual gain and reduced retinal thickening. Side effects of treatment included scotomas related to the focal laser burns.

## 6.2. Vitrectomy

Vitreous surgery for complications of diabetic retinopathy was proposed in order to achieve visual improvement in patients with severe vitreous hemorrhage (Machemer and Norton, 1972).

## 6.2.1. Diabetic Retinopathy Vitrectomy Study (DRVS)

The Diabetic Retinopathy Vitrectomy Study (DRVS) was a randomized clinical trial that evaluated eyes of patients with complications of diabetic retinopathy, such as severe vitreous hemorrhage or very severe neovascularization. The major objective of the study was to demonstrate the benefits and risks of vitrectomy in those patients.

The DRVS provided guidelines for the most opportune time to perform vitrectomy surgery for patients with types 1 and 2 diabetes mellitus and vitreous hemorrhage or severe proliferative diabetic retinopathy in eyes with good vision.

In the Diabetic Retinopathy Vitrectomy Study (DRVS) the patients included had very severe proliferative diabetic retinopathy. In this clinical trial 616 eyes were included with recent severe vitreous hemorrhage from proliferative diabetic retinopathy or 370 eyes with advanced, active of severe proliferative diabetic retinopathy (270 of them with previous photocoagulation).

This study included three groups of eyes with proliferative diabetic retinopathy (DRVS Research Group, 1985): Group N, Group H and Group NR.

Group N, with 744 eyes included, was established in order to obtain information on the outcome of conventional management in eyes with very severe PDR. Group NR consisted of eyes with severe retinopathy, but with useful vision (Diabetic Retinopathy Vitrectomy Study Research Group, 1988). The patients were randomized to early vitrectomy versus conventional management. The major eligibility criteria were the following: VA $\geq$ 10/200, center of the macula attached, extensive, active neovasular or fibrovascular proliferations. The major design features were the same in group H (except conventional management included vitrectomy after six months waiting period in eyes that had in the meanwhile developed severe vitreous hemorrhage). The major conclusions were that these patients had an increased chance for VA $\geq$ 10/20 by early vitrectomy, at least for eyes with very severe new vessels.

Group H included eyes randomly assigned to early vitrectomy or deferral vitrectomy for one year with severe vitreous hemorrhage of less than five months duration reducing visual acuity to 5/200 or less and obscuring details of posterior fundus (Diabetic Retinopathy Vitrectomy Study Research Group, 1990a; 1990b). Major design features were the following: in most patients only one eye was eligible; eligible eyes or eyes randomly assigned to early vitrectomy or conventional management (vitrectomy if center of macula detached or if vitreous hemorrhage persisted for one year, photocoagulation, as needed and when possible).

The results showed that the chance of recovery of VA $\geq$ 10/20 was increased by early vitrectomy, at least in patients with type 1 diabetes, who were younger and had more PDR (in most severe PDR group $\geq$ 10/20 at 7 year in 50% of early vitrectomy group versus 12% in conventional management group).

Results from DRVS showed that in patients with severe vitreous hemorrhage or until tractional retinal detachment involving the macula, conventional management, deferring vitrectomy for one year reduced the chance of obtaining good vision compared to doing early (< six months) vitrectomy. After two years of follow-up, 25% of the early vitrectomy group had visual acuity of 20/40 or better compared with 15% in the deferral group ($P = 0.01$). This difference at two years was even greater (36% versus 12%, $P = 0.001$) for younger patients with type 1 diabetes with more severe PDR.

Early vitrectomy was also effective in preserving good visual acuity in patients with severe or very severe PDR without severe vitreous hemorrhage.

There were some complications during follow-up of these patients: phtisis, endophthamitis, uveitis, corneal epithelial problems or neovascular glaucoma (Diabetic Retinopathy Vitrectomy Study Research Group, 1988; 1990a; 1990b).

Patients were randomized to early vitrectomy versus conventional management and the results demonstrated that the benefit of early vitrectomy was only seen in eyes with most severe proliferative diabetic retinopathy. Visual acuity 20/40 or better was more evident in the early vitrectomy group in the first six months after baseline visit. So, this clinical trial confirms the value of vitrectomy in eyes with very severe PDR or severe vitreous hemorrhage in order to preserve good vision.

## 6.3. Medical Approaches

Long-term microvascular, neurological and macrovascular complications are well known in Diabetes Mellitus. These complications are more evident after 15–20 years after the onset of disease. The role of the systemic disease, the level of glycemic control, blood pressure levels, etc., in the development of diabetic complications and particularly in diabetic retinopathy, has been examined in two large intervention trials which make the basis of our present knowledge on the relationship between diabetes type 1, type 2 and diabetic retinopathy.

### 6.3.1 Diabetes Control and Complications Trial (DCCT)

The Diabetes Control and Complications Trial (DCCT) was designed to answer two important questions regarding diabetic retinopathy: will intensive control of blood glucose slow the development and subsequent progression of diabetic retinopathy?; will intensive control of blood glucose slow progression of diabetic retinopathy? (Diabetic Control and Complications Trial Research Group, 1986; 1993; 1995).

The DCCT was a multicenter, randomized clinical trial designed to compare the effect of versus conventional insulin therapy in patients with type 1 diabetes and to evaluate their effects on the development and progression of the early vascular and neurological complications of insulin dependent diabetes mellitus.

In this clinical trial 1441 patients with type 1 diabetes were enrolled: 726 patients with insulin-dependent diabetes mellitus with one to five years of duration of the disease without retinopathy and 715 patients with insulin-dependent diabetes mellitus with one to 15 years of duration of the disease and mild-to-moderate diabetic retinopathy. The patients were randomized to either intensive control of blood glucose with multiple daily insulin injections or intensive group versus conventional insulin therapy.

The outcome variables were the development or progression of diabetic retinopathy by three steps using a Modified Airlie House Scale. Nephropathy, neuropathy and cardiovascular outcomes were also analyzed. The intensive therapy regimen was designed to achieve blood glucose values as close to the normal range as possible with three or more injections or treatment with an insulin pump. Conventional therapy consisted of one or two insulin injections per day.

The results of DCCT showed that intensive therapy effectively delays the onset and slows the progression of diabetic retinopathy, nephropathy and neuropathy in insulin-dependent diabetes mellitus.

Intensive therapy showed better results than the group with conventional insulin therapy, reducing the adjusted mean risk for the development of retinopathy by 76% as compared with conventional therapy. The intensive therapy slowed the progression of retinopathy by 54% and reduced the development of proliferative or severe nonproliferative retinopathy by 47%, reduced the occurrence of microalbuminuria (urinary albumin excretion of $\geq$ 40 mg per 24 hours) by 39%, that of albuminuria (urinary albumin excretion of $\geq$ 300 mg per 24 hours) by 54% and reduced the risk of clinical neuropathy by 60%. Mean blood glucose was 155 mg/dl in the intensive therapy group against 230 mg/dl in the conventional therapy groups.

The intensive therapy group achieved the median value of $HbA_{1C}$ of 7.2% versus 9.1% in the conventional group ($p < 0.001$). In each group mean $HbA_{1C}$

during the trial was the dominant predictor of retinopathy progression.

A transient worsening of retinopathy was detected in the first 6 and/or 12 months visit of the study in 13.1% (intensive therapy) and 7.6% (conventional therapy) with recovery and no long-term impact. The probable explanation for this fact was due to the higher levels of $HbA_{1C}$ at screening and rapid reduction of $HbA_{1C}$ in the first six months. This fact points to the need for careful ophthalmological monitoring before initiation of intensive therapy to control blood glucose.

The more frequent adverse event associated with intensive therapy was the increase in severe hypoglycemia.

In other studies (Dahl-Jorgensen *et al.*, 1985; Lauritzen *et al.*, 1983, 1985; Kroc Collaborative Study Group, 1988; Diabetes Control and Complications Trial Research Group, 1985; Klein *et al.*, 1996) the effect of intensive glucose control on the retinopathy demonstrates an initial and paradoxical worsening of retinopathy not associated with vision loss but the long-term benefits of intensive insulin treatment greatly exceed this risk, as was well demonstrated in the DCCT (Diabetes Control and Complications Trial Research Group, 1998).

In conclusion, blood glucose control lowers the risk of long-term microvascular and neurological complications that are the frequent causes of morbility and mortality in patients with diabetes mellitus, with the major clinical impact beginning 15–20 years after the onset of diabetes.

### 6.3.2   United Kingdom Prospective Diabetes Study (UKPDS)

The United Kingdom Prospective Diabetes Study (UKPDS), a randomized, multicenter, controlled clinical trial demonstrated that in type 2 diabetic patients the better glycemic control obtained with intensive treatment leads to a decrease in complications including retinopathy (United Kingdom Prospective Diabetes Study Group, 1990; 1991; 1998).

The study began in 1977 and the enrollment period extended untill 1991 and the end of study was set for 1997. The total number of included patients was 5102 with type 2 diabetes, with 53 years of median age. The primary outcome measures in the UKPDS were three end points: any diabetes-related end point, diabetes-related death, all cause mortality. The control of retinopathy was evaluated using four field fundus photography performed every three years and graded according a modified ETDRS protocol.

Randomization was either intensive treatment (pharmacologic agent) versus conventional treatment (only diet adding pharmacologic agents when plasma glucose exceeded 270 mg/dl or when symptoms are developed). The first group had a median $HbA_{1C}$ of 7.0% and the other group 7.9% ($p < 0.001$). After six years of follow-up, a smaller number of patients in the intensive-treatment group than in the conventional-treatment group had an aggravation of retinopathy. At six and nine years' follow-up the study found that 17% was the rate of reduction of the diabetic retinopathy compared to 21% reduction at 12 years follow-up.

Intensive blood glucose control by either sulphonylureas or insulin substantially decreased the risk of microvascular complications in patients with type 2 diabetes.

Tight blood pressure control in patients with hypertension and type 2 diabetes achieved a clinically important reduction in the progression of diabetic retinopathy.

## References

Dahl-Jorgensen K, Brinchmann-Hansen O, Hanssen KF, *et al.* (1985) Rapid tightening of blood glucose control leads to transient deterioration of retinopathy in insulin dependent diabetes mellitus: The Oslo Study. *Br Med J* **290**: 811–815.

Diabetes Control and Complications Trial Research Group. (1986) The Diabetes Control and Complications Trial (DCCT) design and methodologic considerations for the feasibility phase. *Diabetes* **35**: 530–545.

Diabetes Control and Complications Trial Research Group. (1993) The effect of intensive treatment of diabetes on the development and progression of long term complications in insulin-dependent diabetes mellitus. *N Eng Med* **329**: 977–986.

Diabetes Control and Complications Trial Research Group. (1995) The relationship of glicemic exposure (HbA$_{1C}$) to the risk of development and progression of retinopathy in the Diabetes Control and Complications Trial. *Diabetes* **44**: 968–983.

Diabetes Control and Complications Trial Research Group. (1998) Early worsening of diabetic retinopathy in the Diabetes Control and Complications Trial. *Arch Ophthalmol* **116**: 874–886.

Diabetic Retinopathy Study Research Group. (1976) Preliminary report on effects of photocoagulation therapy. *Am J Ophthalmol* **88**: 383–396.

Diabetic Retinopathy Study Research Group. (1978) Photocoagulation treatment of proliferative diabetic retinopathy: The second report of Diabetic Retinopathy Study findings. *Ophthalmology* **85**: 82–106.

Diabetic Retinopathy Study Research Group. (1979) Four risk factors for severe visual loss in diabetic retinopathy. The third report from the Diabetic Retinopathy Study. *Arch Ophthalmol* **97**: 654–655.

Diabetic Retinopathy Study Research Group. (1981a) Design, methods and baseline results. DRS report number 6. *Invest Ophthalmol* **21**: **149**: 209.

Diabetes Retinopathy Study Research Group. (1981b) Photocoagulation treatment of proliferative diabetic retinopathy: Clinical application of diabetic retinopathy study (DRS) findings. DRS Report Number 8. *Ophthalmology* **88**: 583–600.

Diabetic Retinopathy Vitrectomy Study Research Group. (1988) Early vitrectomy for severe proliferative diabetic retinopathy in eyes with useful vision: Results of a randomized trial. DVRS Report Number 3. *Ophthalmology* **95**: 1307–1320.

Diabetic Retinopathy Vitrectomy Study Research Group. (1990a) Early Vitrectomy for Severe Vitreous Hemorrhage in Diabetic Retinopathy. Two year results of a randomized trial: Diabetic Retinopathy Study Report 2. **103**: 1644–1652.

Diabetic Retinopathy Vitrectomy Study Research Group. (1990b) Early Vitrectomy for Severe Vitreous Hemorrhage in Diabetic Retinopathy. Four year results of a randomized trial: Diabetic Retinopathy Study Report 5. *Arch Ophthalmol* **108**: 958–964.

DRVS Research Group (Appended). (1985) Two year course of visual acuity in severe proliferative diabetic retinopathy with conventional management. Diabetic Retinopathy Vitrectomy Study (DRVS) Report 1. *Ophthalmology* **92**: 492–502.

Early Treatment Diabetic Retinopathy Study Research Group. (1991a) Early Treatment Diabetic Retinopathy design and baseline characteristics, Early Treatment Diabetic Retinopathy Study Report 7. *Ophthalmology* **98**: 741–756.

Early Treatment Diabetic Retinopathy Study Research Group. (1991b) Effects of aspirin treatment on diabetic retinopathy. ETDRS report number 8. *Ophthalmology* **98**: 757–765.

Early Treatment Diabetic Retinopathy Study Research Group. (1991c) Early photocoagulation for diabetic retinopathy. ETDRS report number 9. *Ophthalmology* **98**: 766–785.

Kalin HA, Bradley RF. (1975) Prevalence of diabetic retinopathy: Age, sex and duration of diabetes. *Br J Ophthalmol* **59**: 345–349.

Kalin HA, Hiller R. (1974) Blindness caused by diabetic retinopathy. *Am J Ophthalmol* **78**:**58**: 67.

Klein R, Klein BE, Moss SE Cruickshanks KJ. (1994) Relationship of hyperglycemia to the long term incidence and progression of diabetic retinopathy. *Arch Inter Med* **154**: 2169–2178.

Kroc Collaborative Study Group. (1984) Blood glucose control and the evolution of diabetic retinopathy and albuminuria: A multicenter trial. *N England J Med* **311**: 365–372.

Kroc Collaborative Study Group. (1988) Diabetic Retinopathy after two years of intensified insulin treatment: Follow-up of the Kroc Collaborative Study. *J Am Med Assoc* **260**: 37–41.

Lauritzen T, Fros-Larsen K, Larsen HW, Deckert T. (1983) Effect of 1 year of near-normal blood glucose levels on retinopathy. *Lancet* **1**: 200–204.

Lauritzen T, Fros-Larsen K, Larsen HW, Deckert T. (1985) Two-year experience with continuous subcutaneous insulin infusion in relation to retinopathy and neuropathy. *Diabetes* **34**: 74–79.

Machemer R, Norton EW. (1972) A new concept for vitreous surgery, **3**: Indications and results. *Am J Ophthalmol* **74**: 1034–1056.

UK Prospective Diabetes Study Group. (1990) Complications in newly diagnosed type 2 diabetic patients and their association with clinical and biochemical risk factors (UKPDS6). *Diabetes Res* **13**: 1–11.

UK Prospective Diabetes Study Group. (1991) VIII Study design, progress and performance. *Diabetologia* **34**: 877–890.

UK Prospective Diabetes Study Group. (1998a) Intensive blood-glucose control with sulfonylureas or insulin compared with conventional treatment and risk of complications in patients with type 2 diabetes (UKPDS33). *Lancet* **352**: 837–853.

UK Prospective Diabetes Study Group. (1998b) Effect of intensive blood-glucose control with metmorfin on complications in over weight patients with type 2 diabetes (UKPDS34). *Lancet* **352**: 854–865.

UK Prospective Diabetes Study Group. (1998c) Tight blood pressure control and risk of macrovascular and microvascular complications in type 2 diabetes (UKPDS38). *BMJ* **317**: 703–713.

UK Prospective Diabetes Study Group. (1998d) Efficacy of atenol and captopril in reducing risk of macrovascular and microvascular complications in type 2 diabetes: UKPDS39. *BMJ* **317**: 713–720.

# Chapter 7

# Photocoagulation for Macular Edema and Proliferative Retinopathy

## Francisco Goméz-Ulla

The benefit of laser treatment was established by the results of two large multicentre studies: DRS (Diabetic Retinopathy Study) (DRS, 1981) ETDRS (Early Treatment Diabetic Retinopathy Study) (ETDRS, 1985). Both studies showed that panretinal photocoagulation in proliferative diabetic retinopathy reduced the risk of severe visual loss by more than 50%. This effect was achieved with acceptable side effects, such as a certain degree of peripheral field loss and slight decrease in visual acuity. An important beneficial effect of focal photocoagulation was also demonstrated in situations of well defined clinically significant macular edema, slowing and decreasing the risk of visual loss by approximately 50% (ETDRS, 1985).

## 7.1. Rationale and Results of Photocoagulation

Laser photocoagulation is a phototermal procedure, in which heat is generated by the absorption of laser energy by the tissue, inducing protein coagulation and other biological reactions with the objective of causing a beneficial effect by stopping the disease process. In order to achieve this objective, the laser impact on the retina induces a white-yellowish spot on the retinal tissue, which indicates the increase in tissue temperature of the retina induced by the laser.

In Diabetic Macular Edema (DME) the objective is to maintain vision and prevent progressive visual loss. The main rationale (Table 7.1) of photocoagulation is

the closure of the microvascular leaking sites considered to be responsible for the development of the edema (focal macular edema). Many microaneurysms and other microvascular anomalies are localized in the inner nuclear layer or in the inner side of the outer plexiform layer and a laser impact of enough intensity is necessary to achieve a whitish coloration in the center or a small white circle in the zone of retinal burning as recommended (ETDRS, 1987).

In these circumstances, the microvascular lesions are coagulated stopping the abnormal leakage, whereas less intense laser impacts characterized by a gray center only coagulate the retinal pigment epithelium and photoreceptors without reaching the internal nuclear layer and without achieving its objectives.

The development of large membranes under the retinal pigment epithelium after laser photocoagulation have been described, which can contribute to progressive enlargement of the scar and photoreceptor atrophy (Fig. 7.1) covering up to 900 micra of the center of the impact (Wallow and Bindley, 1988). Special precautions must therefore be taken when treating near the fovea.

Recent studies suggest that it is not necessary to damage all retinal layers in order to obtain maximal therapeutic efficacy. Impacts that are not seen by the slit-lamp examination at the moment of treatment induce lesions around the retinal pigment epithelium and have a therapeutic effect without involving the remaining retinal tissue, confirming recent observations indicating that the beneficial effect of laser photocoagulation is mainly due to the liberation of factors derived from the retinal pigment epithelium (Lanzetta

**Table 7.1. Goals and Mechanisms of Action of Photocoagulation in Diabetic Retinopathy**

**Photocoagulation in Diabetic Macular Edema**

**Goal**: Maintain visual acuity and prevent progressive visual loss

**Mechanisms of action:**

✓ Direct closure of the leaking sites or indirectly by factors derived by the retinal pigment epithelium.
✓ Recovery of the blood-retinal barrier.
✓ Decrease in the need for O2 by the external retina, increasing its availability to the inner retina.

**Photocoagulation in Diabetic Proliferative Retinopathy**

**Goal:** To stop the retinopathy progression and prevent severe visual loss

**Mechanisms of action:**

✓ Destruction of large areas of ischemia tissue.
✓ Decrease of vasoproliferative factors by:
  ○ Decrease of the retinal hypoxia
  ○ Release of anti-angiogenic factors

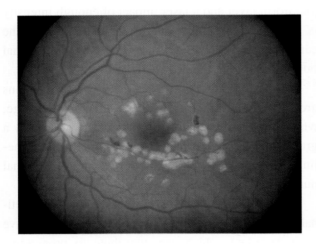

**Fig. 7.1.** Sears of focal photocoagulation, some very intense with marked hyperpigmentation.

*et al.*, 2001). This type of treatment would be particularly appropriate in situations of diffuse macular edema, where fluorescein angiography also shows widespread leakage from the retinal vessels and microaneurysms, indicating that leakage from microaneurysms may not be the sole mechanism of producing macular edema. Other authors using diode laser and subliminal impacts (Friberg and Karatza, 1997; Stanga *et al.*, 1999; Friberg, 1999), difficult to distinguish on ophthalmoscopic examination or even by fluorescein angiography, report stabilization and even improvement in visual acuity in 85% of the treated patients (Luttrull *et al.*, 2005).

Many hypotheses have been proposed to explain the beneficial effect of laser photocoagulation in diabetic macular edema (Tranos *et al.*, 2004). One states that laser lesions in animal models show a temporary breakdown of the blood-retinal barrier followed by a repair process involving the retinal pigment epithelial cells, which proliferate and slide to replace the damaged cells. The new cells develop normal intercellular junctions in a few weeks thus restoring the integrity of the outer blood-retinal barrier (Central Vein Occlusion Study Group, 1994). Other theory (Stefansson *et al.*, 1992) postulates that grid photocoagulation achieves a generalized destruction of the photoreceptors and retinal pigment epithelium, which are the cells that use more oxygen in the retina, leading to less utilization of oxygen by the external layers if the retina allowing its diffusion into the inner retinal layers and lessening the situation of hypoxia in the retinal tissue in diabetes. Higher oxygen tensions induce retinal arteriolar constriction increasing arteriolar resistance and decreasing hydrostatic pressure in venules and capillaries. This decrease in hydrostatic pressure induces vascular constriction (Gottfredottir *et al.*, 1993) according to Laplace law resulting in a decrease in vascular leakage to the surrounding tissues and, according to Starling Law, reducing edema formation.

In Proliferative Diabetic Retinopathy (PDR) the objective of the scatter or pan retinal photocoagulation treatment (PPT) is to stabilize retinopathy progression and prevent severe visual loss. The main rationale is to achieve a decrease in the production of vasoproliferative factors, which are supposedly achieved by eliminating the retinal hypoxia by the mechanisms described previously, associated possibly by liberation of anti-angiogenic factors by the retinal pigment epithelium stimulated by the laser treatment (Stefansson *et al.*, 1992). Scatter photocoagulation destroys large areas of the retina, decreasing the need for oxygen of the retina and improving the conditions of diffusion from the choroid to the retina by decreasing retinal thickness.

In order to achieve this objective, the laser impacts should have a white-yellowish colloration (Diabetic Retinopathy Study Research Group, 1978; Bamroohgsuk *et al.*, 2002; Ferris, 1996; Dastur, 1994; Doft and Blankenship, 1984; O'Donoghue, 1982; Coscas and Chaine, 1979). However, similar levels of efficacy have been reported using less intense laser impacts with lower levels of energy in situations of PDR (Bandello *et al.*, 2001).

## 7.1.1. Diabetic Macular Edema: Results

Diabetic macular edema is one of the main causes of vision loss in developed countries and the main one in diabetic retinopathy (Ferris and Patz, 1984). The prevalence of diabetic macular edema after 15 or more years of duration of the disease is 20% in type 1 diabetic patients, 25% in type 2 diabetic patients receiving insulin and 14% in type 2 diabetic patients not requiring insulin (Klein *et al.*, 1984). It is more when there is Proliferative Diabetic Retinopathy, reaching 71% in this group of eyes (Striph *et al.*, 1988). More than half of the patients with diabetic macular edema will develop loss of visual acuity of two or more lines of vision upon two years of follow-up (Lee and Olk, 1991). These numbers justify by

themselves the need to do everything to treat adequately diabetic macular edema, realizing that the only treatment, that up till now has proven its value, is photocoagulation.

Before the conclusion of the ETDRS, which demonstrated that photocoagulation is effective in the treatment of diabetic macular edema (Early Treatment Diabetic Retinopathy Study Research Group, 1985; Early Treatment Diabetic Retinopathy Study Research Group, 1987; Early Treatment Diabetic Retinopathy Study Research Group, 1991), a number of studies have indicated that photocoagulation treatment could be beneficial both applied as focal photocoagulation (McMeel *et al.*, 1977; Blankenship, 1979; Spalter, 1971; Patz *et al.*, 1973; Rubinstein and Myska, 1974; Cheng, 1975; Wiznia, 1979) or in a grid pattern (Whitelocke *et al.*, 1979; McDonald and Schatz, 1985). Posteriorly, Olk, 1986, in a randomized study of 160 eyes with clinically significant macular edema treated with laser photocoagulation showed a beneficial effect of laser treatment at 12 and 24 months in the treated eyes in contrast with the worsening registered in the control group (45.2% improved, 45.2% remained stable and 9.5% worsened; comparing with 8.1%, 48.5% and 43.2%, respectively registered in the eyes that did not receive photocoagulation).

Diabetic macular edema may be focal or diffuse. Focal macular edema is characterized by an increase in retinal thickening in apparent direct relation with the presence of microaneurysms or focal signs of capillary damage, frequently associated with hard exudates, which are accumulation of plasma lipoproteins. Diffuse macular edema is sometimes associated with the presence of cystic lesions with diffuse leakage, but with less visible focal vascular damage and more scant hard exudates (Bresnick, 1983).

The ETDRS (Early Treatment Diabetic Retinopathy Study, 1985; Early Treatment Diabetic Retinopathy Study, 1987) demonstrated the beneficial effect of focal laser photocoagulation in clinically significant macular edema, but it is important to review its results. The risk of moderate visual loss decreased by 50% as a result of treatment, but 12% of the treated eyes lost vision of three or mores lines in the ETDRS Vision Scale after three years of follow-up and only 3% improved.

Progressive visual loss occurred in 26% of the patients with diabetic macular edema even after photocoagulation. Finally, it is important to recall that the beneficial effect of treatment is better when treating eyes with 20/40 or better visual acuity.

The definition of clinically significant macular edema does not distinguish focal and diffuse edema. In previous studies the eyes with diffuse macular edema showed a relatively poor response to laser treatment (Early Treatment Diabetic Retinopathy Study Group, 1985; Lee and Olk, 1991; Bresnick, 1986). In any case, visual acuity stabilization occurred in 75–85 of the eyes treated (Lee and Olk, 1991; McDonald and Schatz, 1985; Olk, 1990; Akduman and Olk, 1997).

### 7.1.2. Proliferative Diabetic Retinopathy: Results

Proliferative Diabetic Retinopathy (PDR) is responsible for 90% of cases of severe visual loss (visual acuity of 5/200 or less in two or more consecutive visits performed at four months intervals), sometime leading to blindness.

Two large multicenter clinical trials were performed examining the efficacy of scatter laser treatment on diabetic retinopathy: the Diabetic Retinopathy Study (DRS) and the Early Treatment Diabetic Retinopathy Study (ETDRS). The DRS study started in 1981 including 1758 patients with the objective of answering the question: is scatter photocoagulation treatment capable of preventing severe visual loss in patients with PDR and high-risk characteristics (High risk characteristics were considered to be: 1. Disk neovascularization (NVD) involving $\frac{1}{3}$ or more of the disk area; 2. NVD associated with the presence of preretinal or vitreous hemorrhage; 3. Neovascularization away from the disk (NVE) of at least half of the disk area associated with vitreous hemorrhage). The conclusion of the study after five years was that laser scatter treatment was effective in reducing severe visual loss by 50% or more in these eyes (Diabetic

Retinopathy Study Research Group, 1985; Diabetic Retinopathy Study Research Group, 1978).

Because DRS was not designed to evaluate the efficacy of photocoagulation to the eyes with PDR without high risk characteristics or to treat eyes with severe NPDR, another large clinical was designed, addressing specifically these issues. The ETDRS, involved 3828 patients with a minimal follow-up period of three years and one of the three questions addressed was to find out if scatter photocoagulation treatment should be initiated in the presence of PDR or severe NPDR in order to prevent the risk of severe visual loss. The study showed that the risk of severe visual loss decreases by 90% when treating eyes with PDR and high risk characteristics and by 50% when treating severe NPDR (Early Treatment Diabetic Retinopathy Study Research Group, 1978; Early Treatment Diabetic Retinopathy Study Research Group, 1985; Early Treatment Diabetic Retinopathy Study Research Group, 1991).

In a prospective study performed in 50 patients with PDR treated by scatter photocoagulation, 86% showed signs of resolution of the high risk characteristics three weeks after treatment and this beneficial effect remained in 70% of the patients six months after treatment 20. The beneficial effect of photocoagulation treatment on visual acuity appears to be directly related to the regression of the high risk factors of the retinopathy and this response remains for a long time (Vander *et al.*, 1991), even after 15 years of follow-up (Blankenship, 1991). It has been shown that the effect on visual acuity remains in the follow-up between 5 to 12 years (Little, 1985). In 351 eyes treated, 72% maintained a visual acuity of 2/10 or better, whereas, the major causes of very severe visual loss were traccional retinal detachment and neovascular glaucoma.

## 7.2. Clinical Evaluation and Pre-treatment Options

### 7.2.1. Macular Edema

Macular edema is a result of fluid accumulation in the macula due to increased permeability of the

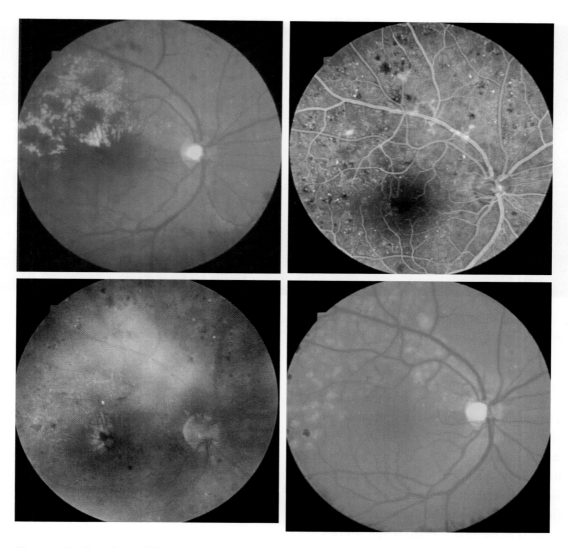

**Fig. 7.2.** *Upper left*: diabetic proliferative retinopathy with low risk characteristics, CSME and hard exudates. *Upper right*: fluorescein angiography showing microaneurysms, IRMAs, zones of focal ischemia and minimal neovascularization. *Lower left*: fluorescein leakage and cystoid macular edema. *Lower right*: disappearance of the exudation after photocoagulating the areas of leakage. It demonstrates the need for fluorescein angiography in order to treat adequately.

microaneurysms and vascular lesions or deficient outward transport of the retinal pigment epithelium, which in the diabetic eyes is not capable of eliminating the fluid accumulated in the retina. The retina appears on ophthalmoscopic examination to be thickened and of a white-greyish color.

To evaluate the severity of the macular edema it is necessary to consider the extension, site and maximum thickness of the affected area of the retina. Macular edema may be present in every stage of the

retinopathy, but is more frequent in the more severe stages of the retinopathy (Fig. 7.2).

The evaluation of macular edema in clinical trials involving photocoagulation has been made by slit-lamp biomicroscopy and stereophotography of the central 30° of the retina, both methods revealing good agreement (Kinyoun *et al.*, 1989). The problem associated with these methods is their poor sensitivity and their subjectivity, allowing for a qualitative evaluation of the macula but needing marked increases in the

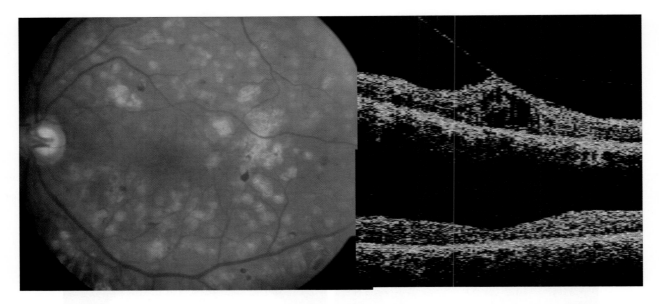

**Fig. 7.3.** *Left*: panretinal photocoagulation and cystoid macular edema. *Upper right*: OCT showing macular thickening and its traccional origin. *Lower right*: recovery of the normal macular profile after vitrectomy.

thickness of the retina in order to be detected by these methods. Since the development of optical coherence tomography (OCT) in 1991 (Huang *et al.*, 1991) and its commercialization in 1995 we have an objective method to evaluate quantitatively retinal thickness.

OCT is more useful for the diagnosis and treatment of diabetic macular edema than fluorescein angiography, because this method identifies the lesions that should be treated but does not demonstrate the changes occurring in the different retinal layers. A numbers of studies have shown that OCT is more sensitive than slit-lamp examination (Hee *et al.*, 1995; Yang *et al.*, 2001; Browning *et al.*, 2004) and, furthermore, helps in distinguishing the eyes that have a vitreal traction component, which is very important for appropriate treatment planning and performing vitrectomy (Lewis *et al.*, 1992; Lewis, 2001). Since the initial observations of Lewis in 1992, a number of clinical studies have confirmed the value of vitrectomy for treatment of diabetic macular edema (Van Effenterre *et al.*, 1993; Harbour *et al.*, 1996; Tachi and Ogino, 1996; Hikichi *et al.*, 1997; Yang, 2000) even in situations when no vitreal traction could be demonstrated before the surgery (Tachi and Ogino,

1996; La Heij *et al.*, 2001; Jahn *et al.*, 2004; Otani and Kishi, 2000).

It is convenient to perform an OCT examination in patients with diabetic macular edema, when considering focal or grid laser treatment (Otani and Kishi, 2000; Otani *et al.*, 1999; Otani and Kishi, 1999) to eliminate the possibility of the presence of an important tractional component (Fig. 7.3).

Fluorescein angiography is useful to identify the sites of leakage before applying the laser treatment and to classify the edema as focal or diffuse (Early Treatment Diabetic Retinopathy Study Group, 1995).

Diabetic macular edema may be classified according to the risk of vision loss in:

1. Macular edema (without clinical significance), requiring close follow-up but no laser treatment characterized by:

   — Localized increased retinal thickness in an area equivalent to an optic disk area from the *center*.
   — Hard exudates located within an optic disk area from the *center* of the macula, but at more than 500 $\mu$m from the *center* (hard exudates may be present at less than 500 $\mu$m from the *center*

but without associates surrounding increased retinal thickness).

2. Macular edema classified has clinical significance (CSME), requiring photocoagulation, because it is considered that the edema is approaching the *center* of the fovea, which is associated with the potential for severe visual loss. CSME is divided in three groups:

   — Retinal thickening located at 500 $\mu$m or less of the *center* of the macula.

   — Hard exudates at 500 $\mu$m or less from the *center* of the macula, with surrounding retinal thickening.

   — Areas of retinal thickening (equal or more of an optic disk area) when at least part of the thickened area is located within an optic disk area from the *center* of the fovea.

It is important to improve metabolic control of the patient before performing laser photocoagulation of diabetic macular edema: glycosilated hemoglobin (HbA$_{1C}$) equal or less than 10 mg/dl, diasolic blood pressure of less than 100 mm Hg and no renal failure. It is considered important to refer poor controlled patients to the endocrinologist in order to achieve these reference values.

It is also important to advise the patient of the objective of the treatment and its consequences. Usually it is necessary to explain what we want to achieve with the photocoagulation treatment and that the main objective is to avoid further loss of vision than to improve vision, that more than one or two sessions may be necessary, that the edema may remain after treatment, needing further treatment later and that there will some degree of decrease in quality of vision immediately after treatment and that this negative effect may not disappear entirely. Finally, laser treatment for macular edema is not a final treatment and revision will be necessary in a period of at least four months.

It is also important to consider other treatment alternatives (Donnelly *et al.*, 2004; Martidis *et al.*, 2002; Jonas *et al.*, 2003; Massin *et al.*, 2004; Ciardella *et al.*,

2004; Sutter *et al.*, 2004; Gómez-Ulla *et al.*, 2004), particularly when laser treatments fail, keeping in mind that vitrectomy should be the first option when there are clear signs of vitreous traction (Lewis *et al.*, 1992).

## 7.2.2. Proliferative Diabetic Retinopathy

Proliferative diabetic retinopathy is the result of generalized retinal ischemia, which acts as a stimulus for neovascularization by vascular growth factors, such as VEGF, and, as noted previously, scatter photocoagulation treatment is capable of arresting the development of new vessels or even prevent their development in eyes at risk, eyes with very severe forms of NPDR, where the risk of developing new vessels during a one year period is more than 50% (Diabetic Retinopathy Study Research Group, 1978).

The main indication of urgent scatter photocoagulation treatment is PDR with high risk characteristics or patients with rubeosis iridis and neovascularization in the anterior chamber angle, even without retinal neovessels. In this situation it is important to make the differential diagnosis with an old occlusion of the central retinal vein or an ocular ischemic syndrome by performing fluorescein angiography and even a carotid doppler examination.

In PDR with lower risk characteristics and in the more severe forms of NPDR the photocoagulation treatment may be performed more slowly. In these cases many surgeons prefer to follow up closely with their patients, improving their metabolic control before considering treatment. They do this based on the results of both studies, DRS and ETDRS, which have showed that some patients do not develop proliferative retinopathy and high risk characteristics even after five years of follow-up. However, our option is to treat these patients. Particularly if we are not sure of the patient compliance to close follow-up, if they had already a serious form of PDR in the other eye or severe maculopathy with poor visual result, if they are expecting to need cataract surgery in the near future or are envisaging a pregnancy.

Before submitting the patient to photocoagulation we should explain the objective of treatment, what we expect to achieve, the possibility of continued progression of retinopathy, the possible need of further treatments and even that the treatment may induce some degree of vision loss. The main objective is to stabilize the progression of the disease and delay the vision loss. The possibility of a vitreous hemorrhage occurring after treatment must be discussed with the patient and explained as a consequence of the disease rather than a direct result of the treatment.

The patients must be advised of the need for improved metabolic control. Their levels of glycemia should adjust progressively and slowly, as well as, their blood pressure levels. In any case it is not wise to wait until PDR has high risk characteristics.

It is also necessary to tell the patient that the treatment may be painful and that peribulbar anesthesia may be given if considered necessary to achieve full treatment. The pain is usually due to the laser impacts in mid periphery and the horizontal meridians. In these situations it is acceptable to decrease the duration of the exposure while increasing the laser power. It is also appropriate to tell the patients that it will be some time before vision returns to normal after treatment and that scatter photocoagulation decreases peripheral and night vision, sometimes inducing problems for driving.

## 7.3. Laser Treatment Techniques

It is fundamental to obtain maximal pupillary dilatation, particularly when performing pan-retinal scatter laser photocoagulation, using repeated topical administrations of midriatics every 5 to 10 minutes during half an hour before the laser treatment. Usually topical anesthesia is adequate for scatter photocoagulation, but in some patients and when performing retreatments it may be necessary to perform peribulbar anesthesia.

There is a great variety of lenses which may be used depending if the photocoagulation is to be applied in the posterior pole, the equator or the periphery. The lenses may be of direct or reversed image. The first are more useful when photocoagulating the posterior pole or for grid treatment. The ones using reversed images allow greater field of vision, but caution must be taken regarding their magnification or minimization effects on the laser spot and the size of each burn (Mainster *et al.*, 1990). In Table 7.2 the magnification of the laser impact and its final size on the retina is listed. For instance, if a Mainster Ultrafield lens is used, one laser spot of 100 $\mu$m induces a final burn spot in the retina of 189 $\mu$m.

The more frequently used laser source is argon, especially the green wavelength, but at present solid state lasers are quite common. Many studies have been performed using different wavelengths (Olk, 1990; Fernandez-Vigo *et al.*, 1989; Khairallah *et al.*, 1996). However, no significant differences have been registered in clinical situations between different laser sources, such as between argon laser and kripton laser (Krypton Argon Regression Neovascularization Study Research Group, 1993). This one could be preferably used, however, if it is considered necessary to initiate treatment in the presence of a vitreous hemorrhage or if there is an important lens opacity.

### 7.3.1. Macular Edema

The recommendation of the ETDRS when in presence of Clinically Significant Macular Edema is to treat the lesions, which are within two optic disk areas from the *center* of the fovea:

(a) Sites of discrete retinal hyperfluorescence or leakage located at a distance of 500 $\mu$m or more of the *center* of the fovea.
(b) Areas of diffuse leakage in the retina

   i.   microaneurysms
   ii.  intraretinal vascular anomalies
   iii. hyperpermeable capillary bed

**Table 7.2.    Contact Lenses for Fundus Photocoagulation (from Bloom and Brucker, 1997)**

| Contact Lens | Uses | Image | Lateral Magnification | Axial Magnification | Relative Magnification | Spot Magnification | Field of View |
|---|---|---|---|---|---|---|---|
| Goldmann | Macula Equator Periphery | Virtual Erect | 0.93 | 0.86 | 1.00 | 1.08 | 36° |
| Mainster High Magnification | Macula | Real Inverted | 1.25 | 1.56 | 1.34 | 0.81 | 75° |
| Volk Area Centralis | Macula Equator | Real Inverted | 1.05 | 1.10 | 1.13 | 0.95 | 82° |
| Mainster Standard | Macula Equator | Real Standard | 0.96 | 0.92 | 1.03 | 1.05 | 90° |
| Panfunduscope | Equator Periphery | Real Inverted | 0.71 | 0.51 | 0.76 | 1.41 | 120° |
| Volk TransEquator | Equator Periphery | Real Inverted | 0.70 | 0.49 | 0.75 | 1.43 | 122° |
| Mainster Wide-Field | Equator Periphery | Real Inverted | 0.68 | 0.46 | 0.73 | 1.47 | 125° |
| Volk QuadPediatric | Equator Periphery | Real Inverted | 0.55 | 0.30 | 0.59 | 1.82 | 100° |
| Mainster Ultra Field PRP | Equator Periphery | Real Inverted | 0.53 | 0.28 | 0.57 | 1.89 | 140° |
| Volk QuadAspheric | Equator Periphery | Real Inverted | 0.52 | 0.27 | 0.56 | 1.92 | 130° |
| Volk SuperQuad 160 | Equator Periphery | Real Real | 0.52 | 0.27 | 0.56 | 1.92 | 160° |
| Mainster PRP 165 | Equator Periphery | Real Real | 0.51 | 0.26 | 0.54 | 1.96 | 165° |
| Volk Equator Plis | Equator Periphery | Real Real | 0.45 | 0.20 | 0.48 | 2.22 | 114° |

(c)  Avascular zones of the retina

(d)  Focal areas of leakage located between 300 and 500 $\mu$m of the *center* of the fovea if the eye bad received previous treatment and there is persisting CSME, when there are areas of perifoveal capillary loss that may be enlarged by the treatment.

The treatment should be different according to the type of edema that is present at the time of treatment; focal or diffuse. In order to make an appropriate planning a fluorescein angiography may be necessary in order to identify the areas of increased leakage and the areas of capillary loss.

The fluorescein angiography is less necessary because the lesions causing the exudation are located in the *center* of the circinate lesions and they may treated directly (Fig. 7.4). Focal treatment (Table 7.3) involves individual photocoagulation of all microaneurysms between 500 $\mu$m and 300 $\mu$m of the *center* of the macula (Fig. 7.5). The objective is to induce occlusion of the leaking sites causing the edema, looking for whitening of the vascular lesions with laser. The size if the spots should be 100 $\mu$m and the exposure time 0.1 s. When the diabetic macular edema is diffused it is recommended to perform a grid treatment, covering all the areas of diffuse leakage or showing no perfusion within the central 3000 $\mu$m. The

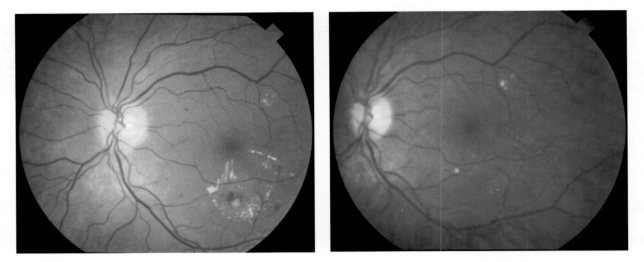

**Fig. 7.4.**  *Left*: clinically significant macular edema with circinate hard exudates. *Right*: 6 months after focal photocoagulation there is almost complete reabsorption of the exudates. In this case fluorescein angiography is not necessary and treatment should be directed to the *center* of the area of exudation.

**Table 7.3.  Photocoagulation of Diabetic Macular Edema**

| **Photocoagulation of Diabetic Macular Edema** | | |
|---|---|---|
| | **Focal** | **Grid** |
| Wavelength | Green | Green |
| Size (micras) | 100 | 100–150 |
| Exposure (sec.) | 0.1 | 0.1 |
| Power (mW) | Whitening or darkening | Soft |
| N° of burns | variable | Treatment of the nonperfused and edema |
| Distance from the centre of the fovea | > 500 $\mu$ | 500–3000 $\mu$ and 500 $\mu$ to the optic disk |
| Number of sessions | 1 | 1 |
| Interval of treatment | 3–4 months | 3–4 months |
| Additional treatment | 1 to 3 sessions | 1 to 3 sessions |

laser impacts should be 100–150 $\mu$m each separated by at least one burn diameter. The burns should be soft and just visible (Table 7.3).

To perform these treatments it is necessary, after explaining the procedure, dilating the pupil and placing the topical anesthesia and the contact lens, to identify clearly the fovea, for which it is useful to have a fluorescein angiography in front of us. If there are any doubts it is possible to use the dought of the aiming

beam with the laser at zero level and the slit-lamp light off and to ask the patient to follow the aiming light. After that the slit lamp is turned on and the fixation point and *center* of fovea identified. It is important to tell the patient to keep the eye steady and to fixate the recommended fixation reference.

To achieve the adequate power for focal photocoagulation it is useful to perform a few trial burns on lesions located well away from the *center* of the

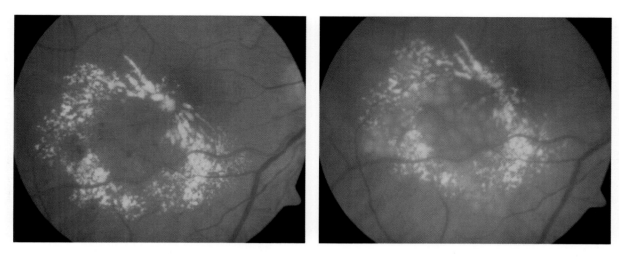

**Fig. 7.5.**   *Left*: diabetic macular edema with circinate hard exudates. *Right*: photocoagulation spots after focal treatment.

macula, starting with low power levels and increasing the power progressively until whitening or darkening of the vascular lesion is achieved.

Usually a microaneurysm or area of diffuse edema that is slightly distant from the fovea is treated first. The power is increased in controlled increments until the desired end point is reached: a burn of mild or light intensity that is off-white but definitely visible. The clinician then locates the fovea and decides how close to it the treatment should be applied. In general, the first session of laser treatment of diabetic macular edema should not be at or near the foveal avascular zone.

A focal leak is usually due to a microaneurysm and one medium-intensity burn is placed over it. If the microaneurysm does not darken or whiten or if the burn was off-*center*, another burn is placed. After the second burn, as long as the retinal pigment epithelium beneath the microaneurysm is moderately white, even if the microaneurysm has not changed color, the clinician moves on to the next lesion. White burns are usually applied to particularly prominent and leaky microaneurysms that appear to be a major source of the macular edema.

A grid pattern is placed using 100 $\mu$m burns in areas of diffuse macular edema without focal leaks (Figs. 7.6 and 7.7). Large areas of diffuse macular edema (1500 $\mu$m or more from the fovea) may be

treated with 200 $\mu$m burns. Burns are placed one and a half or two burns apart or closer if the leakage and edema are severe. Burns for grid treatment are usually slightly less prominent than burns for focal leaks, but should be easily visible.

More power is needed to achieve a burn in more edematous areas than in less edematous ones. Burns may become too intense as the clinician moves from swollen area to an area with minimal or no edema. Treatment of areas of intraretinal hemorrhage are usually avoided, because energy absorption in the inner retinas layers may cause substantial damage to the nerve fiber layer.

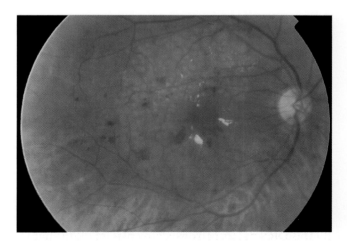

**Fig. 7.6.**   Grid treatment of the macular area.

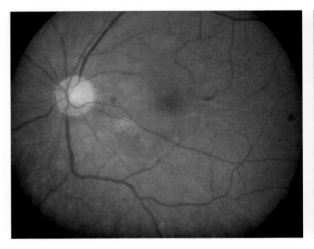 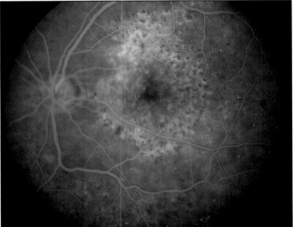

**Fig. 7.7.** *Left*: grid treatment four months after the photocoagulation. *Right*: fluorescein angiography of the same case.

**Table 7.4.  Panretinal Photocoagulation**

| Panretinal Photocoagulation | |
| --- | --- |
| Wavelength | Green (red if there is cataract or vitreous hemorrhage) |
| Size | 300 with Mainster Ultrafield or similar) |
| Exposure | 0.1 |
| Power | Grey-yellow |
| Number of burns | 1500 to 2000 initially |
| Number of sessions | 3–4 |
| Interval for retreatment | $1\frac{1}{2}$ a 2 months |
| Additional treatment | Directly over the retinal new vessels or between previous photocoagulation scars. |

## 7.3.2.  Proliferative Retinopathy

Scatter photocoagulation (Table 7.4) implies the treatment of the entire retinal surface between the posterior pole and equator, respecting generally an outline of a disk diameter nasal to the optic disk up to the temporal arcades and a distance of 4 disk diameters temporal to the fovea. However, in certain cases it may be necessary to photocoagulate within this central area (Fig. 7.8).

The DRS protocol consists of placing 1200 burns, spaced one-half burn width apart from posterior pole

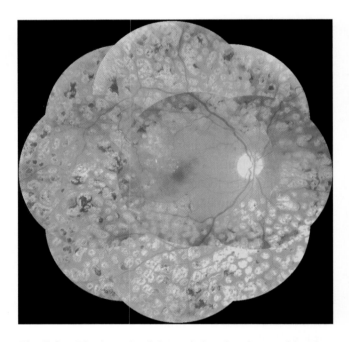

**Fig. 7.8.**  Final result of the peripheral and central borders of a panretinal photocoagulation when it was decided to treat within the temporal arcades.

to equator. Scatter burns should be of medium intensity or grey-white. The laser spot size usually used is 500 $\mu$m with the Goldman lenses and smaller with wide-angle lenses that magnify the spot (see Tables). We use the Mainster Widefield Ultrafield or equivalent, with a spot size of 300 $\mu$m.

The number of impacts necessary for regression and atrophy of retinal neovascularization is not known

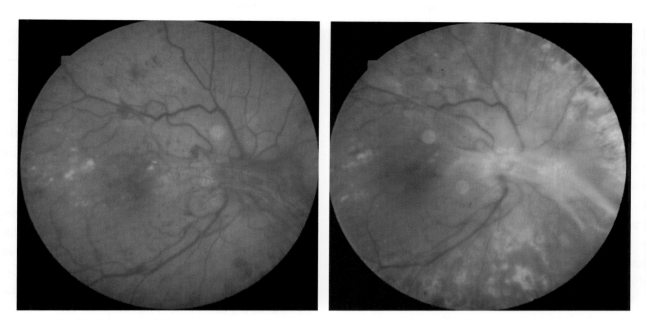

**Fig. 7.9.** *Left*: diabetic proliferative retinopathy with high-risk characteristics. Neovascular proliferation in the optic disk. *Right*: regression of the new vessels leaving only the fibroglial front after panretinal photocoagulation.

(Fig. 7.9) and this will depend of a variety of factors. In a study of 294 eyes an attempt has been made to calculate the amount of retina that needs to be ablated in order to achieve regression of the neovascularization (Reddy *et al.*, 1995).

Sometimes it is necessary to make a large number of confluent impacts in order to achieve the elimination of the new vessels, but the treatment must be continued and repeated (Aylward *et al.*, 1989).

The exposure time used is usually 0.1s, because longer exposure times induce pain and may be too aggressive to Bruch's membrane. The power (Fig.7.10) is necessary to achieve a grey-yellowish burn. Usually we perform scatter photocoagulation in four sessions separated by 10 days, although when there are particularly high risks, such as high intraocular pressure and neovascularization of the anterior chamber angle, it is performed in two sessions and, exceptionally, in one. This last situation, however, should be avoided because it may lead to exudative detachment of the retina and choroid with closed angle glaucoma (McDonald and Schatz, 1985). When absolutely necessary, it is advisable to administer 1 mg predinisone/Kg body weight during

3–5 days, paying particular attention to metabolic control.

Recently, the intravitreal administration of triamcinolone (Bandello *et al.*, 2004) has been proposed as an adjuvant of scatter photocoagulation in

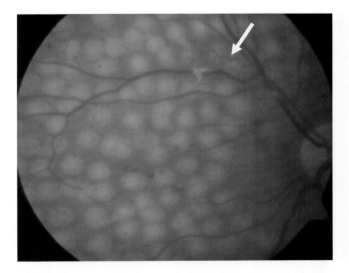

**Fig. 7.10.** Showing the placement of the laser spots. Treatment parameters: Mainster Wide Field lens, size 300 micras, power 210 mw, exposure 0.1 sec, number of burns, 290. We surround the vascular proliferations with laser avoiding direct treatment (arrow).

special cases. A report has been published describing four cases in which intravitreal injection of triamcinolone was given in association with scatter photocoagulation thus avoiding the expected worsening of the macular edema (Zacks and Johnson, 2005).

When the PDR shows low risk characteristics or in severe forms of NPDR it is preferable to allow larger time intervals between the photocoagulation sessions in order to avoid an excessive macular response. Studies performed with OCT showed better recovery of the retinal thickening when scatter photocoagulation is performed with intervals of two weeks instead of one (Shimura *et al.*, 2003).

We give the laser applications by quadrant, starting with the inferior nasal and followed by the inferior temporal. In order to avoid any undesirable photocoagulation in the macula it is useful to initiate scatter laser photocoagulation by applying two rows of laser impacts temporally to the fovea establishing the limit for the ensuing treatments (Fig. 7.11). We treat first the inferior quadrants in order to facilitate continuation of the treatment if a vitreous hemorrhage develops.

It is important to avoid treating fibrous or fibrovascular proliferations, placing photocoagulations only around these proliferations.

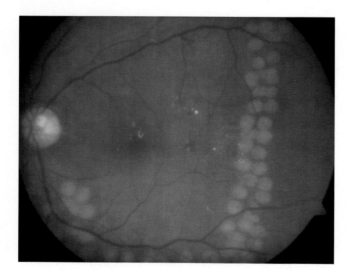

**Fig. 7.11.** Laser burns defining the posterior limit of a panretinal photocoagulation.

## 7.4. Post-operative Follow-up and Complications

### 7.4.1. Macular Edema

The patient should be seen every three to four months. If there is residual CSME, which is a frequent finding, there is indication for a repeat fluorescein angiography and further laser treatment following the guidelines described previously. The treatment now must pay particular attention to the regions that had not been treated before, realizing that persistent macular edema will remain in approximately 20%.

A variety of complications may result from laser treatments applied in the posterior pole. The most serious is, of course, the extremely rare occurrence of involuntary photocoagulation of the fovea, associated with unexpected movements of the eye of the patients, particularly when treating superiorly to the fovea, because the retinal reflex to the intense light application is to move the eye upwards. It is always fundamental to initiate the treatment by explaining well the possible dangers and the need for extreme attention by the patient.

Another important consideration is to avoid confluent laser impacts in order the minimize the risk of paracentral scotomes.

Another complication is the progressive enlargement if the scars, which near the fovea may lead to progressive visual loss, an observation well described in a series of 203 eyes in which this progressive enlargement of the treatment scar was registered in 5.4% of the eyes submitted to grid treatment (Schatz *et al.*, 1991). This may be due to the development of fibrotic membranes under the retinal pigment epithelium (Rutledge *et al.*, 1993).

The laser damage involving the deeper layers of the retina include subretinal fibrosis (Han *et al.*, 1992), defined as the formation of a grey-white tissue layer under the retina and extending to the *centre* of the macula (Fong *et al.*, 1997; Guyer *et al.*, 1992; Varley *et al.*, 1988; Lewis *et al.*, 1990).

In a study of 109 eyes with subretinal fibrosis, its development could be associated with the laser impacts in only nine eyes, whereas, an excessive presence of hard exudates was present in 74% of these 109 eyes (Fong *et al.*, 1997).

## 7.4.2.  Proliferative Retinopathy

After scatter laser photocoagulation it is not necessary, in general, to prescribe any specific treatment unless there is a history of repeated intraocular inflammations or the session involved more than 1000 impacts.

In this last situation topical application of anti-inflammatory and ciclopegic drugs may be appropriate.

The pain and moderate visual loss that follows the treatment go away in a relatively short period of time, but it is advisable to tell the patient that he should report

any unexpected events occurring immediately after the laser lesions. In general, scatter photocoagulation reduces intraocular pressure (Kaufman *et al.*, 1987).

It is advisable to see the patient again within one or two months after the treatment in order to check the effective regression of the retinal neovascularization. We use a panfundoscopic contact lens for this purpose. If there is regression but the neovascularization is still present the next visit should be scheduled four months after the initial treatment and additional photocoagulation considered on that occasion.

Additional photocoagulation in the presence of persisting neovascularization should involve direct photocoagulation of the neovessels when located elsewhere in the retina, away from the disk (Figs. 7.12 and 7.13) and in areas of the retina that were not treated previously.

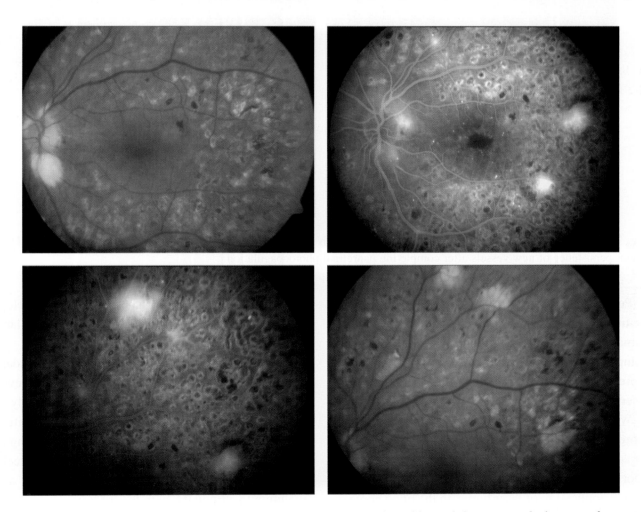

**Fig. 7.12.**  *Upper left*: complete panretinal photocoagulation. *Upper right and lower left*: new vessels that caused repeated vitreous hemmorrhages. *Lower right*: Direct photocoagulation of the new vessels.

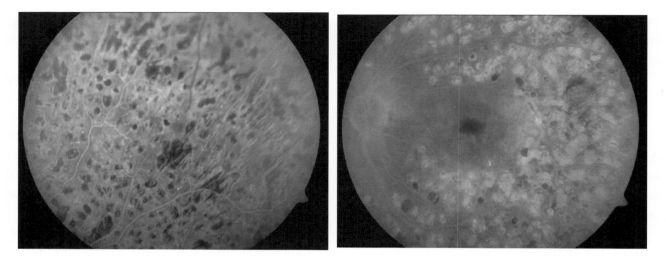

**Fig. 7.13.**   Follow-up of Fig. 7.12, showing on fluorescein angiography the regression of the new vessels. There are no signs of macular edema.

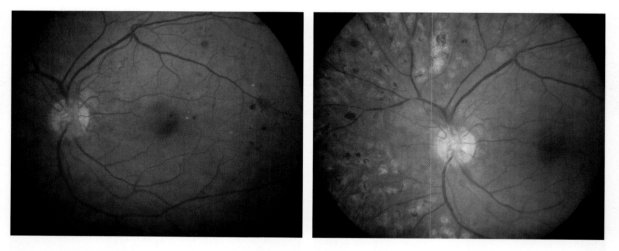

**Fig. 7.14.**   *Left*: proliferative diabetic retinopathy with high risk characteristics (disk new vessels of more than ½ DD). *Right*: persistence of new vessels after completing panretinal photocoagulation.

Persisting new vessels in the optic disk should not be treated directly, because there is a real danger of damaging the optic nerve fibers. The alternative is to complete the scatter photocoagulation by applying more impacts in the intervals between the previous laser scars (Fig. 7.14).

When performing scatter photocoagulation there is more risk for complications than when treating macular edema. Some of these complications may be due to poor focusing leading to corneal and iris burns undesirable application of laser burns, in the optic nerve or excessive laser power causing ruptures of Bruch's membrane, retinal hemorrhages and even development of choroidal neovascularization (particularly when spots small with high power levels).

Scatter photocoagulation may induce a secondary worsening of the pre-existing macular edema or even lead to development of macular edema. In a study of 175 eyes submitted to scatter photocoagulation (McDonald and Schatz, 1985) there was worsening of the macular edema in 43% of the eyes, 6 to 12 weeks after treatment, with persisting edema in 27% and evolution to chronicity, with loss of two or more lines of vision.

Other complications include alterations in color vision, poor night vision and marked losses of the peripheral visual field.

## 7.5.   Special Cases

### 7.5.1.   Proliferative Retinopathy and Macular Edema

When diabetic macular edema coexists with PDR, especially in type 1 diabetic patients, scatter laser treatment may exacerbate the macular edema and cause vision loss (Early Treatment Diabetic Retinopathy Study Group, 1991; McDonald and Schatz, 1985; Ferris *et al.*, 1985).

In these cases, the macular edema should be treated first, followed by a short period of close observation before the scatter photocoagulation (Figs. 7.15 and 7.16).

When it is necessary to perform macular treatment and scatter photocoagulation simultaneously then it is advisable to treat the nasal retina in the first session and the macular edema afterwards, in two sessions the temporal retina, although some degree of vision loss will be expected initially and the patient should be informed of this probable development (Early Treatment for Diabetic Retinopathy Research Group, 1987).

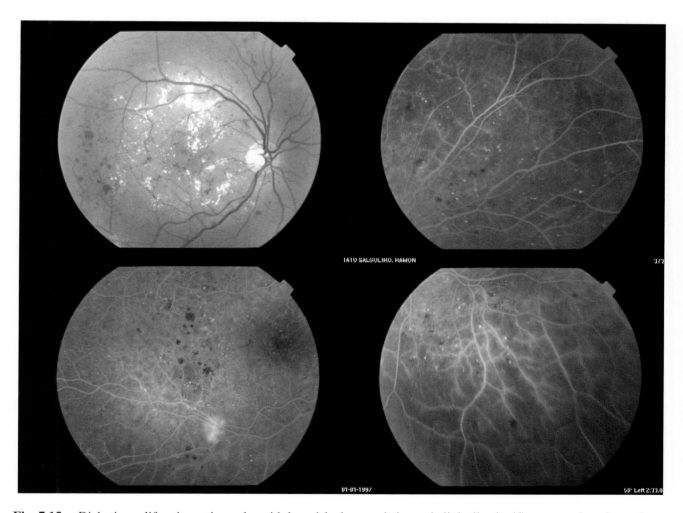

**Fig. 7.15.**   Diabetic proliferative retinopathy with low risk characteristics and clinically significant macular edema showing many hard exudates (red free image — *upper left*). There are areas of peripheral ischemia in the superior and inferior nasal regions (*right*) and new vessels of peripheral ischemia in the superior temporal arcade (*lower left*).

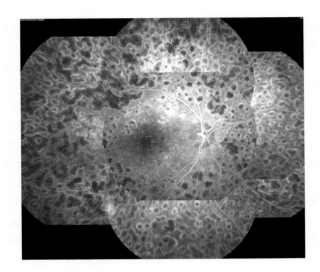

**Fig. 7.16.** Angiographic images of the panretinal photo-coagulation performed in the eye represented in Fig. 7.14, showing regression of the new vessels.

### 7.5.2. Macular Edema and Traction

Separation between the vitreous and the macula may promote spontaneous resolution of the diabetic macular edema. This separation was observed in 27% of 82 patients with type 2 diabetes and CSME, with spontaneous resolution of the edema in 57%, whereas resolution of the edema only occurred in 25% of the eyes that did not have edema. Visual acuity improved two or more lines in 36% and 15%, respectively (Hickichi *et al.*, 1997).

A relatively small number of eyes with diabetic macular edema have a prominent posterior hyaloid attachment at the macula. The fovea may be pulled forward by the hyaloid and is often cystic in appearance. Diabetic macular edema may decrease after vitrectomy when this traction is surgically removed (Lewis *et al.*, 1992; Lewis, 2001; Van Effenterre *et al.*, 1993; Harbour *et al.*, 1996; Tachi and Ogino, 1996).

In order to detect situations of macular edema secondary to vitreous traction it is advisable to perform an Optical Coherence Tomography examination whenever there is CSME and a possibility of vitreous traction.

Macular pucker, distortion or displacement is caused by a partial vitreous detachment or by fibrovascular membranes from PDR. These patients often have blurred vision with metamorphopsia. A vitrectomy should be considered if visual acuity has decreased to 20/50 or less.

### 7.5.3. Diabetic Retinopathy and Cataract Surgery

In diabetic patients with cataract and diabetic retinopathy two situations may be considered:

(a) Cataract and PDR: if possible it is better to perform scatter photocoagulation before the cataract surgery, because of the risk of rubeosis iridis and neovascular glaucoma, which is important after cataract surgery and intraocular lens implantation (Pavese and Insler, 1987; Poliner *et al.*, 1985), particularly if there is rupture of the posterior capsule. If the lens opacity is too dense for argon laser then diode laser should be tried. If it is impossible to perform scatter photocoagulation before surgery, then our preference is for lens phacoemulsification with intraocular lens implant using one suture (sometimes associating an intravitreal injection of triamcinolone at the end of the surgery) followed one week later by the scatter photocoagulation, paying particular attention to the pressure applied to the eye by the contact lens.

(b) Cataract and diabetic macular edema: diabetic macular edema may worsen following cataract surgery (Jaffe and Burton, 1988). The diabetic macular edema sometimes progresses rapidly and responds poorly to laser treatment in this setting. Therefore, it is advisable to treat the edema, if possible, before cataract surgery. After treatment, it is advisable to wait three months or more before undertaking cataract surgery (Figs. 7.17 and 7.18). If necessary it is possible to perform the intraocular implant surgery followed by an intravitreal

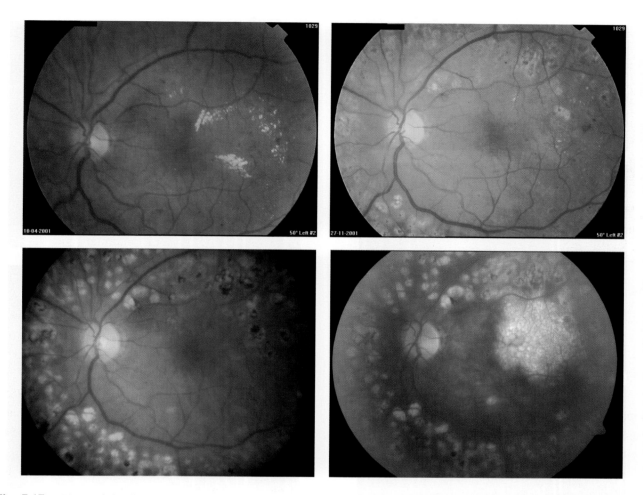

**Fig. 7.17.**   *Upper left*: diabetic proliferative retinopathy, with clinically significant macular edema and hard exudates. *Upper right*: regression of the new vessels and hard exudates a few months after panretinal photocoagulation. *Lower left and right*: six months after, development of cystoid macular edema.

tricomcinolone injection at the end of the surgery (Lam *et al.*, 2004).

### 7.5.4. Proliferative Retinopathy and Traction on Vitreous Hemorrhage

When there is PDR and evidence of fibrovascular proliferation, laser treatments are still indicated (Diabetic Retinopathy Study Research Group, 1981), but the scatter photocoagulation should be performed paying particular attention to avoid treatment of the proliferation in order not to induce secondary contraction of the fibrovascular tissue, which may lead to retinal hole formation.

Whenever treating patients that had a partial vitreous hemorrhage and an acceptable view of the fundus it is important to check for the occurrence of a peripheral retinal detachment associated with retinal neovascularization and localized traction (Fig. 7.19).

When there is a subhyaloid hemorrhage it is necessary to perform scatter photocoagulation as soon as possible, because the hemorrhage will sooner or later involve the entire vitreous making the laser treatment more difficult. If the subhyaloid hemorrhage does not

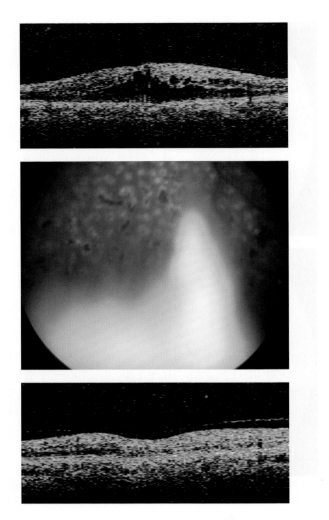

**Fig. 7.18.** Same patient of Fig. 7.17. *Upper*: OCT showing loss of the normal foveal profile and poor reflectivity. *Center*: deposit of triamcinolome acetonide injected 48 hours before (4 mg/0,1 ml.). *Lower*: three months later the macular edema disappeared and there was a normal foveal profile. Visual acuity went from 20/200 to 20/60.

allow the laser treatment a vitrectomy should be considered, particularly in young patients.

## 7.6. Conclusions and General Guidelines

Diabetes mellitus is the leading cause of blindness in the western world in people of less than 65 years of

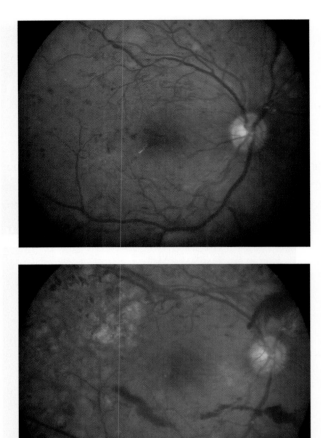

**Fig. 7.19.** *Left*: 23-year-old patient with Diabetes Mellitus Tipo 1 and high risk proliferative retinopathy. *Right*: after panretinal photocoagulation there is vitreous hemorrhage there are active new vessels and cystoid vascular edema. Vitrectomy is indicated.

age. The DRS and the ETDRS have given clinicians useful guidelines for the management of diabetic macular edema and proliferative retinopathy. It must be realized, however, that not all patients are alike, and the evolution of the retinopathy varies markedly between different patients. Furthermore, the guidelines of the DRS and ETDRS are very specific and are particularly appropriate to the eyes that are considered in the design of the studies. Clinicians must always balance information on the systemic metabolic control, guidelines for laser treatment and the specific situation of each patient and then use their own informed clinical judgement.

Laser treatment is an extreme situation for the diabetic patient and the treatment of the retinopathy. Prevention by good metabolic control and close follow-up remains fundamental.

New fundus imaging techniques, such as the OCT, have contributed to an improved evaluation of the retinopathy, helping the clinician in the decision to treat, when and how. New therapies are expected to become available in the near future to complement the generally well accepted laser photocoagulation.

# References

Akduman L, Olk RJ. (1997) Diode laser (810 nm) versus argon green (514 nm) modified grid photocoagulation for diffuse diabetic macular edema. *Ophthalmology* **104**(9): 1433–1441.

Aylward GW, Pearson RV, Jagger JD, Hamilton AM. (1989) Extensive argon laser photocoagulation in the treatment of proliferative diabetic retinopathy. *Br J Ophthalmol* **73**(3): 197–201.

Bamroongsuk P, Yi Q, Harper CA, MoCarty D. (2002) Delivery of photocoagulation treatment for diabetic retinopathy at a large Australian ophthalmic hospital: Comparisons with national clinical practice guidelines. *Clin Experiment Ophthalmol* Apr; **30**(2): 115–119.

Bandello F, Brancato R, Menchini U, *et al.* (2001) Light panretinal photocoagulation (LPRP) versus classic panretinal photocoagulation (CPRP) in proliferative diabetic retinopathy. *Semin Ophthalmol* **16**(1): 12–18.

Bandello F, Pognuz DR, Pirracchio A, Polito A. (2004) Intravitreal triamcinolone acetonide for florid proliferative diabetic retinopathy. *Graefes Arch Clin Exp Ophthalmol* **242**(12): 1024–1027.

Blankenship GW. (1979) Diabetic macular edema and argon laser photocoagulation: A prospective randomized study. *Ophthalmology* **86**(1): 69–78.

Blankenship GW. (1991) Fifteen-year argon laser and xenon photocoagulation results of Bascom Palmer Eye Institute's patients participating in the diabetic retinopathy study. *Ophthalmology* **98**(2): 125–128.

Bonafonte S, García ChA. (1996) Fotocoagulación del edema macular diabético. In: *Retinopatía Diabética*. Sergio Bonafonte, Charles García eds.; Local of Publication-Madrid pp. 127–144.

Bresnick GH. (1986) Diabetic macular edema. A review. *Ophthalmology* **7**: 989–997.

Bresnick GH. (1983) Diabetic maculopathy. A critical review highlighting diffuse macular edema. *Ophthalmology* **90**(11): 1301–1317.

Browning DJ, McOwen MD, Bowen RM, O'Marah TL. (2004) Comparison of the clinical diagnosis of diabetic macular edema with diagnosis by optical coherence tomography. *Ophthalmology* **11**(4): 712–715.

Central Vein Occlusion Study Group. (1994) Evaluation of grif patterns photocoagulation for macular edema in central vein occlusion. *Ophthalmology* **102**: 1425–1433.

Cheng H. (1975) Multicentre trial of xenon-arc photocoagulation in the treatment of diabetic retinopathy. A randomized controlled study. Interim report. *Trans Ophthalmol Soc UK* **95**(2): 351–357.

Ciardella AP, Klancnik J, Schihh W, *et al.* (2004) Intravitreal traimcinolone for the treatment of refractory diabetic macular edema with hard exudates: An optical coherence tomography study. *Br J Ophthalmol* **88**: 1131–1136.

Coscas G, Chaine G. (1979) Treatment of diabetic retinopathy with laser photocoagulation (author's transl. *Diabete Metab.* **5**(3): 247–259.

Dastur YK. (1994) The rationale of argon green laser photocoagulation for diabetic maculopathy. *J Postgrad Med* **40**(1): 13–17.

Diabetes Control and Complications Trial Research Group. (1995) The relationship of glycemic exposure (HbA$_{1C}$) to the risk of development and progression of retinopathy in the Diabetes Control and Complications Trial. *Diabetes* **44**: 968–983.

Diabetic Retinopathy Study Research Group. (1978) Photocoagulation treatment of proliferative diabetic retinopathy: The second report of diabetic retinopathy vitrectomy study findings. *Am J Ophthalmol* **85**: 82–106.

Diabetic Retinopathy Study Research Group. (1981) Photocoagulation treatment of proliferative diabetic retinopathy: Clinical application of Diabetic Retinopathy Study (DRS) findings. DRS Report Number 8. *Ophthalmology* **88**: 583–600.

Diabetic Retinopathy Study Research Group. (1978) Photocoagulation treatment of proliferative diabetic retinopathy: The second report of Diabetic Retinopathy Study (DRS) findings. *Ophthalmology* **85**: 82–106.

Diabetic Retinopathy Study Research Group. (1981) Photocoagulation treatment of proliferative diabetic retinopathy: Relationship of adverse treatment effects to retinopathy severity. DRS Report Number 5. *Dev Ophthalmol* **2**: 248–261.

Doft BH, Blankenship G. (1984) Retinopathy risk factor regression after laser panretinal photocoagulation for proliferative diabetic retinopathy. *Ophthalmology* **91**: 1453–1457.

Donnelly R, Idris I, Forrester JV. (2004) Proteinkinase C inhibition and diabetic retinopathy: A shot in the dark at translational research. *Br J Ophthalmol* **88**: 145–151.

Early Treatment Diabetic Retinopathy Study Research Group. (1991) Early photocoagulation for diabetic retinopathy. ETDRS report number 9. *Ophthalmology* **98**: 766–785.

Early Treatment Diabetic Retinopathy Study Group (1995) Focal photocoagulation treatment of diabetic macular edema: Relationship of treatment effect to fluorescein angiographic and other retinal characteristics at baseline. ETDRS Report Number 19. *Arch Ophthalmol* **113**: 1144–1145.

Early Treatment Diabetic Retinopathy Study Research Group. (1985) Photocoagulation for diabetic macular edema: Early Treatment Diabetic Retinopathy Study report number 1. *Arch Ophthalmol* **12**: 1796–1806.

Early Treatment Diabetic Retinopathy Study Research Group. (1987) Treatment techniques and clinical guidelines for photocoagulation of diabetic macular edema. ETDRS Report Number 2. *Ophthalmology* **94**: 761–774.

Early Treatment for Diabetic Retinopathy Study Research Group. (1987) Techniques for scatter and local photocoagulation treatment of diabetic retinopathy: ETDRS report no. 3. *Int Ophthalmol Clin* **27**: 254–264.

Fernandez-Vigo J, Fandino J, Fernandez MI, Solario MS. (1989) Comparative study of efficacy of focal photocoagulation in diabetic macular edema according to the wave length used. *J Fr Ophthalmol* **12**(11): 785–789.

Ferris F. (1996) Early photocoagulation in patients with either type I or type II diabetes. *Trans Am Ophthalmol Soc* **94**: 505–537.

Ferris FL 3rd, Podgor MJ, Davis MD. (1987) Macular edema in Diabetic Retinopathy Study patients. Diabetic Retinopathy Study Report Number 12. *Ophthalmology* **94**(7): 754–760.

Ferris FL III, Patz A. (1984) Macular Edema. A complication of diabetic retinopathy. *Surv Ophthalmol* **28**(Suppl): 452–461.

Fong DS, Segal PP, Myers F, *et al.* (1997) Subretinal fibrosis in diabetic macular edema. ETDRS report 23. Early Treatment Diabetic Retinopathy Study Research Group. *Arch Ophthalmol* **115**(7): 873–877.

Friberg TR, Karatza EC. (1997) The treatment of macular disease using a micropulsed and continuous wave 810-nm diode laser. *Ophthalmology* **104**(12): 2030–2038.

Friberg TR. (1999) Subthreshold (invisible) modified grid diode laser photocoagulation and diffuse diabetic macular edema (DDME). *Ophthalmic Surg Lasers* **30**(9): 705.

Gómez-Ulla F, Marticorena J, Fernández M, Rodríguez Cid MJ. (2004) Tratamiento del edema macular diabético persistente con triamcinolona intravítrea. Sociedad Española de Oftalmología. In Antiinflamatorios y antiangiogénicos intraoculares. Madrid. *Sociedad Española de Oftalmología* 83–92.

Gottfredsdottir MS, Stefansson E, Jonasson F, *et al.* (1993) Retinal vasoconstriction after laser treatment for diabetic macular edema. *Am J Ophthalmol* **115**(1): 64–67.

Guyer DR, D'Amico DJ, Smith CW. (1992) Subretinal fibrosis after laser photocoagulation for diabetic macular edema. *Am J Ophthalmol* **113**(6): 652–656.

Han DP, Mieler WF, Burton TC. (1992) Submacular fibrosis after photocoagulation for diabetic macular edema. *Am J Ophthalmol* **113**(5): 513–521.

Harbour JW, Smiddy WE, Flynn HW Jr., Rubsamen PE. (1996) Vitrectomy for diabetic macular edema associated with a thickened and taut posterior hyaloid membrane. *Am J Ophthalmol* **121**: 405–413.

Hee MR, Puliafito CA, Wong C, *et al.* (1995) Quantitative assessment of macular edema with optical coherence tomography. *Arch Ophthalmol* **113**(8): 1019–1029.

Hikichi T, Fujio N, Akiba J, *et al.* (1997) Association between the short-term natural history of diabetic macular edema and the vitreomacular relationship in type II diabetes mellitus. *Ophthalmology* **104**: 473–478.

Huang D, Swanson EA, Lin CP, *et al.* (1991) Optical Coherence Tomography. *Science* **2545**: 1178–1181.

Jaffe GJ, Burton TC. (1988) Progression of nonproliferative diabetic retinopathy following cataract extraction. *Arch Ophthalmol* **106**(6): 745–749.

Jahn CE, Topfner von Schutz K, Richter J, *et al.* (2004) Improvement of visual acuity in eyes with diabetic macular edema after treatment with pars plana vitrectomy. *Ophthalmologica* **218**(6): 378–384.

Jonas JB, Kreissig I, Sofker A, Degenring RF. (2003) Intravitreal injection of triamcinolone for diffuse diabetic macular edema. *Arch Ophthalmol* **1**: 57–61.

Kaufman SC, Ferris FL 3rd, Swartz M. (1987) Intraocular pressure following panretinal photocoagulation for diabetic retinopathy. Diabetic Retinopathy Report No. 11. *Arch Ophthalmol* **105**(6): 807–809.

Khairallah M, Brahim R, Allagui M, Chachia N. (1996) Comparative effects of argon green and krypton red laser photocoagulation for patients with diabetic exudative maculopathy. *Br J Ophthalmol* **80**(4): 319–322.

Kinyoun J, Barton F, Fischer M, *et al.* (1989) Detection of diabetic macular edema: Ophthalmoscopy versus photography. Early Treatment Diabetic Retinopathy Study. Report number 5. *Ophthalmology* **96**: 746–750.

Klein R, Klein BE, Moss SE. (1984) Visual impairment in diabetes. *Ophthalmology* **91**: 1–9.

Klein R, Klein BE, Moss SE, *et al.* (1984) The Wisconsin epidemiologic study of diabetic retinopathy. IV. Diabetic macular edema. *Ophthalmology* **12**: 1464–1474.

La Heij EC, Hendrikse F, Kessels AG, Derhaag PJ. (2001) Vitrectomy results in diabetic macular oedema without evident vitreomacular traction. *Graefes Arch Clin Exp Ophthalmol* **239**(4): 264–270.

Lam DS, Chan CK, Mohamed S, *et al.* (2004) Phacoemulsification with intravitreal triamcinolone in patients with cataract and coexisting diabetic macular oedema: A 6-month prospective pilot study. *Eye* Sep 24.

Lanzetta P, Dorin G, Pirracchio A, Bandello F. (2001) Theoretical bases of non-ophthalmoscopically visible endpoint photocoagulation. *Semin Ophthalmol* **16**(1): 8–11.

Lee CM, Olk RJ1. (1991) Modified grid laser photocoagulation for diffuse diabetic macular edema. Long-term visual results. *Ophthalmology* **10**: 1594–1502.

Lewis H, Abrams GW, Blumenkranz MS, Campo RV. (1992) Vitrectomy for diabetic macular traction and edema associated with posterior hyaloidal traction. *Ophthalmology*. **99**(5): 753–759.

Lewis H, Schachat AP, Haimann MH, Haller JA. (1990) Choroidal neovascularization after laser photocoagulation for diabetic macular edema. *Ophthalmology* **97**(4): 503–510.

Lewis H. (2001) The role of vitrectomy in the treatment of diabetic macular edema. *Am J Ophthalmol* **131**(1): 123–125.

Littel HL. (1985) Treatment of proliferative diabetic retinopathy. Long-term results of argon laser photocoagulation. *Ophthalmology* **92**(2): 279–283.

Luttrull JK, Musch DC, Mainster MA. (2005) Subthreshold diode micropulse photocoagulation for the treatment of clinically significant diabetic macular oedema. *Br J Ophthalmol* **89**(1): 74–80.

Mainster MA, Crossman JL, Erickson PJ, Heacock GL. (1990) Retinal laser lenses: Magnification, spot size, and field of view. *Br J Ophthalmol* **74**(3): 177–179.

Martidis A, Duker JS, Greenberg PB, *et al.* (2002) Intravitreal triamcinolone for refractory diabetic macular edema. *Ophthalmology* **5**: 920–927.

Massin P, Audren F, Haouchine B, *et al.* (2004) Intravitreal triamcinolone acetonide for diabetic diffuse macular edema: Preliminary results of a prospective controlled trial. *Ophthalmology* **2**: 218–224.

McDonald HR, Schatz H. (1985) Grid photocoagulation for diffuse macular edema. *Retina* **5**(2): 65–72.

McDonald HR, Schatz H. (1985) Visual loss following panretinal photocoagulation for proliferative diabetic retinopathy. *Ophthalmology* **92**(3): 388–393.

McMeel L, Trempe CL, Franks EB. (1977) Diabetic maculopathy. *Trans Am Acad Ophthalmol Otolaryngol* **83**: 476–487.

O'Donoghue HN. (1982) Laser treatment in diabetic retinopathy. *Trans Ophthalmol Soc UK* **102**: 468–470.

Olk RJ. (1986) Modified grid argon (blue-green) laser photocoagulation for diffuse diabetic macular edema. *Ophthalmology* **93**(7): 938–950.

Olk RJ. (1990) Argon green (514 nm) versus krypton red (647 nm) modified grid laser photocoagulation for diffuse diabetic macular edema. *Ophthalmology* **97**(9): 1101–1112.

Otani T, Kishi S, Maruyama Y. (1999) Patterns of diabetic macular edema with optical coherence tomography. *Am J Ophthalmol* **127**: 688–693.

Otani T, Kishi S. (2000) Tomographic assessment of vitreous surgery for diabetic macular edema. *Am J Ophthalmol* **129**(4): 487–494.

Otani T, Kishi S. (2001) Tomographic findings of foveal hard exudates in diabetic macular edema. *Am J Ophthalmol* **131**(1): 50–54.

Patz A, Schatz H, Berkow JW, *et al.* (1973) Macular edema — an overlooked complication of diabetic retinopathy. *Trans Am Acad Ophthalmol Otolaryngol* **77**(1): 34–42.

Pavese T, Insler MS. (1987) Effects of extracapsular cataract extraction with posterior chamber lens implantation on the development of neovascular glaucoma in diabetes. *J Cataract Refract Surg* **13**: 197–201.

Poliner LS, Christianson DJ, Escoffery RF, *et al.* (1985) Neovascullar glaucoma after intracapsular and extracapsular cataract extraction in diabetic patients. *Amer J Ophthalmol* **100**: 637–643.

Reddy VM, Zamora RL, Olk RJ. (1995) Quantitation of retinal ablation in proliferative diabetic retinopathy. *Am J Ophthalmol* **119**(6): 760–766.

Rubinstein K, Myska V. (1974) Pathogenesis and treatment of diabetic maculopathy. *Br J Ophthalmol* **58**(2): 76–84.

Rutledge BK, Wallow IH, Poulsen GL. (1993) Sub-pigment epithelial membranes after photocoagulation for diabetic macular edema. *Arch Ophthalmol* **111**(5): 608–613.

Schatz H, Madeira D, McDonald HR, Johnson RN. (1991) Progressive enlargement of laser scars following grid laser photocoagulation for diffuse diabetic macular edema. *Arch Ophthalmol* **109**(11): 1549–1551.

Shimura M, Yasuda K, Nakazawa T, *et al.* (2003) Quantifying alterations of macular thickness before and after panretinal photocoagulation in patients with severe diabetic retinopathy and good vision. *Ophthalmology* **110**(12): 2386–2394.

Spalter HF. (1971) Photocoagulation of circinate maculopathy in diabetic retinopathy. *Am J Ophthalmol* **1**: 242–250.

Stanga PE, Reck AC, Hamilton AM. (1999) Micropulse laser in the treatment of diabetic macular edema. *Semin Ophthalmol* **14**(4): 210–213.

Stefansson E, Machemer R, de Juan E, *et al.* (1992) Retinal oxygenation and laser treatment in patients with diabetic retinopathy. *Am J Ophthalmol* **113**: 36–38.

Striph GG, Hart WM Jr, Olk RJ. (1988) Modified grid laser photocoagulation for diabetic macular edema. The effect on the central visual field. *Ophthalmology* **95**(12): 1673–1679.

Sutter FKP, Simpson JM, Gillies MC. (2004) Intravitreal triamcinolone for diabetic macular edema that persists after laser treatment. Three-month efficacy and safety results of a prospective, randomized, doubled-masked, placebo-controlled clinical trial. *Ophthalmology* **111**: 2044–2049.

Tachi N, Ogino N. (1996) Vitrectomy for diffuse macular edema in cases of diabetic retinopathy. *Am J Ophthalmol* **122**: 258–260.

The Krypton Argon Regresión Neovascularization Study Research Group. (1993) Randomized comparison of krypton versus argon scatter photocoagulation for diabetic disc neovascularization. *Ophthalmology* **100**: 1655–1664.

Tranos PG, Wickremasinghe SS, Stangos NT, *et al.* (2004) Macular edema. Major review. *Surv Ophthalmol* **49**: 470–490.

United Kingdom Prospective Diabetes Study Group. (1998) Intensive blood-glucose control with sulphonylureas or insulin compared with conventional treatment and risk of complication in patients with type 2 diabetes. UPKDS 33. *Lancet* **352**: 837–853.

van Effenterre G, Guyot-Argenton C, Guiberteau B, *et al.* (1993) Macular edema caused by contraction of the posterior hyaloid in diabetic retinopathy. Surgical treatment of a series of 22 cases. *J Fr Ophthalmol* **16**(11): 602–610.

Vander JF, Duker JS, Benson WE, *et al.* (1991) Long-term stability and visual outcome after favorable initial response of proliferative diabetic retinopathy to panretinal photocoagulation. *Ophthalmology* **98**(10): 1575–1579.

Varley MP, Frank E, Purnell EW. (1988) Subretinal neovascularization after focal argon laser for diabetic macular edema. *Ophthalmology* **95**(5): 567–573.

Wallow IHL, Bindley CD. (1988) Focal photocoagulation of diabetic macular edema. *Retina* **8**: 261–269.

Whitelocke RA, Kearns M, Blach RK, Hamilton AM. (1979) The diabetic maculopathies. *Trans Ophthalmol Soc UK* **99**(2): 314–320.

Wiznia RA. (1979) Photocoagulation of nonproliferative exudative diabetic retinopathy. *Am J Ophthalmol* **88**(1): 22–27.

Yang CM. (2000) Surgical treatment for severe diabetic macular edema with massive hard exudates. *Retina* **20**(2): 121–125.

Yang CS, Cheng CY, Lee FL, *et al.* (2001) Quantitative assessment of retinal thickness in diabetic patients with and without clinically significant macular edema using optical coherence tomography. *Acta Ophthalmol Scand* **79**(3): 266–270.

Zacks DN, Johnson MW. (2005) Combined intravitreal injection of triamcinolone acetonide and panretinal photocoagulation for concomitant diabetic macular edema and proliferative diabetic retinopathy. *Retina* **25**(2): 135–140.

# Chapter 8

# Vitrectomy for Diabetic Retinopathy

**José Carlos Pastor**

## 8.1. Surgical Indications

The indications for surgical intervention for diabetic retinopathy (DR) were established during the mid-1980s (Aaberg and Abrams, 1987; Blankenship, 1989; Michels, 1981; Michels *et al.*, 1981; DRVS, 1985a,b; DVRS, 1988). As newer instrumentation evolved along with improved surgical technique and further clinical experience, these indications have been refined. The Diabetic Retinopathy Vitrectomy Study (DRVS) is considered a reference milestone for the establishment of new and more accurate indications (1985). It consisted of three studies that evaluated the natural course of severe proliferative diabetic retinopathy (PDR) and the effects of surgical intervention and its complications. After these clinical trials additional work in basic and clinical sciences contributed to the development of new and refined indications. Among these are new indications for treating diabetic macular edema that are extremely important because of the devastating impact of this complication on visual function. Consequently, the outcomes of surgical intervention in DR are now much better than twenty years ago. Many cases that were considered inoperable in the 1990s are now candidates for surgical intervention. For instance, patients with total tractional retinal detachment and rubeosis iridis (Helbig, 1996) now have better chances of achieving at least a moderate improvement in visual function (Ishida and Takeuchi, 2001). As a result of these advances, indications for vitrectomy in

diabetic patients fall into three categories: clearing media opacities, tractional complications and other indications.

### 8.1.1. Clearing Media Opacities

#### 8.1.1.1. *Non-clearing vitreous hemorrhage*

Historically non-clearing vitreous hemorrhage was the first indication for pars plana vitrectomy. The incidence of spontaneous vitreous hemorrhage is approximately seven new cases per 100,000 population per year. The commonest cause is PDR, accounting for 32% of all cases (Spraul and Grossniklaus, 1997). Based on the DRVS studies of type 1 diabetes patients, vitrectomy should be considered if there is no clearance of the dense vitreous hemorrhage within one month. For type 2 diabetics, waiting two to three months for spontaneous clearing is reasonable if there is no evidence of retinal detachment (RD).

Ultrasound examination is mandatory if a satisfactory view of the fundus cannot be obtained. Ultrasound may also provide useful information that could be associated with non-spontaneous reabsorption of vitreous hemorrhage in type 2 diabetics. For instance, ultrasound may reveal the presence of an extramacular tractional RD, the presence of fibrovascular membranes or the location of blood in the subhyaloidal space. In these cases vitrectomy should not be delayed (Capeans *et al.*, 1997). Obviously all other causes of vitreous hemorrhage must be ruled out

**238** *Diabetic Retinopathy*

before the hemorrhage is attributed to DR, especially if the other eye has mild to moderate nonproliferative diabetic retinopathy (NPDR).

Other conditions may modify the surgical decision. Earlier vitrectomy is recommended when no previous laser has been applied or when the fellow eye is blind or has rapidly progressing visual loss. Rubeosis iridis in the eye with recent vitreous hemorrhage can be considered a relatively urgent indication, especially if panretinophotocoagulation (PRP) has not been applied. On the other hand, surgical intervention can be cautiously deferred if a posterior vitreous detachment is present and when extensive PRP has been delivered previously.

### 8.1.1.2. *Dense premacular hemorrhages*

The existence of a dense premacular hemorrhage causes severe visual loss in patients with DR. Tractional forces along the vitreoretinal interface can result in a localized posterior vitreous detachment. Tension on the new vessels can cause hemorrhage in the subhyaloid space or under the internal limiting membrane. The confinement of blood in the subhyaloidal space indicates that the posterior hyaloid has not fully separated and the remains can act as a scaffold for progressive fibrovascular proliferation. Thus, these hemorrhages are associated with worsened anatomical and functional prognosis. They are loculated because of the presence of strong adhesions of the posterior hyaloid to the retina surface. This is especially true if the hemorrhage is dense and has fibrosis at the edges. Most premacular hemorrhages clear spontaneously or through the vitreous. In some cases a vitrectomy or a Nd:YAG laser membranotomy is mandatory. In these cases peripheral scatter photocoagulation must be performed at the time of the initial examination so that a vitrectomy can be performed within one month if the hemorrhage has not improved. If these hemorrhages are not treated, an intense fibrotic reaction will occur in the posterior hyaloid and serve as a scaffold for fibrovascular proliferation and subsequent tractional macular detachment.

In 1986, Tokui *et al.* reported the spontaneous outcome of a series of massive premacular hemorrhages. Those cases, in which new vessels were in fibrovascular stage (with apparent fibrous tissue), tended to be larger than four disc diameters and showed a clear tendency to be complicated with tractional RD. Thus, they are candidates for prompt vitrectomy. Their results showed that vision improves in up to 75% of operated eyes.

Some authors (Faulborn, 1988; Gabel *et al.*, 1989; Ezra *et al.*, 1996) have advocated the use of Nd:YAG laser membranotomy for diabetic premacular hemorrhage to drain the blood into the vitreous. There are no randomized prospective series to support this approach and indications of this technique remain unclear. Dense premacular hemorrhage without active fibrovascular proliferation could be a good indication. On the other hand, Nd:YAG laser application in patients with active fibrovascular proliferation can precipitate tractional macular detachment. Thus Nd:YAG laser hyaloidotomy may be useful in a few selected cases (Celebi and Kukner, 2001; Puthalath *et al.*, 2003).

### 8.1.1.3. *Dense asteroid hyalosis*

Occasionally, dense asteroid hyalosis may preclude fundus visualization. This condition, characterized by deposition of calcium-lipid complexes in the collagen meshwork of the vitreous, affects from 0.5% to 0.9% of the general population. In patients with dense asteroid hyalosis, the diagnosis and treatment of underlying posterior segment diseases may be complicated (Feist *et al.*, 1990). If the fellow eye has severe DR, that may be a reason for a vitrectomy (Lambrou *et al.*, 1989; Ikeda *et al.*, 1989).

### 8.1.2. Tractional Complications

The second category of indications for vitrectomy in diabetic patients is the presence of epiretinal and preretinal tractional components. These indications constitute the majority of patients undergoing vitrectomy for complications of DR.

### 8.1.2.1. *Tractional retinal detachment and tractional macular detachment*

Tractional retinal and macular detachments are at present the commonest indication for vitrectomy. They are the consequences of severe and active fibrovascular proliferation and the DRVS found that without intervention the natural history was very poor. The existence of a posterior vitreous detachment is an important factor for the prognosis of this complication. If a posterior hyaloid is still attached and has broad-based vitreoretinal connections, a tractional RD may occur. If traction is located at the periphery, a localized detachment can develop. In these cases, caution is advised in recommending vitrectomy because peripheral or midperipheral tractional detachments progress to involve the macula in only 15% of the cases (Charles and Flinn, 1981). Vitrectomy is generally reserved for those cases, in which the macula is involved or is clearly threatened.

As in the case of non-clearing vitreous hemorrhage, other factors influence the final surgical decision. Patients with media opacities in whom an adequate PRP has not been applied, those with a rapidly progressive course in the fellow eye and some others should be considered for earlier vitrectomy.

As mentioned, involvement of the macula requires surgical intervention. The existence of a tractional macular detachment is a definite indication for vitrectomy as long as the eye has any visual potential. Chronic macular detachment leads to a thinner, atrophic retina with more tightly adherent fibrovascular membranes. Therefore, when macular detachment has been present for six months or more, surgery is usually not recommended.

The pathological of this entity is very complex and depends on the relationship between the posterior vitreous, the fibrovascular tissue and the retina. The reason the macula tends to be affected is that the posterior vitreous is especially adherent to the macula, the retinal vessels and the optic disk. With anterior-posterior contraction of the hyaloid, the traction detaches the retina in these areas.

The general goals of vitrectomy include the removal of the posterior vitreous surface in which the fibrovascular tissue grows and the release of anterior-posterior and tangential vitreoretinal traction (Lewis and Sanchez, 1993). Expert surgeons achieve long-term retinal reattachment in more than 85% of the cases, although functional results are variable. Several studies have tried to determine the correlation between preoperative measurements and postoperative visual outcome. Unfortunately, only preoperative ultrasound gives useful information, especially if ophthalmoscopy is not possible (Meier and Wiedemann, 1997).

### *Progressive macular traction and macular heterotopia*

Progressive macular traction is characterized by partial vitreous detachment with vitreoretinal traction along the temporal arcades and the optic nerve head (Packer, 1994). It causes retinal traction extending through the fovea and, if progression is allowed, it will lead to macular heterotopia or to tractional RD of the macula. Several authors have suggested that these changes are features of PDR (Okun *et al.*, 1971; McMeel, 1977).

The indications for surgery are based on the impairment of visual acuity associated with metamorphopsia in many cases. Several factors predispose to poor visual outcome. These include the presence of iris or angle neovascularization, poor visual acuity in fellow eye, many active vessels in preretinal membranes, ischemic maculopathy demonstrated by fluorescein angiography and aphakia (Packer, 1987).

Other authors have demonstrated that cases with iris neovascularization and normal or low intraocular pressure (IOP) can regress after vitrectomy and intra- or postoperative laser photocoagulation. The visual status of the fellow eye was not definitively predictive for visual outcome. Lens extraction made at the time of vitrectomy did not significantly increase the amount of postoperative complications. Almost 50% of the cases had improvement of visual acuity (Sato *et al.*, 1994).

### 8.1.2.2. *Combined tractional and rhegmatogenous retinal detachment*

In patients with previous tractional detachment a sudden and profound visual loss must be interpreted as the result of a rhegmatogenous combination. The traction exerted by the posterior vitreous surface will cause a retinal break, frequently adjacent to fibrovascular epicenters and lead to combined tractional and rhegmatogenous RD. In contrast to pure tractional detachments, the combined detachments tend to be more bullous and may extend into the periphery (Lewis and Sanchez, 1993). Retinal breaks typically occur posterior to the equator and sometimes are not detected during the preoperative examination. Prompt surgery is indicated even if the macula is still attached. Anatomic results may be similar to the ones obtained in pure tractional detachments, but functional results are very often disappointing.

### 8.1.2.3. *Severe equatorial fibrovascular proliferation*

Severe equatorial fibrovascular proliferation is an uncommon situation, in which the neovascularization grows along hyaloidal attachments in the mid-periphery, causing peripheral traction, vitreous hemorrhage and/or hypotony. This unusual situation results in peripheral traction or tractional rhegmatogenous RD in eyes that have not necessarily been operated previously. A complex surgery is mandatory to reattach the retina. This surgery consists of lensectomy, encircling scleral buckle, delamination or segmentation of membranes and relaxing retinotomies. Visual outcome is not very good (Han *et al.*, 1995).

### 8.1.2.4. *Anterior hyaloidal fibrovascular proliferation*

Anterior hyaloidal fibrovascular proliferation usually occurs after previous vitrectomy surgery in both phakic and pseudophakic diabetic eyes. It is characterized by the development of neovascularization and fibrous proliferation from the anterior retina extending along the anterior hyaloid to the posterior lens surface. This condition should be suspected in previously vitrectomized patients suffering acute onset or exacerbation of rubeosis iridis (Boop *et al.*, 1992). Because the vitreous has been removed except at the base, recurrent retinal neovascularization is limited to the far periphery near the ora serrata and the pars plana. Features of hyaloidal fibrovascular proliferation include recurrent vitreous hemorrhages, presence of fibrovascular tissue on the posterior lens capsule and anterior extraretinal vascularization extending towards the lens on the anterior hyaloid. The natural history is a rapid progression to ciliary body detachment, rubeosis iridis, peripheral RD and phthisis. Patients, who develop this complication, tend to be young males with severe retinal neovascularization and extensive retinal ischemia that do not respond to photocoagulation. They also tend to have a tractional macular detachment that constitutes the indication for vitrectomy and placement of a scleral buckle. This condition frequently occurs within the first 12 weeks after vitrectomy (Lewis *et al.*, 1987).

As fibrous proliferation develops, anterior retinal and ciliary body detachments occur causing hypotony, cyclitic membrane formation and eventually atrophy of the eyeball with shrinkage. High-resolution contact B-scan echography may detect the anterior tractional detachment associated with this condition (Han *et al.*, 1991). Management of this complication requires aggressive surgery, despite which some cases progress to atrophia bulbi, especially if the eye has already developed a ciliary body detachment. Immediate reattachment surgery in combination with anterior peripheral coagulation therapy is an effective measure for controling neovascular activity, but function is usually limited to a low level (Bopp *et al.*, 1992). Extensive PRP before and during vitrectomy and removal of the clear lens and anterior vitreous in eyes at great risk of developing this complication can prevent its appearance (Lewis and Sanchez, 1993).

## 8.1.3. Other Indications

### 8.1.3.1. *Severe neovascular proliferation*

Eyes that develop iris and/or angle neovascularization, in which transpupillary PRP cannot be delivered, are candidates for vitrectomy. Removal of media opacities and extensive endophotocoagulation and/or cryopexy may induce regression of the anterior segment neovascularization. Additionally, this can prevent the development of neovascular glaucoma.

### 8.1.3.2. *Red blood cell-induced glaucomas*

Intraocular blood may result in different types of secondary glaucomas (Spraul and Grossniklaus, 1997). Among these, the most frequent are the hemolytic (erythroclastic) and the ghost cell glaucomas. Red cells debris (haemolytic) or degenerate red cells in the vitreous (ghost cell) can obstruct the trabecular meshwork and increase IOP. These complications are more commonly seen in aphakic eyes and may developed in previously vitrectomized eyes. Even though ghost cells are very common after vitreous hemorrhage, glaucomas induced by these cells occur only infrequently (Bailez *et al.*, 2002). While topical medications usually fail in lowering IOP, vitrectomy usually solves the problem. In previous vitrectomized eyes with a residual hemorrhagic basal vitreous, a new and total vitrectomy should be performed. However, if the eye has been completely vitrectomized, an outpatient fluid/air exchange might be enough to solve the problem.

### 8.1.3.3. *Macular edema*

In DR, involvement of the macula may occur in different ways. In tractional complications the macula can be occasionally affected through progressive traction and heterotopia. DR may cause dense premacular hemorhages and ultimately diabetic macular edema (DME). Macular edema is a principal cause of visual loss in diabetic patients (Moss *et al.*, 1998). Today the most interesting and controversial indication for vitrectomy in DR is the treatment of diffuse DME.

In 1992 Lewis *et al.* reported the results of a small series of eyes with DME associated with macular traction caused by dense premacular, posterior hyaloid membranes. While this condition is infrequent, vitrectomy resolves it and improves visual acuity in more than 80% of the cases.

In 1996 Tachi and Ogino reported successful results for diffuse macular edema in cases with attached premacular posterior hyaloid, but without a thickened hyaloid membrane. Traction exerted by the posterior hyaloid membrane on retinal vessels may cause extravasation in addition to the breakdown of the inner and outer blood-retinal barriers. Vitrectomy, by relieving this traction, may ameliorate diffuse DME. This initial series demonstrated the resolution of the edema in more than 90% of the cases but a visual improvement in only 50% of treated eyes (Tachi and Ogino, 1996). Today, the presence of a taut premacular posterior hyaloid is considered an indication for vitrectomy. In selected cases, removal of the posterior hyaloid improves macular edema and visual function in up to 90% of eyes, if macular ischemia is not present (Pendergast *et al.*, 2000).

Also in the mid-1990s objective assessments of DME were introduced in clinical practice. Fluorescein angiography has been traditionally used in conjunction with biomicroscopy to evaluate the diabetic macula, but more recently, optical coherent tomography (OCT) and retinal thickness analysis have become critical adjuncts in the management of diabetic patients. OCT, a non-invasive and non-contact system commercially available since 1995, works like B-scan ultrasonography but uses near infrared light. It is based on Michaelson's principle of low coherence interferometry and provides high resolution (10 $\mu$m axial and 20 $\mu$m transverse) cross-sectional images of optical reflectivity. Retinal thickness measurements with OCT have excellent intraobserver, interobserver and intervisit reproducibility.

OCT not only allows the quantification of macular thickness and volume, but in the scan profile mode has the great advantage of showing vitreoretinal relationships, at least when the posterior hyaloid is partially detached from the macula surface. In fact OCT has become a standard evaluation tool for most clinical trials for treatment of macular edema (Browning *et al.*, 2004). Now the so called ultrahigh-speed, ultrahigh-resolution OCT is available with an axial resolution of about 3 $\mu$m. Its real value in the management of DME is currently being evaluated.

One of the important limitations of OCT is that it is unable to evaluate ischemia. Retinal capillary non-perfusion is a feature commonly associated with progressive NPDR. Evidence of foveal avascular zones greater than 1000 $\mu$m in diameter generally means visual loss and must be recognized before surgery.

Since the end of the 1990's many clinicians have tried to establish the real value of vitrectomy in treating DME. In spite of these efforts, the efficacy of vitrectomy in cases where a taut posterior hyaloid is the only finding is not clear. It is certain that the presence of an epimacular membrane associated with diffuse edema is a clear indication of vitrectomy. However, the effect of other factors, such as the presence or absence of posterior vitreous detachment, remains unclear (Yamamoto *et al.*, 2001). Despite some papers on the efficacy of vitrectomy (Otani and Kishi, 2002) there is still controversy over the criteria for selecting surgical cases if clinical examination does not demonstrate a significant tractional effect of the posterior hyaloid or the presence of a epiretinal membrane.

Recently the value of internal limiting membrane (ILM) peeling to improve the results of visual outcome in DME surgery has been evaluated (Gandorfer *et al.*, 2000). It is accepted that the ILM may contribute to the permanence of the edema because of its rigidity and its removal may release all tractional forces. Some papers have advocated for systematic ILM peeling, but further studies are necessary (Stefaniotou *et al.*, 2004).

An interesting issue in patients with diabetic maculopathy has been the direct removal of submacular hard exudates by using subretinal forceps inserted through paramacular retinotomies. The idea was presented several years ago, in combination with posterior hyaloid removal, focal endolaser treatment and PRP. Despite some positive cases, based on the overall absence of long-term improvement in visual acuity, the results do not justify this kind of technique (Takaya *et al.*, 2004).

Finally, intravitreal injection of triamcinolone acetonide has been tested to treat cystoid macular edema that is resistant to vitreous surgery. With or without vitrectomy, intraocular triamcinolone injection can result in an improvement in visual acuity and in macular thickness, although these positive effects are temporary (Inoue *et al.*, 2004). Thus new drugs and new delivery systems are under investigation.

### 8.1.3.4. *Complications of previous vitrectomies*

The presence of one or more complications from a previous vitrectomy constitutes another important indication for performing vitrectomy again. Severe, recurrent vitreous hemorrhage, tractional or rhegmatogenous RD, anterior hyaloidal fibrovascular proliferation and fibrinoid syndrome are some of these complications. Fibrinoid syndrome is a rare postvitrectomy complication that involves extensive fibrinous membrane cross-linking of the vitreous (Sebestyen, 1982). It may represent the response of an ischemic retina and increased vascular permeability induced by vitrectomy. Minor degrees of postoperative fibrin formation occur in about 10% of vitrectomy patients, but they usually resolve spontaneously. However, severe fibrin deposition can lead to papillary or cyclitic membranes, pupillary-block glaucoma, ciliary body detachment with hypotony and recurrent tractional RD. With severe fibrin formation, the use of tissue plasminogen activator or streptokinase has been advocated. Tissue plasminogen activator, a fibrin-specific thrombolytic agent, is very useful in the clearance of postvitrectomy fibrin formation. However, in some cases with severe neovascularization, intraocular bleeding occurs (Esser *et al.*, 1997). A second vitrectomy must be considered in the more severe cases. The visual prognosis is very poor in eyes with severe postoperative fibrin formation.

## 8.2. Managing Vitrectomy-Associated Cataracts

The coexistence of cataract and DR is a common finding in clinical practice. Undoubtedly a relationship exists with the posterior development of cataract in a previously vitrectomized eye. It is accepted that almost 30% of adult vitrectomized eyes develop cataracts within one year and the percentage rises to 66% in two years in some series (Smiddy and Feuer, 2004).

Traditionally, intraocular lenses were not implanted during diabetic vitrectomy due to the risk of severe complications, such as postoperative anterior segment neovascularization. In the mid-1980s extracapsular cataract extraction showed several problems, and implantation of a lens was considered only in select cases where there was adequate control of retinal disease. Certainly iris neovascularization was considered a strict contraindication to intraocular lens implantation. Despite these reservations, the combined surgery gained popularity (Amino and Tanihara, 2002) and since the earliest 1990s some surgeons have performed cataract and vitrectomy surgeries in a single operation (Benson *et al.*, 1990).

In the late 1990s studies demonstrated that if adequate control of the underlying DR was achieved prior to cataract surgery, this technique was not associated with unacceptable intraoperative or early postoperative complications in cases with rubeosis iridis. Other major concerns were related to the inflammatory reaction caused by cataract procedure, which is higher in patients with PDR or branch retinal vein occlusion, than in other pathologies without a retinal vascular component (Sawa *et al.*, 1995). Thus two options were developed. The first option was to perform a phacoemulsification through a scleral tunnel. The alternative option involved a pars plana lensectomy, leaving the anterior capsule and zonules intact and then introducing the lens through a superior limbal incision at the end of vitrectomy.

Some authors pointed out that cataract removal after vitrectomy was associated with several complications,

such as inadequate pupillary mydriasis, superior conjunctival scarring, intraoperative anterior chamber depth, pupil size and iris lens excursions. Posterior capsules were excessively flaccid, prone to rapid anterior and posterior excursions and occasionally had plaques that were resistant to intraoperative removal. Thus in the mid-1990s extracapsular cataract extraction was replaced by phacoemulsification. Comparisons of extracapsular extraction versus phacoemulsification (Biro and Kovacs, 2002) demonstrated better results and fewer complications with phacoemulsification in previously vitrectomized eyes.

Despite that, phacoemulsification following vitrectomy had increased complications, especially due to zonular instability that caused abnormal deepening of the anterior chamber (Ahfat *et al.*, 2003). Thus in recent years many surgeons have advocated combining the phacoemulsification and vitrectomy procedures into a single operation termed phacovitrectomy. The aim is to simplify surgery and reduce complications. Indeed, the results and complications rate of this combination seem appropriate in selected patients (Jun *et al.*, 2001; Demetriades *et al.*, 2003; Honjo and Ogura, 1998). This procedure has the advantage of facilitating the removal of peripheral vitreous and, thereby, preventing important postvitrectomy complications (Suzuki *et al.*, 2001). For instance, the larger amount of removed vitreous may reduce foveal thickness in eyes that undergo concurrent vitrectomy, phacoemulsification and intraocular lens implantation (Kojima *et al.*, 2003). In some series the incidence of post-surgical iris neovascularization is lower with combined procedures, 2%, than with vitrectomy alone, 15% (Kadonosono *et al.*, 2001). Combining procedures allows an early rehabilitation, but the techniques must be evaluated and possibly refined, because rates of RD, DME, cystoid macular edema and rebleeding are still high (Lahey *et al.*, 2003).

Despite the advantages of the combined procedure, there are some complications still not solved, such as the presence of fibrin reaction and the development of posterior synechia (Honjo and Ogura, 1998;

Shinoda *et al.*, 2001) especially in cases with severe PDR. The presence and extent of these complications may be related to the use of gas tamponade and the amount of photocoagulation delivered during surgery. Even in severe cases of PDR with tractional detachment, it is possible to perform a combined phacoemulsification and vitrectomy with injection of silicone oil tamponade and obtain relatively good results (Douglas *et al.*, 2003; Kim *et al.*, 2004).

Finally removal of a clear lens might be considered in eyes with high risk of developing anterior hyaloidal fibrovascular proliferation or eyes with tractional RD extending into periphery. No clear indications for inserting an intraocular lens in these eyes are available in the literature.

## 8.3. Surgical Objectives and Techniques

Among the numerous surgical objectives of vitrectomy for complications of DR, the most relevant are to neutralize and, if possible, eliminate the factors leading to vision loss. The objectives can be summarized as the removal of media opacities, relieving retinal traction and delivering appropriate laser treatment.

### 8.3.1. Media Opacities

Standard 3 port pars plana vitrectomy is used, associated sometimes with lensectomy or phacoemulsification instruments. Non-complicated cases can be safely and reliably treated with the new 25G instrumentation (see Section 8.5: New Instrumentation).

### 8.3.2. Vitreoretinal Traction

The surgical repair of complex diabetic traction detachment requires the removal of the vitreous and the release of anterior and tangential forces from the retina. This was originally accomplished by vitrectomy with segmentation of the posterior membranes (Michels, 1981) and by vitrectomy with delamination and complete removal of the vitreous proliferation (Charles, 1971). However, one of the major complications in repairing diabetic tractional retinal detachment is the production of inadvertent retinal breaks and tears. Several techniques have been developed to minimize this risk. These modifications, termed "en bloc techniques" rely more on bimanual surgery. A multiport illumination system has been developed (Koch *et al.*, 1991) to allow the surgeon complete bimanual capability and total flexibility.

#### 8.3.2.1. *Techniques*

The removal of both antero-posterior and tangential traction, as well as membranes, requires four basic techniques: membrane, peeling, segmentation, delamination and "en bloc" membrane removal. Most surgeons use a combination, depending on the nature of each case and their own experience.

Membrane peeling consists of grasping membranes with forceps and peeling them tangentially across the surface. It may be assisted by the bimanual approach. It is a quick technique that can be used for atrophic and avascular membranes. The major disadvantage is the risk of tearing the retina and increased risk of bleeding.

The segmentation technique consists of traction removal by isolating islands of membranes through dissecting and cutting bridges of tissue between strong fibrovascular connections. Little or no attempt is made to remove the centers from the retinal surface. Picks and scissors are used to segment preretinal membranes. Theoretically, segmentation may have a lower rate of iatrogenic break formation. However, it is difficult to determine if all traction has been relieved and residual membranes may lead to residual or recurrent traction.

In the delamination technique the anomalous newly formed tissue is removed at the plane of the retina. Scissors are usually supplemented by illuminated instruments, such as picks and/or forceps. When successfully performed, all traction is removed and normal anatomy is restored. However, this is a more time consuming technique and has a high risk of iatrogenic hole formation and bleeding when vascular attachments are cut.

The "en bloc" technique consists of using horizontal scissors to remove epiretinal tissue from the posterior pole. This is followed with the vitrectomy probe to remove remaining vitreous. The preservation of the posterior hyaloid facilitates the separation of the membranes from the retina. In some cases, fibrovascular proliferation is more completely removed and bleeding less frequent than with membrane sectioning techniques. The major surgical complication of this technique is the production of retinal breaks (Abrams and Williams, 1987).

Some papers have compared membrane dissection and "en bloc" technique and found no differences in visual results and complications rate (Li *et al.*, 2004). It must be realized, however, that it is very difficult to design these types of studies so as to avoid bias and the influence of the learning curve of the surgeons. Thus, true differences in results and complications may exist and become apparent with time and experience.

Despite the refinement of the previously mentioned techniques, complications are still so high that new procedures continue to be developed. For instance, viscodissection uses viscomaterial for peeling the epiretinal membranes. When the viscoelastic material is pulsed between the retina and surface membranes, it improves the visibility of epicentres and allows a larger work area for scissors. Even more, when stretched, the viscoelastic material puts tension on the tissue and provides countertraction to maximize cutting. It facilitates the stabilization of the tissue and it is the only technique that pushes the retina down as the membrane is elevated. Problems with this technique include the additional cost of the viscoelastic material itself and the ancillary equipment. Furthermore, there is the potential for subretinal injection, higher incidence of hole formation, postoperative pressure rise, bleeding and increased risk of epiretinal membrane formation. Some clinical studies have reported

that the incidence of retinal breaks is not increased during viscodissection and those authors state that viscodissection appears to be a safe and effective alternative (Grigorian *et al.*, 2003).

### 8.3.3. Control of Hemorrhage and Vascular Proliferation

#### 8.3.3.1. *Hemorrhage*

In some cases intraoperative hemorrhages are a major complication and may result in severe postoperative intraocular fibrin formation. Certain procedures, such as the Valsalva maneuver, can cause acute peaks of IOP and are associated with massive suprachoroidal hemorrhage during pars plana vitrectomy (Pollack *et al.*, 2001). The prevalence of this complication varies among different series, probably due to patient selection. Overall, some degree of hemorrhage is expected in 20%–50% of vitrectomies.

Intraocular diathermy, increasing the infusion pressure and intraoperative PRP are strategies developed to minimize the effects of hemorrhaging. In 1986 intravitreal bovine thrombin was proposed to control intraoperative bleeding (Thompson *et al.*, 1986). Despite some positive results, there was increased postoperative intraocular inflammation and the technique has been abandoned. Mechanical measures, such as the use of intravitreal sodium hyaluronate (Packer *et al.*, 1989 (Joondeph and Blankenship, 1989; Schulze *et al.*, 2000) and $SF_6$, (Koutsandrea *et al.*, 2001) have been applied to the posterior segment to control hemorrhage following vitrectomy. Air did not reduce the postoperative hemorrhage rate in an experimental model, but had a positive effect in a short clinical series (Schulze *et al.*, 2000). $SF_6$ was also ineffective in reducing the incidence of vitreous hemorrhage when compared with BSS (Koutsandrea *et al.*, 2001). Systemic blood pressure control may also lessen intraoperative and postoperative bleeding.

Patients at risk for thromboembolic events must be managed very carefully. Aspirin and warfarin can significantly increase the risk of bleeding complications during ocular surgery. Thus, if the patient's thromboembolic risk is low, these treatments should be stopped (Narendran and Williamson, 2003).

### 8.3.3.2. *Vascular Proliferation*

Post-surgical vascular reproliferation is a complication that frequently occurs. Endolaser PRP is usually delivered intraoperatively to reduce the risk of anterior segment neovascularization. When media opacities prevent this application or a very peripheral treatment is needed, panretinal cryopexy is also an option.

After successful vitrectomy, vascular reproliferation may cause severe complications, such as RD. Reproliferation is a major complication of vitrectomy, occurring 47% of ocular injuries and in 23% of patients with PDR (Kroll *et al.*, 1989). The incidence of reproliferation was highest during the first three postoperative months, however, there are interesting differences between these two conditions. For ocular injuries the rate of reproliferation was highest during the first month, while in cases of PDR the incidence peaked during the second and third months.

Adjunctive treatment with intravitreal triamcinolone (25 mg) has been advocated to control reproliferation after vitrectomy for PDR (Jonas *et al.*, 2003). However, intraocular injection of silicone oil continues to be the first choice in these cases (Castellarin *et al.*, 2003; Douglas *et al.*, 2003) even though it must be removed between the third and sixth postoperative month (Kroll *et al.*, 1989). Removal may be followed by complications, such as redetachments, severe hypotony and severe postoperative hemorrhages (Pearson *et al.*, 1993).

## 8.4. Outcomes and Complications of Vitrectomy in Diabetic Retinopathy

### 8.4.1. Outcomes

While the DRVS demonstrated that early vitrectomy improves the overall chances of better visual acuity after two years of follow up, the results are not so clear in type 2 diabetes. Anatomic and functional outcomes depend on the nature of the complications that indicate vitrectomy, the degree of retinal traction, area of capillary nonperfusion, retinal detachment and existence of macular edema among other factors. Many series have been published over the last 30 years on the outcome of vitrectomy in DR complications, but usually they are composed of a heterogeneous group of patients. Thus, it is difficult to summarize the anatomic and functional results. The classification of vitrectomy patients by Kroll was a significant step towards developing criteria that has prognostic value (Hesse *et al.*, 2002). This classification defines four stages of PDR based upon the status of the macula. It has demonstrated a prognostic value for postoperative outcomes, but unfortunately it has not been widely accepted. Consequently, much of the recent work has been made without any type of classification.

Studies published ten years ago established the anatomical and functional results in cases of PDR and basically these have not changed. In cases of vitreous hemorrhage and other media opacities, an improvement of vision in the range of 59% to 83% occurs. However, in cases of combined tractional and rhegmatogenous retinal detachment, the improvement declines to 32% to 53%.

Patients with only vitreous hemorrhage improve visual acuity in nearly 90% of the cases, but if a tractional RD is present, the improvement declines to only 50% of the patients. Major complications include neovascular glaucoma that develops postoperatively in 7% of the cases and secondary retinal detachment in 8% (Sima and Zoran, 1994).

Results and complications depend on the complexity of the underlying disease, the existence of tractional retinal detachment and the existence of a previous PRP. Hajji *et al.* published a series of 137 eyes treated with a combination of segmentation-delamination technique. A third of the cases had a preoperative complete PRP and 27% had tractional RD. Anatomical success was obtained in 69% of the patients, with 55% having improved vision. Common complications included iatrogenic breaks (8%), single intravitreous hemorrhage (8%), with recurrent vitreous hemorrhage (8%) and developed neovascular glaucoma (5%) (Hajji *et al.*, 2003). Even patients with multiple vitrectomies for recurrent diabetic vitreous hemorrhages can have a favorable anatomic outcome while maintaining ambulatory vision (Cooper *et al.*, 2004).

Several attempts have been made to predict the visual outcomes after vitrectomy in patients with tractional RD for DR. Based on multivariate logistic regression analysis, the status of the macula and the existence of rubeosis are considered important risk factors for poor functional results (Helbig *et al.*, 1998). Less than 25% of patients who underwent vitrectomy for complications of DR had a visual acuity of 20/60 or better. In a recent study (La Heij *et al.*, 2004) age and iris neovascularization were considered the strongest predictors of a worse visual outcome. Single flash electroretinogram and some other electrophysiological tests have been used to predict the functional outcome in patients with massive vitreous hemorrhage, but its use has not been widely accepted (Hiraiwa *et al.*, 2003).

Recently the predictive value of measuring vitreous fluid levels of vascular endothelial growth factor (VEGF) and angiotensin was reported (Funatsu *et al.*, 2004). Only high levels of VEGF showed an association with a significant risk of postoperative progression of PDR. But high VEGF levels were also found in RD and other proliferative vitreoretinopathies of nondiabetic patients (Hattenbach *et al.*, 1999; Nicoletti *et al.*, 2003). Thus VEGF plays a fundamental but not specific role in diabetic retinal neovascularization and proliferation.

## 8.4.2. Complications

Pars plana vitrectomy can be associated with numerous complications, such as cataract, secondary glaucoma, retinal and/or vitreous incarcerations,

endophthalmitis, postoperative massive intraocular fibrin accumulation and recurrent vitreous hemorrhage. The principal complications of vitrectomy in diabetic patients are recurrent vitreous hemorrhage, retinal detachment and rubeosis iridis with or without neovascular glaucoma. Other complications include retinal breaks, cataract development, corneal epithelial complications and others.

### 8.4.2.1. *Recurrent vitreous hemorrhage*

Some degree of postoperative vitreous hemorrhage occurs in virtually all case but is visually significant in about 30% of them (Schachat *et al.*, 1983). Some authors have advocated the use of air endotamponade to reduce this rate, though this technique, as mentioned above, remains controversial (Schulze *et al.*, 2000). Management options, after a waiting period of weeks to allow spontaneous clearing, include office-based fluid-gas exchange, vitreous lavage or a new vitrectomy (Millar *et al.*, 1986; Martin and McCuen, 1992).

One important complication that can be a source of rebleeding after vitrectomy is fibrovascular ingrowth in the sclerotomy sites. Histopathology has demonstrated considerable disruption of tissues around incisions, vitreous incarceration in the wound and infiltration of the vitreous base by granulation tissue (Koch *et al.*, 1995). Rebleeding in these cases develops at an average of nine weeks after initial surgery (Sawa *et al.*, 2000). Because of the anatomic locations of these sites, they are frequently difficult, if not impossible, to visualize ophthalmoscopically or biomicroscopically. This fibrous ingrowth may be suspected in eyes richly vascularized in the pars plana entry sites where there is dilation of subconjunctival vessels (Krieger, 1993; West and Koch *et al.*, 2000). Other factors associated with this fibrovascular ingrowth are incomplete posterior vitrectomy, larger sclerotomy incisions, pronounced postoperative inflammation at the sites and poor surgical closure of the scleral wounds (Sawa *et al.*, 2000).

Ultrasound biomicroscopy (UBM) has been used to assess changes at the sclerotomies (Bhende *et al.*, 2000).

Vitreous incarceration was demonstrated in 19% of infusion ports and fibrovascular proliferation was seen in 9% of active ports, 13% of light ports and 15% of infusion ports. Those cases with recurrent vitreous hemorrhage, in which UBM demonstrated fibrovascular ingrowth, required more extensive surgery than a simple fluid-air exchange. A more recent study using UBM showed that fibrovascular ingrowth is more frequent in eyes that experience recurrent non-clearing vitreous hemorrhage. This information may aid in reoperative planning (Hershberger *et al.*, 2004). One clinical study suggested that in addition to the factors mentioned above, fibrovascular ingrowths are more frequent in eyes without peripheral laser or cryotherapy (Krieger, 1993) and the use of cryopexy around the scleral wounds at the end of vitrectomy has been advocated to prevent its appearance.

### 8.4.2.2. *Retinal breaks*

Retinal breaks are a common complication of vitreoretinal surgery, but they are significantly more frequent in vitrectomies for PDR. Retinal breaks occur in up to 20% of vitrectomies for DR and may lead to a RD with a very poor prognosis. Some of the intraoperative breaks can be treated with fluid-gas exchange and retinopexy. In some other cases tamponade with silicone oil is mandatory. Some authors have advocated systematic extensive PRP to prevent RD, but others prefer to reserve intra-and/or postoperative photocoagulation for management of iatrogenic retinal breaks (Hajji *et al.*, 2003).

In our own experience (Rola *et al.*, 2003) retinal breaks develop in 6.6% of all vitrectomies studied, but the rate increases to 13% in diabetic vitrectomies. They are more often located in the posterior pole than in periphery. These results are slightly higher than the 8% iatrogenic breaks reported by other authors (Hajji *et al.*, 2003). More than 50% of undetected breaks during surgery develop a postoperative retinal detachment, with poor anatomic prognosis. There is no protocol to manage these retinal breaks, but according to our experience, it is mandatory to explore carefully the posterior pole and the retinal periphery by indirect ophthalmoscopy or wide-angle system and indentation at the end of surgery for localizing them. Breaks in the periphery must be treated with gas injection and an encircling procedure. In the posterior pole breaks, the use of silicone oil tamponade should be considered. Obviously intra-and/or postoperative photocoagulation should be applied.

### 8.4.2.3. *Retinal detachment*

Retinal detachment is one of the major complications of vitrectomy. As with all postoperative problems, the incidence depends on the severity of the underlying disease. Rates of postoperative RD vary with the preoperative diagnosis and may occur in up to 20% of the PDR cases and only in 5% of simple vitreous hemorrhages (Helbig *et al.*, 1998).

### 8.4.2.4. *Iris rubeosis and neovascular glaucoma*

Iris rubeosis and neovascular glaucoma (NVG) are frequent complications of vitrectomy for PDR. From a clinical point of view, retinal areas of nonperfusion in the midperiphery and occlusion of capillaries in the peripapillary region, temporal raphe and optic disk are risk factors for angle neovascularization (Hamanaka *et al.*, 2001). Following vitrectomy more than 8% of the eyes developed stromal iris rubeosis and NVG occurred in 5% (Helbig *et al.*, 1998). In aphakic eyes the incidence is higher than in phakic eyes (Blankenship, 1980). The absence of vitreous gel may allow anterior diffusion of vasoproliferative factors and lensectomy may reduce this barrier further. Rubeosis iridis and NVG are associated with high concentrations of intraocular VEGF. The aqueous humor VEGF level is elevated in patients with NVG (Tripathi *et al.*, 1998) and intravitreal injection of VEGF can experimentally produce iris neovascularization and NVG in primates (Tolentino *et al.*, 1996).

Recently Itakura *et al.* reported high levels of VEGF in the vitreous cavity after vitrectomy for PDR (Itakura *et al.*, 2004). The main source of VEGF is the ischemic retina. Retinal photocoagulation may reduce the production of VEGF (Aiello *et al.*, 1994) and prevent development of rubeosis. If postoperative rubeosis occurs, fluid-air exchange may transiently reduce intravitreal VEGF (Itakura *et al.*, 2004).

Once developed, NVG is difficult to control and several attempts have been made to solve the situation. Aggressive treatments, such as pars plana vitrectomy, PRP, laser coagulation of the ciliary processes and silicone oil tamponade controlled pressure in 72% of the patients after one year, but almost 30% lost vision and 15% had hypotony (Bartz-Schmidt *et al.*, 1999; Valmaggia *et al.*, 2004). Drainage implants associated with pars plana vitrectomy have been evaluated to control NVG. Molteno devices used in combination with pars plana vitrectomy had severe complications (Lloyd *et al.*, 1991).

More recently a new technique in which aqueous humor is diverted from the anterior chamber to the suprachoroidal space by a Seton device seems to be effective in lowering intraocular pressure in refractory NVG (Ozdamar *et al.*, 2003). At one year post-surgery 72% of selected patients with or without antiglaucoma medications had IOP under 21 mm Hg. However, visual outcomes were poor because of severe underlying ocular disease and postoperative complications (Scott *et al.*, 2000). The development of new trans-scleral diode lasers has open a new approach to the treatment of NVG that needs to be evaluated (Nabili and Kirkness, 2004).

### 8.4.2.5.  *Corneal epithelial complications*

Corneal epithelial complications were very common at the beginning of vitrectomy (Foulks *et al.*, 1979), but the incidence has decreased significantly. Nevertheless they still develop in about 10% of our cases (Chiambo *et al.*, 2004). Most are due to persistent epithelial defects. However, we have identified cases of presumably necrotizing herpetic keratitis, probably related to surgical trauma and the postoperative use of topical corticosteroids.

In some cases a corneal epithelial debridement is necessary to perform the vitrectomy. Irrigating contact lenses appear to increase the need for epithelial debridement compared with other alternatives, such

as sew-on lenses, non-contact lenses. In most cases the healing process restores the corneal integrity without any problem, but in some patients, epithelial defects persist over weeks.

### 8.4.2.6.  *Fibrin formation*

As mentioned, intravitreal fibrin formation frequently occurs after vitrectomy for DR and intravitreal tissue plasminogen activator can resolve this postoperative complication in some cases (Esser *et al.*, 1997; Wu *et al.*, 2001). Also dexamethasone phosphate (0.8 mg intravitreal) may reduce the postoperative intraocular inflammatory process and fibrin formation (Blankenship, 1991). Even though this treatment reduced inflammation and fibrin formation to 15% of the treated eyes compared to 27% of controls, it has not been routinely accepted.

## 8.5. New Instrumentation

Improvement of instrumentation has been continuous since the 1970s. These advances have reduced the complications of DR by enabling removal of axial opacities, release of anteroposterior and/or tangential traction, segmentation or peeling of epiretinal membranes, achieving efficient hemostasis and delivering appropriate laser treatment. New instruments continue to be developed. Several high-speed vitreotomes allow for a more controlled vitreous removal. These high-speed cutters can be used to remove membranes from the retinal surface (Gallemore *et al.*, 2004). After the completion of vitrectomy many cases need endolaser, prompting the development of curved-tipped probes to facilitate treatment of the entire peripheral retina.

To reduce the risk of inadvertent retinal traction at the vitreous base that causes retinal tears, a modified "en bloc" technique was developed in 2002 (Steinmetz *et al.*, 2002). This technique relies more on bimanual surgery with an illuminated membrane pick and a multiport illumination system. It allows the surgeon complete bimanual capability and total flexibility. Short retrospective, non-comparative interventional series have shown good anatomic and functional results.

Another option is the use of systems that avoid the use of fiberoptics for endo-illumination, using instead the light source of the operating microscope (Horiguchi *et al.*, 2002). These systems seem to facilitate bimanual techniques, but still need further and more extensive evaluation.

Recently the use of 25-gauge instruments for vitrectomy, termed "transconjunctival sutureless vitrectomy," have been developed to operate with less invasive techniques. Small gauge vitrectomy instrumentation is now available allowing no-stitch surgery. This technique seems to have some potential benefits in selected cases of DR by hastening the recovery period and minimizing surgically induced trauma (Fuji *et al.*, 2002). Nevertheless, it has several disadvantages including practical limitations of flow for removal of dense hemorrhages and membranes and a limited choice of ancillary instrumentation. Its real value in complicated cases of DR needs further study.

During vitrectomy it is necessary in some cases to create a posterior vitreous separation for a complete removal of the posterior hyaloid from the retinal plane. The surgical implications of posterior vitreous removal in diabetic eyes are obvious. Failure to recognize true posterior vitreous hyaloid may contribute to continued morbidity in patients after vitrectomy. If the inner wall of the vitreoschisis cavity is mistaken for the posterior vitreous wall or if the residual vitreous cortex on the retina is left untreated during vitrectomy, this tissue serves as a scaffold for continued proliferation of cells and may also contribute to persistent tangential tractional force on the retinal surface. Even more, in eyes with diabetic macular edema, the residual vitreous cortex after vitrectomy could be a factor that may hinder visual recovery.

The surgical separation of posterior vitreous is usually created by high vacuum levels created by the vitreotome probe or the silicone-tipped extrusion needle. However, this manoeuvre may be difficult to perform in some patients, in part due to the inability to visualize adequately the posterior vitreous cortex. Recently Peyman *et al.* reported that a triamcinolone-assisted vitrectomy greatly improved the visibility of the posterior vitreous cortex (Peyman *et al.*, 2000). Several patterns of residual vitreous cortex have been identified (Sonoda *et al.*, 2004). The commonest type in diabetic patients is the diffuse, being the vitreous cortex present in all the temporal vascular arcade area. Triamcinolone acetonide used in this way seems not to have any adverse effects.

Some complications of vitrectomy are related to adherences of the vitreous body to the retina and several attempts have been made to dissolve or liquefy the vitreous. Purified ovine hyaluronidase (Vitrase®) has now been evaluated in a randomized, controlled clinical trail for its effectiveness in managing nonclearing diabetic vitreous hemorrhage (Boyer *et al.*, 1998). In addition to this primary use, hyaluronidase and some others agents, such as plasmin or chondroinase, have been evaluated to promote the development of posterior vitreous detachment, which can simplify diabetic vitrectomy. Few reports have been published, but the results do not seem very enthusiastic (Le Mer *et al.*, 1999).

As in some other vitreo-retinal surgeries, the use of heavy liquids for endotamponade has been tested. The usefulness of these compounds as retinal tools to reattach the retina in severe cases of PDR is now without doubt (Maturi *et al.*, 1999). However, the use of these agents for long-term tamponade is very controversial due to their numerous side effects, mainly related to inflammation (Schatz *et al.*, 2004). Silicone oil continues to be the preferred long-term tamponade. It may reduce anterior segment neovascularization and may be better than gas in patients with severe rubeosis, anterior hyaloidal fibrovascular proliferation, multiple recurrent vitreous hemorrhages and complex cases combining rhegmatogenous and tractional retinal detachments (Castellarin *et al.*, 2003).

## 8.6. Conclusions

Vitrectomy remains an essential tool in the management of severe complications from DR. While postvitrectomy visual acuity outcomes are favorable compared to the natural history of DR, they are still poor when compared to the efficacy of preventive measures.

## References

Aaberg TM, Abrams GW. (1987) Changing indications and techniques for vitrectomy in the management of complications in diabetic retinopathy. *Ophthalmology* **94**: 775–779.

Abrams GW, Williams GA. (1987) "En bloc" excision of diabetic membranes. *Am J Ophthalmol* **103**: 302–308.

Ahfat FG, Yuen CH, Groenewald CP. (2003) Phacoemulsification and intraocular lens implantation following pars plana vitrectomy: A prospective study. *Eye* **17**: 16–20.

Aiello LP, Avery RL, Arrigg PG, *et al.* (1994) Vascular endothelial growth factor in ocular fluid of patients with diabetic retinopathy and other retinal disorders. *N Eng J Med* **331**: 1480–1487.

Amino K, Tanihara H. (2002) Vitrectomy combined with phacoemulsification and intraocular lens implantation for diabetic macular edema. *Jpn J Ophthalmol* **46**: 455–459.

Bailez C, Pastor JC, Martin F, Saornil MA. (2002) Ghost cell detection in vitreous cytology: Clinico-pathological correlation. *Arch Soc Esp Oftalmol* **77**: 369–375.

Bartz-Scmidt KU, Thumannn G, Psichias A, *et al.* (1999) Pars plana vitrectomy, endolaser coagulation of the retina and ciliary body combined with silicone oil endotamponade in the treatment of uncontrolled neovascular glaucoma. *Graefes Arch Clin Exp Ophthalmol* **237**: 969–975.

Benson WE, Brown GC, Tasman W, McNamara J. (1990) Extracapsular cataract extraction, posterior chamber lens insertion, and pars plana vitrectomy in one operation. *Ophthalmology* **97**: 918–921.

Bhende M, Agraharm SG, Gopal L, *et al.* (2000) Ultrasound biomicroscopy of sclerectomy sites after pars plana vitrectomy for diabetic vitreous hemorrhage. *Ophthalmology* **107**: 1729–1736.

Biro Z, Kovacs B. (2002) Results of cataract surgery in previously vitrectomized eyes. *J Cataract Refract Surg* **28**: 1003–1006.

Blankenship GW. (1991) Evaluation of a single intravitreal injection of dexamethasone phosphate in vitrectomy surgery for diabetic retinopathy complications. *Graefes Arch Clin Exp Ophthalmol* **229**: 62–65.

Blankenship GW. (1980) The lens influence on diabetic vitrectomy results. Report of a prospective randomized study. *Arch Ophthalmol* **98**: 2196–2198.

Blankenship GW. (1989) Proliferative diabetic retinopathy: principles and techniques of surgical treatment. In: Ryan SJ. (ed.), *Retina*, Vol. 3, CV Mosby, St Louis, pp. 515–539.

Bopp S, Lucke K, Laqua H. (1992) Acute onset of rubeosis iridis after diabetic vitrectomy can increase peripheral traction retinal detachment. *Ger J Ophthalmol* **1**: 375–381.

Boyer DS, Thomas EL, Novack RL. (1998) Intravitreal injection of ACS-005 hyaluronidase produces clearing of vitreous hemorrhage. *Invest Ophthalmol Vis Sci* **39**: 2345–2347.

Browning DJ, McOwen MD, Bowen RM, O'Marah TL. (2004) Comparison of the clinical diagnosis of diabetic macular edema with diagnosis by optical coherence tomography. *Ophthalmology* **111**: 712–715.

Capeans C, Santos L, Tourino R, *et al.* (1997) Ocular echography in the prognosis of vitreous haemorrhage in type II diabetes mellitus. *Int Ophthalmol* **21**: 269–275.

Castellarin A, Grigorian R, Bhagat N, *et al.* (2003) Vitrectomy with silicone oil infusion in severe diabetic retinopathy. *Br J Ophthalmol* **87**: 318–321.

Celebi S, Kukner AS. (2001) Photodisruptive Nd:YAG laser in the management of premacular subhyaloid hemorrhage. *Eur J Ophthalmol* **11**: 281–286.

Charles S, Flinn CE. (1981) The natural history of diabetic extramacular traction detachment. *Arch Ophthalmol* **99**: 66–68.

Charles S. (1971) *Vitreous Microsurgery*, 2nd ed. Williams and Wilkins, Baltimore, pp. 107–120.

Chiambo S, Bailez C, Pastor JC, *et al.* (2004) [Corneal epithelial complications alter vitrectomy: A retrospective study]. *Arch Soc Esp Oftalmol* **79**: 155–162.

Cooper B, Shah GK, Grand MG, *et al.* (2004) Visual outcomes and complications after multiple vitrectomies for diabetic vitreous hemorrhage. *Retina* **24**: 19–22.

Demetriades AM, Gottsch JD, Thomsen R, *et al.* (2003) Combined phacoemulsification, intraocular lens implantation and vitrectomy for eyes with coexisting cataract and vitreoretinal pathology. *Am J Ophthalmol* **135**: 291–296.

Diabetic Retinopathy Vitrectomy Study Research Group. (1985) Early vitrectomy for severe vitreous hemorrhage in diabetic retinopathy. Diabetic Retinopathy Vitrectomy Study Report 2. *Arch Ophthalmol* **103**: 1644–1651.

Diabetic Retinopathy Vitrectomy Study Research Group. (1988) Early vitrectomy for severe proliferative diabetic retinopathy in eyes with useful vision. Results of a randomized trial. Diabetic Retinopathy Vitrectomy Study Report 3. *Ophthalmology* **95**: 1307–1320.

Diabetic Retinopathy Vitrectomy Study Research Group. (1985) Two-year course of visual acuity in severe proliferative diabetic retinopathy with conventional management. Diabetic Retinopathy Vitrectomy Study Report 1. *Ophthalmology* **92**: 492–501.

Douglas MJ, Scott IU, Flynn HW. (2003) Pars plana lensectomy, pars plana vitrectomy, and silicone oil tamponade as initial management of cataract and combined traction/rhegmatogenous retinal detachment involving the macula associated with severe proliferative diabetic retinopathy. *Ophthalmic Surg Lasers Imaging* **34**: 270–278.

Esser P, Heimann K, Bartz-Schmidt KU, *et al.* (1997) Plasminogen in proliferative vitreoretinal disorders. *Br J Ophthalmol* **81**: 590–594.

Ezra E, Dowler JGF, Burges F, *et al.* (1996) Identifying maculopathy after neodymium:YAG membranotomy for dense premacular hemorrhage. *Ophthalmology* **103**: 1568–1574.

Faulborn J. (1988) Behandlung einer diabetischen pramakularn Blutung mit dem Q-swched Neodym:YAG laser. *Spektrum Augenheilkd* **2**: 33–35.

Feist RM, Morris RE, Witherspoon CD, *et al.* (1990) Vitrectomy in asteroid hyalosis. *Retina* **10**: 173–177.

Foulks GN, Thoft RA, Perry HD, Tolentino FI. (1979) Factors related to corneal epithelial complications after closed vitrectomy in diabetics. *Arch Ophthalmol* **97**: 1076–1078.

Friberg TR, Ohji M, Scherer JJ, Tano Y. (2003) Frequency of epithelial debridement during diabetic vitrectomy. *Am J Ophthalmol* **135**: 553–554.

Fujii G, de Juan E, Humayun M, *et al.* (2002) Inicial experience using the transconjunctival sutúreles vitrectomy system for vitreoretinal surgery. *Ophthalmology* **109**: 1814–1820.

Funatsu H, Yamashita H, Noma H, *et al.* (2004) Risk evaluation of outcome of vitreous surgery for proliferative diabetic retinopathy based on vitreous level of vascular endothelial growth factor and angiotensin II. *Br J Ophthalmol* **88**: 1064–1068.

Gabel VP, Birngryber R, Gunter-Koazka H, *et al.* (1989) Nd:YAG laser photodisruption of hemorrhagic detachment of the internal limiting membrane. *Am J Ophthalmol* **107**: 33–37.

Gallemore R, Boyer D, Thomas E. (2004) Evolving treatment strategies for diabetic retinopathy. *Retinal Physician* **1**: 24–60.

Gandorfer A, Messmer EM, Ulbig MW, Kampik A. (2000) Resolution of diabetic macular edema after surgical removal of the posterior hyaloid and the inner limiting membrane. *Retina* **20**: 126–133.

Grigorian RA, Castellarin A, Fegan R, Grange JD. (2003) Epiretinal membrane removal in diabetic eyes: Comparison of viscodissection with conventional methods of membrane peeling. *Br J Ophthalmol* **87**: 737–741.

Hajji Z, Rouillot JS, Roth P, Grange JD. (2003) Should associated intraoperative and/or postoperative photocoagulation be systematic during or after vitrectomy for proliferative diabetic retinopathy. *J Fr Ophthalmol* **26**: 47–53.

Hamanaka T, Akabane N, Yajima T, *et al.* (2001) Retinal ischemia and angle neovascularization in proliferative diabetic retinopathy. *Am J Ophthalmol* **132**: 648–658.

Han DP, Lewandowski M, Mieler WF. (1991) Echographic diagnosis of anterior hyaloidal fibrovascular proliferation. *Arch Ophthalmol* **109**: 842–846.

Han DP, Pulido JS, Mieler WF, Johnson MW. (1995) Vitrectomy for proliferative diabetic retinopathy with severe equatorial fibrovascular proliferation. *Am J Ophthalmol* **119**: 563–570.

Hattenbach LO, Allers A, Gumbel HO, *et al.* (1999) Vitreous concentrations of TPA and plasminogen activator inhibitor are associated with VEGF in proliferative diabetic vitreoretinopathy. *Retina* **19**: 383–389.

Helbig H, Kellner U, Bornfeld N, Foerster MH. (1996) Limits and possibilities of vitreous body surgery in diabetic retinopathy. *Ophthalmology* **93**: 647–654.

Helbig H, Kellener U, Bornfeld N, Foerster MH. (1998a) Vitrectomy in diabetic retinopathy: Outcome, risk factors and complications. *Klin Monatsbl Augenheilkd* **212**: 339–342.

Helbig H, Kellener U, Bornfeld N, Foerster MH. (1998b) Rubeosis iridis after vitrectomy for diabetic retinopathy. *Graefes Arch Clin Exp Ophthalmol* **236**: 730–733.

Hershberger VS, Augsburger JJ, Hutchings RK, *et al.* (2004) Fibrovascular ingrowth at sclerotomy sites in vitrectomized diabetic eyes with recurrent vitreous hemorrhage: Ultrasound biomicroscopy findings. *Ophthalmology* **111**: 1215–1221.

Hesse L, Heller G, Kraushaar N, *et al.* (2002) The predictive value of a classification for proliferative diabetic retinopathy. *Klin Monatsbl Augenheilkd* **219**: 46–49.

Hiraiwa T, Horio N, Terasaki H, *et al.* (2003) Preoperative electroretinogram and postoperative visual outcome in patients with diabetic vitreous hemorrhage. *Jpn J Ophthalmol* **47**: 307–311.

Honjo M, Ogura Y. (1998) Surgical results of pars plana vitrectomy combined with phacoemulsification and intraocular lens implantation for complications of proliferative diabetic retinopathy. *Ophthalmic Surg Lasers* **29**: 99–105.

Horiguchi M, Kojima Y, Shimada Y. (2002) New system for fiberoptic-free bimanula vitreous surgery. *Arch Ophthalmol* **120**: 491–494.

Ikeda T, Sawa H, Koizumi K, *et al.* (1998) Vitrectomy for proliferative diabetic retinopathy with asteroid hyalosis. *Retina* **18**: 410–414.

Inoue M, Nagai N, Shinoda H, *et al.* (2004) Intravitreal injection of triamcinolone acetonide for cystoid macular edema resistant to vitreous surgery. *Nippon Ganka Gakkai Zasshi* **108**: 92–97.

Ishida M, Takeuchi S. (2001) Long-term results of vitrectomy for complications of proliferative diabetic retinopathy. *Nippon Ganka Gakkai Zasshi* **105**: 457–462.

Itakura H, Kishi S, Kotajima N, Murakami M. (2004) Persistent secretion of vascular endothelial growth factor into the vitreous cavity in proliferative diabetic retinopathy after vitrectomy. *Ophthalmology* **111**:1880–1884.

Jonas JB, Sofker A, Degenring R. (2003) Intravitreal triamcinolone acetonide as an additional tool in pars plana vitrectomy for proliferative diabetic retinopathy. *Eur J Ophthalmol* **13**: 468–473.

Joondeph BC, Blankenship GW. (1989) Hemostatic effects of air versus fluid in diabetic vitrectomy. *Ophthalmology* **96**: 1701–1706.

Jun Z, Pavlovic S, Jacobi KW. (2001) Results of combined vitreoretinal surgery and phacoemulsification with intraocular lens implantation. *Clin Experiment Ophthalmol* **29**: 307–311.

Kadonosono K, Matsumoto S, Uchio E, *et al.* (2001) Iris neovascularization alter vitrectomy combined with phacoemulsification and intraocular lens implantation for proliferative diabetic retinopathy. *Ophthalmic Surg Lasers* **32**: 19–24.

Kim SH, Chung JW, Chung H, Yu HG. (2004) Phacoemulsification and foldable intraocular lens implantation combined with vitrectomy and silicone oil tamponade for severe proliferative diabetic retinopathy. *J Cataract Refract Surg* **30**: 1721–1726.

Koch FH, Kreiger AE, Spitznas M, *et al.* (1995) Pars plana incisions of four patients: Histopathology and electron microscopy. *Br J Ophthalmol* **79**: 486–493.

Koch FHJ, Pawlowski D, Spiznas M. (1991) A multiport illumination system for panoramic bi-manual vitreous surgery. *Graefes Arch Clin Exp Ophthalmol* **229**: 425–429.

Kojima T, Terasaki H, Nomura H, *et al.* (2003) Vitrectomy for diabetic macular edema: Effect of glycemic control (HbA(1c)), renal function (creatinine) and other local factors. *Ophthalmic Res* **35**: 192–198.

Koutsandrea CN, Apostolopoulos MN, Chatzoulis DZ, *et al.* (2001). Hemostatic effects of SF6 after vitrectomy for vitreous hemorrhage. *Acta Ophthalmol Scand* **79**: 34–38.

Krieger A. (1993) Wound complications in pars plana vitrectomy. *Retina* **13**: 335–344.

Kroll P, Gerding H, Busse H. (1989) [Occurrence of retinal complications by reproliferation following vitreoretinal silicone surgery]. *Klin Monatsbl Augenheilkd* **195**: 145–149.

Kuchle M, Handel A, Naumann GO. (1998) Cataract extraction in eyes with diabetic iris neovascularization. *Ophthalmic Surg Lasers* **29**: 28–32.

La Heij EC, Tecim S, Kessels AG, *et al.* (2004) Clinical variables and their relation to visual outcome after vitrectomy in eyes with diabetic retinal traction detachment. *Graefes Arch Clin Exp Ophthalmol* **242**: 210–217.

Lahey JM, Francis RR, Kearney JJ. (2003) Combining phacoemulsification with pars plana vitrectomy in patients with proliferative diabetic retinopathy: A series of 223 cases. *Ophthalmology* **110**: 1335–1339.

Lambrou FH, Sternberg P, Meredith TA, *et al.* (1989) Vitrectomy when asteroid hyalosis prevents laser photocoagulation. *Ophthalmic Surg* **20**:100–102.

Le Mer Y, Korobelnik JF, Morel C, *et al.* (1999) TPA-assisted vitrectomy for proliferative diabetic retinopathy: Results of a double-masked, multicenter trial. *Retina* **19**: 378–382.

Lewis H, Abrams GW, Williams GA. (1987) Anterior hyaloidal fibrovascular proliferation after diabetic retinopathy vitrectomy. *Am J Ophthalmol* **104**: 607–613.

Lewis H, Sanchez G. (1993) Vitreoretinal surgery for complications of diabetic retinopathy. In: Freeman WR, (ed.), *Practical Atlas of Retinal Disease and Therapy*. Raven Press, New York, pp. 195–209.

Lewis HL, Abrams GW, Blumenkranz MS, *et al.* (1992) Vitrectomy for diabetic macular traction and edema associated with posterior hyaloid traction. *Ophthalmology* **99**: 753–759.

Li XX, Jiang YR, Yin H, Zhao MW. (2004) [Influence of membrane dissection and en bloc excision on the outcome of vitreous surgery in proliferative diabetic retinopathy]. *Zhonghua Yan Ke Za Zhi* **40**: 439–442.

Lloyd MA, Heuer DK, Baerveldt G, *et al.* (1991) Combined Molteno implantation and pars plana vitrectomy for neovascular glaucoma. *Ophthalmology* **98**: 1401–1405.

Martin DF, McCuen BW. (1992) Efficacy of fluid-air exchange for postvitrectomy diabetes vitreous hemorrhage. *Am J Ophthalmol* **114**: 457–463.

Maturi RK, Merrill PT, Lomeo MD, *et al.* (1999). Perfluoro-N-octane (PFO) in the repair of complicated retinal detachments due to severe proliferative diabetic retinopathy. *Ophthalmic Surg Lasers* **30**: 715–720.

McDermott ML, Puklin JE, Abrams GW, Eliott D. (1997) Phacoemulsification for cataract following pars plana vitrectomy. *Ophthalmic Surg Lasers* **28**: 558–564.

McMeel JW. (1977) Photocoagulation approach with various vitreoretinal problems. In: L'Ésperance FA (ed). *Current Diagnosis and Management of Chorioretinal Diseases*. CV Mosby, St Louis, Chap. 22.

Meier P, Wiedemann P. (1997) Vitrectomy for traction macular detachment in diabetic retinopathy. *Graefes Arch Clin Exp Ophthalmol* **235**: 569–574.

Michels RG, Rice TA, Rice EF. (1983) Vitrectomy for diabetic vitreous hemorrhage. *Am J Ophthalmol* **95**: 12–21.

Michels RG. (1981) Proliferative diabetic retinopathy. Pathophysiology of extraretinal complications and principles of vitreous surgery. *Retina* **1**: 1–17.

Millar JA, Chandra SR, Stevens TS. (1986) A modified technique for performing outpatient fluid-air exchange following vitrectomy surgery. *Am J Ophthalmol* **101**: 116–117.

Moss SE, Klein R, Klein BE. (1998) The 14-year incidence of visual loss in a diabetic population. *Ophthalmology* **105**: 998–1003.

Nabili S, Kirkness CM. (2004) Trans-scleral diode laser cyclophoto-coagulation in the treatment of diabetic neovascular glaucoma. *Eye* **18**: 352–356.

Narendran N, Williamson TH. (2003) The effects of aspirin and warfarin therapy on hemorrhage after vitreoretinal surgery. *Acta Ophthalmol Scand* **81**: 38–40.

Nicoletti VG, Nicoletti R, Ferrara N, *et al.* (2003) Diabetic patients and retinal proliferation: An evaluation of the role of vascular endothelial growth factor (VEGF). *Exp Clin Endocrinol Diabetes* **111**: 209–214.

Okun E, Johnston GP, Boniuk I. (1971) Management of diabetic retinopathy: A stereoscopic presentation. CV Mosby, St Louis, pp. 18–92.

Otani T, Kishi S. (2002) A controlled study of vitrectomy for diabetic macular edema. *Am J Ophthalmol* **134**: 214–219.

Ozdamar A, Aras C, Karacorlu M. (2003) Suprachoroidal seton implantation in refractory glaucoma: A new surgical technique. *J Glaucoma* **12**: 354–359.

Packer AJ, McCuen BW, Hutton WL, Ramsay RC. (1989) Procoagulant effects of intraocular sodium hyaluronate (Healon) after phakic diabetic vitrectomy. A prospective, randomized study. *Ophthalmology* **96**: 1491–1494.

Packer AJ. (1994) Diabetic macular traction detachment. In: Bovino JA (ed.), *Macular Surgery*. Appleton & Lange, Norwalk, pp. 27–39.

Packer AJ. (1987) Vitrectomy for progressive macular traction associated with proliferative diabetic retinopathy. *Arch Ophthalmol* **105**: 1679–1687.

Pearson RV, McLeod D, Gragor ZJ. (1993) Removal of silicone oil following diabetic vitrectomy. *Br J Ophthalmol* **77**: 204–207.

Pendergast SD, Hassan TS, Williams GA, *et al.* (2000) Vitrectomy for diffuse diabetic macular edema associated with a taut premacular posterior hyaloid. *Am J Ophthalmol* **130**: 178–186.

Peyman GA, Cheema R, Conway MD, Fang T. (2000) Triamcinolone acetonide as an aid to visualization of the vitreous and the posterior hyaloid during pars plana vitrectomy. *Retina* **20**: 554–555.

Pollack AL, McDonald HR, Ai E, *et al.* (2001) Massive suprachoroidal hemorrhage during pars plana vitrectomy associated with Valsalva maneuver. *Am J Ophthalmol* **132**: 383–387.

Puthalath S, Chirayath A, Shermila MV, *et al.* (2003) Frequency-doubled Nd:YAG laser treatment for premacular hemorrhage. *Ophthalmic Surg Lasers Imaging* **34**: 284–290.

Rola A, Baílez C, Pastor JC, *et al.* (2003) [Iatrogenic retinal breaks during vitrectomy: Retrospective study]. *Arch Soc Esp Oftalmol* **78**: 487–492.

Sato Y, Shimada H, Aso S, Matsui M. (1994) Vitrectomy for diabetic macular heterotopia. *Ophthalmology* **101**: 63–67.

Sawa H, Ikeda T, Matsumoto Y, *et al.* (2000) Neovascularization from scleral wound as cause of vitreous rebleeding alter vitrectomy for proliferative diabetic retinopathy. *Jpn J Ophthalmol* **44**: 154–160.

Sawa M, Kondo M, Ogino N. (1995) [Anterior chamber inflammation alter cataract intraocular lens surgery in postvitrectomy eyes]. *Nippon Ganka Gakkai Zasshi* **99**: 687–691.

Schachat AP, Oyakawa TR, Michels RG, Rice TA. (1983) Complications of vitreous surgery for diabetic retinopathy. II: Postoperative complications. *Ophthalmology* **90**: 522–530.

Schatz B, El-Shabrawi Y, Haas A, Langmann G. (2004) Adverse side effects with perfluorohexyloctane as a long-term tamponade agent in complicated vitreoretinal surgery. *Retina* **24**: 567–573.

Schulze S, Schulze S, Schmidt J, Kroll P. (2000) [Air endotamponade in 52 vitrectomies due to proliferative diabetic retinopathy-retrospective comparison with 40 vitrectomies without endotamponade]. *Klin Monatsbl Augenheilkd* **217**: 329–333.

Scott IU, Alexandrakis G, Flynn HW, *et al.* (2000) Combined pars plana vitrectomy and glaucoma drainage implants placement for refractory glaucoma. *Am J Ophthalmol* **129**: 334–341.

Sebestyen JG. (1982) Fibrinoid syndrome: A severe complication of vitrectomy surgery in diabetics. *Ann Ophthalmol* **14**: 853–856.

Shinoda K, O'hira A, Ishida S, *et al.* (2001) Posterior synechia of the iris after combined pars plana vitrectomy, phacoemulsification, and intraocular lens implantation. *Jpn J Ophthalmol* **45**: 276–280.

Sima P, Zoran T. (1994) Long-term results of vitreous surgery for proliferative vitreoretinopathy. *Doc Ophthalmol* **87**: 223–232.

Smiddy WE, Feuer W. (2004) Incidence of cataract extraction after diabetic vitrectomy. *Retina* **24**: 574–581.

Sonoda KH, Sakamoto T, Enaida H, *et al.* (2004) Residual vitreous cortex after surgical posterior vitreous separation visualized by intravitreous triamcinolone acetonide. *Ophthalmology* **111**: 226–230.

Spraul CW, Grossniklaus HE. (1997) Vitreous hemorrhage. *Surv Ophthalmol* **42**: 3–39.

Stefaniotou M, Aspiotis M, Kalogeropoulos C, *et al.* (2004) Vitrectomy results for diffuse diabetic macular edema with and without inner limiting membrane removal. *Eur J Ophthalmol* **14**: 137–143.

Steinmetz RL, Grizzard S, Hammer ME. (2002) Vitrectomy fir diabetic traction retinal detachment using the multiport illumination system. *Ophthalmology* **109**: 2303–2307.

Suzuki Y, Sakuraba T, Mizutani H, *et al.* (2001) Postoperative complications after simultaneous vitrectomy and cataract surgery. *Ophthalmic Surg Lasers* **32**: 391–396.

Tachi N, Ogino N. (1996) Vitrectomy for diffuse macular edema in cases of diabetic retinopathy. *Am J Ophthalmol* **122**: 258–260.

Takaya K, Suzuki Y, Mizutani H, *et al.* (2004) Long-term results of vitrectomy for removal of submacular hard exudates in patients with diabetic maculopathy. *Retina* **24**: 23–29.

Thompson JT, Glaser BM, Michels RG, de Bustros S. (1986) The use of intravitreal thrombin to control hemorrhage during vitrectomy. *Ophthalmology* **93**: 279–282.

Tokui K, Kitgawa M, Niki T, *et al.* (1986) Massive preretinal hemorrhage in diabetic retinopathy. *Jpn Clin Ophthalmol* **40**: 641–647.

Tolentino MJ, Miller JW, Gragoudas ES, *et al.* (1996) Vascular endothelial growth factor is sufficient to produce iris neovascularization and neovascular glaucoma in a nonhuman primate. *Arch Ophthalmol* **114**: 964–970.

Tripathi RC, Li J, Tripathi BJ, *et al.* (1998) Increased level of vascular endothelial growth factor in aqueous humor of patients with neovascular glaucoma. *Ophthalmology* **105**: 232–237.

Valmaggia C, de Smet M. (2004) Endoscopic laser coagulation of the ciliary processes in patients with severe chronic glaucoma. *Klin Monatsbl Augenheilkd* **221**: 343–346.

West JF, Gregor Zj. (2000) Fibrovascular ingrowth and recurrent haemorrhage following diabetic vitrectomy. *Br J Ophthalmol* **84**: 822–825.

Wu WC, Chang SM, Chen JY, Chang CW. (2001) Management of postvitrectomy diabetic vitreous hemorrhage with tissue plasminogen activator (t-PA) and volume homeostatic fluid exchanger. *J Ocul Pharmacol Ther* **17**: 363–371.

Yamamoto T, Akabane N, Takeuchi S. (2001) Vitrectomy for diabetic macular edema: The role of posterior vitreous detachment and epimacular membrane. *Am J Ophthalmol* **132**: 369–377.

# Chapter 9

# Medical Management of Diabetic Retinopathy

## José Rui Faria Abreu and José Cunha-Vaz

Diabetic retinopathy (DR) remains the leading cause of visual disability and blindness among professionally active adults in economically developed societies. This is of even greater concern now that a sharp increase in diabetes mellitus is expected in the next decade.

Laser photocoagulation remains the only tested method for treating DR (Table 9.1). However, laser photocoagulation is advised only for patients with advanced retinal disease, either high-risk proliferative retinopathy or clinically significant macular edema. Vitrectomy has also been shown to be beneficial in even more advanced stages of retinopathy.

It is clear that the ophthalmologist views the accepted treatment of DR to include mainly surgical and ablative procedures. In general, these forms of treatment are given independent of the diabetes disease itself and metabolic status. However, recent developments in the medical management of diabetes have indicated that it may play a major role in preventing the macro and microvascular complications of diabetes. The appropriate management of diabetes is particularly useful and effective in the earliest stages of retinal disease, when the disease process may still be reversible and before visual loss is already present.

Medical therapy may be targeted to control DR at three levels: the first level should be directed at achieving near physiological levels of glycemia as soon as the diagnosis of diabetes mellitus is made. This approach is particularly effective if applied when retinopathy is in its initial stages.

The second and third levels are still at the developmental stage. Their potential, however, is tremendous and the ophthalmologist must be aware of this and their rapid development.

The second level includes drugs aimed at controlling the biochemical events occurring in the retina as a result of the excessive availability of glucose: good candidates include aldose reductase inhibitors, inhibitors of protein kinase C activation and inhibitors of advanced glycation end-products. Evidence, mostly experimental, but also clinical, is accumulating of their potentially favorable effects on the stabilization of the early stages of diabetic retinal disease.

Finally, the third level, at which medical therapy may be targeted in order to halt the progression of diabetic retinal disease, is at the lesion site, both at the neuronal and vascular levels. Treatment of the initial sites of cytotoxic and vasogenic retinal edema may be considered an appropriate goal, because there are now techniques available to monitor these initial retinal changes clinically (Cunha-Vaz *et al.*, 2004).

## 9.1. Glycemic Control

Analysis from a number of epidemiologic studies and randomized controlled clinical trials suggest a significant relationship between glycemia and retinopathy. In these studies, integrated glycemic control is measured by glycosylated hemoglobin either HbA1c or HbA1 (which includes $HbA_{1C}$ as well as HbA1a and HbA1b) or total glycosylated hemoglobin.

Table 9.1. **Management Recommendations for Patients with Diabetes (AAO Guidelines, 2003)**

| Severity of Retinopathy | Follow-up (months) | Focal Laser | Panretinal Photocoagulation |
|---|---|---|---|
| Mild on Minimal PDR | 12 | No | No |
| Mild to Moderate NPDR | 6–12 | No | No |
| Mild to Moderate NPDR c/CSME | 2–4 | Usually | Sometimes |
| Severe or very severe NPDR | 2–4 | No | Sometimes |
| Severe or very severe c/CSME | 2–4 | Usually | Sometimes |
| Non High-risk PDR | 2–4 | No | Sometimes |
| Non High-risk PDR c/SME | 2–4 | Usually | Sometimes |
| High-risk PDR | 3–4 | No | Usually |
| High-risk PDR c/CSME | 3–4 | Usually | Usually |

NPDR — Nonproliferative diabetic retinopathy.
PDR — Proliferative diabetic retinopathy.
CSME — Clinically significant macular edema.

At both 4 and 10 year follow-up in the Wisconsin Epidemiologic Study of Diabetic Retinopathy there was a statically significant relationship between baseline HbA1 and the incidence of retinopathy, progression of retinopathy by two or more steps on a modified scale developed by the Early Treatment Diabetic Retinopathy Study (ETDRS) and progression to proliferative DR (PDR).

## 9.1.1. Glycemic Control and Diabetic Retinopathy

### 9.1.1.1. *Type 1 diabetes*

The DCCT, a multicenter intervention study, showed that intervening to obtain a good metabolic control reduces the incidence and gravity of retinal lesions.

Intensive management, aimed at achieving glycemic levels as close to the normal range as possible, including three or more daily injection or continuous subcutaneous insulin infusion was compared with "conventional treatment" — one or two daily injections.

Intensive management over an average of 6.5 years reduced the mean risk of retinopathy incidence in 76%, 85% in those with less than 2.5 years duration of diabetes and 70% in those with duration of more

than 2.5 years ($p < 0.001$); reduced in 54% the risk of progression; reduced in 47% the risk in the development of severe nonproliferative diabetic retinopathy (NPDR) or proliferative diabetic retinopathy (PDR); reduced in 23% the risk of clinically significant macular edema (CSME) and reduced in 6% the need for laser treatment (The DCCT, 1993; 1995).

Intensive treatment had a substantial effect over time (8–9 years) but the difference from conventional treatment did not become apparent until 2–3 years after beginning treatment (DCCT, 2000). About 10% of the patients with preexisting retinopathy had a transient worsening of their retinopathy after the institution of tight blood glucose control (The DCCT, 1998).

The DCCT was stopped after a mean follow-up time of 6.5 years when the benefits of intensive treatment were deemed incontrovertible and participants, who had been assigned to conventional treatment, were advised to change to intensive treatment. Further progression of retinopathy showed that the benefit derived from intensive therapy did not wane.

The incidence of worsening of retinopathy between the end of the DCCT and after four years is significantly lower for those with intensive treatment during the DCCT. The odds reduction was 66% for 3-step progression from no retinopathy, 76% for severe

nonproliferative retinopathy or worse, 74% for proliferative retinopathy, 77% for clinically significant
macular edema and 77% for laser therapy (focal or
scatter). The long-term benefits of the DCCT intensive treatment when compared with conventional
treatment have persisted and increase further (The
DCCT/EDIC, 2000).

### 9.1.1.2. *Type 2 Diabetes*

Control of glycemia in type 2 diabetes may include
insuline secretagogues, sulfonylureas and repaglinide,
insulin sensitizers, which enhance muscle glucose
uptake and decrease hepatic glucose production,
inhibitors of carbohydrate absorption, alfa-glucosi-
dade inhibitors and finally, when necessary, insulin or
insulin analogs.

Sato *et al.* (2001) in a longitudinal study of
Japanese patients with "mild preproliferative diabetic
retinopathy," presence of scattered soft exudates without large nonperfused areas or venous beading
showed that 27% of all patients developed proliferative diabetic retinopathy and they had a mean value of
$HbA_{1c}$ of 9.4%. The remaining 73% did not develop
proliferative diabetic retinopathy and the mean $HbA_{1C}$
was 7.6% ($p < 0.0004$).

The proportion developing PDR was 48% among
those with $HbA_{1C}$ of 8.6% or more by comparison
with 8% among those with mean $HbA_{1C}$ value below
8.6% ($p < 0.04$). The proportion developing PDR was
estimated to approximately double with each 1%
increase in the mean $HbA_{1C}$ value.

A study from Kumamoto University in Japan
involved 110 non-obese patients with type 2 diabetes
(Ohkubo *et al.*, 1995). Of these, 102 subjects completed the 6-year study, which was designed to be similar to the DCCT except for the inclusion of subjects
with type 2 diabetes. Over the six years of follow-up,
glycemic outcomes and risk reductions were almost
identical to those found in the DCCT. The intensive-
therapy group achieved a mean $HbA_{1C}$ over the six
years of the study of 7.1% versus a value in the con-
ventional-therapy group of 9.4%. Progression to
severe nonproliferative DR (NPDR) or to PDR was

reduced by 40%, as well as the need for laser photocoagulation in the intensive therapy group.

Finally, the United Kingdom Prospective Diabetes
Study (UKPDS, 1998), a randomized, multicenter, controlled clinical trial demonstrated that an intensive treatment policy in type 2 diabetes with the goal of
meticulous glycemic control decreased diabetic complications including retinopathy. A total of 5102 subjects
with newly diagnosed type 2 diabetes were enrolled.
Retinopathy was assessed by four-field fundus photography performed at baseline and every three years. The
intensive-treatment group achieved a median $HbA_{1C}$ of
7.0 versus 7.9% in the conventional-treatment group.
Patients assigned to intensive treatment had a significant
25% risk reduction in microvascular endpoints compared with conventional treatment, most of which was
due to fewer cases of retinal photocoagulation for which
there was a significant 29% risk reduction.

The current glycemic recommendations of the
American Diabetes Association (ADA) appear in their
*Standards of Medical Care for Patients with Diabetes
Mellitus.* The goal is, ideally, for a fasting plasma glucose
of < 110 mg/dl and a $HbA_{1C}$ of < 7% (normal range about
3.0–6.0%). The ADA uses the term "action suggested" to
define another category which might also be defined as
"unacceptable glycemic control," that is a fasting plasma
glucose of > 140 mg/dl and a $HbA_{1C}$ of > 8%.

## 9.2. Blood Pressure Control

For a long time epidemiologic studies have suggested
a relationship between blood pressure elevation and
progression of retinopathy. Demonstration of this
relationship is, however, recent and, at last, based on
large randomized studies.

### 9.2.1. Type 1 Diabetes

Parving *et al.* (1989) showed that treatment with an
angiotensin, converting enzyme (ACE) inhibitor significantly reduced the permeability of blood-retinal

barrier in patients with nonproliferative diabetic retinopathy.

ACE converts Angiotensin 1 to Angiotensin 2 and subsequent increase in intracellular calcium and stimulates the production of endothelin-1 (ET-1) implicated in retinal vessels constriction (Takagi *et al.*, 1996). ACE inhibitors could block calcium influx into cells decreasing ET-1 expression (Tadesse *et al.*, 2001).

The EURODIAB Controlled Trial of Lisinopril in insulin-dependent diabetes mellitus, a randomized, multicenter, controlled clinical trial was conducted in 354 patients with type 1 diabetes aged 20–59 years in 15 European centers (Chatuverdi *et al.*, 1998). Patients were not hypertensive and were either normoabuminuric (85%) or microalbuminuric (15%). Patients were randomized at baseline and followed up for 24 months. Lisinopril decreased retinopathy progression by two or more grades (73% risk reduction, $p < 0.05$) and progression to PDR (82% risk reduction, $p < 0.03$). In this study, patients with better glycemia control had the most benefit from ACE inhibitors, suggesting that the combination may be the best therapeutic approach.

### 9.2.2. Type 2 Diabetes

The Hypertension in Diabetes Study (HDS) was embedded in the UKPDS by using a factorial design (UKPDS, 1998).

The HDS was conducted in 20 centers with 1148 patients who had type 2 diabetes and coexisting hypertension. The design was a randomized controlled trial comparing "tight" blood pressure control aiming for a blood pressure of < 150/85 mm Hg with the use of an angiotensin-converting enzyme inhibitor (captopril) or a $\beta$-blocker (atenolol) as the main treatment and "less tight" control aiming for a blood pressure of < 180/105 mm Hg. Median follow-up was 8.4 years. The tight control group achieved a mean blood pressure of 144/82 versus 154/87 mm Hg in the less tight control group ($p < 0.0001$). Patients assigned to the tight control group had a significant 37% risk

reduction in microvascular end points compared with the less tight control group.

Blood pressure lowering with captopril or atenolol was similarly effective in reducing the incidence of diabetic complications. There was no evidence that either drug has any specific beneficial or deleterious effect, suggesting that blood pressure reduction in itself may be more important.

Calcium-channel blockers should also be considered because their multiple effect: antihypertensive, neuroprotection and correction of ATP synthesis (Cunha-Vaz, 2004).

However, another trial, the Appropriated Blood Pressure Control in Diabetes (ABCD) a randomized trial of 470 hypertensive patients (baseline diastolic pressure >90 mm Hg) did not find any difference, over a mean 5.3 years follow-up period, between intensive control (diastolic < 75 mm Hg) and moderate control (80–89 mm Hg) with regard to progression of diabetic retinopathy (Estacio *et al.*, 2000).

In patients with diabetes, current blood pressure recommendations of the ADA appear in their "*Standards of Medical Care for Patients with Diabetes Mellitus*" and in a consensus statement on "*Treatment of Hypertension in Diabetes.*" Similar recommendations are contained in *The 6$^{th}$ Report of the Joint National Committee on Prevention, Detection, Evaluation, and Treatment of High Blood Pressure* (1997).

The primary goal of therapy for nonpregnant adults >18 years of age with diabetes is to decrease blood pressure and to maintain it at < 130 mm Hg the initial goal of treatment is a reduction of 20 mm Hg. If these goals are achieved and well tolerated, further lowering to < 140 mm Hg may be appropriate.

## 9.3. Dyslipidemic Control

Diabetic dyslipidemia, particularly in patients with poor glycemic control, is characterized by increased levels of total cholesterol, low density lipoproteins

(LDLs) and triglycerides and by decreased levels of high-density lopoproteins (HDLs).

The Wisconsin epidemiologic study of diabetic retinopathy found that elevated serum cholesterol levels were associated with increased severity of hard exudates (Klein *et al.*, 1991). This was also confirmed by the ETDRS. Higher serum lipids were associated with a greater risk of developing high-risk proliferative diabetic retinopathy, as well as with a greater risk of developing visual loss from diabetic macular edema and associated hard exudates (Chew *et al.*, 1996).

Dyslipidemia may cause or exacerbate diabetic retinopathy by damaging the endothelial cells and pericytes through oxidized LDL (Chowdhury *et al.*, 2002) by increasing blood viscosity and by alteration of the fibrinolytic system (Freyberger *et al.*, 1994). Incorporation of triglycerides in the cell membrane cause retinal leakage (Ebeling *et al.*, 1997).

Chowdhury *et al.* (2002, 2003) pointed out to a positive association of any grade of diabetic retinopathy with levels of total cholesterol and triglycerides and another author has found an association of diabetic retinopathy with low levels of HDL (Kordounouri *et al.*, 1996).

Sen *et al.* (2002) in a double blind placebo-control randomized trial in type 2 hypercholesterolaemic diabetic patients reported that sinvastatin reduced visual loss ($p < 0.009$) and the severity of retinopathy, evaluated by fundus photography and fluorescein angiography ($p < 0.009$). Gupta *et al.* (2004) found that diabetic patients with abnormal lipid profiles taking a lipid lowering drug, atorvastatin, showed decreased occurrence in subfoveal lipid migration after laser photocoagulation ($p = 0.04$) when compared with controls.

Current recommendations for the management of dyslipidemia in persons with diabetes are based on the increased risk of cardiovascular disease in those patients (ADA, 2002). Cusik *et al.* (2003) published two cases of regression of hard exudates secondary to aggressive lipid lowering, suggesting the utility of its use reabsorb hard exudates.

Data available suggest that treatment of hyperlipidemia may help stabilize the retinal status and possibly visual acuity. However, there are no data indicating that visual acuity can be improved by treatment of hyperlipidemia. Moreover, whether such treatment has long-term beneficial effect on visual outcome is unknown.

## 9.4.  Treatment of Anemia

In a cross-sectional study involving 1691 diabetic patients, a twofold increased risk of retinopathy was reported in patients with hemoglobin less than 12 gr/dl when controlled for other known risk factors and the severity of retinopathy correlated with the severity of anemia (Qiao *et al.*, 1997).

Anemia is a common accompaniment in diabetic patients during the stage of overt proteinuria, even before the onset of severe impairment of kidney function (Winkler *et al.*, 1999). The reduced erythropoietin results in a secondary normocytic anemia.

Studies of anemia treatment with erythropoietin reported an associated improvement in the retinopathy (Friedman *et al.*, 1995; Calles-Escandon *et al.*, 2001; Shorb, 1985).

In summary, the anemia and relative hypoxia aggravate or accelerate the rate of progression of retinopathy.

Improving hemoglobin concentration improves tissue oxygenation and may result in reduced VEGF production resulting in a decrease of the hyperpermeability and a reduction in the stimulus for neovascularization. In addition, erythropoietin crosses the blood-retinal barrier and has direct antiapoptotic (Grimm *et al.*, 2002).

At the current time, there are no large studies specifically addressing diabetic retinopathy and correction of anemia but Sinclair *et al.* (2003), recommended as target for erythropoietin treatment to raise hemoglobin levels to 12.5 gr/dl. Care must be taken, however, with secondary hypertensive effects.

## 9.5. Experimental Therapies

At present it must be realized that medical management of diabetic retinopathy is largely that of prevention. Controlled clinical trials have demonstrated that aggressive glycemic control reduces the risk of retinopathy. The same occurs with blood pressure control and special attention must be given to maintain low levels of blood pressure in our diabetic patients. Control of dyslipidemia and anemia should also be considered, particularly, if they reach markedly abnormal levels.

It must be realized, however, that the mushrooming incidence of type 2 diabetes, which often goes undiagnosed for years, and increasing evidence that retinal damage begins early underscore the difficulty of preventing diabetic retinopathy altogether.

Our present understanding of the effect of "tight" metabolic control on the prognosis of diabetic retinopathy has clearly established new goals for improved therapy of diabetic retinal disease but vision loss continues to occur.

It is also clear that not all patients behave in the same way and the progression of the retinopathy varies between patients showing different degrees of responses to "tight" metabolic control.

Furthermore, our understanding of the molecular and cellular alterations that occur in the retina in diabetes has opened new perspectives for a more targeted therapy, directed to the specific retinal alteration that may characterize different retinopathy phenotypes (Cunha-Vaz and Bernardes, 2005).

Advances in cellular and molecular biology have identified several key pathways that may play important roles in the different types of diabetic retinopathy: the polyol pathway oxidative stress and free radicals, nonenzymatic glycation, microthrombotic mechanisms, inflammation, growth factors, protein kinase C inhibition, etc. The identification of these different abnormalities in the diabetic retina has offered exciting perspectives for a variety of experimental therapies. There is much expectation for their possible contribution in the near future to reduce vision loss from diabetes.

There are still major problems for the development and demonstration of efficacy of the many drugs that are being tested to correct the abnormalities occurring in the retina as a result of diabetes. One is the generalized reliance on clinical method of evaluation, such as a visual acuity and fundus photography, which have extremely poor sensitivity in the initials stages of diabetic retinal disease. General acceptance of more sensitive methods of clinical evaluation is clearly needed. The second problem lies in the lack of good animal models of diabetic retinopathy.

However, because the future of diabetic retinopathy treatment lies in the development of new therapies still considered experimental, we will review briefly the data presently available on these different therapeutic approaches.

### 9.5.1. Modulation of Antithrombotic Function of the Endothelium: Platelet Function Inhibitors

Diabetic retinopathy is associated with an increased number and size of platelet-fibrin thrombin in retinal capillaries when compared with nondiabetic patients (Spirin *et al.*, 1999; Boeri *et al.*, 2001). Microthrombosis is clearly a feature in the retinal vascular bed of diabetic patients and may be the precursor of capillary closure. The endothelial cells have an antithrombotic action by releasing antiaggregants, such as prostacyclin and nitric oxide, anticoagulants, such as thrombomoduline or by stimulating fibrinolysis. All these functions are decreased in diabetes.

Similarly diabetic patients show alterations in platelet function with increased production of the platelet activating factor (PAF) which, in turn, induces hyperaggregability, increases thromboxane levels and poor response to prostaglandin release (Moreno *et al.*, 1995).

All these mechanisms contribute to increased thrombus formation. Other mechanisms that can contribute to increased thrombus formation include: synthesis of inositoltriphosphate by activation of the phosphoinositol pathway, increase in dyacetylglyc-erol, which may reduce prostacyclin synthesis and increase synthesis of thromboxane. Drugs, such as acetylsalicylic acid and dipyramidol may, therefore, be useful in diabetic patients.

In experimental models De la Cruz *et al.* (2004) demonstrated that antiaggregants inhibit by 20–80% diabetes-induced retinal ischemia.

Clinically, a number of studies have been reported indicating a benefical effect of antithrombotic agents.

A 2-year follow-up study evaluating triflusal showed that nine patients that took 900 mg/day of tri-flusal had lower rate of exudates ($p < 0.02$) and lower number of microaneurysms ($p < 0.05$) as compared with eight patients in the control group (Esmatjes *et al.*, 1989).

A 36-month follow-up study of 31 type 1 diabetic patients testing dipyramidol showed that the 16 patients that received dipyramidol (375 mg/day) did not show significant differences until 30 weeks of fol-low-up, but after that period, they showed a lower "score" which included less microaneurysms, exu-dates and ischemia compared with 15 patients in the placebo group ($p = 0.0025$) (Pagani *et al.*, 1989).

However, large randomized, prospective double-blind studies testing powerful inhibitors of platelet aggregation showed contradictory results:

The DAMAD (1989) showed that high doses of aspirin (990 mg/day) alone or associated to dipyrami-dol (225 mg/day) resulted in a lower annual increase in the number of microaneurysms in fluorescein angiograms as compared to placebo ($p < 0.02$).

The TIMAD (1990), a 3-year study, showed in nonproliferative diabetic retinopathy that ticlopidine (500 mg/day) decreased annually the number of microaneurysms ($p < 0.03$) but with no differences in the appearance of new vessels, exudates, edema and hemorrhages. The Belgian Ticlopidine Retinopathy Study Group (1992) performed a multicenter, double-blind, randomized prospective study assessing the evolution of retinopathy by fluorescein angiography, which showed no statistical difference between ticlo-pidine (250 mg) and placebo after a 3-year period of

treatment. Finally, the ETDRS (1991) found that aspirin (650 mg/day) did not change the evolution of mild to severe nonproliferative diabetic retinopathy or early proliferative diabetic retinopathy.

The efficacy of these drugs for diabetic retinopathy is still controversial but they should be considered to pre-vent cardiovascular complications in diabetic patients.

## 9.5.2. Angiotensin-Converting Enzyme Inhibitors

ACE convert Angiotensin 1 to Angiotensin 2 inducing subsequent increase in intracellular calcium and stim-ulating the production of endothelin-1 (ET-1) impli-cated in retinal vascular constriction (Takagi *et al.*, 1996). ACE inhibitors may block calcium influx into cells decreasing ET-1 expression (Tadesse *et al.*, 2001). Angiotensin 2 is elevated in diabetic macular edema (Funatsu *et al.*, 2003). Angiotensin-converting enzyme (ACE) has been reported to show a correlation with the severity of retinopathy and diabetic macular edema (Danser *et al.*, 1989; 1994; Funastu, 2002).

In a large interventional 2-year multicenter, ran-domized, double-blind placebo-controlled trial, one inhibitor of angiotensin-converting enzyme (ACE), Lisinopril, reduced in 50% the progression of retinopathy in 530 non hypertensive or mildly hyper-tensive patients when compared to the placebo group even after adjusting for glycemic control. There was also a reduction in the incidence of retinopathy, but this effect did not reach statistical significance (Chaturvedi *et al.*, 1998).

ACE inhibition may interfere in diabetic retinopa-thy by mechanisms other than blood pressure control.

## 9.5.3. Inhibitors of the Inducible Form of Nitric Oxide Synthase

Normally endothelial cells can regulate capillary and pre-capillary arteriolar tone and caliber elaborating vasodilators such as nitric oxide (NO), adenosine and prostanoids and vasoconstrictors, e.g. endothelin-1 and Angiotensin 2. There is evidence for a constant release of NO in the retinal bed maintaining the retinal circulation in a constant state of vasodilation and NO also stabilizes platelet function. Endothelial cells, in response to platelet-derived products, hormones and mechanical changes may release more or less NO into the surrounding milieu. NO is synthesized in cells from L-arginine to L-citrulline via activation of Ca++ dependent nitric oxidase synthases (NOS).

Increased glycemic levels cause protein kinase C (PKC) activation with diminished NO synthesis (Inoguchi *et al.*, 1994), increase quenching of NO due to over expression of superoxide (Giugliano *et al.*, 1996) and increases advanced glycated endoproduct (AGEs) formation (Ceriello, 1999; Bucala *et al.*, 1991).

A number of drugs may have a beneficial effect on diabetic retinopathy by preventing activation of PKC, AGEs formation (aminoguanidine) and free radical formation aldose reductase activity, (antioxidants) by stimulating NO synthesis through NOS. Calcium dobesilate has been reported to stimulate the production and effect of NO (Tejerina *et al.*, 1999).

Aspirin also stimulates NO formation and that is a potential pathway for its role in the treatment of diabetic retinopathy (De La Cruz *et al.*, 2004).

### 9.5.4. Antioxidants

Free radicals are atoms or molecules that have one or more unpaired electrons in their atomic structure and this makes them intrinsically unstable and highly reactive. They are continuously formed in all aerobic cells. In the organism the creation of free radicals is generally due to capture of hydrogen atoms (electron plus protons) from surrounding organic molecules. There is a rupture of the covalent link between an atom of carbon and an atom of hydrogen. To convert to a stable state, free radicals must take an electron from another molecule, and in most cases, this process changes the molecule from which the electron was taken to a free radical.

The sequential stealing of electrons by free radicals often induces a cascade of biochemical chain reactions that can leave many molecules permanently altered or damaged by consuming valuable polyunsatured fatty acids that become lipid peroxyl (LPO) radicals by lipid peroxidation with destabilization of cell membrane and causing denaturation of sulfur-containing enzymes and other key cellular components, through cross-linking and fragmentation until they are neutralized or quenched by antioxidants.

Free radicals also catalyze a series of prostaglandins F2-like compounds (isoprostanes) produced from arachinoid acid that induce vasoconstriction and modulate the function of human platelets.

The most damaging free radicals are those derived from Reactive Oxygen Species (ROS), superoxide, hydroperoxil, hydrogen peroxide, hydroxyl and lipid peroxyl radicals. The singlet oxygen although not technically a free radical, is produced when molecular oxygen absorbs energy causing the spin of one of the electrons to invert and can cause similar damage in the body as it converts back to normal oxygen.

The levels of ROS are controlled by various cellular defence mechanisms: enzymatic (superoxide dismutase, catalase and glutation peroxidase) and nonenzymatic (glutation, vitamin E, vitamin C and betacarotene).

Oxydative stress may play a role in diabetic retinopathy from increased production and/or ineffective scavenging of reactive oxygen species.

Sources of ROS in diabetes may include autoxidation of glucose, AGEs formation, binding of AGEs to AGEs-receptors, increased substrate flux through the polyol pathway, stimulation of eicosanoid metabolism and increased cyclooxygenase activity (De La Cruz *et al.*, 1997).

Plasma LPO levels of diabetic patients are higher than in normal controls (Kaji *et al.*, 1985). Similarly, LPO levels of diabetics with angiopathy are higher than in diabetics without any complications (Sato *et al.*, 1979; Baynes, 1991; Augustin *et al.*, 1993; Losada *et al.*, 1996; Verdejo *et al.*, 1999; Gurler *et al.*, 2000; Uzel *et al.*, 1987). Diabetic patients show a decrease in ascorbic acid levels as compared to normal controls (Gurler *et al.*, 2000).

In diabetes mellitus, hypoxia due to impaired blood flow and the pseudohypoxia (increased NADH/NAD+ ratio due to hyperglycemia) may generate free radicals and there is evidence of an excessive consumption of antioxidants in diabetic patients (Watanable *et al.*, 1984).

A vicious cycle might be envisaged in which free radicals are both cause and consequence of ischemia (Giugliano *et al.*, 1996).

The human body does not produce antioxidants and minerals so it must be continuously supplied either in the diet or from supplementation. Under normal circumstances, free radicals are rapidly quenched by antioxidants that must be used in dietary supplementation. Vitamins C and E may favorably influence the natural course of disease process (Kowluru *et al.*, 1996).

### 9.5.5. Inhibitors of Protein Kinase C (PKC)

Protein kinase C beta 2 is involved in modulation of the VEGF receptor signal transduction cascade.

Adding and removing $PO_4$ groups to intracellular proteins, via kinases and phosphatase respectively, is an important regulatory system for activating and deactivating tissue enzymes, receptor pathways and transcription factors controling gene expression.

Hyperglycemia stimulates the "*de novo*" synthesis of diacylglycerol, the endogenous activator of PKC activity in vascular tissues (Inoguchi *et al.*, 1992; Xia *et al.*, 1994). In humans, PKC activity in circulating monocytes correlates with plasma glucose concentration in both diabetic and nondiabetic subjects (Ceollotto *et al.*, 1999). Inositol triphosphate (IP3) activation and NADH/NAD+ ratio imbalance due to overactivity of the sorbitol pathway also increase the activity of PKC (Williamson *et al.*, 1993; Le Good *et al.*, 1982).

PKC, specially the beta 2 isoform appears to be activated in retina. In diabetic animals it has been found that PKC activation can affect vascular permeability,

basement membrane synthesis, vessel contractility, blood flow and coagulation (Archer, 1998). PKC activation also contributes to loss of capillary pericytes (Pomero *et al.*, 2003). Hyperactivity of PKC sensitises vascular smooth muscle cells to vasoconstrictors and involved in the modulation of VEGF and its "downstream" actions and induces platelet aggregation.

PKC-beta 2 isoform specific inhibitor (LY333531), a macrocyclic bisindolymaleimide compound, has been shown to attenuate diabetic complications of retinopathy (Koya *et al.*, 1998).

Two international randomized placebo controlled trials of Ruboxistaurin a PKC-beta 2 inhibitor are now in progress to evaluate progression in patients with moderate to severe nonproliferative diabetic retinopathy at baseline and diabetic macular edema.

### 9.5.6. Inhibition of Nonenzymatic Glycation of Proteins and Advanced Glycation End Products

Extracellular glucose and other intracellular sugars, like fructose, can bind nonenzymatically to free amino groups of proteins (beta 2 microglobulin and immunoglobulins) and lipids (vg LDLs), a process that gives rise to reversible Shiff bases and Amadori products, which over time, by complex reactions, such as rearrangement, dehydration and condensation, produce a irreversible class of products, termed advanced-glycation end-products (AGEs) that can alter cell/matrix functions.

Normally AGEs increase with age, but this increase is accelerated in diabetes mellitus in direct proportion to levels of glycemia. Enzyme-linked immunosorbent assays (ELISAs) using AGE-specific antibodies show that diabetics have 10–45 times more AGEs than nondiabetic in tissue samples (Brownlee, 1993).

In a DCCT ancillary cross sectional study, the risk of retinopathy was associated with the level of AGEs in skin collagen (Monnier *et al.*, 1999).

In experimental diabetes, the biochemical abnormalities induced by AGEs are numerous and include: reaction with a variety of cytosol proteins, whose function is, thereby, altered (Vlassara, 1997); reaction with the extracellular matrix, such as subendothelial matrix of capillaries, with structural alterations in the vessels (Haitoglou *et al.*, 1992) and functional alterations on collagen, vitreonectin, laminine with increased quenching of nitric oxide and arterial wall fluid filtration and decreased wall elasticity.

Interaction with endothelial receptors results in procoagulatory changes in the endothelial surface (Esposito *et al.*, 1992; Bucala *et al.*, 1991; Brownlee, 1993) and increased angiogenesis by up-regulating the level of mRNAs for VEGF (Archer, 1998). Futhermore, an inhibitory effect on pericytes (Yamagishi *et al.*, 1997), production of endothelin-1 (Nawroth *et al.*, 1992) and increased sensitivity of blood vessels to free radicals with damage of nuclear DNA (Esposito *et al.*, 1992).

A number of therapeutic agents aminoguanidine, amadorins and peridoxal phosphate have been studied in animal models (Brownlee *et al.*, 1986; Chen *et al.*, 1993).

### 9.5.6.1. *Aminoguanidine*

Aminoguanidine is structurally similar to L-arginine and can block AGEs formation by producing nonreactive Amadori products that block the sequence of reactions that lead to AGEs formation (Huijberts *et al.*, 1994).

Aminoguanidine has some beneficial effect on the breakdown of the blood-retinal barrier, as shown in a vitreous fluorometry study in rats with streptozotocin-induced diabetes (Cho *et al.*, 1991). Its administration prevents the development of microaneurysms, acellular capillaries and markedly reduces pericyte drop-out (Hammes *et al.*, 1991).

### 9.5.6.2. *Amadorins*

Amadorins are products than can block, through a mechanism different from that described to aminoguanidine, the conversion of Amadori products into AGes. Pyridonine, a Vitamin B6 analog and Pyridoxamine have been shown to prevent morphological abnormalities in experimental diabetic retinopathy (Stitt *et al.*, 2002).

### 9.5.6.3. *Pyridoxal phosphate*

Pyridoxal phosphate, a vital metabolite, forms a Schiff base with proteins, as does glucose, induces glucose-induced nonenzymatic glycosylation inhibition and may be a preferable drug over aminoguanidine (Khatami *et al.*, 1988).

## 9.5.7. Aldose Reductase Inhibitors

The retina like other nervous tissues does not require insulin for cellular glucose uptake. Hyperglycemia leads to accumulation of glucose in these tissues and the excess of glucose is reduced by aldose reductase (AR), coupled to oxidation of NADPH to $NADP^+$ to the sugar alcohol sorbitol. Excessive AR activity has been postulated to be responsible for diabetic retinopathy (Beaumont *et al.*, 1971).

The accumulation of sorbitol in tissues causes several events: osmotic damage (Cogan *et al.*, 1984), pseudohypoxia (Williamson *et al.*, 1993), $Na^+K^+$ Atpase depression (Sweeadner *et al.*, 1980). In diabetic and galactosemic animals Aldose Reductase Inhibitors (ARIs) prevent sorbitol accumulation and the cascade of associated events. Use of ARIs has been shown to retard the onset and progression of histopathologic changes in diabetic animal models.

ARIs act as antioxidants, decreasing the production of free radicals produced by glucose autooxidation (Greene *et al.*, 1984), inhibit the high glucose-induced death of retinal capillary cells (Goldfarb *et al.*, 1991), diminish basement membrane thickening (Robison *et al.*, 1995) and prevent to some degree expression of VEGF (Frank *et al.*, 1997). Cusick *et al.* (2003) using fluorescein angiography, found that an ARi-M79175 can prevent or retard the development of large areas of nonperfusion in a galacosemic dog model.

A variety of unrelated compounds have aldose redutase inhibiting properties, most acting by non-competitive or uncompetitive inhibition. In three small randomized clinical trials our group (Cunha-Vaz et al., 1977; 1985; Leite et al., 1990) has shown that drugs with AR inhibiting activity, cyclandelate, sulindac and calcium dobesilate, exert a significantly beneficial effect on the early breakdown of the blood-retinal barrier using vitreous fluorometry measurements in diabetic patients with nonproliferative diabetic retinopathy.

However, the relationship between the early breakdown of blood-retinal barrier, as assessed by vitreous fluorometry and the progression to more severe retinopathy, has not been fully established.

Aldose redutase inhibitors (ARI) that contain a chromone ring, such as alrestatin, ponalrestat, tolrestat, fidarestat and zenalestat, were tried with limited success in clinical trials (Pfeifer et al., 1997).

The Sorbinil Retinopathy Study Trial (1990), a multicenter randomized trial of 497 patients, showed at the end of 3-year follow-up that sorbinil, an ARI, had no clinically significant effect on the course of diabetic retinopathy in adults with insulin-dependent diabetes of moderate duration (1–15 years). Furthermore, 7% of the patients developed a hypersensitivity reaction, sometimes severe in the first three months. The failure to influence diabetic retinopathy may reflect the nature and concentrations of the inhibitor used, the length of time of trial and its incapacity to cross the blood-retinal barrier.

## 9.5.8. Rheological Agents

Various rheological abnormalities have been found in diabetic patients suggesting a role in capillary closure.

Increased leukostasis, leukocytes attached to the endothelial wall, is a common pathological event both in human disease (McLeod et al., 1995; Lutty et al., 1997) and in experimental models (Miyamoto et al., 1999; Cannas et al., 2000).

The filterability of polymorphonuclear leucocytes is reduced in diabetic patients compared with age-matched controls (DeVaro et al., 1988; Ernest et al., 1986), leucocytes in diabetes are less deformable and have increased viscosity (Kubes et al., 1991; Chien et al., 1983; Myamoto, 1997) and monocytes and granulocytes have been found to cause capillary occlusion in a rat model of diabetic retinopathy (Schröder et al., 1991).

In diabetes there is increased plasma and whole blood viscosity (Kurose et al., 1994), increased aggregation of platelets (Sagel et al., 1975) and erythrocytes (Schmid-Schonbein et al., 1976). There is also a decreased filterability of erythrocytes (McMillan et al., 1978) in diabetes.

It has been suggested that the diabetic environment produces a "sticky" vascular endothelial phenotype, in which increased adhesion plays a role in the mechanisms that lead to increased leukostasis (Miyamoto et al., 1999). Hughes et al. (2004), however, did not find an increased expression of E-selectin, P-selectin and ICAM-1 in post-mortem diabetic eyes when compared to controls.

Pentoxyfilin is a rheological agent that has been tested with some success. Pentoxyfilin is a methylxantine derivative and acts as a phosphodiesterase inhibitor improving, in normal humans, retinal capillary blood flow velocity and whole blood viscosity due to an improvement in leukocyte fluidity, increasing filtration rate of whole blood, red blood cell deformability and decreasing red blood cell and platelet aggregation (Sonkin et al., 1993). Sonkin et al. (1993) showed using blue-field entopic phenomenon (computer simulation technique) that three months after pentoxyfilin therapy there was an increase in retinal capillary blood flow velocity ($p = 0.005$) from baseline with a return to baseline after discontinuation of therapy.

## 9.5.9. Antiinflammatory Agents

Vascular endothelium controls transcellular migration of blood-born leucocytes to the neuropile by regulation of adhesion molecules, such as Selectines and ICAM-1/VCAM-1 in response to inflammatory stimuli. Leucocytes have been shown to adhere to the retinal vascular endothelium early in experimental diabetic retinopathy (Haimovich *et al.*, 1993). In diabetes, PKC promotes activation of platelet-activating factor (PAF) via PAF synthesis and stimulation of PAF receptors with production of leucotrienes (Triggiani *et al.*, 1999; Komatsu *et al.*, 1999). Integrines and Leukocyte adhesion molecules to the endothelial cells via the intercellular adhesion molecule 1-(ICAM-1) that is also upregulated by endothelial PKC. Increased adherence of leukocytes to capillary endothelium decreases blood flow with hypoxia and may also increase breakdown of blood-retinal barrier.

A variety of antiinflammatory agents have, at one point or another, been tested for its effect on diabetic retinal disease. Although aspirin was shown to be ineffective (ETDRS, 1991), corticoids in intravitreal injections or slow release implants are currently under investigation for diabetic macular edema.

Martidis *et al.* (2002), in diabetic patients with refractory diffuse diabetic macular edema, in a prospective open study, reported a 58% reduction in macular thickness three months after intravitreal triamcinolone. Jonas *et al.* (2003), in a prospective study in 26 eyes with diffuse macular edema, showed that intravitreal triamcinolone improved visual acuity ($p < 0.01$) with 81% of eyes with a follow-up period of more than one month, improving visual acuity. Massin *et al.* (2004) in a prospective controlled short term study with a follow-up of at least three months for refractory diffuse diabetic macular edema, using optical coherence tomography to evaluate the anatomic results, found that intravitreal injection of triamcinolone effectively reduced macular thickening ($p < 0.001$), but at no time the difference between ETDRS visual scores was significant.

Nonsteroid antiinflammatory agents have also been tested. Cunha-Vaz *et al.* (1985) in a group of insulin-dependent diabetic patients with minimal or no retinopathy showed that sulindac, a nonsteroidal antiinflammatory drug capable of inhibiting prostaglandin, after six months of treatment, produces a significant beneficial effect on the breakdown of the blood-retinal barrier, as shown by vitreous fluorophotometry. A trial with an oral COX2 inhibitor (celebrex) to treat macular edema is now ongoing (Aiello, 2003).

Histamine H1 receptors antagonists have also been shown to stabilize alterations of the blood-retinal barrier in experimental animals (Hollis *et al.*, 1992). Gardner *et al.* (1995) showed by vitreous fluorophotometry a significant reduction ($p < 0.05$) in blood-retinal barrier permeability in type 1 diabetic patients with mild nonproliferative retinopathy treated with astemizole and ranitidine, as compared with similar control patients six months after treatment.

## 9.5.10. Angiogenesis Signaling Inhibitors

Perivascular glial cells and the composite vascular matrix immobilise various heparin-binding paracrine growth factors, VRGF and bFGF, and pericytes secrete an inhibiting growth factor TGF-$\beta$.

Angiogenesis, the development of new vessels from existing ones, is a requirement for new organ development and for differentiation during embryogenesis, during tissue growth and repair and during the female reproductive cycle.

Compensatory angiogenesis is demonstrated in the formation of collateral blood vessels when there is oxygen or nutrient deprivation in normal tissues (Dor *et al.*, 1997). Angiogenic growth factors are released by diseased or injured cells in response to hypoxia, hypoglycemia, mechanical stress, release of inflammatory proteins and also by genetic alterations (Rosen, 2001).

Angiogenesis is regulated by pro and antiangiogenesis growth factors. Some of these factors are more specific for the endothelium. They may be proangiogenic, basic fibroblast growth factor (bFGF), leptin, platelet-derived growth factor (PDGF), transforming growth factor (TGF), vascular endothelial growth factor (VEGF) and antiangiogenic, angiostatin, antithrombin III, interferon alpha beta gama, interleukin 12, plasminogen activator inhibitor and transforming growth factor beta (TGF-$\beta$).

Activated endothelial cells signal their nucleus to produce enzymes, such as metalloproteinases (MMPs) that break down the extracellular matrix of the blood vessel, allowing proliferating endothelial cells to migrate in response to VEGF through the holes made in the matrix. Adhesion molecules mediate the migration of the new endothelial cells organized into hollow tubes, new vessels, towards the growth stimulus.

### 9.5.10.1.  *VEGF*

VEGF isoforms are cell-specific mitogenes for vascular endothelial cells, increase permeability at blood-tissue barriers, maybe by interfering with interendothelial cell junctions (Kevil *et al.*, 1998) and also an antiapoptotic factor for endothelial cells in newly formed vessels (Alon *et al.*, 1995).

Normally, VEGF expression substantially decreases after birth, but some cells, like those in the neural retina, in the choroid and retinal epithelium, constitutively secret picomolar amounts.

The most important mechanism that regulates VEGF is hypoxia. The biological effects of VEGF are mediated by two receptors, tyrosine kinase VEGFr-1 and VEGFr-2. When VEGF binds to its receptor, a proangiogenic signal is transmitted to downstream proteins initiating a cascade of events leading to proliferation, migration and differentiation of endothelial cells.

VEGF injected into the vitreous of the eyes of monkeys induced neovascularization of the iris (Tolentino *et al.*, 1996) and retina (Tolentino *et al.*, 2002) and has produced some clinical features of non-proliferative diabetic retinopathy (Tolentino *et al.*, 1996).

Antisense oligodeoxynucleotide technology provides an approach for inhibiting gene expression with target specificity by modifying oligodeoxynucleotide synthesis with production of molecules that are stable for several days and are relatively nontoxic at effective concentrations (Field *et al.*, 1995). Intravitreal injection of two antisense oligodeoxynucleotides (PS-ODNs) prior to the onset of a murine model of proliferative diabetic retinopathy appeared to inhibit protein expression of VEGF. Intravitreal injection of anti VEGF antibodies also appeared to prevent neovascularization (Adamis *et al.*, 1996; Robinson *et al.*, 1996) and soluble VEGF-receptors also prevented neovascularization (Aiello *et al.*, 1995).

Vitreous samples from patients with diabetic macular edema contain elevated VEGF levels (Brooks *et al.*, 2004). More recently, experiments in animals have suggested a central role for the 165 isoform of VEGF specifically in the pathogenesis of diabetic macular edema (Tolentino *et al.*, 1916; Qaum *et al.*, 2001; Ishida *et al.*, 2003). Moreover, increased retinal VEGF 164 levels (the rodent equivalent to primate VEGF 165) in this model coincide temporally with breakdown of the blood-retinal barrier (Ishida *et al.*, 2003). When VEGF 164 bioactivity is selectively blocked using pegaptanib sodium injection (Macugen), the blood-retinal barrier is re-established in animals with induced diabetes (Ishida *et al.*, 2003).

Results from a phase II randomized double-masked, multicenter, controlled efficacy of pegaptanib sodium injection in the treatment of diabetic macular edema, showed that subjects assigned to pegaptanib had better visual acuity outcomes, were more likely to show reduction in central retinal thickness and were less likely to need additional therapy with photocoagulation at follow-up (Macugen Diabetic Retinopathy Study Group, 2005).

### 9.5.10.2.  *Pigment-epithelium derived factor*

In the eye pigment-epithelium derived factor (PEDF) is secreted from the apical surface of retinal pigment epithelium (Becerra *et al.*, 2001).

PEDF is downregulated in hypoxic tissues and this is observed in eyes with active proliferative diabetic retinopathy, possibly, for promoting apoptosis of endothelial cells (Williams, 1989; Dawson *et al.*, 1999).

Systemic administration of PEDF inhibits neovascularization in the hyperoxygenated neonatal mouse, a model of human retinopathy of prematurity (Stellmach *et al.*, 2001).

PEDF and VEGF appear to have a reciprocal relation in the eye. There is evidence that in proliferative diabetic retinopathy, levels of VEGF increase (Aiello *et al.*, 1994), whereas those of PEDF decrease (Gao *et al.*, 2001).

Adenovirus transfection opens the possibility for gene therapy to upregulate PEDF and inhibition of neoangiogenesis. Intravitreal injection of a replication-deficient adenovirus containing the PEDF gene has been shown to inhibit retinal and choroidal neovascularization (Mori *et al.*, 2001). A phase 1 study of this approach in patients with wet ARMD is under way.

### 9.5.10.3. *Growth hormone*

Diabetic patients even under adequate glucose control show excess growth hormone (GH) levels (Feinstein *et al.*, 1998) and diabetic retinopathy correlates with the magnitude of GH hypersecretion (Sundvist *et al.*, 1988). Spontaneous resolution of PDR in a woman with acute panhypopituitarism (Poulsen, 1953) and stabilization of diabetic retinopathy was observed after infiltrative destruction of the pituitary in patients with hemochromatosis (Sonksen *et al.*, 1993) formed the basis for the interest pituitary ablation as treatment for vision threatening retinopathy (Lundbaek *et al.*, 1989).

A pilot study in patients with severe nonproliferative diabetic retinopathy or non-high-risk proliferative showed that a growth hormone inhibitor, somastatin, may delay development of high-risk proliferative diabetic retinopathy (Grant *et al.*, 2000).

Now, a multicentric open large-scale trial with a subcutaneous somatostatin analogue (octreotide) is in progress. Over a 15 months period the percentage of eyes treated with octreotide that required panretinal photocoagulation (4.5%), as compared with those that did not receive treatment (41%), is significant (*p* < 0.0006) (Grant *et al.*, 2000).

## 9.6. Conclusions

At present it must be realized that medical management of diabetic retinopathy must focus on prevention with aggressive glycemic control to aim at a $HbA_{1C}$ of less than 7% and blood pressure of levels lower than 130/85 mm Hg.

In the future, medical therapy for DR will probably involve the association of drugs that include:

a. Euglycemic control by insulin or oral antidiabetic drugs.
b. Drugs to correct the altered metabolism of the retina associated with excess glucose availability (*ex*: aldose redutase inhibitors, protein kinase C inhibitors and antioxidants).
c. Neuroprotective drugs if clinical examination shows the predominance of cytotoxic edema or vasoprotective drugs in case of vasogenic edema.

Diabetic retinopathy must be envisaged as a long-term therapy that must be initiated well before visual loss or irreversible retinal lesions develop, which means that side effects should be minimal and medications must have a good benefit to risk ratio.

## References

Adamis AP, Shima DT, Tolentino MJ, *et al.* (1996) Inhibition of vascular endothelial growth factors prevents retinal ischaemia-associated iris neovascularization in nonhuman primate. *Arch Ophthalmol* **114**: 66–71.

Aiello LM. (2003) Perspectives on diabetic retinopathy. *Am J Ophthalmol.* **136**: 122–135.

Aiello LP, Avery RL, Arrigg PG, *et al.* (1994) Vascular endothelial growth factor in ocular fluid of patients with diabetic retinopathy and other retinal disorder. *N Eng J Med* **331**: 1480–1487.

Aiello LP, Northrup JM, Keyt BA, *et al.* (1995) Hypoxic regulation of vascular endothelial growth factor in retinal cells. *Arch Ophthalmol* **113**: 1538–1544.

Aiello LP, Pierce EA, Foley ED, *et al.* (1995) Suppression of retinal neovascularization *in vivo* by inhibition of vascular endothelial growth factor (VEGF) using soluble VEGF-receptor chimeric proteins. *Proc Natl Acad Sci USA* **92**: 10457–10461.

Aiello LP, Davis MD, Sheetz MJ. (2002) The PKC inhibitor diabetic retinopathy study group. Designed, baseline patient characteristics and high prevalence of clinically significant macular edema (CSME) in patients with moderately severe to very severe nonproliferative diabetic retinopathy (NPDR) in the Protein Kinase C diabetic retinopathy study (PKC-DRS). *Diabetes* **51**(2): A-209.

Alon T, Hemo I, Itn A, *et al.* (1995) Vascular endothelial growth factor acts as a survival factor for newly formed retinal vessels and has implications for retinopathy of prematurity. *Nature Med* **1**: 1024–1028.

American Diabetes Association. (2002) Clinical practice recommendations. *Diabetes Care* **25**(1): S1–S147.

American Diabetes Association. (2002) Management of dyslipidemia in adults with diabetes. *Diabetes Care* **25**: S74–S77.

Archer DB. (1999) Diabetic retinopathy: Some cellular, molecular and therapeutic considerations. *Eye* **13**: 497–523.

Augustin AJ, Breipohl W, Boker T, *et al.* (1995) Increased lipid peroxide levels and myeloperoxidase activity in the vitreous of patients suffering from proliferative diabetic retinopathy. *Graefes Arch Ophthalmol* **231**: 647–650.

Aydin A, Orhan H, Sayal A, *et al.* (2001) Oxidative stress and nitric oxide related parameters in type 2 diabetes: Effect of glycemic control. *Clin Biochem* **34**: 65–70.

Barouch FC, Miyamoto K, Allport JR, *et al.* (2000) Integrin-mediated neutrophil adhesion and retinal leukostasis in diabetes. *Invest Ophthalmol Vis Sci* **31**: 1153–1158.

Bashkin P, Doctrow S, Klagsbrun CM, *et al.* (1989) Basic fibroblast growth factor binds to subendothelial extracellular matrix and is released by heparitinase and heparin-like molecules. *Biochemistry* **28**: 1737–1743.

Baynes JW. (1991) Perspective in diabetes. Role of oxidative stress in development of complications in diabetes (review) *Diabetes* **40**: 405–412.

Beaumont P, Schofield PJ, Hollows FC, *et al.* (1974) Growth hormone, sorbitol and diabetic capillary disease. *Lancet* **1**(7699): 579–581.

Becerra SP, Wu YQ, Montuenga L, *et al.* (2001) Pigment epithelium-derived factor (PEDF) in monkey eye: Apical secretion from the retinal pigment epithelium. *Invest Ophthalmol Vis Sci* **42**: S772.

Brooks HL Jr, Caballero S Jr, Newell CK, *et al.* (2004) Vitreous levels of vascular endothelial growth factor and stromal-derived factor 1 in patients with diabetic retinopathy and cystoid macular edema before and after intraocular injection of triamcinolome. *Arch Ophthalmol* **122**(12): 1801–1887.

Belgian Ticlopidine Retinopathy Study Group. (1992) Clinical study of Ticlopidine in diabetic retinopathy. *Ophthalmologica* **204**: 4–12.

Boeri D, Maiello M, Lorenzi M. (2001) Increase prevalence of microthromboses in retinal capillaries of diabetic individuals. *Diabetes* **50**: 1432–1439.

Brownlee M. (1993) Lilly lecture 1993: 1994; **43**: 836–841. Glycation and diabetes complications. Diabetes 1.

Brownlee M, Vlassara H, Kooney A, *et al.* (1986) Aminoguanidine prevents diabetes-induced arterial wall protein cross-linking. *Science* **232**: 1629–1632.

Brownlee M. (1994) Glycation and diabetic complications. *Diabetes* **43**: 836–841.

Brownlee M. (1996) Advanced glycation end products in diabetic complications. *Curr Opin Endocrin Diabetes* **3**: 291–297.

Bucala R, Tracey KJ, Cerami A. (1991) Advanced glycosylation products quench nitric oxide ad mediate defective endothelium-dependent vasodilatation in experimental diabetes. *J Clin Invest* **87**: 432–438.

Bunting S, Moncada S, Vane JR. (1983) The prostacyclin-thromboxane A2 balance; pathophysiological and therapeutics implications. *Br Med Bull* **39**: 271–276.

Bursell SE, King GL. (1999) Can protein kinase C inhibition and vitamine E prevent the development of diabetic vascular complications? *Diabetes Res Clin Pract* **45**: 169–172.

Calles-Escandon J, Cipolla M. (2001) Diabetes and endothelial dysfunction: A clinical perspective. *Endocrine Rev* **22**: 36–52.

Carroll WJ, Hollis TM, Gardner TW. (1988) Retinal histidine decarboxylase activity is elevated in experimental diabetes. *Invest Ophthalmol Vis Sci* **29**: 1201–1204.

Ceolotto G, Gallo A, Miola M, *et al.* (1999) Protein kinase C activity is acutely regulate by plasma glucose concentration in human monocytes *in vivo. Diabetes* **48**: 1316–1322.

Ceriello A. (1999) Hyperglicemia: A bridge between nonenzymatic glycation and oxidative stress in the pathogenesis of diabetic complications. *Diabetes Nutr Metab* **12**: 42–46.

Chaturvedi N, Sjolie A-K, Stephenson JM, *et al.* (1998) Effect of lisinopril on progression of retinopathy in normotensive people with type 1 diabetes. *Lancet* **351**: 28:31.

Chen H, Cerami A. (1993) Mechanism of inhibition of advanced glycosylation by aminoguanidine *in vitro. J Carbohydrate Chem* **12**: 731–742.

Chew EY, Klein ML, Feris FL 3rd, *et al.* (1996) Association of elevated serum lipid levels with retinal hard exudate in diabetic retinopathy. ETDRS report number 22. *Arch Ophthalmol* **114**: 1079–1084.

Chien S, Schmalzer EA, Lee MM, *et al.* (1983) Role of white blood cells in filtration of blood cell suspension. *Biorheology* **20**: 11–27.

Cho HK, Kozu H, Peyman GA, *et al.* (1991) The effect of aminoguanidine on the blood-retinal barrier in streptozotocin-induced diabetic rats. *Ophthalmic Surg* **22**: 44–47.

Chowdhury TA, Hopkins D, Dodson PM, Vafidis GC. (2002) The role of serum lipids in exudative diabetic maculopathy: Is there a place for lipid lowering therapy? *Eye* **6**: 689–693.

Cogan DG, Kinoshita JH, Kador PF, *et al.* (1984) Aldose redutase inhibition improves nerve conduction velocity in diabetic patients. *Ann Intern Med* **101**: 82–91.

Cox SN, Hay E, Bird AC. (1988) Treatment of chronic macular edema with acetazolamide. *Arch Ophthalmol* **106**: 1190–1195.

Crabtree DV, Adler AJ, Snodderly EM. (1996) Radial distribution of tocoferol in rhesus monkey retina and retinal pigment epithelium-choroid. *Invest Ophthalmol Vis Sci* **37**: 61–76.

Crabtree DV, Snodderly EM, Adler AJ. (1997) Retinyl palmitate in macaque retina-retinal pigment epithelium-choroid: Distribution and correlation with age and vitamine E. *Exp Eye Res* **64**: 455–463.

Cunha-Vaz JG, Reis Fonseca J, Hagenouw JRB. (1977) Treatment of early diabetic retinopathy with cyclandelate. *Br J Ophthalmol* **61**: 399–404.

Cunha-Vaz JG, Mota MC, Leite EC, *et al.* (1985) Effect of sulindac on the permeability of the blood-retinal barrier in early diabetic retinopathy. *Arch Ophthalmol* **103**: 1307–1311.

Cunha-Vaz JG. (2000) Diabetic retinopathy: Surrogate outcomes for drug development for diabetic retinopathy. *Ophthalmologica* **214**: 377–380.

Cunha-Vaz JG. (2004) Medical treatment of retinopathy of type-2 diabetes. *Ophthalmologica* **218**: 291–296.

Cusick M, Chew EY, Ferris III F, *et al.* (2003) Effects of aldose reductase inhibitors and galactose withdrawl on fluorescein angiographic lesions in galactose — fed dogs. *Arch Ophthalmol* **121**: 1745–1751.

Cusick M, Chew EY, Chan C-C, *et al.* (2003) Histopathology and regression of retinal hard exudates in diabetic retinopathy after reduction of elevated serum lipid levels. *Ophthalmology* **110**: 2126–2133.

Danis RP, Bingaman DP. (1997) Insulin-like growth factor — 1 retinal microangiopathy in the pig eye. *Ophthalmology* **104**: 1661–1669.

Danser AHJ, van den Dorpel MA, Deinum J, *et al.* (1989) Renin, protein, and immunoreactive renin in vitreous fluid from eyes with and without diabetic retinopathy. *J Clin Endocrinol Metab* **68**: 160–167.

Danser AHJ, Derkx FHM, Admiraal PJJ, *et al.* (1994) Angiotensin levels in the eye. *Invest Ophthalmol Vis Sci* **35**: 1008–1018.

Dawson DW, Volpert OV, Gillis P, *et al.* (1999) Pigment epithelium-derived factor: A potent inhibitor of angiogenesis. *Science* **285**: 245–248.

De La Cruz JP, Maximo MA, Blanco E, *et al.* (1997) Effect of erythrocytes and prostacyclin 'production in the effect of fructose and sorbitol on platelet activation in human whole blood *in vitro*'. *Thromb Res* **86**: 515–524.

De La Cruz JP, Gonzalez-Correa, Guerrero A, la Cuesta FS. (2004) Pharmacological approach to diabetic retinopathy. *Diabetes Metab Res Ver* **20**: 91–113.

De Varo J, Chumdermpodetsuk R, Edelman R, *et al.* (1988) Polymorphonuclear filterability in diabetes mellitus. *Inves Ophthalmol Vis Sci* **29**: 181.

Dills DG, Moss SE, Klein R, Klein BE. (1991) Association of elevated ILGF 1 with increased retinopathy in late-onset diabetes. *Diabetes* **40**: 1725–1730.

Dor Y, Keshet E. (1997) Ischemia-driven angiogenesis: therapeutic implications. *Trends Cardiovasc Med* **7**: 289–294.

Ebeling P, Koivisto VA. (1997) Occurence and interrelationships of complications in insulin-dependent diabetes in Finland. *Acta Diabetol* **34**: 33–38.

Enea NA, Hollis TM, Kern JÁ, Gardner TW. (1989) Histamine H1 receptors mediate increased blood-retinal permeability in experimental diabetes. *Arch Ophthalmol* **107**: 270–274.

Ernest E, Matrai A. (1986) Altered red and white blood cell rheology in type II diabetes. *Diabetes* **35**: 1412–1415.

Esmatjes E, Maseras M, Gallelo M, *et al.* (1989) Effect of treatment with an inhibitor of platelet aggregation on the evolution of background retinopathy: 2 years follow-up. *Diabetes Res Clin Pract* **7**: 285–291.

Esposito C, Gerlach H, Brett J. (1992) Endothelial receptor mediated binding of glucose modified albumine is associated with increased monolayer permeability and modulation of cell surface coagulant properties. *J Exp Med* **170**: 1387–1397.

Estacio RO, Jeffers BW, Gifford N, Schrier RW. (2000) Effect of blood pressure control on diabetic microvascular complications in patients with hypertension and type 2 diabetes. *Diabetes Care* **23**(2): B54–B64.

Feinstein D, Fagin JA, Litwak LE, *et al.* (1998) Growth hormone insulin-like growth factor-I axis in adult insulin-dependent diabetes patients: Evidence for central hypersensitivity to growth hormone-releasing hormone and peripheral resistance to growth hormone. *Hom Metab Res* **30**: 737–742.

Field AK, Goodchild J. (1995) *Expert Opin Drugs* **9**: 799–821.

Fong DS, Ferris FL. (2003) Practical management of diabetic retinopathy. *Focal points. American Academy of Ophthalmology* March 2003, Section 3.

Frank RN. (2004) Diabetic retinopathy. *N Engl J Med* **350**: 48–58.

Frank RN, Amin R, Kennedy A, Huhman TC. (1997) An aldose reductase inhibitor and aminoguanidine prevent vascular endothelial growth factor expression in rats with long-term galactosemia. *Arch Ophthalmol* **115**: 1036–1047.

Franzone M, Molinatti A, Indemini P, *et al.* (1987) Fluoroangiographic and fluorophotometric evaluation of chromocarbo-diethylamine therapy in diabetic retinopathy. In: *Ocular Fluorophotometry. Proceedings International Society of Ocular Fluorophotometry — ISOF.* Kugler Publications, Amsterdam, pp. 69–76.

Freyberger H, Schifferdecker E, Schaltz H. (1994) Regression of hard exudates in diabetic background retinopathy in therapy with etofibrate antilipemic agent. *Med Klin* **89**: 594–597.

Friedman E, Brown C, Berman D. (1995) Erythropoietin in diabetic macular edema and renal insufficiency. *Am J Kidney Dis* **26**: 202–208.

Funatsu H, Yamashita H, Ikeda T, *et al.* (2002) Angiotensine II and vascular endothelial growth factor in the vitreous fluid of patients with diabetic macular edema and other retinal disorders. *Am J Ophthalmol* **133**: 537–543.

Funatsu H, Yamashita H, Ikeda T, *et al.* (2003) Relation of diabetic macular edema to cytokines and posterior vitreous detachment. *Am J Ophthalmol* **135**: 321–327.

Gao G, Li Y, Zhang D, *et al.* (2001) Unbalanced expression of VEGF and PEDF in ischemia-induced retinal neovascularization. *FEBS Lett* **489**(2–3) 270–276.

Gardner TW, Eller AW, Friberg TR, *et al.* (1995) Antihistamines reduce blood retinal barrier permeability in type 1 (insulin-dependent) diabetic patients with non-proliferative retinopathy. *Retina* **15**: 134–140.

Giardino I, Edelstein D, Brownlee D. (1994) Nonenzymatic glycosylation *in vitro* and in bovine endothelial cells alters basic fibroblast growth factor activity. *J Clin Invest* **94**: 110–117.

Giardino I, Fard AK, Hatchell DL, Brownice M. (1998) Aminoguanidine inhibits reactive oxygen species formation, lipid peroxidation and oxidant-induced apoptosis. *Diabetes* **47**: 1114–1120.

Gilbert RE, Kelly DJ, Cox AJ, *et al.* (2000) Angiotensin converting enzyme inhibition reduces retinal overexpression of vascular endothelial growth factor and hyperpermeability in experimental diabetes. *Diabetologia* **43**: 1360–1367.

Giugliano D, Ceriello A, Paolisso G. (1996) Oxidative stress and diabetic vascular complications. *Diabetes Care* **19**: 257–267.

Goldfarb S, Ziyadeh FN, Kern EF, Simmons DA. (1991) Effects of polyol-pathway inhibition and dietary myoinositol on glomerular hemodynamic function in experimental diabetes mellitus in rats. *Diabetes* **40**: 465–471.

Grant M, Russel B, Fitzgerald C, Merimee TJ. (1986) Insulin-like growth factors in vitreous; studies in control and diabetic subjects with neovascularization. *Diabetes* **35**: 416–420.

Grant MB, Mames RN, Fitzgerald C, *et al.* (2000) The efficacy of octreotide in the therapy of severe nonproliferative and early proliferative diabetic retinopathy; a randomized controlled study. *Diabetes Care* **23**: 504–509.

Grattagliano I, Vendemiale G, Micelli-Ferrari T, *et al.* (1995) Abnormal protein redox status and impairment of antioxidant defence in lens and vitreous of diabetic subjects (Abstract). *Diabetologia* **38**(1): A276.

Greene DA, DeJesus PV, Winegrad AI. (1975) Effects of insulin and dietary myoinositol on impaired peripheral motor nerve conduction velocity in acute streptozotocin diabetes. *J Clin Invest* **55**: 1326–1336.

Greene DA, Lattimer SA. (1984) Action of sorbinil in diabetic peripheral nerve: Relationship of polyol (sorbitol) pathway inhibition to myo-inositol-mediated defect in sodium-potassium ATPase activity. *Diabetes* **33**: 712–716.

Gries FA. (1995) Alternative therapeutic principles in the prevention of microvascular and neuropatic complications. *Diab Res Clin Pract* **28**(1): S201–S207.

Growth Hormone Antagonists for Proliferative Diabetic Retinopathy Study Group. (2001) The effect of a growth hormone receptor antagonist drug on proliferative diabetic retinopathy. *Am. J. Ophthalmol* **108**: 2266–2272.

Grimm C, Wenzel A, Groszer M, *et al.* (2002) HIF-1 induced erythropoietin in the hypoxic retina protects against light-induced retinal degeneration. *Nature Med* **8**: 718–722.

Gupta A, Gupta V, Thapar S, Bhansali A. (2004) Lipid-lowering drug atorvastatin as an adjunct in the management of diabetic macular edema. *Am J Ophthalmol* **137**: 675–682.

Gurler B, Vural H, Yilmaz N, *et al.* (2000) The role of oxidative stress in diabetic retinopathy. *Eye* **14**: 730–735.

Haimovich B, Lipfert L, Brugge JS, Shattil SJ. (1993) Tyrosine phosphorylation and cytoskeletal reorganization in platelets are triggered by interaction of integrin receptors with their immobilized ligands. *J Biol Chem* **268**: 15868–15877.

Haitoglou CS, Tsilibari EC, Brownlee M, Charonis AS. (1992) Altered cellular interactions between endothelial cells and nonenzymatically glucosilated laminin/type IV collagen. *J Biol Chem* **1267**: 12404–12407.

Hammes H-P, Martin S, Federlin K, *et al.* (1991) Aminoguanidine treatment inhibits the development of experimental diabetic retinopathy. *Proc Natl Acad Sci USA* **88**: 11555–11558.

Hasebe Y, Thomsom LR, Dorey CK. (2000) Pentoxifylline inhibition of vasculogenesis in the neonatal rat retina. *Invest Ophthalmol Vis Sci* **41**: 2774–2778.

Hogeboom van Buggernum IMH, Polack BCP, Reichert-Thoen JWM, *et al.* (2002) Angiotensin converting enzyme inhibitor therapy is associated with lower vitreous vascular endothelial growth factor concentrations in patients with proliferative diabetic retinopathy. *Diabetologia* **45**: 203–209.

Hollis TM, Campos MJ, Butler C, Gardner TW. (1992) Astemizole reduces blood retinal barrier permeability in experimental diabetes. *J Diabetes Complicat* **6**: 230–235.

Hughes JM, Brink A, Witmer AN, *et al.* (2004) Vascular leucocyte adhesion molecules unaltered in human retina in diabetes. *Br J Ophthalmol* **88**: 566–572.

Huijberts MSP, Wolffenbuttel BHR, Crijins FR, *et al.* (1994) Aminoguanidine reduces regional albumin clearance but not urinary albumin excretion in streptozotocin-diabetic rats. *Diabetologia* **37**: 10–14.

Hyer SL, Sharp PS, Brooks RA, *et al.* (1989) A two-year follow-up study of serum insulin-like growth factor — I in diabetics with retinopathy. *Metabolism* **38**: 586–589.

Inoguchi T, Battan R, Handler E, *et al.* (1992) Preferential elevation of protein kinase C isoform Beta II and diacyglycerol levels in aorta and heart of diabetic rats: Differential reversibility to glycemic control by islet cell transplantation. *Proc Natl Acad Sci USA* **89**: 11059–11063.

Inoguchi T, Xia P, Kunisaki M, *et al.* (1994) Insulin's effect on protein kinase C and diacylglycerol induced by diabetes and glucose in vascular tissues. *Am J Physiol* **267**: E369–E379.

Ishii H, Jirousek MR, Koya D, *et al.* (1996) Amelioration of vascular dysfunctions in diabetic rats by oral PKC inhibitor. *Science* **272**: 728–731.

Ishida S, Usui T, Yamashiro K, *et al.* (2003) VEGF164 is proinflammatory in the diabetic retina. *Invest Ophthalmol Vis Sci* **44**(5): 2155–2162.

Jain SK, McVie R. (1994) Effect of glycemic control, race, and duration of diabetes on reduced glutathione content in erythrocytes of diabetic patients. *Metabolism* **43**: 306–309.

Jonas JB, Kreissig I, Sofker A, Degenring RF. (2003) Intravitreal injection of triamcinolone for diffuse macular edema. *Arch Ophthalmol* **121**: 57–61.

Kaji H, Hurasak M, Ito K. (1985) Increased lipoperoxide value and glutathione peroxidase activity in blood plasma of type 2 (non-insulin dependent) diabetic human. *Klin Wochenschcr* **643**: 765–768.

Khatami M, Suldan Z, David I, *et al.* (1998) Inhibitory effects of pyridoxal phosphate, ascorbate and amino-guanidine on nonenzymatic glycosylation. *Life Sci* **43**: 1725–1731.

Kern TS, Engerman RL. (2001) Pharmacological inhibition of diabetic retinopathy, aminoguanine and aspirin. *Diabetes* **50**: 1636–1642.

Kevil CG, Payne DK, Mire E, Alexander JS. (1998) Vascular permeability factor/vascular endothelial cell growth factor-mediated permeability occurs through disorganization of endothelial junctional proteins. *J Biol Chem* **273**: 15099–15103.

Klein BE, Moss SE, Klein R, Sarawicz TS. (1991) The Wisconsin Epidemiologic Study of Diabetic retinopathy. XIII. Relationship of serum cholesterol to retinopathy and hard exudates. *Ophthalmology* **98**: 1261–1265.

Komatsu H, Amano M, Yamaguchi S, Sugahara K. (1999) Inhibition of activation of human peripheral blood eosinophils by Y-24180 an antagonist to platelet activating factor receptor. *Life Sci* **65**: PL171–PL176.

Kordonouri O, Danne T, Hopfenmuller W, *et al.* (1996) Lipid profiles and blood pressure: Are they risk factors for the development of early background retinopathy and incipient nephropathy in children with insulin-dependent diabetes mellitus? *Acta Paediatr* **85**: 43–48.

Koya D, King GL. (1998) Protein kinase C activation and the development of diabetic complications. *Diabetes* **47**: 859–866.

Kowluru RA, Kern TS, Engerman RL, Armstrong D. (1996) Abnormalities of retinal metabolism in diabetes or experimental galactosemia. III. Effects of antioxidants. *Diabetes* **45**: 1233–1237.

Kubes P, Suzuki M, Granger DN. (1991) Nitric oxide: An endogenous modulator of leucocytes adhesion. *Proc Natl Acad Sci USA* **88**: 4651–4655.

Kurose I, Anderson DC, Miyasaka M, *et al.* (1994) Molecular determinants of reperfusion-induced leuco-cytes adhesion and vascular protein leakage. *Cir Res* **74**: 336–343.

Le Good JA, Ziegler WH, Parekh DB, *et al.* (1998) Protein kinase C isoptypes controlled by phosphoinositide 3-kinase through the protein kinase PDK1. *Science* **281**: 2042–2045.

Leite EB, Mota MC, de Abreu JR, Cunha-Vaz JG. (1990) Effect of calcium dobesilate on the blood-retinal barrier in early diabetic retinopathy. *Int Ophthalmol* **14**: 81–88.

Losada M, Alio LJ. (1996) Melondialdehyde serum concentration in type 1 diabetes with and without retinopathy. *Doc Ophthalmol* **93**: 223–229.

Lundbaek K, Malmros R, Anderson HC. (1989) Hypophisectomy for diabetic retinopathy: A controlled clinical trial. In: Golberg MF, Fine SL (eds.), *Symposium on the Treatment of Diabetic Retinopathy*. Public Health Service Pub, Washington DC.

Lutty GA, Cao J, McLeod DS. (1997) Relationship of polymorphonuclear leukocytes to capillary drop-out in the human diabetic choroids. *Am J Patol* **151**: 707–714.

Macugern Diabetic Retinopathy Study Group. (2005) A phase II Randomized Double-Masked Trial of Pegaptanib and Anti-Vascular Endothelial Growth Factor Aptamer, for Diabetic Macular Edema. *Ophthalmology* **112**: 1747–1757.

Martidis A, Duker JS, Greenberg PB, *et al.* (2002) Intravitreal triamcinolone for refractory diabetic macular edema. *Ophthalmology* **109**: 920–927.

Massin A, Audren F, Haouchine B, *et al.* (2004) Intravitreal triamcinolone acetinide for diabetic diffuse macular edema. Preliminary results of a prospective controlled trial. *Ophthalmology* **111**: 218–225.

McLeod DS, Lefer DJ, Merges C, Lutty GA. (1995) Enhanced expression of intercellular adhesion molecule-1 and p-selectin in the diabetic human retina and choroid. *Am J Pathol* **147**: 642–653.

McMillan DE. (1978) Rheological and related factors in diabetic retinopathy. In: Kohner EM (ed.), *Diabetic Retinopathy*. International Ophthalmology Clinics, Vol. 18, Little, Brown & Co Boston, pp. 35–53.

Merimee TJ, Zapf J, Froesch ER. (1993) Insulin-like growth factors: Studies in diabetics with and without retinopathy. *N Engl J Med* **309**: 527–530.

Miyamoto K, Ogura Y, Kenmochi S, Honda Y. (1997) Role of leucocytes in diabetic microcirculatory disturbances. *Microvasc Res* **54**: 43–48.

Miyamoto K, Khosrof S, Bursell S-E, *et al.* (1999) Prevention of leukostasis and vascular leakage in streptozotocin-induced diabetic retinopathy via intercellular adhesion molecule-1 inhibition. *Proc Natl Acad Sci* **96**: 10836–10841.

Monnier VM, Bautista O, Kenny D, *et al.* (1999) Skin collagen glycation, glycoxidation, and crosslinking are lower in subjects with long-term intensive versus conventional therapy of type 1 diabetes relevance of glycate collagen products versus $HbA_{1C}$ as marker of diabetic complications. *Diabetes* **48**: 870–880.

Moreno A, De La Cruz JP, Campos JG, De la Cuesta FS. (1995) Prostacyclin-thromboxane balance and retinal vascular pattern in rats with experimental induced diabetes. *Can J Ophthalmol* **30**: 117–123.

Mori K, Duh E, Gehlbach P, *et al.* (2001) Pigment epithelium-derived factor inhibits retinal and choroidal neovascularization. *J Cell Physiol* **188**: 253–263.

Mota MC, Leite E, Ruas MA, *et al.* (1987) Effect of cyclospasmol on early diabetic retinopathy. *Intern Ophthalmol* **10**: 3–9.

Nawroth PP, Stern D, Bierhaus A, *et al.* (1992). AGE-Albumin Stimulierte Endothelzelten-ein *in-vitro* Modell diabetischer spätschäden. *Diabetes Stoffwechs* **1** (Suppl. 1): 153A.

O'Brien RC, Kuo M, Balazs N, Mercuri J. (2000) *In vitro* and *in vivo* antioxidant properties of glicazide. *J Diabetes Complicat* **14**: 201–206.

Ohkubo Y, Kishikawa H, Araki E, *et al.* (1995) Intensive insulin therapy prevents the progression of diabetic microvascular complications in Japanese patients with non-insulin-dependent diabetes mellitus: A randomized prospective 6-year study. *Diabetes Res Clin Pract* **28**: 103–117.

Pagani A, Greco G, Tagliaferro V, *et al.* (1989) Dipyridamole administration in insulin-dependent diabetics with background retinopathy: A 36 month follow-up. *Curr Ther Res* **45**: 409–415.

Parving HH, Larsen M, Hommel E, Lund-Andersen H. (1989) Effect of antihypertensive treatment on blood-retinal barrier permeability to fluorescein in hypertensive type 1 (insulin-dependent) diabetic patients with background retinopathy. *Diabetologia* **32**: 440–444.

Pfeifer MA, Shumer MP, Gelber DA. (1997) Aldose reductase inhibitors: The end of an era or the need for different trial designs? *Diabetes* **46**(2): S82–S89.

Pomero F, Allione A, Beltramo E, *et al.* (2003) Effects of protein kinase C inhibition and activation on proliferation and apoptose of bovine retinal pericytes. *Diabetologia* **46**: 416–419.

Poulsen JE. (1953) Recovery from retinopathy in a case of diabetes with Simmonds' disease. *Diabetes* **2**: 7–12.

Qiao Q, Keinanen-Kiukaanniemi S, Laara E. (1997) The relation between hemoglobin levels and diabetic retinopathy. *J Clin Epidemiol* **50**: 153–158.

Quam T, Xu Q, Joussen AM, *et al.* (2001) VEGF-initiated blood-retinal barrier breakdown in early diabetes. *Invest Ophthalmol Vis Sci* **42**(10): 2408–2413.

Robison GS, Pierce EA, Rook SL, *et al.* (1996) Oligodenoxynucleotides inhibit retinal neovascularization in a murine model of proliferative retinopathy. *Proc Natl Acad Sci USA* **93**: 4851–4856.

Robinson WG Jr, Laver NM, Jacot JL, *et al.* (1996) Diabetic-like retinopathy ameliorate with the aldose reductase inhibitor WAY-121, 509. *Invest Ophthalmol Vis Sci* **37**: 1149–1156.

Rosen LS. (2002) Clinical experiences with angiogenesis signalling inhibitors; focus on vascular endothelial growth factor (VEGF) blockers. *Cancer Control* 9(2): 36–44.

Sagel J, Colwell JA, Crook L, Laimins M. (1975) Increased platelet aggregation in early diabetes mellitus. *Ann Intern Med* **82**: 733–738.

Sato Y, Hotta N, Sakamoto N, *et al.* (1979) Lipid peroxide level in plasma of diabetic patients. *Bioch Med* **21**: 104–107.

Sato Y, Lee Z, Hayashi Y. (2001) Subclassification of pre-proliferative diabetic retinopathy and glycemic control: Relationship between mean hemoglobin $A_{1C}$ value and development of proliferative diabetic retinopathy. *Jp J Ophthalmol* **45**: 523–527.

Schmid-Schonbein H, Volger E. (1976) Red cell aggregation and red cell-deformability in diabetes. *Diabetes* **25**: 897–902.

Schröder S, Palinski W, Schmid-Schonbein GW. (1991) Activated monocytes and granulocytes, capillary non-perfusion, and neovascularization in diabetic retinopathy. *Am J Pathopl* **139**: 81–100.

Schweiki D, Itin A, Soffer D, Keshet E. (1992) Vascular endothelial growth factor induced by hypoxia may mediate hypoxia-initiated angiogenesis. *Nature* **359**: 843–845.

Sem K, Misra A, Kumar A, Pandey RM. (2002) Simvastatin retards progression of retinopathy in diabetic patients with hypercholesterolemia. *Diabetes Res Clin Pract* **56**: 1–11.

Shiba T, Inoguci T, Sportsman R, *et al.* (1993) Correlation of diacylglycerol level and protein kinase C activity in rat retina to retinal circulation. *Am J Physiol* **265**: E783–E793.

Shorb S. (1985) Anemia and diabetic retinopathy. *Am J Ophthalmol* **100**: 434–436.

Siemeister G, Schirner M, Reusch P, *et al.* (1998) An antagonistic vascular endothelial growth factor (VEGF) variant inhibits VEGF-stimulated receptor autophosphorylation and proliferation of human endothelial cells. *Proc Natl Acad Sci* **95**: 4625–4629.

Smith LEH, Kopchick JJ, Chen W, *et al.* (1997) Essential role of growth hormone in ischemia-induced retinal neovascularization. *Science* **27**(6): 1706–1709.

Sonkin PL, Sinclair SH, Hatchell DL. (1993) Pentoxifylline improves retinal capillary flow velocity and whole blood viscosity. *Am J Ophthalmol* **115**: 775–780.

Sonkin PL, Kelly LW, Sinclair SH, Hatchell DL. (1993) Pentoxifylline increase retinal capillary flow velocity in patients with diabetes. *Arch Ophthalmol* **111**: 1647–1652.

Sonksen PH, Russel-Jones D, Jones RH. (1993) Growth hormone and diabetes mellitus: A review of sixty-three years of medical research and a glimpse into the future? *Hom Res* **40**: 68–79.

Sorbinil Retinopathy Trial Research Group. (1990) A randomised trial of sorbinil, an aldose reductase inhibitor, in diabetic retinopathy. *Arch Ophthalmol* **108**: 1234–1244.

Spirin KS, Saghizadeh M, Lewin SL, *et al.* (1999) Basement membrane and growth factor gene expression in normal and diabetic human retinas. *Curr Eye Res* **18**: 490–499.

Stavri GT, Zachary IC, Baskerville PA, *et al.* (1995) Basic fibroblast growth factor in vascular smooth muscle cells. Synergistic interaction with hypoxia. *Circulation* **92**: 11–14.

Stellmach V, Crawford SE, Zhou W, Bouck N. (2001) Prevention of ischemia-induced retinopathy by the natural ocular antiangiogenic agent pigment epithelium-derived factor. *Proc Natl Acad Sci USA* **98**: 2593–2597.

Stevens MJ, Dananberg J, Feldman EL, *et al.* (1994) The linked roles of nitric oxide, aldose reductase and (Na$^+$, K$^{+-}$) ATPase in the slowing of nerve conduction in the streptozoptocin diabetic rat. *J Clin Invest* **94**: 853–859.

Sinclair SH, DelVecchio C, Levin A. (2003) Treatment of anemia in the diabetic patient with retinopathy and kidney disease. *Am J Ophthalmol* **135**: 740–743.

Stitt A, Gardiner TA, Alderson NL, *et al.* (2002) The AGE inhibitor piridoxamine inhibits development of retinopathy in experimental diabetes. *Diabetes* **51**: 2826–2832.

Sundkvist G, Lilia B, Almer LO. (1988) Absent elevations in growth hormone, factor VIII elevated antigen and plasminogen activation during exercise in diabetic patients resistant to retinopathy. *Diabetes Res* **7**: 25–30.

Sweadner KJ, Godlin SM. (1980) Active transport of sodium and potassium ions: Mechanism, function and regulation. *N Engl J Med* **302**: 777–783.

Tadesse M, Yan Y, Yossuck P, Higgins RD. (2001) Captopril improves retinal neovascularization via endothelin 1. *Invest Ophthalmol Vis Sci* **42**: 1867–1872.

Takagi C, King GL, Hotoshi T, *et al.* (1996) Endothelin-1 action via receptors in a primary mechanism modulating retinal circulatory response of hypoxia. *Invest Ophthalmol Vis Sci* **37**: 2099–2109.

Tejerina T, Ruiz E, Sanz M, Ganado P. (1999) Study of calcium dobesilate in diabetic rats. *Int J Angiol* **8**: 16–20.

The DAMAD Study Group. (1989) Effect of aspirin alone and aspirin plus dipyramidole in early diabetic retinopathy. A multicentric randomised controlled clinical trial. *Diabetes* **38**: 491–498.

The DCCT Research Group. (1993) The effect of intensive treatment of diabetes on the development and progression of long-term complications in insulin-dependent diabetes mellitus. *N Engl J Med* **329**: 977–986.

The DCCT Research Group. (1995) Progression of retinopathy with intensive versus conventional treatment in the diabetes Control and Complications Trial. *Ophthalmology* **102**: 647–661.

The DCCT Research Group. (1998) Early worsening of diabetic retinopathy in the diabetes Control and Complications Trial. *Arch Ophthalmol* **116**: 874–886.

The DCCT/EDIC Research Group. (2000) Retinopathy and nephropathy in patients with type 1 diabetes four years after a trial of intensive therapy. *N Engl J Med* **342**: 381–389.

The ETDRS Study Group. (1991) Effects of aspirin treatment on diabetic retinopathy. ETDRS report number 8. *Ophthalmology* **98**(5): 757–765.

The Lancet Editorial. (1997) A curious stopping rule from Hoechst Marion Russel. *The Lancet* **350**: 155.

The Sixth Report of the Joint National Committee on Prevention, Detection, Evaluation and Treatment of High Blood Pressure. (1997) *Arch Intern Med* **157**: 2413–2446.

The TIMAD Study Group. (1990) Ticlopidine treatment reduces the progression of nonproliferative diabetic retinopathy. *Arch Ophthalmol* **108**: 1577–1583.

Thornalley PJ, Wolff SP, Crabe MJ, Stern A. (1984) The oxidation of oxyhemoglobin by glyceraldehyde and other simple monosaccharides. *Biochem J* **217**: 615–622.

Tilton RG, Chang K, Hasan KS, *et al.* (1993) Prevention of diabetic vascular dysfunction by guanidines: Inhibition of nitric oxide synthase versus advanced glycation end-product formation. *Diabetes* **42**: 221–232.

Tolentino MJ, Miller JW, Gragoudas ES, *et al.* (1996) Intravitreous injection of vascular endothelial growth factor produce retinal ischemia and microangiopathy in adult primate. *Ophthalmol* **103**: 1820–1828.

Tolentino MJ, Miller JW, Gragoudas ES, *et al.* (1996) Vascular endothelial growth factor is sufficient to produce iris neovascularization and neovascular glaucoma in nonhuman primate. *Arch Ophthalmol* **114**: 964–970.

Tolentino MJ, McLeod DS, Taomoto M, *et al.* (2002) Pathologic features of vascular endothelial growth factor-induced retinopathy in the nonhuman primate. *Arch Ophthalmol* **133**: 373–385.

Triggiani M, Oriente A, Golino P, *et al.* (1999) Inhibition of platelet-activating factor synthesis in human neutrophils and platelets by propionyl-L-carnitine. *Biochem Pharmacol* **58**: 1341–1348.

UK Prospective Diabetes Study Group. (1998) Intensive blood-glucose control with sulphonyureas or insulin compared with conventional treatment and the risk of complications in patients with type 2 diabetes (UKPDS 33) *Lancet* **352**: 837–853.

UK Prospective Diabetes Study Group. (1998a) Intensive blood-glucose control with metformin on complications in overweight patients wit type 2 diabetes (UKPDS 34) *Lancet* **352**: 854–865.

UK Prospective Diabetes Study Group. (1998b) Tight blood-glucose control and risk of macrovascular and microvascular complications in type 2 diabetes (UKPDS 38) *BMJ* **317**: 703–713.

UK Prospective Diabetes Study Group. (1998c) Efficacy of atenolol and captopril in reducing the risk of macrovascular and microvascular complications in type 2 diabetes (UKPDS 39) *BMJ* **317**: 713–720.

Uzel N, Sivas A, Uysal M, Oz H. (1987) Erythrocyte lipid peroxidation and glyutathione peroxidase activities in patients with diabetes mellitus. *Horm Metab Res* **19**: 89–90.

Vasan S, Zhang X, Zhang X, *et al.* (1996) An agent cleaving glucose-derived protein crosslinks *in vitro* and *in vivo*. *Nature* **382**: 275–278.

Verdejo C, Marco P, Renau-Piqueras J, Pinazo-Duran MD. (1999) Lipid peroxidation in proliferative vitreoretinopathies. *Eye* **13**: 183–188.

Vlassara H. (1997) Recent progress in advanced glycation end products and diabetic complications. *Diabetes* **46**(l): S19–S25.

Watanabe J, Umeda F, Wakasugi H, Ibayashi H. (1984) Effect of vitamin E on platelet aggregation in diabetes mellitus. *Thromb Haemost* **51**: 313–316.

Williams LT. (1989) Signal transduction by platelet-derived growth factor receptor. *Science* **243**: 1564–1570.

Williamson JR, Chang K, Frangos M, *et al.* (1993) Prespectives in Diabetes. Hyperglycaemic pseudohypoxia and diabetes complications. *Diabetes* **42**: 801–813.

Williamson JR, Chang K, Frangos M, *et al.* (1997) Prespectives in Diabetes. Hyperglycaemic pseudohypoxia and diabetes complications. *Diabetes* **46**: S19–S25.

Winkler AS, Mardsen J, Chauduria KR, *et al.* (1999) Erythropoietin depletion and anaemia in diabetes mellitus. *Diabetic Med* **16**: 813–819.

Xia P, Inoguchi T, Kern TS, *et al.* (1994) Characterization of the mechanism for the chronic activation of diacylglycerol-protein kinase C pathway in diabetes and hypergalactosemia. *Diabetes* **43**: 1122–1129.

Yamagishi S, Yonekura H, Yamamoto Y, *et al.* (1997) Advanced glycation end products-driven angiogenesis *in vitro*. Induction of the growth and tube formation of human microvascular endothelial cells through autocrine vascular endothelial growth factor. *J Biol Chem* **272**: 8723–8730.

# Chapter 10

# An Integrated Perspective on Diabetic Retinopathy in Type 2 Diabetes

## José Cunha-Vaz

The natural history of the initial lesions occurring in the diabetic retina has particular relevance for our understanding and management of diabetic retinal disease, one of the major causes of vision loss in the Western world.

Four main alterations characterize the initial stages of diabetic retinopathy: the appearance of microaneurysms/hemorrhages, alteration of the Blood-Retinal Barrier demonstrated by fluorescein leakage, capillary closure and alterations in the neuronal and glial cells of the retina. These alterations may be monitored by a variety of methods, namely, fundus images, fluorescein angiography, fluorescein leakage and retinal thickness measurements and psicophysical and electrophysiological tests.

A combination of these methods using Multimodal Imaging of the Macula has contributed by identifying three different phenotypes of diabetic retinopathy. They show different types and rates of progression independent of levels of metabolic control, which suggest the involvement of different susceptibility genes. The identification of different phenotypes opens the door for genotype characterization, different management strategies and targeted treatments. Characterization of risk profiles and risk markers is a fundamental step for improved management of the disease.

A new paradigm of diabetic retinopathy management is developing. Diabetic retinopathy must be detected and diagnosed earlier and treatment must commence earlier. The ultimate goal should not be merely to prevent blindness, but to help patients enjoy their lives to the fullest potential and to provide a clearer indication of when more active treatment, either systemic or local or both, is justified.

Diabetic retinopathy is a chronic retinal disorder that eventually develops, to some degree, in nearly all patients with diabetes mellitus. Diabetic retinopathy is characterized by gradually progressive alterations in the retinal microvasculature and is the leading cause of new cases of legal blindness among Americans between the ages of 20 and 74 years of age (Aiello *et al.*, 1998).

Diabetic retinopathy occurs in both type 1 (also known as juvenile-onset or insulin-dependent diabetes) and type 2 (also known as adult-onset or non-insulin-dependent diabetes) diabetes. All the features of diabetic retinopathy may be found in both types of diabetes but the incidence of the main causes of vision loss, macular edema and retinal neovascularization, is different for each type of diabetes (Aiello *et al.*, 1998).

Diabetic retinopathy in type 1 diabetes induces vision loss mainly due to the formation of new vessels in the eye fundus and development of proliferative retinopathy, whereas in type 2 diabetes vision loss is most commonly due to macular edema and proliferative retinopathy is relatively rare.

It is apparent, from the data available from a variety of large longitudinal studies and from clinical experience, that the evolution and progression of diabetic retinopathy vary, not only according to the types of diabetes involved, but showing dissimilarities among different patients even when belonging to the same type of diabetes and does not necessarily progress in every patient to the terminal stage of proliferative retinopathy.

There is accumulated evidence indicating that only the nonproliferative stage of DR is directly due to the systemic disease and associated hyperglycemia and other metabolic alterations. Proliferative retinopathy occurs in diabetic eyes only after the development of widespread ischemia due to capillary closure. Neovessels in the retina are a direct result of retinal ischemia and when present their evolution is beyond the influence of diabetic metabolic control. Its course and management is not different from other clinical situations in the retina where there is abnormal new vessel formation. Retinal neovascularization is a natural consequence of retinal ischemia. Diabetes causes retinal changes, involving primarily the retinal blood vessels and the progression of these changes lead in many cases to intense and widespread capillary closure and retinal ischemia. When this occurs neovascularization and proliferative retinopathy develops.

Following closely these concepts we can state that in diabetes a retinopathy develops that ultimately may result in extensive retinal ischemia. When that occurs, and independently of diabetic metabolic control, neovascularization may, in turn, develop. Proliferative retinopathy is really a complication of diabetic retinopathy as much as retinal detachment occurs as a complication of proliferative retinopathy. Both occur independently of the course of the systemic diabetic disease and are not influenced by changes in metabolic control.

We will, therefore, attempt to characterize background diabetic retinopathy, i.e. the alterations occurring in the retina as a direct result of the systemic diabetic disease. In this way, diabetic retinopathy includes only the preclinical and nonproliferative stages of diabetic retinopathy.

## 10.1. Limitations of Present Classifications of Nonproliferative Diabetic Retinopathy

There have been many attempts to classify the lesions observed in the retina in diabetes. The first such classification that resulted from consensus and was accepted internationally was the Airlie House Classification.

The Airlie House Classification was developed by a 12-member committee during a Symposium on the Treatment of Diabetic Retinopathy held at Airlie House in Warrington, VA, in September 1968 (Goldberg and Fine, 1969). The goal of its authors was to provide a simple scheme for expressing the presence and severity of the fundus lesions commonly seen in this disorder that were suitable for ophthalmoscopy or fundus photography.

Like most other classifications of diabetic retinopathy, the Early Treatment Diabetic Retinopathy Study (ETDRS) (Early Treatment Diabetic Retinopathy Study Research Group, 1991) modification of the Airlie House Classification is limited to assessing the severity and/or extent of various characteristic abnormalities but does not provide an overall severity scale and has been tested solely for evaluation of progression to proliferative diabetic retinopathy.

In the Diabetic Retinopathy Study (DRS) (Diabetic Retinopathy Study Research Group, 1981), a useful definition was proposed for only one part of the picture, the severe stage of nonproliferative diabetic retinopathy (NPDR). In this definition, which was based on clinical impression and quantitative clinical descriptions, four abnormalities were considered: hemorrhages and/or microaneurysms, cotton-wool spots (soft exudates), intraretinal microvascular abnormalities (IRMA's) and venous beading. Additional DRS analyses demonstrated that hemorrhages and/or microaneurysms and venous beading were the more powerful predictors of visual loss.

The ETDRS adopted the DRS definitions of severe NPDR and contributed by defining moderate NPDR in a more detailed scale. It is interesting that these scales and classifications were all based in a variety of complex statistical analyses all focused on the percentage of eyes with progression to proliferative diabetic retinopathy. The ETDRS-based classification of severity and progression of diabetic retinopathy is entirely based on the assumption that the retinopathy is homogeneous in every diabetic patient and will ultimately progress to proliferative retinopathy. Detailed information constructed on the segment of the final scale dealing with mild-to-severe NPDR is related to 1-, 3- and 5-year rates of development proliferative diabetic retinopathy.

The ETDRS research group in their Report number 12 clearly states that "because few eyes were included in the ETDRS that had very mild retinopathy the definitions of the final scale regarding the lower range of NPDR could not be examined" (Early Treatment Diabetic Retinopathy Study Research Group, 1991). For example, it could not determine whether presence of mild retinal hemorrhages in addition to microaneurysms was sufficiently less severe than the presence of hard or soft exudates to merit designation of separate levels for these two groups (i.e. division of level 35 into two parts).

The available classifications of diabetic retinopathy give very useful information but have two major problems.

One is the lack of information on the mild stage of the disease, which is clearly the most interesting stage because it is the one that shows some degree of reversibility and may respond to improved medical treatment or new forms of treatment.

The second is the fact that the ETDRS classification, which is considered the reference classification, was constructed on the basis that diabetic retinopathy, given time, uniformly progresses to proliferative retinopathy. It assumes that retinal neovascularization and proliferative retinopathy are consequences of the diabetic metabolic syndrome. There are, on the contrary, many arguments to support the thesis that proliferative retinopathy occurs in diabetes as a result of

the extensive capillary closure and ischemia and is, in itself, relatively independent of the diabetic general metabolic status (Cunha-Vaz, 1978).

One classification has been proposed recently in an effort to simplify the ETDRS final scale (Wilkinson *et al.*, 2003). Its main goal has been to establish references for large clinical studies and to facilitate more uniform clinical follow-up of diabetic retinopathy. It does not address the need for more detailed characterization of initial stages of diabetic retinal disease and does not bring any added value if the quest is for improved understanding and management of diabetic retinal disease.

## 10.2.  Natural History of the Initial Stages of NPDR

The fundus abnormalities that are identified on clinical examination of mild to moderate NPDR include microaneurysms and/or hemorrhages, i.e. which appear as small red-dots in the fundus images and exudates.

The initial stages of NPDR are, therefore, characterized by the presence of red-dots (microaneurysms and/or hemorrhages) and indirect signs of vascular hypermeability and capillary closure, i.e. both hard and soft exudates or cotton-wool spots, respectively.

These are the alterations that dominate the initial stages of NPDR and are the only ones used for characterization of levels 15 and 20 of ETDRS classifications. We will analyze their development and progression, in order to clarify their relative importance in the progression of diabetic retinopathy. It is recognized that they are not present in every patient in the same way nor do they form or disappear at the same rate in every patient.

It is particularly important to realize that the course and rates of progression of the retinopathy vary between patients. Microaneurysms, for example, may come and go. Once you get a microaneurysm you do not necessarily continue to have that microaneurysm. Microaneurysms may disappear due to vessel closure, which is an indication of worsening of the retinopathy because of progressive vascular closure (Cunha-Vaz, 1992). Hemorrhages will obviously come and go as the body heals them. Clinical improvement may be apparent but in reality may mask the worsening of the disease.

The initial pathological changes occurring in the diabetic retina are characteristically located in the small retinal vessels of the posterior pole of the retina, that is, in the macular area. The structural changes in the small vessels include endothelial cell and pericyte damage and thickening of basement membrane (Cunha-Vaz, 1978).

Normally, retinal vascular endothelium is a fundamental part of the blood-retinal barrier (BRB), which has many similarities with the Blood-Brain Barrier. It functions as a selective barrier, which has shown to be altered in experimental and human diabetes (Cunha-Vaz *et al.*, 1975).

Pericyte damage has been reported as one of the earliest findings in diabetic retinal disease since the introduction of retinal digest studies (Cogan and Kwabara, 1963). However, pericyte apoptosis is more readily detectable than endothelial cell apoptosis, most probably because the pericytes are encased in basement membrane and thus, less accessible to clearing mechanisms, whereas apoptotic endothelial cells slough off into the capillary lumen and are cleared by blood flow.

The simplest paradigm that explains capillary permeability and closure centers on the vascular endothelium. In the retina endothelial cells are the site of the BRB, a specific blood-tissue barrier, and, as in all vessels, provide a nonthrombogenic surface for blood flow. Both these properties are eventually compromised by diabetes.

On the other hand, diabetes also affects the neural and glial cells of the retina. Consequently, we have an initial pathological picture characterized by endothelial and pericyte alterations associated with basement membrane thickening and microaneurysm formation. These alterations are characteristic for the retina, particularly the alteration of the BRB, the pericyte damage and the microaneurysm formation, but occur in a variety of diseases unrelated to diabetes. There is clear site specificity, not disease specificity (Cunha-Vaz, 1978).

Which are then the features of the retinal circulation, which are specific to the retina and may be responsible for the site specificity of diabetic retinopathy? They are the BRB and the autoregulation of retinal blood flow. Both serve the needs of the neuronal and glial cells of the retina, by protecting the retinal tissue to drastic changes in the retinal circulation and nutrition.

An abnormality of the BRB, demonstrated both by vitreous fluorometry and fluorescein angiography is an early finding both in human and experimental diabetes (Cunha-Vaz *et al.*, 1975; Waltman *et al.*, 1978a, b).

Fluorescein leakage demonstrating the alteration of the BRB is one of the earliest findings in diabetic retinal disease. It appears to lead directly to macular edema, which remains the most frequent cause of vision loss in diabetes.

Another important characteristic of the retinal circulation is its capacity to autoregulate and compensate variations in blood pressure, ocular tension, etc., maintaining a relatively uniform blood flow. Changes in retinal blood flow have, indeed, been reported in both human and experimental diabetes (Kohner, 1977).

Altered autoregulation and progressively decreased retinal blood flow associated with retinal vascular alterations (endothelial cells and pericytes) facilitate development of progressive capillary closure, an hallmark of progression of diabetic retinal disease. Finally, capillary closure leads to retinal ischemia, which creates the conditions for the development of the most dreaded complications of proliferative retinopathy. This complication, proliferative retinopathy, leads to the most tragic outcomes for visual loss: vitreous hemorrhage, rubeosis iridis, retinal detachment, etc. It is now generally accepted that at least three processes can contribute to retinal capillary occlusion and obliteration in diabetes: proinflammatory changes, microthrombosis and apoptosis

(Gardner and Aiello, 2000). These processes have been documented in both human and experimental diabetes. There are indications taken from experimental studies that proinflammatory changes and leukostasis may be important triggering events and that microthrombosis and apoptosis occur subsequently.

## 10.3.  Markers of Diabetic Retinal Disease

The major problems in early detection and development of new forms of medical treatment lie in the limitations that characterize the accepted methods of retinopathy assessment, which are based on poorly sensitive methods, such as visual acuity changes and fundus photography. There is a clear need to discuss the accepted clinical endpoints, which are used to evaluate the progression of diabetic retinopathy.

The problems are many and the controversy remains. The course of retinopathy is not linear and we do not know to predict progression of diabetic retinopathy step by step. The risk factors appear to be different in different stages of retinopathy. For instance, it is not accepted by everyone that capillary closure leading to retinal tissue ischemia is the main factor causing proliferative retinopathy.

The clinical signs are not constant. Microaneurysms, for example, may come and go. Once you get a microaneurysm you do not necessarily continue to have that microaneurysm. It may disappear due to vessel closure, which is an indication of worsening of the retinopathy because of progressive vascular closure. Hemorrhages obviously will come and go as the body heals them. Apparent clinical improvement may be apparent and in reality mask worsening of the disease.

A prominent feature of diabetic retinopathy, diabetic macular edema, can spontaneously resolve. Indeed, approximately a third of patients have it resolved in a period of six months without any intervention.

It must be realized at this point that fundus photography is still widely considered as the method of choice to follow diabetic retinopathy, although it is not capable of demonstrating the main indicators of progression of diabetic retinopathy, capillary closure and fluorescein leakage. Capillary closure leading to retinal ischemia and inducing neovascularization and proliferative retinopathy, a stage of the disease that is characteristically associated with the most tragic outcomes for visual loss: vitreous hemorrhage, rubeosis iridis and retinal detachment. Fluorescein leakage is an indicator of breakdown of the blood-retinal barrier, which leads to macular edema, the most frequent cause of visual loss in diabetes and the reason for 78% of all photocoagulation treatments performed for diabetic retinopathy.

With all these limitations and shortcomings, we have a picture characterized by the need to define what is clinically important and which are the generally accepted meaningful clinical endpoints, and, finally, the real challenge of identifying the surrogate endpoints that may demonstrate efficacy of a drug in realistic and feasible period of time.

### 10.3.1.  Microaneurysms/Hemorrhages. Red-dots Formation and Disappearance Rates

Microaneurysms (MA) and hemorrhages (HEM) identified as red-dots are the initial changes seen on ophthalmoscopic examination and fundus photography. They may be counted and red-dot counting has been suggested as an appropriate marker of retinopathy progression (Klein *et al.*, 1995a, b).

It must be realized that red-dot formation and disappearance are dynamic processes. During a 2-year follow-up of 24 type 1 diabetics with mild background diabetic retinopathy using fluorescein angiography, Hellstedt and Immonen (1996) observed 395 new MA and the disappearance of 258 previously identified.

Generally, the disappearance of a MA is not a reversible process and indicates vessel closure and progressive vascular damage. Therefore, to assess progression of retinopathy, red-dot counting should take into account every newly developed red-dot identified in a new location.

We have developed proprietary software for assisted red-dot counting in fundus-digitized images where the location of each red-dot is taken into account and registered. In this way, in a follow-up study with repeated fundus images obtained at regular intervals, all red-dots in the fundus were counted and added as they became visible in new locations in the retina. The results of red-dot counting using this method, in a 2-year follow-up study of a series of eyes with mild nonproliferative retinopathy in subjects with type 2 diabetes maintaining a stable metabolic control during the period of the study suggest that red-dot counting may be a good marker of disease progression in the initial stages of NPDR (Torrent-Solans *et al.*, 2004).

Fifty eyes from 50 patients with type 2 diabetes mellitus and mild nonproliferative retinopathy were prospectively followed. These were consecutive patients that fulfilled the inclusion criteria. Treated with oral hypoglycemic agents, they maintained a stable metabolic control.

One selection criterion was the presence of at least one red-dot at the first visit in field 2 of the 7-field stereo fundus photography assessed by two independent readers.

Fundus photographs were taken every six months. Field 2 (centered in the macula) was chosen for the analysis of the presence of red-dots since this is the most important area in terms of potential visual impairment.

In order to improve human grader reliability in the identification and counting of red-dots on color fundus images, the software included algorithms for eye movement compensation, color correction and identification of each red-dot by its coordinates.

Using the software's ability to identify each red-dot as a single entity in a specific location with identifiable coordinates, the following parameters were assessed:

1. Cumulative number of red-dots. This number is achieved using the main advantage of the new software, its ability to consider each red-dot as a single entity, identified by its specific location. Therefore, a red-dot identified on a new location is recognized as a new red-dot and added.

2. Red-dot formation rate. Red-dot formation rate is the annual rate of change over the study period. It is computed dividing the difference of the cumulative number of red-dots between the last and first visits by the years of follow-up.

3. Red-dot disappearance rate. Red-dot disappearance rate is the sum of the red-dots that disappeared during the study period divided by the number of years of follow-up. A disappeared red-dot is one missing red-dot from a previous visit that will not show up again (during the study period).

Using the traditional procedure, the total amount of red-dots detected at every visit remained stable. However, the cumulative number of red-dots raised from 115 at the first visit to 505 at the last visit, showing a marked increase in new red-dots. These figures emerged because of the software's potential for counting every red-dot as a single entity once it was identified by its specific location. It is now obvious that there were many more new red-dots in the fundus, i.e. microaneurysms and small hemorrhages, in this 2-year time period than expected using data for each examination separately.

One of the advantages of the Retmaker used is the ability to count the number of real new red-dots appearing at every visit (red-dot formation rate). The rate of formation (red-dots/year) ranged from 0 to 22. The results showed that eyes in the same retinopathy stage from different patients show very different red-dot formation rates. Values for red-dot formation rate higher than 3/year at this stage of mild NPDR correlated well with increased fluorescein leakage measured by vitreous fluorometry ($p < 0.001$) and capillary closure identified by a damaged foveal avascular zone (FAZ) ($p > 0.038$).

The red-dot disappearance rate (red-dots per year) ranged from 0 to 16. Red-dot disappearance rates also varied quite markedly in eyes from different patients and showed similar correlations.

In a recently developed International Clinical Diabetic Retinopathy Disease Severity Scale, developed under the auspices of the American Academy of Ophthalmology, the identification of microaneurysms and hemorrhages are indicated as the only alterations that are present in the initial mild stage of diabetic retinopathy (Wilkinson *et al.*, 2003).

Microaneurysms and hemorrhages identified by fundus photography as red-dots are considered the first clinical sign of retinopathy. Microaneurysm formation has been associated with localized proliferation of endothelial cells, loss of pericytes and alterations of the capillary basement membrane, alterations that occur in the initial stages of diabetic retinal disease and have been considered to be directly involved in its pathophysiology (Ashton, 1963, 1974; Cunha-Vaz, 1978).

Microaneurysm closure and disappearance is most probably due to thrombotic phenomena leading to subsequent rerouting of capillary blood flow and progressive remodeling of the retinal vasculature in diabetes (Boeri *et al.*, 2001). These thrombotic changes are probably enhanced by changes in the red and white cells occurring as a result of diabetes. The presence and number of microaneurysms and their rates of formation and disappearance are, therefore, good candidates as markers of retinal vascular remodeling and may be good indicators of retinopathy progression.

Red-dot counting on fundus photographies and microaneurysm counting on fluorescein angiography have been proposed as predictive indicators for progression of diabetic retinopathy (Kohner *et al.*, 1986). Our specially developed software allows the identification of the exact location of each red-dot in successive fundus photographs performed in each eye. Identification of the exact location of an individual red-dot is considered particularly important, because a new microaneurysm is considered to develop only once in a specific location, its disappearance being generally associated with capillary closure, leaving in its place mainly remnants of basement membrane (Ashton, 1974; Cunha-Vaz, 1978).

Our study demonstrated a steady turnover of red-dots in the diabetic retina, even in the initial stages of retinopathy. In fact, most red-dots show a lifetime of less than one year, with new ones being formed and disappearing at rates, which vary between different patients, confirming previous reports (Kohner and Dollery, 1970).

Most interestingly, however, is the observation that some patients show much higher rates of red-dot formation and disappearance, suggesting that they may represent specific phenotypes of diabetic retinopathy. These eyes showed also faster progression in other retinal lesions, with increased fluorescein leakage, i.e. alterations of BRB and progression in capillary closure.

Our group has shown that microaneurysm formation and disappearance rates (microaneurysm turnover) obtained from color fundus photographs using proprietary software, the MA-Tracker, show a very good agreement between graders in the initial stages of the DR.

Using this new methodology, we analyzed data from a group of 113 type 2 diabetic patients with mild-to-moderate nonproliferative DR (NPDR), followed up for two years as controls in DR clinical trials and thereafter by usual care at the same institution.

Microaneurysm turnover from the initial two years and the occurrence from the initial two years and the occurrence of clinically significant macular edema (CSME) during the following eight years were analyzed in the retrospective 10-year follow-up study.

One hundred and thirty-four patients with type 2 diabetes and NPDR were followed up for two years as controls of DR clinical trials (81 men and 53 women with ages ranging from 41 to 70 years, mean $\pm$ SD: $55.6 \pm 6.3$ years, and with a diabetes duration ranging from 1 to 20 years, mean $\pm$ SD: $7.9 \pm 4.4$ years). Patients were maintained under acceptable metabolic control during this period and underwent ophthalmological examinations (including color fundus photography) every month.

At baseline, all patients showed mild-to-moderate retinopathy and were classified as levels 20 (microaneurysms only) or 35 (microaneurysms/hemorrhages and/or hard exudates) according to the Early Treatment of Diabetic Retinopathy Study (ETDRS) grading scale.

At the end of the 10-year follow-up period, 17 out of the 113 patients developed CSME needing photocoagulation.

At baseline, patients that developed CSME presented $HbA_{1C}$ levels significantly higher (mean ± SD: 8.5 ± 1.2%) than the group of patients that did not develop CSME (mean ± SD: 7.3 ± 1.2%, $p = 0.001$; table 2). No statistically significant differences were found beween CSME and non-CSME eyes for blood pressure, cholesterol, HDL, LDL and triglyceride levels at baseline.

When counting the total number of microaneurysms over the first two years of the follow-up, a significant increase in the number of microaneurysms was found for the CSME eyes ($p = 0.002$), while for the non-CSME eyes the number of microaneurysms remained relatively constant ($p = 0.647$).

When computing the microaneurysm turnover for the same period of time, a higher microaneurysm turnover was found in the group of patients/eyes that developed CSME (higher microaneurysm formation and disappearance rates). Formation and disappearance rates of 9.2 ± 18.2 and 7.5 ± 16.6 microaneurysms/year, respectively, were found for the eyes that developed CSME, while rates of 0.5 ± 1.2 and 0.5 ± 1.2 microaneurysm/year were found for the non-CSME eyes ($p < 0.001$).

A microaneurysm turnover of at least two microaneurysms/year was found in 12 of the 17 eyes that developed CSME (70.6%), whereas this was only found in 8 of the 96 eyes that did not develop CSME during the 10-year follow-up period (8.3%).

This study shows that in the initial stages of DR higher microaneurysm counts and microaneurysm counts and microaneurysm turnover obtained from color fundus photography are good indicators of retinopathy progression and development of CSME needing photocoagulation.

In summary, we found that differences between successive visits using microaneurysm counts are, therefore, less reliable than microaneurysm formation rates, which take into account mainly newly formed microaneurysms and give more accurate information on activity of the retinopathy. Futhermore, we previously found much better agreement between graders when determining microaneurysm turnover than microaneurysm counts.

Recently, Sharp *et al.* found that the microaneurysm turnover varied widely between eyes of the same retinopathy level. This is also consistent with our findings. Microaneurysm turnover has been shown in this study to vary between patients that were classified with the same retinopathy level. Particularly relevant is the finding that the patients who have higher microaneurysm turnover values are the ones that go on to develop CSME within a period of 10 years and show a more rapid retinopathy progression, particularly in association with poor metabolic control demonstrated by higher HbA1C values.

It appears that it is possible to use microaneurysm turnover computed from noninvasive color fundus photographs as a biomarker to identify eyes/patients at risk of progression to CSME.

Microaneurysm counting on fundus photography instead of microaneurysm counting on fluorescein angiography is particularly promising because fundus photography is noninvasive and well accepted by the patients, particularly when involving repeated examinations.

In conclusion, our results, based on precise identification of the location of each red-dot on fundus photograph of diabetic eyes, suggest that red-dot formation and disappearance rates may be appropriate indicators of retinopathy progression, identifying in this simple way eyes that are at more risk for progression and may represent specific retinopathy phenotypes.

## 10.3.2. Alteration of the BRB. Fluorescein Leakage Measurements

Since the early 1950s, two research groups have contributed significantly to our understanding of the pathological picture of diabetic retinopathy: Ashton and co-workers in London (Ashton, 1963) and Cogan and his co-workers in Boston (Cogan and Kuwabara, 1963).

From their observations the endothelial cells and the pericytes were seen to be affected from the earlier stages of diabetic retinopathy. When the BRB was found to be located primarily at the level of the endothelial membrane of retinal vessels (Shakib and Cunha-Vaz, 1966) it was only natural to assume that an alteration of the endothelial cells could play a major role in diabetic retinal diseases. Ashton in his 1965 Bowman Lecture stated that early lesions of diabetic retinopathy are "focal breakdowns of the BRB" (Ashton, 1965).

The advent of fluorescein angiography confirmed most of what was known about the initial pathological picture of diabetic retinopathy and showed in the initial stages of the disease focal leaks of fluorescein, demonstrating, in a clinical setting, the existence of focal breakdowns of the BRB.

In 1975, vitreous fluorometry, a clinical quantitative method for the study of the BRB, was introduced by our group (Cunha-Vaz *et al.*, 1975), showing that an alteration of the BRB could be detected and measured in some diabetic eyes with apparently normal fundi. These results were confirmed by Waltman *et al.* (1978b).

Thereafter, many experimental and clinical studies have examined the alteration of the BRB in diabetes with conflicting results at times, but showing in general that an alteration of the BRB is present in the diabetic retina and may have an important role in its development and progression (Cunha-Vaz, 2000a, b).

The damaged capillaries leak their contents intraretinally, resulting in the formation of hard yellow exudates (confluents of lipids and lipoproteins) in the nerve fiber layer and edema. Localized hemorrhages also result from the excessive vascular porosity. If present hemorrhages take the form of dots and blots, an appearance attributable to their deep location and sequestration of blood in an anatomically compact retina.

Breakdown of the BRB plays, therefore, an important initiating role in the development of the pathological picture of diabetic retinopathy.

An alteration of the BRB has, indeed, been documented in a variety of studies using different models of experimental diabetes. These studies, initiated by Waltman and co-workers, (Waltman *et al.*, 1978a) showed an alteration of the BRB in rats with streptozotocin-induced diabetes, well demonstrated by vitreous fluorometry, soon after the induction of chronic hyperglycemia. Futhermore, this alteration of the BRB was reversed by the administration of insulin and regularization of glycemia.

The alteration of the BRB in the rat with streptozotocin-induced diabetes occurs only one week after the administration of streptozotocin. There have been, however, contradicting reports regarding the site of this BRB breakdown. Studies using horseradish peroxidase as a tracer for electron microscopic investigation, pointed to the retinal pigmented epithelium as the main structure affected (Tso *et al.*, 1980). However, studies using histochemical localization of naturally occurring albumin, performed by Murata *et al.*, 1993 and Viñores *et al.*, 1990 have clearly shown that the main site of increased permeability of the BRB is located at the level of the inner BRB involving the retinal vessels. More recently, our group in Coimbra have demonstrated using confocal microscopy that the breakdown of the BRB occurring in rats one week after onset of streptozotocin-induced diabetes is localized preferentially in the inner BRB (Carmo *et al.*, 1998).

In alloxan-induced diabetes, Engerman was able to demonstrate in the dog the development of a retinopathy presenting many of the features seen in man (Engerman, 1976). Ultrastructural studies, using horseradish peroxidase, a relatively large protein, demonstrated breakdown of the BRB in eyes showing signs of microvascular alterations. The breakdown of the inner BRB was manifested by the presence of the tracer in the cytoplasm of the endothelial cells and in ruptured junctions. It is noteworthy that the breakdown of the BRB was observed preferentially in vessels showing signs of endothelial proliferation.

Clinical studies on the application of vitreous fluorometry to diabetes were reported for the first time in

1975 (Cunha-Vaz *et al.*, 1975). The examination of a series of predominantly adult-onset diabetics with apparently normal fundi revealed the frequent presence of an alteration of the BRB. The fluorescein concentration curves in the vitreous in the diabetic patients followed a gradient indicating penetration of fluorescein across the BRB.

During the following years many research efforts were directed at improving the instrumentation and standardization of the method. An ocular fluorometer described by Zeimer *et al.* finally became available commercially, thus making it possible to repeat studies at different centers avoiding much of the variability in instrumentation that played some of the earlier studies (Zeimer *et al.*, 1983).

An European multicenter study involving six different research groups showed that vitreous fluorometry, performed using the Fluorotron Master and following a well-defined protocol, is a highly sensitive and reliable method for measuring the permeability of the BRB (Van Schaik *et al.*, 1997). Values for the BRB permeability coefficient obtained by different authors have shown good agreement. The European Community Network of Ocular Fluorometry found a mean value of $1.97 \pm 0.93 \times 10^{-7}$ cm/s on data collected from six centers for a total of 81 healthy volunteers.

A general review of the many studies performed using vitreous fluorometry in both type 1 and 2 diabetes shows that there is, in both types of diabetes, an alteration, which is always present after development of ophthalmoscopically visible retinopathy and present in some eyes even before the development of clinically visible retinopathy. Although affecting preferentially a subset of patients, this breakdown of the BRB when considering all patients increases with duration of the disease and is associated with poor metabolic control.

We have followed in a 7-year prospective follow-up study a group of 40 patients with adult-onset diabetes mellitus, with retinopathy no greater than level 35 of the modified Airlie House Classification of diabetic retinopathy at the commencement of the study

(Cunha-Vaz *et al.*, 1998). They were examined by fundus photography, fluorescein angiography and vitreous fluorometry, at entry into the study and 1, 4 and 7 years after the initial examination. After a 7-year follow-up period a total of 22 of the 40 eyes had received photocoagulation. The eyes that needed photocoagulation were those that had higher vitreous fluorometry values at entry to the study and showed higher rates of deterioration. Abnormally high vitreous fluorometry values and their rapid increase over time were shown to be good indicators of progression and worsening of the retinopathy with need for photocoagulation.

Similar findings have been reported by Engler *et al.*, 1991 in an 8-year follow-up study of type 1 diabetic patients. Initially, the patients were submitted to fundus photography and vitreous fluorometry for determination of the BRB permeability. After eight years the patients were re-examined. A positive correlation between a high initial permeability value and an unfavorable clinical course, using photocoagulation as the outcome parameter, was found. In summary, in patients showing the same retinal morphology, high permeability of the BRB appears to indicate a particular phenotype characterized by an unfavorable course of disease.

It appears, therefore, that an alteration of the BRB, measured by vitreous fluorometry, is an early finding in diabetic retinal disease and correlates well with progression and worsening of the retinopathy.

One major limitation of the available commercial instrumentation for vitreous fluorometry was associated with the fact that the permeability of the BRB is measured as an average over the macular area. Accurate mapping of localized changes in the permeability of the BRB would be beneficial for early diagnosis, to explain the natural history of retinal disease and to predict its effect on visual acuity.

We have recently developed a new method of retinal leakage mapping, the Retinal Leakage Analyzer (RLA), that is capable of measuring localized changes in fluorescein leakage across the BRB while simultaneously imaging the retina. The instrument is based on a confocal scanning laser ophthalmoscope that was modified into a confocal scanning laser fluorometer (Lobo *et al.*, 1999).

Two types of information are obtained simultaneously, distribution of fluorescein concentration (retina and vitreous) and fundus image. This simultaneous acquisition is crucial because it allows a direct correlation to be established between the maps of permeability and the morphological information.

It is now possible to follow the natural history of focal alterations of the BRB occurring in the initial stages of the disease and to identify their location and measure the changes over time, while examining their association with the main morphological changes occurring in the diabetic retina, such as microaneurysms, capillary closure and retinal edema.

## 10.3.3. Macular Edema. Retinal Thickness Measurements

Diabetic macular edema is an important alteration occurring in the initial stages of diabetic retinal disease. Its importance is due to its association with loss of vision. Based on WESDR data, it was estimated (as of 1993) that of approximately 7,800,000 people with diabetes about 84,000 North Americans would develop proliferation retinopathy and about 95,000 would develop sight loss from macular edema over a 10-year period (Klein *et al.*, 1995a, b).

Edema of the retina is any increase of water of the retinal tissue resulting in an increase in its volume, i.e. because of the structural organization of the retina, an increase in its thickness. Macular edema is, therefore, edema of the retinal tissue located in the macular area.

This increase in water content of the retinal tissue may be initially intracellular or extracellular. In the first case, also called cytotoxic edema, there is an alteration of the cellular ionic exchanges with an excess of $Na^+$ inside the cell. In the second case, also called vasogenic edema, there is predominantly extracellular accumulation of fluid directly associated with an alteration of the BRB (Cunha-Vaz and Travassos, 1984).

The clinical evaluation of macular edema has been characterized by its subjectivity. Direct ophthalmoscopy may show only an alteration of the foveal reflexes. Stereoscopic fundus photography and slit-lamp biomicroscopy play an important role demonstrating changes in retinal volume in the macular area but they are dependent on the observer experience and the results do not offer a true measurement of the volume change. Furthermore, the interpretation of the extent and type of macular edema varies markedly between different observers (Klystra *et al.*, 1999).

Recently new techniques have become available that measure objectively retinal thickness.

Optical imaging instruments, like the retinal thickness analyzer (RTA, Talia Technology, Ltd) and optical coherence tomography (OCT, Humphrey Instruments), have been proposed as powerful tools for the objective assessment of macular edema. Both techniques, which are able to measure retinal thickness and rapidly generate thickness maps at the posterior pole, are noninvasive and noncontact procedures. Another instrument, the Heidelberg retina tomograph (HRT, Heidelberg Engineering) is a scanning laser ophthalmoscope that is able to measure retinal edema indirectly by performing a topographic assessment of an unevenly raised "retina" thus offering a map of relative increases in retinal thickness (Ang *et al.*, 2000).

The RTA is a quantitative and reproducible method to evaluate retinal thickness. The variability in the measurements obtained in normal subjects was reported as 8% by Shahidi and co-workers (Shahidi *et al.*, 1990).

The principle of the RTA is based on projecting a thin He–Ne laser (543 nm) slit obliquely on the retina and viewing it at an angle. The separation between the reflections (and scatter) from the vitreoretinal interface and the chorioretinal interface is a measure of the retinal thickness. On the other hand, OCT provides cross-sectional tomographs of the retinal structure *in vivo*, in which optical interferometry is used to resolve the distances of reflective structures within the eye. Low coherence light from a superluminescent diode source, operating at 840 nm (infrared light), is divided into two beams: one incident on the retina and the other incident on a translating mirror. The two reflected beams, one on the mirror and the other on retinal structures, are recombined and optical interference detected by a photodiode.

The reproducibility of the method in normal subjects was reported as 7% by Ang and co-workers (Ang *et al.*, 2000).

In recent studies performed with the RTA and OCT we chose to compare five regional measurements of retinal thickness (Pires *et al.*, 2002). Two normal populations volunteered to participate as age matched control groups for RTA and OCT and reference maps were computed using the mean + 2SD. Measurements of retinal thickness obtained with the RTA or the OCT, which were higher than the ones in these reference maps, were expressed as % increases over the reference normal values (Lobo *et al.*, 2000).

We examined three groups of eyes from subjects with type 2 diabetes: (1) with preclinical retinopathy; (2) with mild to moderate nonproliferative retinopathy; (3) with mild clinically significant macular edema according to the ETDRS guidelines, edema identified by stereo fundus photography.

In group 1 RTA detected abnormal increases in 86% of the diabetic eyes examined with increases ranging from 0.3% to 73.5% over the normal mean value + 2SD. OCT detected retinal thickness increases in only 11% of the same series of eyes.

This study showed that there are localized areas of retinal edema, i.e. areas of abnormal increase in retinal thickness, occurring in the macula in the initial stages of diabetic retinal disease. The RTA in this study appeared to be able to detect localized increases in retinal thickness in the diabetic retina well before OCT.

Comparable results have been reported by Shahidi *et al.* (1991) and Hee *et al.* (1998). Shahidi *et al.* (1991) observed that stereo fundus photography did not identify locations with mild or localized thickening demonstrated by the RTA. Hee *et al.* (1998) using the OCT only detected increases in foveal thickness in 3.6% of a series of 55 eyes with no visible retinopathy.

In another group of patients with mild to moderate nonproliferative diabetic retinopathy the RTA again detected larger increases, reaching values as high as 56.5% and 73.5% over the normal value + 2SD in eyes graded 20 and 35 of the Wisconsin grading scale, respectively. It was also clear from this study that the presence of localized areas of retinal edema identified by the RTA is not a constant finding in the diabetic retina, as 14% of eyes remained edema-free. It is to be noted that no clear correlation could be found between the extent of the edema and the retinopathy grading, at least in these initial stages of the retinopathy.

In the third study we examined with the RTA and OCT a series of eyes of patients with type 2 diabetes presenting clinically significant macular edema as defined by stereo fundus photography according to ETDRS characteristics.

In the central macula the RTA measured increases in retinal thickness higher than the mean + 2SD of a healthy control population in 21 of the 25 eyes with CSME characteristics (84%). There were, therefore, four eyes with a diagnosis of retinal edema on stereo fundus photography, which did not show increase in retinal thickness with the RTA. These four eyes, however, showed the presence of isolated hard exudates, confirming the recent observations of Storm *et al.* (2002) indicating that the presence of hard exudates may mislead fundus photography graders into assuming the presence of retinal edema. If these four eyes were excluded, the RTA detected increases in retinal thickness in 21 of the 21 eyes (100%) identified by fundus photography, whereas the OCT measured increases in retinal thickness in only 12 of the 21 eyes that had edema identified by fundus photography in the central macular area (57%). These findings are in agreement with the observations of Zeimer (1998), who reported an agreement of 78% between the RTA and stereo photography with disagreements generally associated with the presence of hard exudates.

The eyes included in this study had characteristically good visual acuity and belonged to the category of relatively mild CSME. The OCT examination did not show the presence of cyst-like structures, large collections of fluid or signs of disorganization of the retinal structure in any of these eyes, thus confirming the mild nature of the retinal edema.

Measurements of retinal thickness are particularly promising because of their quantitative nature and provision of permanent records of the location and degree of thickening.

Comparing the two techniques to measure retinal thickness, the RTA appears to be particularly appropriate to measure changes in retinal thickness in eyes with clear media and when these changes are minimal. We consider it to be an extremely promising tool in evaluating quantitatively the changes in retinal thickness before the development of cystoid macular edema and when an early therapeutic intervention may be more effective. OCT, on the other hand, uses a unique cross-sectional scanning mode offering highly accurate anatomic representation of the retina, which is particularly useful when the retinal edema is associated with other pathologies. OCT, in our experience, is particularly informative when there are changes in the retinal architecture, namely through the formation of cyst-like spaces due to localized intraretinal fluid accumulation or vitreous traction is suspected. OCT is also to be preferred when there is some degree of cataract formation or the eyes have an implanted intraocular lens. In our experience both methods are well accepted by the patients and can be performed with little discomfort giving reliable quantitative information on the size and location of macular edema.

Measurements of retinal thickness offer an objective evaluation of retinal edema and show that localized areas of retinal edema are a frequent finding in the diabetic retina in the initial stages of nonproliferative retinopathy in subjects with type 2 diabetes.

In one study published in 2000 (Lobo, Bernardes and Cunha-Vaz, 2000) we examined a series of 10 eyes from 10 patients with type 2 diabetes and no lesions visible on fundus photography (level 10 of ETDRS-Winsconsin grading), using advanced imaging techniques: the retinal leakage analyzer and the retinal thickness analyzer. Both these imaging techniques are particularly useful to identify minimal

alterations in fluorescein leakage and retinal thickness and their exact location in the macula. The maps of retinal leakage and retinal thickness were aligned and integrated in the same image to correlate changes in leakage with changes in thickness.

Localized sites of increased fluorescein leakage and zones of increased retinal thickness were found in most eyes of the 10 eyes examined. The metabolic control of the patients included was relatively well controlled (average $HbA_{1C}$, 0.07). Abnormal increases in fluorescein leakage were frequent in 90% of examined eyes and abnormal increases in retinal thickness were found in 70% of the eyes examined even though no other abnormalities were visible in the retina or detected by ophthalmoscopy or 7-field stereo fundus photography.

These findings have clear clinical value, since increased retinal fluorescein leakage identifies an alteration of the BRB and increased retinal thickness characterizes the presence of retinal edema. Retinal edema, the more frequent cause of visual loss in type 2 diabetes, is often associated with an alteration of the BRB. In this study this finding occurred in only 6 of 10 eyes examined and only when the alteration of the BRB was most marked. In the other four eyes, however, there was no direct correlation between the location of zones of increased retinal thickness and the sites of abnormal fluorescein leakage. Furthermore, areas of increased retinal thickness were detected in the absence of abnormal fluorescein leakage.

In summary, this study indicates that in the initial stages of diabetic retinal disease, breakdown of the BRB and retinal tissue thickening may occur simultaneously, either in association with each other or independently. The BRB damage may modulate and play a role in the development of retinal tissue thickening, but it is clearly not the only mechanism involved in the development of retinal edema. There are, therefore, more than one mechanism involved in retinal edema formation in the earliest stages of diabetic retinal disease.

More recently, our group reviewed the data obtained on 35 eyes with mild nonproliferative retinopathy of 35 patients with type 2 diabetes followed for two years and examined with the RTA at

6-month intervals, for a total of five examinations for each eye. Focal areas of abnormally increased retinal thickness were detected in the perifoveal ring in at least one examination in 26 of the 35 eyes (74%). Ten of the 35 eyes (29%) showed increases in retinal thickness in the perifoveal ring (500–1500 $\mu$m) in every one of the five visits performed at 6-month intervals. It is of particular interest that in none of these eyes macular edema was detected by ophthalmoscopy or fundus photography.

We have, therefore, in diabetes, a situation of subclinical macular edema that occurs very early in the retina and appears to be relatively common. This subclinical macular edema is also observed in eyes that do not show, with the techniques presently available, measurable fluorescein leakage. This subclinical diabetic macular edema may, in fact, correspond to a situation of neuroglial damage and intracellular swelling, directly resulting from the altered metabolic state of diabetes. In eyes where the BRB is altered the increases in thickness become more marked, reaching values higher than 300 $\mu$m. These higher values of increased retinal thickness are associated with situations of macular edema that are detected clinically, by ophthalmoscopy, stereo fundus photography and slit-lamp examination.

Macular edema in diabetes may present as a continuum as the diabetic retinal disease progresses and may represent a good marker of disease progression. Furthermore, its measurement is performed by a noninvasive procedure.

Diabetic macular edema involves initially the perifoveal ring and is present quite early in the disease process. It may be detected before other signs of retinopathy and indicates both involvement of the neuroretina and the progressive alteration of the BRB as the diabetic retinal progresses.

Finally progression of macular edema leads to clinically significant macular edema and severe visual dysfunction.

Retinal thickness increases in diabetes may constitute an appropriate target for treatment. An appropriate goal of the treatment would be arrest delay or limit progression of abnormal macular thickness to significant visual impairment.

## 10.3.4. Retinal Blood Flow and Capillary Closure

Retinal ischemia due to vascular closure develops relatively early in the course of diabetic retinopathy and is attributed to changes in vascular autoregulation and microthrombosis formation. Retinal blood flow changes are considered to lead to the development of poor perfusion facilitating microthrombosis formation (Boeri *et al.*, 2001).

The control of blood flow through the retina depends on changes in the ophthalmic artery caliber, which has sympathetic innervation, or humoral and local factors. Retinal vessels have no sympathetic nerve supply (Malmfors, 1965). Therefore, local factors play a dominant role. Retinal vessels are particularly responsive to changes in arterial $pO_2$ and to a lesser extent, to changes in $pCO_2$ (Kohner *et al.*, 1975; Kohner, 1977). The response to altered demand by the tissues is mediated through the "autoregulatory" adaptation of the blood vessels and blood flow.

Alterations in retinal blood flow have been identified in the different stages of the progression of retinopathy. In patients with mild retinopathy and using a two-point fluorophotometry technique, we found an increase in retinal arteriolar velocity (Cunha-Vaz *et al.*, 1978). This finding was confirmed by Cuypers *et al.* (2000) using laser Doppler flowmetry. Other authors have, however, registered a decrease in retinal blood flow. Sullivan and associates (Sullivan *et al.*, 1990) found reduced blood flow when the glucose levels remained low and stable, increasing only in association with high glucose levels. In more advanced stages of retinopathy the results also conflict with some authors reporting decreases in retinal blood flow (Michelson *et al.*, 2001) and others reporting increases (Bursell *et al.*, 1996).

One of the major problems associated with these measurements is their technical complexity and variability.

Cuypers *et al.* (2000) used the Heidelberg Retina Flowmeter (HRF; Heidelberg Engineering, Dossenheim, Germany) on a series of eyes from patients with either type 1 or type 2 diabetes. They included in the study patients with all grades of retinopathy. They considered the methodology to be reliable. We have examined with the HRF a series of eyes without clinical signs of retinopathy of subjects with type 2 diabetes and compared our findings with a control healthy population, after examining the reproducibility of the different softwares available and different examination methodologies (Ludovico *et al.*, 2003).

In this study, we have used the HRF realizing that this technique is technically restricted to perform reliable measurements of blood flow in small vessels of the retinal capillary superficial layers. Retinal capillary blood flow measurements performed in the papillomacular area using the whole-scan analysis and the automated full-field perfusion image analysis proposed by Michelson *et al.* (1998) showed acceptable reproducibility in both healthy and diabetic eyes. This methodology involves automatic subtraction of large vessels and takes into account the heartbeat associated pulsation, artificial movements and local variations in brightness of the fundus.

When comparing the retinal capillary blood flow measurements obtained from the papillomacular area with the HRF using the automated full-field perfusion image analysis method in diabetic eyes with preclinical retinopathy and healthy control eyes, the retinal blood flow was increased in the diabetic eyes. However, when analyzing the results obtained in each eye it became clear that this increase in retinal blood flow varied markedly between different patients. Five of the 10 diabetic patients clearly showed abnormal increases in retinal capillary blood flow, i.e. with four of them presenting values higher than the mean + 2SD of the values registered for all parameters (volume, flow and velocity) in the normal control group. The other five diabetic patients showed values within the normal range.

These findings have particular relevance. They may explain the conflicting reports in the literature and indicate that changes in retinal capillary blood flow are an early alteration in the diabetic retina but do not occur in the same degree or at the same time in every retina. They may develop as a result of other retinal alterations and may be of particular value by identifying the eyes that are at risk for progression of the retinopathy and this way indicating different phenotypes of diabetic retinopathy.

In this study, the increases in retinal capillary blood flow registered in 5 of the 10 diabetic eyes with preclinical retinopathy did not show any clear correlations with level of metabolic control ($HbA_{1C}$), blood glucose values on the day of the examination, duration of the disease, blood pressure levels or other systemic variables, in agreement with the observations of Cuypers *et al.* (2000).

There are several possible explanations for an increase in capillary blood flow in diabetes (Kohner *et al.*, 1975). It could indicate shunting, an increase in capillary diameter or capillary recruitment.

The flow of red blood cells through retinal capillaries is modulated by intravascular and extravascular factors. The intravascular pressure gradient between the precapillary arteriole and the postcapillary venule is considered the most important regulator of capillary flow. In our study all patients with type 2 diabetes had similar and acceptable levels of blood pressure. On the other hand, an increase in capillary diameter is considered to have a relatively small effect on the pressure gradient and, therefore, results in a small decrease in capillary flow. Shunting phenomena or capillary recruitment are the most likely candidates to explain the marked increase in capillary red blood cell flow observed in 5 of the 10 eyes of patients.

It is thought that under normal physiological conditions most retinal capillaries are perfused by both plasma and red blood cells. Fluorescein angiographic studies indicate that retinal capillaries are continuously perfused. However, the fluorescein method does not distinguish between flow of plasma and red cells together. It is accepted that in the brain in a small fraction of capillaries, red blood cell perfusion may stop for brief periods (not longer than a few seconds) indicating some degree of intermittence of red blood flow in the capillaries, i.e. plasma skimming.

Whether capillaries open and close at rest and during adaptation of capillary blood flow to changing metabolic needs is still a matter of controversy. Functional "thoroughfare channels" or preferential capillaries with high resting flow have been proposed to play a central role in microcirculation of the brain, surrounded by other capillaries, characterized by slow resting flow, which could be recruited when the tissue blood supply is challenged (Hasegawa *et al.*, 1967).

Finally, another possible alternative is that in the retinal capillaries plasma flow is continuous but red cells travel through only some capillaries at all times. In this case, capillary recruitment would be a natural response to increased metabolic demands by the retinal tissue in diabetes (Kageman *et al.*, 1999) or a situation of relative hypoxia as proposed for the diabetic retina (Keen and Chlouverakis, 1965).

It is possible that the eyes which show increased capillary blood flow, thus apparently creating conditions for more rapid and progressive damage of the capillary walls, are at a special risk of progression to retinopathy.

Our observations indicate that in some diabetic eyes even before the development of visible retinopathy there is (probably due to local factors) a marked increase in retinal capillary blood flow with the maximal utilization of the retinal capillary net, whereas others do not show this circulatory response.

This increase in blood flow may contribute to endothelial damage and establish the appropriate conditions for microthrombosis formation.

In diabetes plasma constituents are also affected and red cells may be altered. Changes in blood viscosity increase the chances of microthrombosis formation, vessel damage and capillary closure.

Through abnormalities in clotting and the fibronolytic system in diabetes play certainly a role in retinal capillary closure it is unlikely that they initiate the process of diabetic retinal vasculature disease. The posterior pole of the retina is affected initially in diabetes in clear contrast to the peripheral involvement, which characterizes the retinopathies resulting from blood disorders, like sickle-cell disease, macroglobulinemia and multiple myeloma (Cunha-Vaz, 1978).

## 10.3.5. Neuronal and Glial Cells Changes

We have stated previously that the simplest paradigm to explain increased capillary permeability and the advent of capillary closure centers on vascular endothelium and pericytes. There are, however, a number of reports showing changes in the neuronal and glial cells of the retina very early in the course of the disease (Lorenzi and Gerhardinger, 2001). This is clearly of major potential importance and it may indicate at least a contributory role in the development of the microangiopathy.

Reports of electroretinographic changes in diabetic patients with demonstrable vascular lesions date back to the 1960s and have been confirmed by several authors (Ghirlanda *et al.*, 1997), who found the electroretinographic abnormalities to originate in the ganglion and inner nuclear layers. Studies mostly performed in streptozotocin-induced diabetic rats have identified changes in the neuroglial elements of the inner two thirds of the retina. Whether the neuroglial abnormalities induced by diabetes eventually contribute to the development of vascular pathology is still not known at present.

Hard and soft exudates are frequent components of the clinical picture of diabetic retinopathy. Hard exudates are abnormal depostitions in the retina of lipids and proteins originating from the blood circulation, crossing an abnormal BRB. Soft "exudates" or cotton-wool spots are recognized as localized ischemic impacts of the nerve fiber layer of the retina. They are considered to result from increased vascular permeability and capillary closure, respectively, but are definitely associated with neuronal and glial damage.

In the rat retina most of the neurons containing neuronal nitric oxide synthase (NOs) appear to be from amacrine cells, which are closely related to the retinal vasculature. The number of these n-NOs containing cells was found to decrease by 32% as early as one week after the induction of STZ-diabetes (Darius *et al.*, 1995). This reduced availability of nitric oxide may play a role by inducing localized changes in blood flow. Such alterations may also be compounded by increased endothelin-1 and endothelin-3 levels, which have been observed in the neural cells of the inner retina 2–4 weeks after STZ-diabetes (Deng *et al.*, 1999). It is noteworthy that increased endothelin levels may be induced by high glucose through activation of protein kinase C (PKC) (Takagi *et al.*, 1996).

In the retina of diabetic rats another major alteration observed only one month after STZ-diabetes is a 10-fold increase in the frequency of apoptosis (Takagi *et al.*, 1996). The majority of apoptotic cells appeared to be ganglion cells.

Although the extent of abnormalities in the neural retinal cells in human diabetes appears to be less conspicuous, there is also clear evidence of their occurrence.

Namely, the phenomenon of early neuroretinal apoptosis appears to be less prominent in human diabetes than in the STZ-diabetic rats. However, the issues of early and extensive neural apoptosis in human diabetes and whether it precedes microangiopathy remains to be settled.

Regarding the involvement of the glial cells in diabetes there is also a wealth of information. Both Muller cells and astrocytes envelope neurons the initial segments of the ganglion cell axons and blood vessels. Specifically, the inner layer of retinal capillaries is enveloped by both astrocytic and Muller cell processes, while only the latter provide most of the glial wrapping to the outer layer of the retinal vasculature (Holländer *et al.*, 1991).

Muller cells have, indeed, characteristics that make them potential targets of diabetes and potential contributors to retinopathy. Muller cells are the primary site of glucose uptake and phosphorylation in the retina (Poitry-Yamate *et al.*, 1965). They are endowed with Glut 1 and metabolize glucose intensely through glycolysis to produce lactates that fuel neuronal metabolism and are the primary site of glycogen storage and metabolism in the retina. Muller cells are also primarily involved in the transformation of glutamate in the retina and in the acquisition of barrier properties by the endothelial cells of the BRB.

Recent evidence suggests that retinal glial and Muller cells in particular are affected early in the course of both experimental and human diabetes. There are reports demonstrating increased expression of glial fibrillary acidic protein (GFAP) and reduced ability to convert glutamate into glutamine in diabetic rat retinas. Glutamate excitotoxicity may occur in the diabetic retina as a consequence of Muller cell dysfunction (Lieth *et al.*, 1998). It is still a matter of controversy if these changes are preceded by an increase in capillary permeability (Rungger-Brändle *et al.*, 2000) and the early alteration of the BRB.

It is interesting to note that the overexpression of GFAP appears to be selective and is not likely to reflect an increased number of Muller cells. Thus, in both human and experimental diabetes, the circumstances of increased retinal GFAP point to altered regulation of gene expression. This could be due to selective transcriptional effects of high glucose or other metabolic abnormalities on the GFAP gene or be an element of more generalized changes in Muller cells fielding a specific "reactive" phenotype.

The focal increases in retinal thickness observed in the initial stages of diabetic retinal disease also indicate that some degree of intracellular neuronal or glials swelling must be present. Very early in the disease process this subclinical macular edema may be a good marker for neuronal or glial damage, particularly in the absence of a clear alteration of the BRB. More work is needed in this area of research, paying particular attention to the potential direct correlation between neuroglial swelling, measured by retinal thickness measurements and alterations in visual function.

### 10.3.6. Multimodal Imaging of the Retina

Our research group has been developing methods to combine and integrate data from fundus photography, angiographic images (scanning laser ophthalmoscope-fluorescein angiography), maps of fluorescein leakage into the vitreous (scanning laser ophthalmoscope-retinal leakage analyzer), maps of retinal thickness and maps of visual function (automated perimetry-humphrey field analyzer HFA II 750) of the macular area to achieve multimodal macula mapping (Lobo *et al.*, 1999, 2000; Bernardes *et al.*, 2002). Scanning laser ophthalmoscopy (SLO) produces high-resolution images using much less light for illumination of the fundus than used for conventional photography. High contrast images of the foveal and perifoveal structures are produced with this technique using directly reflected light. In confocal scanning laser ophthalmoscopy (CSLO), a laser beam illuminates an area of the eye fundus. A confocal stop placed in front of the detector rejects most of the light coming from both anterior and posterior planes. A set of moving mirrors allows the scanning of an area of interest. The light reflected from each retinal point is captured by the detector. Thus, a point-by-point video image is constructed with each retinal point corresponding to a point on the monitor screen. SLO, because of its monochromatic wavelength emission, minimizes scattering and chromatic aberration. This feature of SLO increases contrast and improves visibility as compared with slit-lamp biomicroscopy and fundus photography.

We have been able to develop the Retinal Leakage Analyzer for measuring and mapping the permeability of the BRB based on CSLO system (Lobo *et al.*, 1999). The combination of two data sets, angiographic and permeability mapping, obtained simultaneously using the same instrumentation, provided a good definition of landmark references of the macula, giving simultaneously functional and morphological information and in this way was an important step in the development of multimodal mapping. We have been able to combine in multimodal macula mapping, information on structure and function by integrating data from fluorescein angiography, retinal leakage analysis and retinal thickness analysis. Other available detection devices that may be used for multimodal imaging include laser Doppler retinal flowmetry using the Heidelberg Retina Flowmeter, indocyanine angiography, multifocal

electroretinography (mfERG), autofluorescence mapping and retinal thickness measurements using either the Retinal Thickness Analyzer or Optical Coherence Tomography. Each one of these methods adds more information and appears as potentially valuable tools for evaluating the structure and function of the retina in diabetes.

Electrophysiological methods have been recently proposed for retinal mapping with the introduction of the multifocal electroretinography (mERG). The multifocal ERG technique was developed by Sutter (2001) and can produce 100 or more focal responses from the cone-driven retina. The display usually contains either 61 or 103 hexagons, although 241 hexagons have been used in a few experiments to obtain higher spatial resolution. With the 103 elements display there is no guarantee that a hexagon will fall entirely within the optic disk. With a display of 241 elements at least one hexagon should fall entirely within the disk if steady fixation is maintained. In conclusion, the mERG method offers attractive information on the electrical functions of the retina, but improved spatial resolution is necessary for useful macula mapping. The combination of these different methods of retinal imaging is a tool with tremendous potential to uncover hidden correlations between the different alterations occurring simultaneously in the diabetic retina.

## 10.4. Characterization of Retinopathy Phenotypes

### 10.4.1. Follow-up Studies of the Initial Stages of Diabetic Retinopathy by Multimodal Retinal Imaging

It is well recognized that duration of diabetes and levels of metabolic control and blood pressure are major risk factors for development of diabetic retinopathy.

However, these risk factors do not explain the great variability that characterizes the evolution and rate of progression of the retinopathy in different diabetic individuals. There is clearly great individual variation in the presentation and course of diabetic retinopathy. There are many diabetic patients who after many years with diabetes never develop sight-threatening retinal changes and maintain good visual acuity. There are also other patients that even after only a few years of diabetes show a retinopathy that progresses rapidly and may not even respond to laser photocoagulation treatment.

We have recently performed a prospective 3-year follow-up study of the macular region in 14 patients with type 2 diabetes mellitus and mild nonproliferative retinopathy, using multimodal macula mapping (Lobo *et al.*, 2004).

In a span of three years eyes with minimal changes at the start of the study (levels 20 and 35 of ETDRS-Wisconsin grading) were followed up at 6-month intervals in order to monitor progression of the retinal changes.

The most frequent alterations observed were, by decreasing order of frequency, leaking sites, areas of increased retinal thickness and microaneurysms/hemorrhages.

Leaking sites were a very frequent finding and reached very high BRB permeability values in some eyes. These sites of alteration of the BRB, well identified in RLA-maps, maintained, in most cases, the same location on successive examinations, but their BRB permeability values fluctuated greatly between examinations, indicating reversibility of this alteration.

There was, in general, a correlation between the BRB permeability values and the changes in $HbA_{1C}$ levels occurring in each patient. This correlation was particularly clear when looking at eyes that showed, at some time during the follow-up period, BRB permeability values within the normal range. A return to normal levels of BRB permeability was, in this study and in each patient, always associated with a stabilization or decrease in $HbA_{1C}$ values.

The frequent finding of leaking sites in these 14 eyes confirms previous reports using fluorescein angiography (Wise *et al.*, 1971), vitreous fluorometry (Cunha-Vaz *et al.*, 1985a, b) and retinal leakage analysis (Lobo *et al.*, 1999), which show that alteration of vascular permeability is one of the most frequent alterations occurring in the initial stages of diabetic retinal disease.

Areas of increased retinal thickness were another frequent finding in these eyes. They were present in every eye at some time during the follow-up and were absent, at baseline, in only two of the 14 eyes. This confirms previous observations by our group (Lobo *et al.*, 1999) and by others (Fritsche *et al.*, 2002).

However, the areas of increased retinal thickness varied in their location over subsequent examinations and did not correlate with changes in $HbA_{1C}$ levels. They may represent a delayed response in time to other changes occurring in the retina, such as increased leakage, as suggested previously (Lobo *et al.*, 1999).

The number of red-dots increased in most eyes during the 3-year period of follow-up. This was particularly well demonstrated when the location of each red-dot was taken into consideration. This increase in the number of red-dots may be the most reliable indicator of retinal vascular damage and remodeling of the retinal circulation, particularly in the initial stages of DR.

Increased rates of red-dot accumulation were registered in eyes that had more red-dots at baseline and higher values of BRB permeability during the study. In summary, the rate of red-dot formation appears in this study to have the potential to be a good indicator of retinopathy progression. We realized that by combining different imaging techniques, i.e. multimodal imaging of the macula, made apparent three major evolving patterns occurring during the follow-up period of three years: Pattern A included eyes with reversible and relatively little abnormal fluorescein leakage, a slow rate of microaneurysm formation and a normal FAZ. This group appeared to represent eyes presenting slowly progressing retinal disease; Pattern B included eyes with persistently high leakage values, indicating an important alteration of the BRB, high rates of microaneurysm accumulation and a normal

FAZ. All these features suggest a rapid and progressive form of the disease. This group may identify a "wet" form of diabetic retinopathy and Pattern C included eyes with variable and reversible leakage and an abnormal FAZ. This group is less well characterized considering the small number of eyes that showed an abnormal FAZ. It may be that abnormalities of the FAZ may occur as a late development of groups A and B or progress rapidly as a specific "ischemic" form (Fig. 10.1).

We have now extended our observations by following 57 patients for seven years with type 2 diabetes with all eyes presenting at the time of enrollment mild NPDR. In this larger study these three different phenotypes were again clearly identified after an initial 2-year period of follow-up with repeated examinations at 6-month intervals. The discriminative markers of these phenotypes were: red-dot formation rate, measurements of fluorescein leakage, and signs of capillary closure in the capillaries surrounding the FAZ.

After an average seven years of follow-up, ten of these 57 eyes had developed clinically significant macular edema with clear indication for photocoagulation treatment. In this series of patients, after the

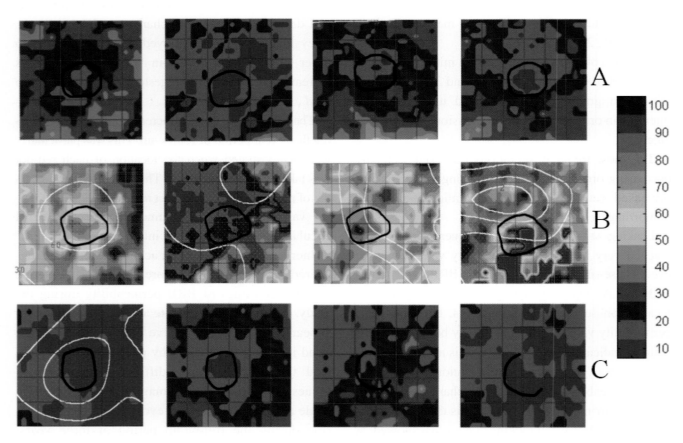

**Fig. 10.1.** Multimodal images taken at 0, 12, 24 and 36 months visits (left to right) showing for each visit the foveal avascular zone (FAZ) — black contour — retinal leakage analyzer results and retinal thickness analyzer results. The retinal leakage analyzer color-coded maps of the blood-retinal barrier permeability indexes are shown; retinal thickness analyzer views show white dot density maps of the percentage increases in retinal thickness. *Top row*: pattern A. Note the little amount of retinal leakage over the 4 represented visits and the normal FAZ contour. This patient showed a slow rate of microaneurysm formation. *Middle row*: pattern B. Note the high retinal leakage showing a certain degree of reversibility and the normal FAZ contour. This patient showed a high rate of microaneurysm accumulation over the 3-year follow-up period. *Bottom row*: pattern C. Note the reversible retinal leakage and the development of an abnormal FAZ contour. This patient showed a high rate of microaneurysms formation.

initial 2-year period of follow-up, 35 eyes (61% of the total) were identified as showing the characteristics a pattern A, slow progression, 12 (21%) were classified as presenting pattern B and the other 10 (18%) had the characteristics of pattern C.

None of the 35 eyes identified initially as pattern A, developed after seven years of follow-up severe macular edema needing laser photocoagulation. This was in clear contrast with the findings registered in the other two retinopathy subtypes, B and C. Five of the 12 eyes classified as having pattern B, (41%) developed severe macular edema needing photocoagulation. Similarly, five of the 10 eyes identified has having pattern C, (50%) developed severe macular edema needing photocoagulation during the 7-year period of follow-up.

In summary, the slow progression type, pattern A, did not progress to severe macular edema during the 7-year period of follow-up confirming that this subtype of DR has good prognosis.

On the other hand, both other DR subtypes, the leaky type or pattern B, characterized initially by particularly high levels of leakage, i.e. alteration of the BRB and the ischemic type, or pattern C, characterized by signs of capillary closure, lead much more frequently to the development of severe macular edema with incidences at seven years of 41% and 50%, respectively.

If diabetic retinopathy is a multifactorial disease — in the sense that different factors or different pathways may predominate in different groups of cases with diabetic retinopathy — then it is crucial that these differences and the possible different phenotypes be identified (Grange, 1995). The characterization of three different phenotypes of DR with different progression patterns opens particularly interesting perspectives to gain more insight into the understanding and management of DR.

Diabetes mellitus is a familial metabolic disorder with strong genetic and environmental etiology. Familial aggregation is more common in type 2 diabetes than in type 1 diabetes. Rema *et al.* (2002) reported that familial clustering of diabetic

retinopathy was three times higher in siblings of type 2 subjects with diabetic retinopathy. Presence or absence of genetic factors may play a fundamental role in determining specific pathways of vascular disease and, as a consequence, different progression patterns of diabetic retinal disease. It could be that certain polymorphisms would make the retinal circulation more susceptible to an early breakdown of the BRB (type B) or microthrombosis and capillary closure (type C). The absence of these specific genetic polymorphisms would lead to an evolving pattern of type A.

It is clear from this study and from previous large studies, such as the Diabetes Control and Complications Trials group (DCCT) (2002) and UKPDS (Stratton *et al.*, 2001), that hyperglycemia plays a determinant role in the progression of retinopathy. It is interesting to note that $HbA_{1C}$ levels are also largely genetically determined (Snieder *et al.*, 2001).

An interesting perspective of our observations, analyzed under the light of available literature, depicts diabetic retinopathy as a microvascular complication of diabetes mellitus conditioned in its progression and prognosis by a variety of different genetic polymorphisms and modulated in its evolution by $HbA_{1C}$ levels, partly genetically determined and partly dependent on individual diabetes management. The interplay of these multiple factors and the duration of this interplay would finally characterize different clinical pictures or phenotypes of diabetic retinopathy (Fig. 10.2).

The ultimate goal, therefore, should be the characterization of relationships between genetic factors (represented by distinct genotypes) and their medically significant expression (distinct diabetic retinopathy phenotypes). Our observations of prospective studies of eyes with mild nonproliferative diabetic retinopathy of patients with type 2 diabetes mellitus suggest three different phenotypes of diabetic retinopathy: a "wet" or "leaky" type, an "ischemic" type and finally, an apparently more common, slow progression type.

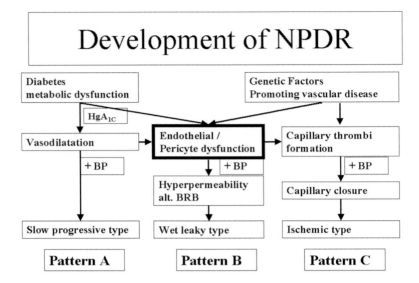

**Fig. 10.2.** Schematic development of nonproliferative diabetic retinopathy leading to the three different patterns proposed: A, B and C.

## 10.4.2. Progression of Nonproliferative Retinopathy Under Stabilized Metabolic Control

It must be realized that levels of hyperglycemia and duration of diabetes, i.e. exposure to hyperglycemia, are expected to influence the evolution and rate of progression classified by our group in three major clinical phenotypes of retinopathy progression.

To determine the natural history of the initial alterations occurring in the retina in subjects with type 2 diabetes under a situation of stable metabolic control, our group performed a 2-year prospective study on eyes with mild nonproliferative retinopathy under intensive oral tritherapy (Ribeiro *et al.*, 2004; Duarte *et al.*, 2005).

In type 2 diabetes very good levels of metabolic control may be achieved using only oral administration of drugs, in the absence of insulin therapy, by associating a sulphonylurea with a biguanide and an alpha-glucosidase inhibitor. Since this was a condition for inclusion in the study. In this study HgA$_{1C}$ levels were stabilized during the entire 2-year study period. Red-dot counts on fundus photographs, inward BRB permeability values and retinal thickness measurements were

determined in the chosen eyes of each patient at 6-month intervals.

The number of red-dots increased steadily throughout the 2-year study period in spite of the patients stabilized metabolic control, with more red-dots counted in the eyes of patients with worse glucose control.

Red-dot progression rates during the 2-year period of the study varied widely among patients. There appeared to be individual red-dot progression rates that may be genetically determined and are basically predetermined and independent of medical management, although influenced by metabolic control. It was interesting to note that higher values of red-dot progression rates were registered also in patients with higher HbA$_{1C}$ levels both throughout the study and at baseline.

HbA$_{1C}$ levels at baseline may indicate previous metabolic control, but they may also indicate that HbA$_{1C}$ levels are genetically determined and independent of the genes influencing fasting glucose values (Smieder *et al.*, 2001).

In this study, different patients showed clearly different rates of red-dots progression, which appeared to be largely independent of stabilized metabolic control, but could be influenced favorably by tight metabolic control.

The increases in the number of red-dots showed statistically significant correlations with the increases in the permeability of the BRB and changes in the FAZ, which are indicative of capillary loss. All these parameters appeared to be indicators of retinopathy progression.

Retinopathy continued to progress under well stabilized metabolic control indicating role for genetic factors but progression appears to accelerate in the eyes of patients under worst metabolic control.

We have now established that DR has different phenotypes characterized by different types and rates of retinopathy progression and that these phenotypes can be identified since the initial stages of the retinopathy, after a period of follow-up of one to two years. The initial vascular lesions that can be identified clinically on slit-lamp or ophthalmoscopic examination are microaneurysms and hemorrhages appearing on the eye fundus as red-dots. These are also the alterations that characterize the first levels of the ETDRS Wisconsin classification. The rate of formation of new red-dots is probably the best indicator of retinopathy progression and the indicator to follow in the initial stages of the retinopathy.

## 10.5. Dominant Pathophysiological Mechanisms of Disease Progression

### 10.5.1. Aging Phenomena

Retina tissue like the brain consists predominantly of neurons and neuroglia. Neurons are post-mitotic cells, which are unable to divide in response to damage or to replace abnormal or dead neurons. The total number of neurons gradually declines with age. Furthermore, some of the commonest causes of neuronal damage are associated with defects in the vascular supply.

Although the human brain is about 2% of the total body weight, it uses about 20% of the total oxygen supply.

The retina can be regarded as an extension of the brain. The two types of photoreceptor cells (cones and rods) transmit signals to the bipolar cells and to the glanglion cells with axons that extend to the brain. Oxygen is supplied by an extensive capillary network. Several features of the retina illustrate, indeed, the inevitability of age-related changes.

Retinal diabetic microangiopathy is characterized by BRB breakdown, basement membrane thickening of retinal vessels, microaneurysms, hemorrhages, cotton-wool spots, capillary obliteration and a cellular capillaries, which may ultimately lead to retinal ischemia and neovascularization. Some of these events occur because retinal vascular cells, namely pericytes and endothelial cells, die prematurely during diabetes. Microvascular cells become dysfunctional and undergo apoptosis as a result of hyperglycemia. It appears that the early apoptosis in retinal microvascular cells predicts the development of the histologic lesions (Kern *et al.*, 2000).

Consistent with the fact that apoptosis of pericytes and endothelial cells appears to be the mechanism of retinal capillary cell loss are the observations made by different authors (Kowbree and Koppolow, 2002; Lecomte *et al.*, 2004 and Podestá *et al.*, 2000) that caspase-3, caspase-10 are present in post-mortem retinas of diabetic donors.

The microvascular cells apoptosis may be triggered or mediated by a variety of mechanisms: accumulation advanced glycation end products, increased activity of aldose reductase, oxidative stress etc. (see Chap. 5).

It is clear, that hyperglycemia causes apoptosis in microvascular cells leading to progressive dysfunction of the retinal capillary architecture and development of retinopathy.

Diabetic retinopathy has been considered a microvascular disease but recent studies have given added importance to associated neuronal dysfunction and death in the pathophysiology of DR. It is accepted now that we are dealing with a neurodegenerative disease of the eye in addition to microvascular disease (Barber, 2003).

Barber and colleagues in 1998 published the first quantitative report showing an increase in neuronal cell apoptosis in the diabetic retina. They demonstrated that the thickness of the inner plexiform and inner nuclear layers are reduced upon 7.5 months of STZ-induced diabetes and that the number of ganglion cells is also decreased.

Several studies have since corroborated these findings suggesting neuronal apoptosis is an early occurrence in the diabetic retina. Similarly astrocytes and Muller cells are affected. Hammes and colleagues (1995) showed that in addition to neurons and microvascular cells Muller cells exhibit apoptic features and increase the expression of the intermediate glial fibrillary acidic protein (GFAP).

In summary, there is a wealth of evidence indicating that the chronic hyperglycemia of diabetes induces apoptosis in all retinal cells, microvascular, neuronal and glial creating a situation that may be identified with accelerated aging.

## 10.5.2. Hemodynamic Phenomena

It is a well recognized "clinical impression" that one of earliest alterations observed in the retinal circulation in diabetes is dilatation of the retinal capillary network in the posterior pole. This increased visibility of the retinal capillary network is probably associated with an increase in retinal capillary blood flow.

In a study performed by our research group, when comparing the retinal capillary blood flow measurements obtained from the papillomacular area using the Heidelberg Retinal Flowmeter in diabetic eyes with preclinical retinopathy and in healthy control eyes, we found an overall statistical significant increase in retinal blood flow in the diabetic eyes. However, it was particularly interesting to find that when analyzing the results obtained in each eye that this increase in retinal capillary blood flow varied

markedly between them. The increases were clearly much higher in five of the ten patients studied. Five of the ten showed clearly abnormal increases, with four of them presenting values higher than the mean +2SD of the values registered in the normal control group. The finding that the other five diabetic patients in this study has retinal capillary blood flow values within the normal control range was also of interest.

These results may have particular relevance. They explain the conflicting results in the literature regarding retinal capillary blood flow values in the initial stages of diabetic retinal disease. They also demonstrate that changes in retinal capillary blood flow are an early alteration in the diabetic retina, but not in the same degree or at the same time in every diabetic retina.

We have now follow-up data on the initial stages of diabetic retinal disease showing that eyes that have an increased retinal capillary blood flow also have more marked alterations of the BRB and increased values of retinal thickness in the macular area (Ribeiro *et al.*, 2004). These changes seem to characterize what has been called by Lobo *et al.* (2002), the pattern B of diabetic retinopathy progression or the "leaky" type.

We have, apparently, in some diabetic patients in the initial stages of the diabetic retinal disease a failure of the retinal blood flow autoregulatory mechanisms. The retinal circulation of diabetic patients with the same level of metabolic control and duration of disease appear to respond differently in some patients, suggesting a specific susceptibility to circulatory changes that demand an autoregulatory response.

The limits of the autoregulatory response of the retinal circulation in pattern B appears to be reached earlier, leading to damage to the retinal endothelium and disruption of the BRB. Disruption of the BRB results in extravasation of plasma proteins into the proteins into the retina, neuronal dysfunction and development of edema.

In this DR phenotype, hemodynamic phenomena seem to underlie the progress of the retinopathy. The mechanisms responsible for this specific situation of abnormal flow autoregulation may be due to one of three hypotheses:

1. A decreased contractility deficiency of the retinal capillary cells, pericytes and/or endothelial cells leading to a passive increase in the diameters of the capacitance microvasculature (capillaries and venules);
2. Alterations in the intercellular communication between glia and retinal vessels leading to a deficient response of the retinal circulation to the abnormal metabolic environment;
3. Decreased liberation of vasoactive substances by the retinal endothelium needed to maintain the autoregulatory response of the retinal circulation to the abnormal hyperglycemic environment.

How this loss of the autoregulatory response of the retinal circulation occurs in a percentage of eyes of patients with diabetes and what is the chain of events remains to be clarified.

It is clear, however, that there appears to be a DR phenotype characterized by the presence of a series of events where hemodynamic changes predominate. An abnormal autoregulatory response characterized initially by an increase in retinal blood flow, focal alterations of the BRB and development of areas of retinal edema appears to be hallmarks of this rapidly progressive DR phenotype.

## 10.5.3. Thrombotic Phenomena

Capillary nonperfusion and capillary closure occur frequently in the diabetic retina and are a characteristic feature in the more advanced stages of DR. They are indicators of retinopathy progression and direct signs of presence of ischemia.

Both capillary nonperfusion and capillary closure are most probably the result of retinal microthrombosis. Increased platelet adhesiveness and aggregation has been documented in diabetic patients since at least three decades (Heath *et al.*, 1971). Microthrombosis

have been demonstrated by election microscopy in experimental diabetes, these microthrombi are mainly composed of aggregated platelets and fibrin strands (Ishibashi *et al.*, 1981).

Recently, Boeri and colleagues (2001) demonstrated in post-mortem specimens from diabetic and nondiabetic donors that diabetic retinas present an increased number of platelet-fibrin thrombi in the retinal capillaries. They demonstrated also a topographical association of microthrombosis with apoptotic cells.

We have recently developed a new software to count red-dots on color images of the eyes fundus capable of identifying the exact topographical location of each red-dot. Comparing the exact location of each red-dot on successive fundus images it was possible to verify that most red-dots are only seen in the same location for periods of less than one year and that they cannot be seen in the same location after disappearance. These observations indicate that the red-dots, mostly microaneurysms, disappear by closing off probably by microthrombosis.

Thrombosis is a dynamic process, which is initiated when the hemostatic system is perturbed by injury to the vessel wall, activation of coagulation and/or flow disturbance. Alterations in endothelial integrity, disturbances in laminar blood flow, thrombin generation and inhibition of endogenous fibrinolytic activities contribute to thrombus formation.

Numerous studies have shown that coagulation abnormalities occur in the course of diabetes mellitus resulting in a state of trombophilia (Cerviello, 1993). The abnormalities observed involve all stages of coagulation, affecting both thrombus formation and its inhibition, fibronolysis, platelet and endothelial function.

We have observed in our follow-up studies of eyes from diabetic patients in the initial stages of retinopathy that in some eyes showing rapid progression characterized by increased rates of microaneurysms formation and disappearance had also particularly low values of retinal blood flow and relatively low values of alteration of the BRB. This is a pattern of retinopathy progression that was identified characterizing a specific DR phenotype, phenotype C or "ischemic."

Thrombi are known to develop in the ischemic microvasculature and are most likely the predominant feature of DR phenotype C. The other features that were identified by our group all appear to concur to thrombi formation and rapid retinopathy progression.

### 10.5.4. Adjuvant Phenomena

There has recently been a renewed interest in the role of inflammation as a relevant factor in the development and progression of the vascular dysfunction of DR. Gardner (2002) and Avanis (2002) have called upon a number of arguments in favor of this hypothesis.

At microscopic level inflammation is associated with vascular dilatation, altered flow, exudation of fluids and leukocyte accumulation and migration. All these features can be identified in the pathological picture of diabetic retinal disease.

It has been shown that within one week of experimental diabetes leukocytes adhere to and accumulate within the vasculature of the retina (Miyamoto *et al.*, 1999). The leukocytes attach to the endothelial cell lining via classic adhesion molecules, including intercellular adhesion molecule-1 (ICAM-1) on the vasculature and B-integrins in the leukocytes. The expression levels for these adhesion molecules increase in early diabetes.

When powerful experimental techniques are applied to detect the earliest changes occurring in the diabetic retina, the initial alterations are the breakdown of the BRB, endothelial cell injury and death and capillary ischemia. Leukocytes may be causal in inducing all of these changes. However, at what point is their role relevant is not clear yet.

It must be kept in mind that a variety of clinical studies have shown that antiinflammatory drugs have a beneficial effect on the alterations of DR. Macular edema may be improved by local administration of steroids and there are a few reports suggesting that this is so.

The available data is not conclusive but at least an adjuvant role may be played by a coexistent low grade inflammatory status in the development and progression of DR.

Abnormalities in the leukocytes and platelets may facilitate the conditions for more rapid progression of the retinopathy and correction of these abnormalities may help stabilize DR.

## 10.6. Biochemical Pathways Involved

Excessive concentration of glucose within cells of the retina as a result of the hyperglycemia of diabetes is a common thread underlying most of the biochemical and molecular mechanisms that have been postulated to play a role in the pathogenesis of diabetic retinopathy.

The observation that not all patients with poor metabolic control develop advanced stages of diabetic retinopathy suggests that other factors, such as genetic predispositions, are likely to determine individual susceptibility to the disease.

Despite virtually all retinal cells and tissues being potentially affected in diabetic retinopathy, an overwhelming amount of data suggests that vascular cells are dramatically affected during development and progression of diabetic retinopathy. There is also some degree of consensus on the importance of endothelial cell dysfunction and that DR is primarily a vascular disorder.

However, the molecular mechanisms that underlie tissue damage are still unknown, although there is agreement that the main factor for development of the disease is hyperglycemia.

Glucose uptake by retinal endothelial cells occurs in excess of metabolic rates. The intracellular level of glucose in retinal endothelial cells is approximately 16 times higher that the amount of glucose that can be metabolized by hexokinase (Berkowitz *et al.*, 1995). This leads to a large pool of intracellular hyperglycemia, which is critical in the conceptualization of many molecular mechanisms associated with glucose toxicity, contributing, finally, to the development of DR. Chronic exposure of the retina to the high levels of glucose is accepted as the upstream event leading to cell damage in diabetes.

A number of major mechanisms have been proposed with strong arguments to explain the toxicity of glucose in diabetes: activation of protein kinase C, activation of glucose reductase, formation of AGE and the hexosamine pathway. These pathways or enzymes have been proposed to act independently, but recent data suggests a common thread between them that could account for the hyperglycemia-induced damage in diabetes. It has, indeed, been shown that hyperglycemia induces overproduction of superoxide by the mitochondrial electron transport chain (Brownlee, 2001) and that this excess production of reactive oxygen species can be the upstream event.

There is also evidence supporting the concept that the main site of production of superoxide in mitochondria of endothelial cells following exposure to high glucose is the mitochondrial complex II (succinate: ubiquinone oxidoreductase).

This unifying hypothesis is consistent with the four main pathways considered to be involved in the development of diabetic complications: activation of aldose reductase, increased formation of AGE's, activation of protein kinase C and increased hexoxamine pathway/flux. This hypothesis further accounts for the relevance of increased production of reactive oxygen species in diabetes and also provides a unifying hypothesis regarding the effects of hyperglycemia on cellular dysfunction.

Furthermore, the activation of the transcription factor NF-kB by superoxide provides an extra link between hyperglycemia and the expression of multiple genes related to vascular stress response (Collins, 1993).

Although the current rise in prevalence of diabetes is most certainly driven by life-style changes, individual differences in susceptibility to the complications associated with diabetes can, at least, in part be attributed to genetic differences in susceptibility to the disease. It is conceivable both that some genes expressed in certain groups individuals make them less prone or more susceptible to retinopathy progression and, on the other hand, that specific genes may be differentially induced in response to hyperglycemia.

## 10.7. Candidate Phenotype/ Genotype Correlations

Hyperglycemia occurs in every patient with diabetes mellitus and it is a fundamental factor for the development of diabetic complications. Several studies have provided evidence that good diabetes control is important to prevent progression of diabetic retinopathy, but it is clear that some patients develop a rapidly progressing retinopathy despite good control, while others escape the development of severe retinopathy despite poor control.

The onset, intensity and progression of diabetic complications show large interindividual variations (Lobo *et al.*, 2002; Rogus *et al.*, 2002). There is, indeed, clear evidence from aggregation in families and specific ethnic groups, together with lack of serious complications in some diabetic patients with poor metabolic control that there is a genetic predisposition to develop some diabetic complications, such as retinopathy (Warpeha and Chakravarthy, 2003).

It is recognized that polymorphic variability in the genetic make-up of an individual can profoundly influence the expression of a gene and its response to environmental factors. As we predict that the impact of single common mutations on RD development will be modest (increasing relative risk (RR) by 20–40% at most), the main issue of clinical relevance is whether the conferred risk of such a mutation is very much higher in some population subgroups. To be clinically useful in a risk algorithm we might require for any factor to have a RR of 2 or greater (Humphries *et al.*, 2001).

Such subgroups might be those carrying a second important mutation in another gene and such individuals might be identified using conventional genetic strategies. Alternatively, one might identify individuals exposed to a given environment which amplifies the risk associated with that gene, i.e. gene-environment interaction.

Diabetic retinopathy shows familial aggregation and variation in disease severity, which is not explained by environmental, biochemical or biological risk factors alone.

There are substantial variations in onset and severity of retinopathy in different patients, which are independent of the duration of diabetes and level of glycemic control. A relatively large number of candidate genes have been examined in patients with diabetes, but clear genotype-phenotype associations have not yet been identified.

One of the major problems is associated with poor characterization of different retinopathy phenotypes. It is fundamental before embarking in a search for candidate genes to define clinical phenotypes characterized by specific patterns of severity and progression of DR. It is clear that it is necessary to identify first and well the DR phenotypes that are associated with rapid progression of the retinopathy to severe forms of the disease, such as macular edema and proliferative retinopathy. Only then studies on candidate genes are worth pursuing, involving appropriately well-defined subgroups of patients (Warpeha and Chakravarthy, 2003).

There are several physiological systems that are involved in maintaining retinal vascular health and disease can be predicted to develop resulting from a failure to maintain hemostasis. One is the endothelial lining of the vessel wall with its role in maintaining the BRB, influencing vessel tone, maintaining normal wall structure and preventing thrombosis. Another is the coagulation cascade. Other possibilities include the normal homeostatic systems, which regulate short-term blood pressure and plasma and intracellular lipid metabolism.

Variations in the genes expressed in the aldose reductase pathway may influence microvascular susceptibility. Aldose reductase is strongly expressed in retinal pericytes and is also found in the vascular endothelium (Viñores *et al.*, 1993). It has been suggested that 7q35 is a susceptibility region for diabetic retinopathy by virtue of the aldose-reductase gene (AR2) (Patel *et al.*, 1996).

In type 1 diabetes the strongest genetic risk component is localized within the major histocompatibility complex. The HLA region that is located on 6p21 has also been implicated as genomic region of interest for susceptibility to retinopathy in both type 1 (Stewart *et al.*, 1993) and type 2 diabetes (Serrano-Rios *et al.*, 1983).

Glut transporter genes have been examined but no association between polymorphisms in the Glut 1 gene and retinopathy status was found.

Other candidate genes involved in cell communication and the extracellular communication have also been investigated without conclusive data (Warpeha and Chakravarthy, 2003). These authors and their group have paid special attention to the genes of endothelins (ET) and nitric oxide synthases (NOS). NOS and ET are counter regulatory and the NO/ET pathway is crucial to maintain the tone of the vasculature, which is delicately controlled by the balance in their expression. They identified microsatelite polymorphic markers in members of ET and NOS families as well as those of endothelin converting enzyme (ECE1).

Subjects with no retinopathy despite 15 years or more of diabetes (controls) and any subject with severe retinopathy regardless of duration (ETDRS level 50 or worse) were prospectively recruited into these studies. None of the polymorphisms studied in the NOS 1 or NOS 3 genes was significantly associated with cases or controls. However, studies on the NSO2A gene showed that a 14-repeat allele of a pentanucleolide polymorphism in the 50UTR of NOS2A gene was protective against developing diabetic retinopathy in both patient populations (Warpeha *et al.*, 1999). The authors suggest that when NOS3 expression is low in the diabetic retina induction of NOS2A may occur in an attempt to achieve homeostasis (Graier *et al.*, 1993), possibly playing a crucial role in preventing or delaying pathological alterations in the microcirculation in diabetes.

There are indications that the vascular complications of diabetes are related with the formation of advanced glycated-end products (AGE). The glycation of proteins and lipids is a result of hyperglycemia and this effect of AGEs is mediated the AGE receptor (RAGE) which is regulated by a gene (Hudson *et al.*, 2001).

Angiotensin-converting enzyme (ACE) is another important mediator of vasoconstriction and homeostasis, however, studies to date on genetic markers of members of this signaling pathway (Matsumoto *et al.*, 2000) have not shown definitive evidence of direct genetic risk. It remains, however, an interesting candidate gene to play a role in DR. Clinical studies have shown that ACE inhibition may play a useful specific role in the management of DR.

Large interindividual differences in plasma ACE levels exist but are similar within families, suggesting a strong genetic influence. The human ACE gene is found on chromosome 17 and contains a restriction fragment length polymorphism consisting of the presence (insertion, I) or absence (deletion, D) of a 287 base pair "ALU" repeat sequence in intron 16 (Rigat *et al.*, 1990). In 1992 the I/D polymorphisms of the ACE gene were reported to be associated with risk of myocardial infarction (Cambien *et al.*, 1992) and this effect, though more modest then originally reported, has been confirmed in larger studies (Keavney *et al.*, 2000).

Glucose may itself be the mitigating environmental factor that induces expression of the polymorphism.

The situation on a complex and multifactorial disease, such as diabetes, favors the presence of gene-environment interactions. A key factor in the identification and study of gene-environment interaction is that an individual carrying such a mutation will develop the phenotype only if and when they enter the high risk environment. Thus, the mutation will cause a specific retinal vascular alteration, i.e. alteration of BRB or blood-flow changes in the presence of a specific environmental challenge. This classical "lack of

penetrance" of a mutation will cause analytical problems and mis-phenotyping, which will be particularly problematic with some sampling analytical designs. This "content dependency" of a mutation, i.e. gene X environment effect, must be taken into consideration when analyzing associations between a candidate gene polymorphism and intermediate phenotypes.

Most of the results published indicate the presence of genetic determinants for resistance or susceptibility to vascular complications. However, there is evidence of problems in replicating results suggesting that the studies performed have been plagued with confounding factors.

The results of our research group on the characterization of different phenotypes of DR confirm that there are distinct morphological manifestations in DR with different subjects presenting different rates of progression and different evolution patterns. (Lobo *et al.*, 2004). There is now evidence indicating that susceptibility to the late vascular complications of diabetes, such as retinopathy, depend at least partly on genetic factors (Wasgenknecht *et al.*, 2001).

The risk of severe DR in the siblings of affected individuals is substantially increased (Leslie and Pyke, 1982). It is possible that the problems associated with identifying susceptibility genes for diabetic retinopathy is mainly due to the still accepted view that diabetic retinopathy is one uniform and homogenous disease. Specific types of more severe retinopathy may need to be identified before progress is achieved in this area of research.

Another factor that must be taken into consideration is duration of diabetes. Problems encountered may be minimized by selecting case subjects with short diabetes duration and control subjects with larger duration or by adjusting to duration during analysis.

It is clear that future studies should focus on the need to characterize more accurately different phenotypes with respect to retinopathy status. We agree entirely with Warpeha and Chakravarthy (2003) when they state that agreed international standards for data collection, particularly agreement on a minimum data set for the phenotyping of retinopathy in subjects with diabetes, would permit the pooling of data from the many studies with enhanced power to detect associations.

A classification of diabetic retinopathy based on both relevant genotypes and disease phenotypes is an ambitious goal. We believe that this route may help identify the particular form that threatens an individual patient and consequently offer an opportunity for specific and more effective therapies.

## 10.8. Relevance for Clinical Trial Design

Studies, such as the Diabetes control and complications trial (Diabetes control and complications trial Group 2002), the United Kingdom prospective diabetes study (United Kingdom Prospective Diabetes Study, 1998), the diabetic retinopathy study research group (Diabetic Research Study Research Group, 1981) and the early treatment diabetic retinopathy study (Early Treatment Diabetic Retinopathy Study, 1991) validated methods now considered standard in treating diabetic retinopathy when it occurs, i.e. tight control of blood glucose levels to prevent retinopathy and laser photocoagulation to halt progression after development of CSME or proliferative retinopathy. However, despite the aim of tight blood glucose control and the use of retinal photocoagulation, blindness still occurs. Other forms of therapy targeted at the earliest stages of retinal disease, involving necessarily the demonstration of efficacy of a new drug are urgently needed and remain a priority for eye research.

One of the major problems lies in the limitations that characterize at present the accepted methods of retinopathy assessment, visual acuity changes and fundus photography. Visual acuity changes are detected too late in the course of the disease and fundus photography, as it has been used, in descriptive manner, is subjective and has been unable to characterize progression in the initial stages of the retinopathy. To make things more difficult it is well known that the course of retinopathy is not linear

and lesions that are seen on fundus photography may come and go. Apparent clinical improvement on fundus photography may, in reality, mask worsening of the disease.

It is crucial in order to design an appropriate clinical trial to test the efficacy of a drug, to identify not only the meaningful clinical endpoints but also the surrogate endpoints that may demonstrate efficacy of a drug in a realistic and feasible period of time (Cunha-Vaz, 2001). Approval of a drug to treat diabetic retinopathy must take into account that it must appeal to clinicians as being useful to their patients, which means that it must show efficacy to clinical endpoints that they can see in their patients and recognize "this is the patient I would use that therapy for."

It must be taken into account that the clinicians must understand what the drug is being used for and in which group of patients, so that they can explain the potential risks and benefits to their patients.

It is immediately clear that such process implies the validation of surrogate endpoints by the associated occurrence of hard clinical outcomes, such as significant visual loss. It is here that the problem lies. Diabetic retinopathy progresses to irreversible stages of the disease with relatively little visual loss and when macular edema or proliferative retinopathy are present it becomes ethically mandatory to perform photocoagulation treatment.

The development of an effective drug must take into account the need to demonstrate efficacy on the earliest and reversible stages of diabetic retinal disease by demonstrating its effect on surrogate endpoints, which can be followed for shorter periods of time. The assumption would be that those surrogate endpoints would ultimately be validated by association with more hard clinical outcomes, but that should not necessarily need to occur before provisional approval.

It is, therefore, an urgent priority to identify endpoints, which people can accept as surrogates that are expected to be later validated in longer natural history studies.

The clinical endpoints that have been accepted in the past are: mean difference between groups in visual acuity of at least three lines in a ETDRS-Type chart, i.e. doubling of the visual angle; mean difference in visual field of at least 10 dB; reduction in percentage of patients with vitreous hemorrhage; reduction in percentage of patients with rubeosis; reduction in occurrence of retinal detachments and need for photocoagulation treatment according to DRS and ETDRS guidelines (DRS, 1981; ETDRS, 1991). All of these are what may be called terminal endpoints. They only give indications about the late irreversible stages of diabetic retinopathy.

One candidate reduction in macular thickening by measuring the changes in retinal thickness with dedicated instrumentation is a promising alternative. The measurements are reliable and changes in retinal thickness are a direct indication of macular edema (Shahidi *et al.*, 1994; Hee *et al.*, 1995).

Finally possibility red-dot counting on fundus photographs taking into account every new microaneurysms/hemorrhage according to their exact specific location in the eye fundus is noninvasive and has the potential to become an extremely informative marker of the overall progression of diabetic retinal vascular disease. The rate of formation of new red-dots appears to be a direct indication of the progression of retinal vascular damage and is statistically correlated with the progression in fluorescein leakage, i.e. the alteration of the BRB and capillary closure (Torrent-Solans *et al.*, 2004). By counting red-dots on digitalized fundus photographies, using appropriate software to identify the specific location of each red-dot, we may be able to measure the rate of progression of the two major factors in diabetic vascular retinal disease: vascular hyperpermeability and capillary closure.

It is now crucial and urgent to validate these two candidates for surrogate endpoints, retinal thickness measurements and/or red-dot formation rates both using noninvasive methodologies. Their use and final validation are expected to contribute decisively to design clinical trials to test the efficacy of new drugs capable of halting diabetic retinal disease in the initial stages of the disease.

Another fundamental step in this procedure is the characterization of the different phenotypes of diabetic retinal disease. The design of future clinical trials should consider only groups of patients characterized by their homogeneity: patients presenting a specific retinopathy phenotype characterized by rapid progression (wet/leaky or ischemic) with similar duration of diabetes and at similar levels of blood pressure and metabolic control (HbA$_{1C}$ values).

## 10.9.  Relevance for Clinical Management

It is accepted that in the initial stages of diabetic retinopathy when the fundus alterations detected by ophthalmoscopy or slit-lamp examination are limited to red-dot and hard or soft exudates, i.e. mild nonproliferative DR, an annual examination is indicated to every patient with five or more years of duration of their diabetes.

This is the recommendation of the American Academy of Ophthalmology Guidelines for Diabetic Retinopathy (Fong and Ferris, 2003). Our observations and the identification of different diabetic retinopathy phenotypes in the initial stages of DR, i.e. mild or moderate NPDR, characterized by different rates of progression of the retinopathy suggest that specific approaches should be used when managing these different retinopathy phenotypes. (Table 10.1)

A patient with mild or moderate NPDR, presenting retinopathy phenotype B (wet/leaky), characterized by marked breakdown of the BRB, identified by highly increased values of fluorescein leakage into the vitreous and a high red-dot formation rate, registered during a period of 1–2 years of follow-up, indicating fast retinopathy progression, should be watched more closely and examined at least at 6-month intervals.

Furthermore, blood pressure values and metabolic control should be closely monitored at least at 3-month intervals and medication given to keep HbA$_{1C}$ levels at $< 7.1\%$, systolic blood pressure at $< 140$ mm Hg and diastolic blood pressure at $< 85$ mm Hg. Communication channels should be

**Table 10.1  Management Recommendations for Nonproliferative Diabetic Retinopathy in the Absence of Severe Macular Edema**

| Phenotypes | A | B | C |
|---|---|---|---|
| Metabolic Control | Regular | Tight HgA$_{1C}$ < 7% | Progressively tighter |
| Blood Pressure | | As low as acceptable | Progressively lower |
| Follow-up intervals | 1–3 years | 6 months | 6 months |

rapidly established between ophthalmologist and their diabetologist, internist or general health care provider. Information should be given indicating that the chances of rapid retinopathy progression to more advanced stages of disease are in these patients relatively high, calling for immediate tighter control of both glycemia and blood pressure.

A patient with mild or moderate nonproliferative diabetic retinopathy presenting retinopathy phenotype C, ischemic, characterized by clear signs of capillary closure and variable red-dot formation rates would similarly indicate the need for shorter observation intervals than one year with particular attention for other systemic signs of microthrombosis. Here, however, control of hyperglycemia and blood pressure must be addressed with some degree of caution. Improved metabolic and blood pressure control must be progressive and less aggressive than with phenotype B. It is realized that the ischemia that characterizes phenotype C may become even more apparent in eyes submitted to rapid changes in metabolic control and lowering rapidly the blood pressure may increase the retinal damage associated with ischemia. Finally, a patient with mild or moderate NPDR, presenting phenotype A, identified by low levels of 1 fluorescein leakage, no signs of capillary closure, low red-dot formation rates and with a diabetes duration of more than ten years, all signs indicating a slowly progression subtype of diabetic retinopathy may be followed at intervals longer than one year. If the examination performed at two years intervals confirms the initial phenotype characterization, the patient and his diabetologist, internist or general health care provider should be informed of the good prognosis associated with this retinopathy phenotype.

## 10.10.  Targeted Treatments

It would be of great benefit to have a drug available which would prevent the need for photocoagulation and particularly one which may remove the other variables that remain a cause of concern. So many of these patients are not well controlled, they do not come to the doctor often and they are going blind because they do not get medical attention in time for photocoagulation. The major large clinical trials have shown that tight glycemic control slows the development and progression of diabetic retinopathy. But the constantly increasing incidence of type 2 diabetes and the evidence that retinal damage begins early on underscore the need for a medical treatment that is targeted to the initial retinal alterations and to specific phenotypes of the retinal diabetic disease. Several key pathways have been incriminated in the process of triggering diabetic retinal disease and they may play specific roles in the development of specific retinopathy phenotypes. Four candidates, the polyol pathway, nonenzymatic glucosylation, growth factors and protein-kinase C may be playing leading roles in the development of diabetic retinal disease. The polyol pathway theory holds that increased glucose metabolism, through the enzyme aldose-reductase interferes with sodium-potassium ATPase, damaging the retina (Greene *et al.*, 1987).

The nonenzymatic glycosylation theory holds that the bonding of sugar molecules to other reactive molecules leads to critical retinal alterations and enhancement of processes of oxidative stress to the retina (Brownlee, 1994).

In the growth factor hypothesis diabetes-induced damage promotes the liberation of growth factors that appear clearly as the best candidates to explain the developments of proliferative retinopathy. However, the potential role of growth factors in the initial stages and in nonproliferative retinopathy remains highly hypothetical (Clermont *et al.*, 1997).

Finally, the protein kinase C theory. Many of the metabolic changes associated with hyperglycemia-induced oxidative stress, advanced glycosylation end-products of diacylglycerol through the polyol pathway, ultimately activate protein kinase C. In the retina, there is evidence that activation of the beta-isoform of PKC (PKC-beta) is associated with retinal vasodilatation and alterations in retinal blood flow, thus making PKC-beta an obvious target for intervention (Ishii *et al.*, 1996).

A role for inflammation has also been proposed and inflammation mediators have been suggested to be responsible for the increased fluorescein leakage observed in the initial stages of diabetes by causing alterations in the tight junctions of the retinal vessels (Antonetti *et al.*, 1998).

It is possible that all these different mechanisms of disease play complementary roles in the progression of diabetic retinal disease. The identification of different retinopathy phenotypes characterized by different rates of progression and different dominant retinal alterations may indicate that different disease processes predominate in specific retinopathy phenotypes probably determined by specific gene mutations. Individuals with a specific gene mutation, which makes them more susceptible to the abnormal metabolic environment of diabetes, will respond by developing a specific retinopathy phenotype. Identification of well-defined retinopathy phenotypes appears to be an essential step in the quest for a successful treatment of diabetic retinopathy. After the characterization of specific retinopathy phenotypes the predominant disease mechanisms involved may be identified and drugs directly targeted at the correction of these disease mechanisms used with greater chances of success.

## 10.11. Determining Risk in the Individual Patient. Preventative Ophthalmology

It is clear now that only a subset of patients with diabetes who develop some form of retinopathy is expected to lose functional vision during their lifetime.

Identification of risk factors to progression to visual loss precise calculations of risk for progression to visual impairment in individual patients over given time periods appears, finally, to these knowledge would be crucial to decide which patients to treat, when to initiate treatment and how ingorously.

A method of assessing risk of progression from mild nonproliferative diabetic retinopathy to severe macular edema and loss of functional vision for individual patients is clearly needed. A successful global risk assessment model that evaluates total disease risk based on the summation of major risk factors has been used for many years in the management of patients with cardiovascular disease. Eventually, a point system was established to facilitate assessment of an individuals global risk of progression to an atherosclerotic cardiovascular event.

More recently Weinreb *et al.* (2004) have initiated attempt to establish estimates for glaucoma risk assessment.

Diabetic retinopathy is a microvascular complication of diabetes mellitus that presents to the practitioner at various stages of a continuum that is characterized by accelerated retinal vascular changes also involving the neuronal and glial retinal tissue with eventual development of severe macular edema and/or abnormal retinal or optic disk neovascularization leading to irreversible functional visual loss.

The initial changes in the retina are often asymptomatic and undetectable with existing diagnostic tests. There is still no complete agreement on criteria for the diagnosis of early damage that predicts visual function loss.

This suggests that awaiting overt signs of disease involves accepting some irreversible damage and probable progression. As disease progresses, severe visual dysfunction and blindness will occur only in a small group of patients. Since many patients may be examined in the early stages of the disease the goal of treatment must be to arrest delay or limit progression of predisposing retinal vascular damage to significant visual impairment.

The continuum of diabetic retinopathy progression may be represented as depicted in Fig. 10.3, taking into consideration the three proposed diabetic retinopathy phenotypes: slow progression, "wet"/leaky and ischemic. Different individuals with diabetes have clearly different rates of progression and these must be identified and taken into account. The wealth of epidemiological data available, particularly the studies performed within the context of the WESDR, should be looked at with the aim of determining risk in the individual patient.

Development of a method to assess patients based on summation of all the major risk factors will allow patients who are most likely to benefit from treatment to be identified and would quantify the combined effect of the risk factors that practitioners should consider in making treatment decisions. In addition, the risks and benefits of various modalities should be considered in making such treatment decisions (Weinreb *et al.*, 2004).

Consolidation and analysis of cardiovascular risk factors from large patient data sets have led to the development of predictive algorithms that allow physicians to estimate individual patient risk of suffering an atherosclerotic cardiovascular event (Wilson *et al.*, 1998). Similarly, an algorithm that would allow ophthalmologists to use a patient's red-dot formation rate and other risk factors, such as retinal thickness progression and HbA$_{1C}$ levels, that is a so-called "risk calculator," to estimate the risk of visual impairment for diabetic would certainly facilitate standardization of treatment and help in determining appropriate treatment for individual patients.

As in the cardiovascular model, a calculator would be a valuable adjunct to and not a substitute for experience and judgement of a well-trained physician.

Finally, it is clear that identifying individual variations in disease progression by characterizing the diabetic retinopathy phenotype that each patients falls in and other modulating risk factors, such as HbA$_{1C}$ levels, may open completely new perspectives for the management of diabetic retinal disease. If the patients with the greatest risk of progression and with the greatest potential to benefit from treatment can be identified by multivariate risk assessment, fewer patients will need to be treated to prevent one case of blindness. This is of extreme importance at a time where search resources must be focused and concentrated on the individual cases that need close follow-up and timely treatment.

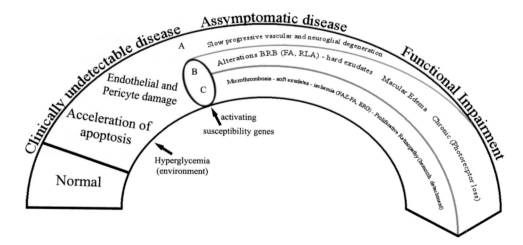

**Fig. 10.3.** Continuum of the progression of diabetic retinopathy.

# References

Aiello LP, Gardner TW, King GL, *et al.* (1998) Diabetic retinopathy. *Diabetes Care* **21**: 143–156.

Ang A, Tong L, Vernon SA. (2000) Improvement of reproducibility of macular volume measurements using the Heidelberg retinal tomograph. *Br J Ophthalmol* **84**: 1194–1197.

Antonetti DA, Barber AJ, Khin S, *et al.* (1998) State Retina Research Group, vascular permeability in experimental diabetes is associated with reduced endothelial occluding content. Vascular endothelial growth factor decreases occludin in retinal endothelial cells. *Diabetes* **47**: 1953–1959.

Ashton N. (1963) Studies of retinal capillaries in relation to diabetic and others retinopathies. *Br J Ophthalmol* **47**: 521–538.

Ashton N. (1965) The blood–retinal barrier and vasoglial relationships in retinal disease. *Trans Ophthalmol Soc UK* **85**: 199–230.

Ashton N. (1974) Vascular basement membrane changes in diabetic retinopathy. Montgomery lecture, 1973. *Br J Ophthalmol* **58**: 344–347.

Bernardes R, Lobo C, Cunha-Vaz JG. (2002) Multimodal macula mapping: A new approach to study diseases of the macula. *Surv Ophthalmol* **47**: 580–589.

Boeri D, Maiello M, Lorenzi M. (2001) Increased prevalence of microthromboses in retinal capillaries of diabetic individuals. *Diabetes* **50**: 1432–1439.

Brownlee M. (1994) Glycation and diabetic complications (Lilly lecture 1993). *Diabetes* **43**: 836–841.

Bursell SE, Clermont AC, Kinsley BT, *et al.* (1996) Retinal blood flow changes in patients with insulin-dependent Diabetes mellitus and no diabetic retinopathy a video fluorescein angiography study. *Invest Ophthalmol* **37**: 886–897.

Cambien F, Poirier O, Lecerf L, *et al.* (1992) Deletion polymorphism in the gene for angiotensin-converting enzyme is a potent risk factor for myocardial infarction. *Nature* **359**: 641–644.

Carmo A, Ramos P, Reis A, *et al.* (1998) Breakdown of the inner and outer blood-retinal barriers in streptozotocin-induced diabetes. *Exp Eye Res* **67**: 569–575.

Clermont AC, Aiello LP, Mori F, *et al.* (1997) Vascular endothelial growth factor and severity of nonproliferative diabetic retinopathy mediate retinal hemodynamics *in vivo*: A potential role for vascular endothelial growth factor in the progression of nonproliferative diabetic retinopathy. *Am J Ophthalmol* **124**: 433–436.

Cogan DG, Kwabara T. (1963) Capillary shunts in the pathogenesis of diabetic retinopathy. *Diabetes* **12**: 293–300.

Cunha-Vaz JG. (1978) Pathophysiology of diabetic retinopathy. *Br J Ophthalmol* **62**: 351–355.

Cunha-Vaz JG. (1992) Perspectives in the treatment of diabetic retinopathy. *Diabetes/Metabolism Rev* **8**: 105–116.

Cunha-Vaz JG. (2000a) Blood-retinal barrier in diabetes. In: van Bijsterveld P. (ed.), *Diabetic Retinopathy*. Taylor & Francis, A Martin Dunitz, London, pp. 155–168.

Cunha-Vaz JG. (2000b) Diabetic retinopathy: Surrogate outcomes for drug development for diabetic retinopathy. *Ophthalmologica* **214**: 377–380.

Cunha-Vaz JG, Travassos A. (1984) Breakdown of the blood-retinal barriers and cystoid macular edema. *Surv Ophthalmol* **28**: 485–492.

Cunha-Vaz JG, Faria de Abreu JR, Campos AJ, Figo GM. (1975) Early breakdown of the blood-retinal barrier in diabetes. *Br J Ophthalmol* **59**: 649–656.

Cunha-Vaz JG, Fonseca JR, Faria de Abreu JF. (1978) Vitreous fluorophotometry and retinal blood flow studies in proliferative retinopathy. *Albrecht Graefe's Arch Klin Exp Ophthalmol* **207**: 71–76.

Cunha-Vaz JG, Gray JR, Zeimer RC, *et al.* (1985) Characterization of the early stages of diabetic retinopathy by vitreous fluorophotometry. *Diabetes* **34**: 53–59.

Cunha-Vaz JG, Mota CC, Leite EC, *et al.* (1985) Effect of sulindac on the permeability of the blood-retinal barrier in early diabetic retinopathy. *Arch Ophthalmol* **103**: 1307–1311.

Cunha-Vaz JG, Mota CC, Leite EC, *et al.* (1986) Effect of sorbinil on blood-retinal barrier in early diabetic retinopathy. *Diabetes* **35**: 574–578.

Cunha-Vaz JG, Lobo C, Castro Sousa JP, *et al.* (1998) Progression of retinopathy and alteration of the blood-retinal barrier in patients with type 2 diabetes: A seven-year prospective follow-up study. *Graefe's Arch Clin Exp Ophthalmol* **236**: 264–268.

Cuypers MHM, Kasanardjo JS, Polak BCP. (2000) Retinal blood flow changes in diabetic retinopathy measured with the Heidelberg scanning laser Doppler flowmeter. *Graefes Clin Arch Exp Ophthalmol* **238**: 935–941.

Darius S, Wolf G, Huang PL, Fishman MC. (1995) Localization of NADPH-diaphorase/nitric oxide synthase in the rat retina: An electron microscopic study. *Brain Res* **690**: 231–235.

Deng D, Evans T, Mukherjee K, *et al.* (1999) Diabetes-induced vascular dysfunction in the retina: Role of endothelins. *Diabetologia* **42**: 1228–1234.

Diabetes Control and Complications Trials Group. (2002) Effect of intensive therapy on the microvascular complications of type 1 diabetes mellitus. *JAMA* **287**: 2563–2569.

Diabetic Retinopathy Study Research Group. (1978) Photocoagulation treatment of proliferative diabetic retinopathy: The second report of diabetic retinopathy study findings. *Ophthalmology* **85**: 82–106.

Diabetic Retinopathy Study Research Group. (1981) A modification of the Airlie House classification of diabetic retinopathy. Report 7. *Invest Ophthalmol Vis Sci* **21**: 210–226.

Early Treatment Diabetic Retinopathy Study Research Group. (1991) Fundus photographic risk factors for progression of diabetic retinopathy. ETDRS Report Number 12. *Ophthalmology* **98**: 823–833.

Engerman RL. (1976) Animal models of diabetic retinopathy. *Trans Am Acad Otolaryngol* **81**: 710–715.

Engler C, Krogsaa B, Lund-Andersen H. (1991) Blood-retinal barrier permeability and its relation to the progression of diabetic retinopathy in type 1 diabetics. *Graefe's Arch Clin Exp Ophthalmol* **229**: 442–446.

Ferris F, Davis M. (1990) Treating 20/20 eyes with diabetic macula edema. *Arch Ophthalmol* **117**: 675–676.

Fong DS, Ferris F. (2003) Practical management of diabetic retinopathy. Focal Points **21**(3): 1–17.

Fritsche P, VanderHeijde R, Suttorp-Schulten MSA, *et al.* (2002) Retinal thickness analysis (RTA). An objective method to assess and quantify the retinal thickness in healthy controls and diabetics without diabetic retinopathy. *Retina* **22**: 768–771.

Gardner TW, Aiello LP. (2000) Pathogenesis of diabetic retinopathy. In: Flynn Jr HW, Smiddy, WE. (eds.), *Diabetes and Ocular Disease: Past, Present, and Future Therapies*. AAO Monograph No. 14. The Foundation of the American Academy of Ophthalmology, San Francisco, pp. 1–17.

Garner A. (1987) Pathogenesis of diabetic retinopathy. *Semin Ophthalmol* **2**: 4–11.

Ghirlanda G, Di Leo MAS, Caputo S, *et al.* (1997) From functional to microvascular abnormalities in early diabetic retinopathy. *Diabetes Metab Rev* **13**: 15–35.

Goldberg MF, Fine SL, (Eds.), (1969) Symposium on treatment of Diabetic Retinopathy. Washington, DC, US Department of Health, Education and Welfare.

Graier WF, Wascher TC, Lockner L, *et al.* (1993) Exposure to elevated D-glucose concentrations modulates vascular endothelial cell vasodilatory responses. *Diabetes* **42**: 1497–1505.

Grange JD. (1995) Retinopathie Diabétique. Rapport à la Société Française d'Ophthalmologie. Masson, Paris.

Greene DA, Lattimer SA, Sima AAF. (1987) Sorbitol, phosphoinositides, and sodium–potassium-ATPase in the pathogenesis of diabetic complications. *N Engl J Med* **316**: 599–606.

Hasegawa T, Ravens JR, Toole JF, Salem W. (1967) Precapillary arteriovenous anastomoses "Thoroughfare channels" in the brain. *Arch Neurol* **16**: 217–224.

Hee MR, Puliafito CA, Duker JC, *et al.* (1998) Topography of diabetic macular edema with optical coherence tomography. *Ophthalmology* **105**: 360–370.

Hellstedt T, Immonen I. (1996) Disappearance and formation rates of microaneurysms in early diabetic retinopathy. *Br J Ophthalmol* **80**: 135–139.

Holländer H, Makarov F, Dreher Z, *et al.* (1991) Structure of the macroglia of the retina: Sharing and division of labour between astrocytes and Müeller cells. *J Comput Neurol* **313**: 587–603.

Hollis TM, Gardner TW, Vergis GJ, *et al.* (1998) Antihistamines reverse blood-ocular barrier breakdown in experimental diabetes. *J Diabet Complications* **2**: 47–49.

Hudson HL, Stickand MH, Futers S, Grant PJ. (2001) Effects of novel polymorphisms in the RAGE gene on transcriptional regulation and their association with diabetic retinopathy. *Diabetes* **50**: 1505–1511.

Humphries SE, Talmud PH, Montgomery H. (2001) Gene-environment interaction: Lipoprotein lipase and smoking and risk of CAD and the ACE and exercise-induced left ventricular hypertrophy as examples. In: Malcom S, Gooship J. (eds.), *Genotype to Phenotype*. Bios Scientific, Oxford, pp. 55–72.

Ishii H, Jirousek MR, Koya D, *et al.* (1996) Amelioration of vascular dysfunctions in diabetic rats by an oral PKC X inhibitor. *Science* **272**: 728–731.

Kageman L, Harris A, Chung HS, *et al.* (1999) Basics and limitations of color Doppler imaging. In: Pillmat LE, Harris A, Anderson DR, Greve EL. (eds.), *Current Concepts on Ocular Blood Flow in Glaucoma*. Kugler, The Hague, pp. 103–110.

Keavney B, McKenzie C, Parish S, *et al.* (2000) International Studies of Infarct Survial (ISIS) Collaborators, Large-scale test of hypothesised associations between the angiotensin-converting-enzyme insertion/deletion polymorphism and myocardial infarction in about 5000 cases and 6000 controls. *Lancet* **355**: 434–442.

Keen H, Chlouverakis C. (1965) Metabolic factors in diabetic retinopathy. In: Graymore CN. (ed.), *Biochemistry of the Retina*. Academic Press, New York, p. 123.

Kern TS, Tang J, Mizutani M, Kowluru RA, *et al.* (2000) Response of capillary cell death to aminoguanidine predicts the development of retinopathy: Comparison of diabetes and galactosemia. *Invest Ophthalmol Vis. Sci.* **41**(12): 3972–3978

Klein R, Klein BEK, Moss SE, Crukschanks KJ. (1995a) The Wisconsin epidemiologic study of diabetic retinopathy. XV the long-term incidence of macular edema. *Ophthalmology* **102**: 7–16.

Klein R, Meuer SM, Moss SE, Klein BEK. (1995b) Retinal microaneurysms counts and 10-year progression of diabetic retinopathy. *Arch Ophthalmol* **113**: 1386–1391.

Klystra JA, Brown JC, Jaffe GJ, *et al.* (1999) The importance of fluorescein angiography in planning laser treatment of diabetic macular edema. *Ophthalmology* **106**: 2068–2073.

Kohner EM. (1977) The problem of retinal blood flow in diabetes. In: *Selected Topics in Diabetes*. Proceedings of Int. Meeting Carlo Erba S.p.A., Milan, Italy, pp. 15–24.

Kohner EM, Dollery CT. (1970) The rate formation and disappearance of microaneurysms in diabetic retinopathy. *Eur J Clin Invest* **1**: 167–171.

Kohner EM, Hamilton AM, Saunders SJ, *et al.* (1975) The retinal blood flow in diabetes. *Diabetologica* **27**: 48–52.

Kohner EM, Sleightholm M. (1986) The KROC collaborative study group. Does microaneurysm count reflect severity of early diabetic retinopathy? *Ophthalmology* **93**: 586–589.

Larsen M, Hammel E, Parving HH, Lund-Andersen H. (1990) Protective effect of captopril on the blood-retina barrier in normotensive insulin-dependent diabetic patients with nephropathy and background retinopathy. *Graefe's Arch Clin Exp Ophthalmol* **228**: 505–509.

Leite E, Mota MC, Faria de Abreu JR, Cunha-Vaz JG. (1990) Effect of calcium dobesilate on the BRB in early diabetic retinopathy. *Int Ophthalmol* **14**: 81–88.

Leslie RDG, Pyke DA. (1982) Diabetic retinopathy in identical twins. *Diabetes* **31**: 19–21.

Lieth E, Barber AJ, Xu B, *et al.* (1998) Penn State Retina Research Group, Glial reactivity and impaired glutamate metabolism in short-term experimental diabetic retinopathy. *Diabetes* **47**: 815–820.

Lobo CL, Bernardes RC, Santos FJ, Cunha-Vaz JG. (1999) Mapping retinal fluorescein leakage with confocal scanning laser fluorometry of the human vitreous. *Arch Ophthalmol* **117**: 631–637.

Lobo CL, Bernardes RC, Cunha-Vaz JG. (2000) Alterations of the blood-retinal barriers and retinal thickness in pre-clinical retinopathy in subjects with type 2 diabetes. *Arch Ophthalmol* **118**: 1664–1669.

Lobo CL, Bernardes RC, Figueira JP, *et al.* (2004) Three-year follow-up of blood-retinal barrier and retinal thickness alterations in patients with type 2 diabetes mellitus and mild nonproliferative diabetic retinopathy. *Arch Ophthalmol* **122**: 211–217.

Lorenzi M, Gerhardinger C. (2001) Early cellular and molecular changes induced by diabetes in the retina. *Diabetologia* **44**: 791–804.

Ludovico J, Bernardes R, Pires I, *et al.* (2003) Alterations of retinal capillary blood flow in preclinical retinopathy in subjects with type 2 diabetes. *Graefe's Arch Clin Exp Ophthalmol* **241**: 181–186.

Malmfors T. (1965) The adrenergic innervation of the eye as demonstrated by fluorescence microscopy. *Acta Physiol Scand* **65**: 259–266.

Matsumoto A, Iwashima Y, Abiko A, *et al.* (2000) Detection of the association between a deletion polymorphism in the gene encoding angiotensin I-converting enzyme and advanced diabetic retinopathy. *Diabetes Res Clin Pract* **50**: 195–202.

Michelson G, Welzenbach J, Pal I, Harazny J. (1998) Automatic full fields analysis of perfusion images gained by scanning laser Doppler flowmetry. *Br J Ophthalmol* **82**: 1294–1300.

Michelson G, Welzenbach J, Pal I, Harazny J. (2001) Functional imaging of the retinal microvasculature by scanning laser Doppler flowmetry. *Int Ophthalmol* **23**: 327–333.

Murata T, Ishibashi T, Inomata H. (1993) Immuno-histochemical detection of blood-retinal barrier break-down in streptozotocindiabetic rats. *Graefe's Arch Clin Exp Ophthalmol* **231**: 175–177.

Patel A, Hibberd ML, Millward BA, Demaine AG. (1996) Chromosome 7q35 and susceptibility to diabetic micro-vascular complications. *J Diabetes Complications* **10**: 62–67.

Pires I, Bernardes RC, Lobo CL, *et al.* (2002) Retinal thick-ness in eyes with mild nonproliferative retinopathy in patients with type 2 diabetes mellitus Comparison of measurements obtained by retinal thickness analysis and optical coherence tomography. *Arch Ophthalmol* **120**: 1301–1306.

Poitry-Yamate CL, Poitry S, Tsacopoulos M. (1965) Lactate released by Müller glial cells is metabolized by photoreceptors from mammalian retina. *J Neurosci* **15**: 5179–5191.

Rigat B, Hubert C, Alhenc-Gelas F, *et al.* (1990) An insertion/deletion polymorphism in the angiotensin I-converting enzyme gene accounting for half the variance of serum enzyme levels. *J Clin Invest* **86**: 1343–1346.

Roufail E, Soulis T, Boel E, *et al.* (1998) Depletion of nitric oxide synthase-containing neurons in the diabetic retina: Reversal by aminoguanidine. *Diabetologia* **41**: 1419–1425.

Rungger-Brändle E, Dosso AA, Leuenberger PM. (2000) Glial reactivity, an early feature of diabetic retinopathy. *Invest Ophthalmol Vis Sci* **41**: 1971–1980.

Serrano-Rios M, Regueiro JR, Serverino R, *et al.* (1983) HLA antigens in insulin dependent and non-insulin dependent Spanish diabetic patients. *Diabetes Metab* **9**: 116–120.

Shahidi M, Zeimer R, Mori M. (1990) Topography of reti-nal thickness in normals. *Ophthalmology* **97**: 1120–1197.

Shahidi M, Ogura Y, Blair NP, *et al.* (1991) Retinal thick-ness analysis for quantitative assessment of diabetic macular edema. *Arch Ophthalmol* **109**: 1115–1119.

Shakib M, Cunha-Vaz JG, (1966) Studies on the perme-ability of the blood-retinal barrier. IV. Junctional complexes of the retinal vessels and their role in the permeability of the blood-retinal barrier. *Exp Eye Res* **5**: 229–234.

Snieder H, Sawtell PA, Ross L, *et al.* (2001) HbA1C levels are genetically determined even in type 1 diabetes. Evidence from healthy and diabetic twins. *Diabetes* **50**: 2858–2863.

Stewart LL, Field LL, Ross S, McArthur RG. (1993) Genetic risk factors in diabetic retinopathy. *Diabeto-logia* **36**: 1293–1298.

Storm C, Sander B, Larsen N, *et al.* (2002) Diabetic macu-lar edema assessed with optical coherence tomography and stereo fundus photography. *Invest Ophthalmol Vis Sci* **43**: 241–245.

Stratton IM, Kohner EM, Aldington SJ, *et al.* (2001) for the UKPDS Group, UKPDS 50: Risk factors for inci-dence and progression of retinopathy in type II diabetes over 6 years from diagnosis. *Diabetologia* **44**: 156–163.

Sullivan PM, Davies GE, Caldwell G, *et al.* (1990) Retinal blood flow during hyperglycemia: A laser dop-pler velocimetry study. *Invest Ophthalmol Vis Sci* **31**: 2041–2045.

Sutter EE. (2001) Imaging visual function with the multifocal sequence techniques. *Vision Res* **41**: 1241–1255.

Takagi C, Bursell SE, Lin YW, *et al.* (1996) Regulation of retinal hemodynamics in diabetic rats by increased expression and action of endothelin-1. *Invest Ophthalmol Vis Sci* **37**: 2504–2518.

Torrent-Solans T, Duarte L, Monteiro R, *et al.* (2004) Red-dots counting on digitalized fundus images of mild non-proliferative retinopathy in Diabetes type 2. *Invest Ophthalmol Vis Sci* **45**: E-Abstract 2985.

Tso MO. (1988) Cystoid macular edema. In: Tso MOM. (ed.), *Retinal Diseases*. Lippincott, Williams and Wilkins, New York, pp. 2215–2241.

Tso MOM, Cunha-Vaz JG, Shih CY, Jones CW. (1980) Clinicopathologic study of blood-retinal barrier in experimental diabetes mellitus. *Arch Ophthalmol* **98**: 2032–2040.

Van Schaik HJ, Heintz B, Larsen M, *et al.* (1997) Permeability of the blood-retinal barrier in healthy humans. European concerted action on ocular fluorom-etry. *Graefe's Arch Clin Exp Ophthalmol* **235**: 639–646.

Viñores SA, McGehee R, Lee A, *et al.* (1990) Ultrastructural localization of blood-retinal barrier breakdown in diabetic and galactosemic rats. *J Histochem Cytochem* **38**: 1341–1352.

Viñores SA, Van Niel E, Swerdloff JL, Campochiaro PA. (1993) Electron microscopic immunocytochemical demonstration of blood-retinal barrier breakdown in human diabetics and its association with aldose reductase in retinal vascular endothelium and retinal pigment epithelium. *Histochem J* **25**: 648–663.

Waltman SR. (1989) Sequential vitreous fluorophotometry in diabtes mellitus: A five year prospective study. *Trans Am Ophthalmol Soc* **82**: 827–940.

Waltman SR, Krupin T, Hanish S, *et al.* (1978a) Alteration of the blood-retinal barrier in experimental diabetes mellitus. *Arch Ophthalmol* **96**: 878–879.

Waltman SR, Oestrich C, Krupin T, *et al.* (1978b) Quantitative vitreous fluorophotometry: A sensitive technique for measuring early breakdown of the blood-retinal barrier in young diabetic patients. *Diabetes* **27**: 85–87.

Warpeha KM, Chakravarthy U. (2003) Molecular genetics of microvascular disease in diabetic retinopathy. Eye **17**: 305–311.

Warpeha KM, Ah-Fat F, Harding S, *et al.* (1999) Dinucleotide repeat polymorphisms in EDN1 and NOS3 are not associated with severe diabetic retinopathy in type 1 or type 2 diabetes. *Eye* **13**: 174–178.

Wasgenknecht LE, Bowden DW, Carr JJ, *et al.* (2001) Familial aggregation of coronary artery calcium in families with type 2 diabetes. *Diabetes* **50**: 861–866.

Wilkinson CP, Ferris III FL, Klein RE, *et al.* (2003) Representing the Global Diabetic Retinopathy Project Group. Proposed international clinical diabetic retinopathy and diabetic macular edema disease severity scales. *Ophthalmology* **101**: 1677–1682.

Wise GN, Dollery CT, Henkid P. (1971) *The Retinal Circulation.* Harper & Row, New York, pp. 421–454.

Zeimer R. (1998) Application of retinal thickness analyzer to the diagnosis and management of ocular diseases. *Ophthalmol Clin North America* **11**: 359–379.

Zeimer RC, Blair NP, Cunha-Vaz JG. (1983) Vitreous fluorophotometry for clinical research. I. Description and evaluation of a new fluorophotometer. *Arch Ophthalmol* **101**: 1753–1756.

# Index